Anterior Segment Complications of Contact Lens Wear

Anterior Segment Complications of Contact Lens Wear

SECOND EDITION

Edited by

JOEL A. SILBERT, O.D., F.A.A.O.

Professor and Director of The Cornea and Specialty Contact Lens Service,
The Eye Institute, Pennsylvania College of Optometry, Philadelphia

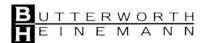

Boston • Oxford • Auckland • Johannesburg • Melbourne • New Delhi

Copyright © 2000 by Butterworth–Heinemann

 A member of the Reed Elsevier group

All rights reserved.

Every effort has been made to ensure that the drug dosage schedules within this text are accurate and conform to standards accepted at the time of publication. However, as treatment recommendations vary in the light of continuing research and clinical experience, the reader is advised to verify drug dosage schedules herein with information found on product information sheets. This is especially true in cases of new or infrequently used drugs.

 Recognizing the importance of preserving what has been written, Butterworth–Heinemann prints its books on acid-free paper whenever possible.

AMERICAN FORESTS
GLOBAL ReLEAF 2000 Butterworth–Heinemann supports the efforts of American Forests and the Global ReLeaf program in its campaign for the betterment of trees, forests, and our environment.

Library of Congress Cataloging-in-Publication Data
Anterior segment complications of contact lens wear / edited by Joel
   A. Silbert. -- 2nd ed.
      p. cm.
    Includes bibliographical references and index.
    ISBN 0-7506-7116-5
    1. Contact lenses--Complications. 2. Anterior segment (Eye)-
-Diseases. I. Silbert, Joel A.
    [DNLM: 1. Contact Lenses--adverse effects. 2. Anterior Eye
Segment--physiopathology. 3. Corneal Diseases—etiology. WW 355
A627 2000]
   RE977.C6A58 2000
   617.7'523--dc21
   DNLM/DLC
   for Library of Congress   99-40664
                                         CIP

British Library Cataloguing-in-Publication Data
A catalogue record for this book is available from the British Library.

The publisher offers special discounts on bulk orders of this book.
For information, please contact:
Manager of Special Sales
Butterworth–Heinemann
225 Wildwood Avenue
Woburn, MA 01801-2041
Tel: 781-904-2500
Fax: 781-904-2620

For information on all Butterworth–Heinemann publications available,
contact our World Wide Web home page at: http://www.bh.com

10 9 8 7 6 5 4 3 2 1

Printed in Canada

This work is dedicated in loving memory of my father, Milton Silbert, who left this world too soon, but not before teaching me about the power of the written word.

This second edition is dedicated to my past and present students:

To those in clinical internships and contact lens residencies;
To those who are now well established in clinical practice;
To those whom I have had the pleasure to instruct through continuing education;
To those practitioners in Europe, in South America, in South Africa, and especially to those in Israel who have been a source of great joy;
And to those who are just beginning their careers in the ophthalmic professions.

Contents

Contributing Authors

Mark P. Andre, F.C.L.S.A.
Director of Contact Lens Services, Casey Eye Institute, Oregon Health Sciences University, Portland
   9. Dermatologic Complications of the Lids and Adnexa

James V. Aquavella, M.D.
Clinical Professor of Ophthalmology and Director, Cornea Research Laboratory, University of Rochester Medical Center, Rochester, New York; Clinical Professor of Ophthalmology and Attending, Strong Memorial Hospital, Rochester
   13. Protozoan and Fungal Keratitis in Contact Lens Wear; 20. Penetrating Keratoplasty

Joseph T. Barr, O.D., M.S., F.A.A.O.
Associate Professor, The Ohio State University College of Optometry, Columbus
   18. Effects of Contact Lenses in Keratoconus

Jimmy D. Bartlett, O.D., F.A.A.O.
Professor of Optometry, University of Alabama at Birmingham School of Optometry; Professor of Pharmacology, University of Alabama at Birmingham School of Medicine
   22. Medications and Contact Lens Wear

Edward S. Bennett, O.D., F.A.A.O.
Associate Professor and Co-Chief, Contact Lens Service, University of Missouri–St. Louis School of Optometry
   16. Contact Lens–Induced Distortion and Corneal Reshaping

Jan P. G. Bergmanson, Ph.D., O.D., FCOptom, F.A.A.O.
Professor and Director, Texas Eye Research and Technology Center, University of Houston College of Optometry
   3. Endothelial Complications

Joseph A. Bonnano, O.D., Ph.D.
Professor, Indiana University School of Optometry, Bloomington
   2. Corneal Edema

Dennis Burger, O.D., F.A.A.O.
Clinical Professor, University of California School of Optometry, Berkeley; Senior Optometrist, Permanente Medical Group, Oakland
   18. Effects of Contact Lenses in Keratoconus

Barbara E. Caffery, O.D., M.S., F.A.A.O.
Private Practice, Toronto, Ontario
   5. Corneal Vascularization; 8. Complications of Lens Care Solutions

Patrick J. Caroline, C.O.T., F.A.A.O.
Associate Professor of Optometry, Contact Lens Department, Pacific University College of Optometry, Forest Grove, Oregon; Assistant Professor of Ophthalmology, Casey Eye Institute, Oregon Health Sciences University, Portland
   9. Dermatologic Complications of the Lids and Adnexa

Connie L. Chronister, O.D., F.A.A.O.
Associate Professor of Basic and Clinical Sciences and Chief of Primary Care, The Eye Institute, Pennsylvania College of Optometry, Philadelphia; Staff Optometrist, Veterans Administration Hospital, Philadelphia
   11. Viral Infections and the Immunocompromised Patient

John G. Classé, O.D., J.D., F.A.A.O.
Professor of Optometry, University of Alabama at Birmingham School of Optometry; Member of the Alabama Bar
   25. Medicolegal Complications of Contact Lens Wear

Larry J. Davis, O.D., F.A.A.O.
Assistant Professor, University of Missouri–St. Louis
School of Optometry
    4. Noninfectious Corneal Staining

Michael D. DePaolis, O.D., F.A.A.O.
Adjunct Professor of Optometry, Pennsylvania College of
Optometry, Philadelphia; Clinical Associate, Department
of Ophthalmology, University of Rochester School of Med-
icine and Dentistry and Strong Memorial Hospital,
Rochester, New York
    *13. Protozoan and Fungal Keratitis in Contact Lens
Wear; 20. Penetrating Keratoplasty*

Timothy B. Edrington, O.D., M.S., F.A.A.O.
Professor and Chief, Cornea and Contact Lens Service,
Southern California College of Optometry, Fullerton
    17. Keratoconus

Michael J. Giese, O.D., Ph.D., F.A.A.O.
Department of Ophthalmology, Jules Stein Eye Institute,
University of California, Los Angeles, UCLA School of
Medicine
    12. Ulcerative Bacterial Keratitis

David T. Gubman, O.D., M.S., F.A.A.O.
Assistant Professor of Clinical and Basic Sciences, Penn-
sylvania College of Optometry, Elkins Park; Director,
Corneal Refractive Eyecare Service, The Eye Institute,
Philadelphia
    19. Complications after Corneal Refractive Surgery

Michael G. Harris, O.D., J.D., M.S., F.A.A.O.
Associate Dean, Clinical Professor, and Chief, Contact
Lens Clinic, University of California School of Optome-
try, Berkeley
    25. Medicolegal Complications of Contact Lens Wear

Vinita Allee Henry, O.D., F.A.A.O.
Clinical Associate Professor of Optometry, University of
Missouri–St. Louis School of Optometry
    *16. Contact Lens–Induced Distortion and Corneal
Reshaping*

Brien A. Holden, Ph.D., D.Sc., OAM
Director, Cooperative Research Centre for Eye Research
and Technology, University of New South Wales, Sydney, Australia
    *14. Complications of Hydrogel Extended-Wear
Lenses*

Joshua E. Josephson, B.Sc., O.D., F.A.A.O.
Josephson Opticians, Toronto, Ontario
    *5. Corneal Vascularization; 8. Complications of Lens
Care Solutions*

Janice M. Jurkus, O.D., M.B.A., F.A.A.O.
Professor of Optometry, Illinois College of Optometry,
Chicago
    7. Contact Lens–Induced Giant Papillary Conjunctivitis

Rodger T. Kame, O.D., F.A.A.O.
Adjunct Associate Professor, Southern California Col-
lege of Optometry, Fullerton; Staff Optometrist, Cedars-
Sinai Medical Center, Los Angeles
    9. Dermatologic Complications of the Lids and Adnexa

Kenneth A. Lebow, O.D., F.A.A.O.
Private Practice, Virginia Beach, Virginia
    *4. Noninfectious Corneal Staining; 24. Corneal Topog-
raphy and Contact Lens Complications*

Bartly J. Mondino, M.D.
Chairman, Department of Ophthalmology, and Director,
Jules Stein Eye Institute, University of California, Los Ange-
les, UCLA School of Medicine and UCLA Medical Center
    12. Ulcerative Bacterial Keratitis

Cristina M. Schnider, O.D., M.Sc., F.A.A.O.
Adjunct Professor, Pacific University College of Optometry, Forest Grove, Oregon
    15. Rigid Gas-Permeable Extended-Wear Lenses

Leo P. Semes, B.S., O.D., F.A.A.O.
Associate Professor of Optometry, University of Alabama
at Birmingham School of Optometry
    10. Keratoconjunctivitis Sicca and Ocular Surface Disease

Joseph P. Shovlin, O.D., F.A.A.O.
Adjunct Clinical Faculty, Pennsylvania College of Optom-
etry, Philadelphia; Senior Optometrist and Director of
Contact Lens Services, Northeastern Eye Institute, Scran-
ton, Pennsylvania
    *13. Protozoan and Fungal Keratitis in Contact Lens
Wear; 20. Penetrating Keratoplasty*

Joel A. Silbert, O.D., F.A.A.O.
Professor and Director of The Cornea and Specialty Contact Lens Service, The Eye Institute, Pennsylvania College of Optometry, Philadelphia
    6. Inflammatory Responses in Contact Lens Wear

Christopher Snyder, O.D., M.S., F.A.A.O.
Professor of Optometry, University of Alabama at Birmingham School of Optometry
   1. Preocular Tear Film Anomalies and Lens-Related Dryness

Michael R. Spinell, O.D., F.A.A.O.
Associate Professor of Clinical Sciences, Pennsylvania College of Optometry, Philadelphia
   23. Contact Lenses for Cosmetic Disfigurement

Helen A. Swarbrick, Ph.D., F.A.A.O.
Senior Lecturer, School of Optometry, The University of New South Wales, Sydney, Australia
   14. Complications of Hydrogel Extended-Wear Lenses

Barry M. Weiner, O.D., F.A.A.O.
Ancillary Faculty, Department of Ophthalmology, Wilmer Eye Institute, Johns Hopkins Hospital, Baltimore
   21. Therapeutic Bandage Lenses

Barry A. Weissman, O.D., Ph.D., F.A.A.O.
Professor of Ophthalmology, Jules Stein Eye Institute, University of California, Los Angeles, UCLA School of Medicine
   12. Ulcerative Bacterial Keratitis

Karla Zadnik, O.D., Ph.D., F.A.A.O.
Associate Professor, The Ohio State University College of Optometry, Columbus
   17. Keratoconus

Preface to the Second Edition

Since the publication of the first edition of *Anterior Segment Complications of Contact Lens Wear*, the number of contact lens wearers in the United States has increased by approximately one-third, to 32 million wearers. This is in no small measure because of improvements in lens design, additional lens-wearing modalities, and remarkable advancements in lens care products. This turnabout follows quite a few years of flat market growth, as there were as many new wearers as there were dropouts. For these numbers to have changed so dramatically, particularly during a time of heavy advertising of refractive surgery, it is clear that the industry is not only producing better lenses and fitting a wider array of spectacle wearers but is also reducing the dropout rate.

Instead of the contact lens practitioner advising his or her patients that they have to discontinue wearing contact lenses because of corneal edema, staining, or vascularization, we now have lenses of high transmissibility that can better meet the physiologic needs of the cornea. Where we once had to advise patients with ocular allergies to stop wearing their lenses, either seasonally or permanently, we now have preservative-free and nontoxic care systems, single use daily-wear lenses, and medications that can control the allergic response and allow the patient to continue to enjoy the benefits of lens wear. Where we had seen many patients develop inflammatory reactions, either from heavily coated lenses or from bacterial adherence, toxins, and metabolic by-products, we now have lenses in a wide array of fitting parameters in disposable or planned replacement modalities that can mitigate many (but not all) of these complications. With the advent of a new breed of hydrogel extended-wear lens polymers that can deliver high levels of oxygen to the cornea, we will likely see many of the high-risk complications of extended-wear greatly reduced. Whereas this development will most assuredly see a resurgence in 30-day extended-wear use, an interesting and viable alternative to refractive surgery, it remains to be seen whether all complications associated with extended wear will disappear. More than likely, the high levels of oxygen will lead to a marked diminution in hypoxic-driven complications, including edema, polymegethism, vascularization, and microbial infection, but inflammatory complications associated with lens coatings, bacterial adherence and the biofilm, and microbial toxins may still adversely affect some lens wearers.

The second edition of *Anterior Segment Complications of Contact Lens Wear* provides the experienced and novice practitioner with a wealth of information about contact lens–related complications. All chapters have been updated to provide the reader with a comprehensive discussion based on the latest clinical and research data, written by contributing authors who are eminent in their fields and who have a wealth of clinical expertise to share with the reader. The Grand Rounds Case Reports provide a typical case that could be seen in one's practice, with a succinct description of clinical assessment and plan. Ocular therapeutics are discussed in considerable depth throughout this volume to provide the clinician with appropriate guidelines in therapeutic management of contact lens complications. New chapters include topics pertinent to management of complications seen in the immuno-compromised patient, in patients experiencing corneal distortion and untoward orthokeratologic changes, and in patients experiencing complications after keratorefractive surgery. In addition, a comprehensive chapter on the use of corneal topography in the diagnosis and management of contact lens complications has been included, as topography becomes an essential diagnostic imaging tool of the contact lens practitioner. In addition to adding color images throughout the text of the second edition, an appendix containing the world-renown CCLRU Grading Scales has been included to help standardize the grading of complications seen in clinical practice.

It is my hope that this volume serves the practitioner with a useful and comprehensive reference on the diagnosis and management of contact lens complications as we cross the threshold of a new millenium.

J.A.S.

Preface to the First Edition

Nearly 25 million people wear contact lenses in the United States alone. Worldwide, this figure mushrooms to nearly 50 million, with much growth anticipated in coming years in Europe and Asia. Whether worn as an alternative to spectacles for correction of refractive errors or as therapeutic devices for a wide variety of ocular conditions, contact lenses serve many important roles.

The success of today's (1994) contact lenses, whether made from hydrogel or gas-permeable polymers, or prescribed in reusable or disposable modalities, is due in great part to the careful observations of clinicians and researchers. Modern advances in lens designs have led to sophisticated manufacturing methods, high reproducibility, and the ability to provide correction for practically any refractive condition, corneal shape, or cosmetic requirement.

Concurrent advances in contact lens polymer chemistry and biocompatibility have led to the ability to minimize corneal hypoxia and its many sequelae. Yet edema still presents serious challenges for the patient desiring extended wear lenses. Much has been learned about contact lens solutions, lens coatings, and solution toxicity and hypersensitivity. Yet patients continue to have complications that can only be resolved through frequent lens or solution replacement. Although the development of rigid gas-permeable lenses of extremely high oxygen transmissibility has been seen, some patients continue to have complications of peripheral corneal desiccation, lens adhesion, and even corneal exhaustion. The dry eye continues to confound the contact lens practitioner. And no matter how excellent contact lenses become or how non-toxic their care solutions, the human condition is such that poor compliance, environmental exposure, concurrent pathology, and the ever-present desire to sleep in contact lenses sets up conditions that predispose the patient to ocular inflammation and infection. Clearly, complications of contact lens wear, although fewer than in years past, continue to limit the success of these remarkable devices.

Although some patients do develop complications, most are quite manageable through the clinical observations and skills of their contact lens practitioners. *Anterior Segment Complications of Contact Lens Wear* has been written not only to bring together into one source what is known about contact lens complications in the widest sense, but also to present to the contact lens practitioner a very clinically useful text. The contributing authors have provided chapters that reflect the latest research findings as well as their considerable experience as clinicians. A special feature in this volume is the incorporation of Grand Rounds Case Reports in each chapter. These are actual case studies taken from the authors' files, which, along with other case reports throughout this book, should be of considerable benefit to the reader in providing a clinical framework for the subject material.

I hope that this volume provides the reader, whether novice or experienced clinician, with the most comprehensive and clinically useful information on anterior segment complications of contact lens wear and their clinical management.

J.A.S.

Acknowledgments

The response to the first edition of *Anterior Segment Complications of Contact Lens Wear* has been gratifying. Since its publication in 1994, however, numerous changes have occurred in the field of contact lenses, as well as in diagnostic and therapeutic management of associated complications. I am indebted to my colleagues, who have taken time out of their busy academic, clinical, and research schedules to update their respective chapters. I am also grateful for the second edition's new authors, who have contributed their expertise so that this text may continue to serve as a comprehensive resource for the contact lens practitioner.

A special thank you goes to my colleague and friend, Dr. Michael Spinell, who has encouraged me to undertake this project and has served as a mentor and sounding board throughout this undertaking.

Of course, this volume would not have been possible without the expertise of the Butterworth–Heinemann editorial staff. In particular, I would like to thank Karen Oberheim for enabling us to provide such a comprehensive resource for contact lens professionals, and Leslie Kramer, who greatly assisted me in the preparation of the manuscript and in seeing the project to fruition.

I

Physiologic Complications of Contact Lens Wear

1

Preocular Tear Film Anomalies and Lens-Related Dryness

CHRISTOPHER SNYDER

GRAND ROUNDS CASE REPORT

Subjective:
A 28-year-old woman wearing disposable hydrogel lenses (58% water content) on a daily-wear basis for past 6 months reports consistent dry, scratchy sensation after 6 hours. Rewetting drops do not help for more than a few minutes. Uses multipurpose lens care system with apparently good compliance. Replaces lenses after 2 weeks of wear. Maximum wearing time with lenses is 12 hours per day. Patient takes no medication and is in good health.

Objective:
- Entering acuity: right eye (OD) $^{20}/_{20}$, left eye (OS) $^{20}/_{20}$ (distance and near)
- Lenses appear clean and fit well
- Biomicroscopy: grade 1 minimal bulbar injection; lid eversion negative for papillary changes
- Tear meniscus: moderate in height
- Tear film breakup time (TBUT): OD 15 seconds, OS 20 seconds
- Vital dyes: No staining with fluorescein or rose bengal
- Blink rate normal and full magnitude
- All other ocular health tests normal each eye (OU)

Assessment:
Marginal dry eye with hydrogel lenses (minimal sicca syndrome); clinically normal tears with stable tear film and well-fitted contact lenses; no evidence of true dry eye or physiologic intolerance from contact lens wear.

Plan:
1. Punctal occlusion with nondissolvable intracanalicular plugs, inferior puncta only, OU.
2. Use lens lubricant drops as required (PRN).
3. Change to hydrogen peroxide lens care system.

Follow-up:
Patient reported that lens-wearing comfort improved and wearing time could now be extended to all waking hours. Combination of change in lens care system and punctal occlusion significantly impacted on her ability to comfortably wear lenses.

TABLE 1-1. *Drugs Affecting Aqueous Production*

Antihistamines
    Chlorpheniramine (Dristan)
    Diphenhydramine (Benadryl)
Anxiolytics
    Chlordiazepoxide (Librium)
    Diazepam (Valium)
β-Adrenergic blockers
    Timolol (Timoptic)
    Levobunolol (Betagan)
Phenothiazides
    Chlorpromazine (Thorazine)
    Thiordazine (Mellaril)
Anticholinergics
    Atropine (Comhist)
    Scopolamine (Donnagel)
Oral contraceptives
    Progesterone/estrogen combinations

The tear fluid and its components originate from the main lacrimal gland and various accessory lacrimal glands. The tears have bulk characteristics, such as tonicity, viscosity, protein levels, electrolyte composition, average volume, and turnover rate. Its functions include supporting the anterior segment surface, washing of metabolic waste and cellular debris from the ocular surface, and providing protection by way of antimicrobial components, such as lysozyme, lactoferrin, and immunoglobulins. The tears of contact lens wearers must also support the physical requirements of the contact lens polymer.

The primary functions of the tears, when organized into the preocular tear film, are to serve as a smooth, regular refracting surface for light incident to the eye and to moisten, maintain, and support the surface cells of the anterior segment. The tear film has physical characteristics such as thickness, stability, quality, and individual layers. It is dynamic, influenced by internal environmental factors, such as tear volume, tear consistency, general nutrition, eyelid anatomy and blink influence, regularity of the corneal surface, and by external environmental factors, such as humidity, air pollution, and air currents. Debate continues concerning the distinction between basic tears and stimulated or reflex tears.[1]

Deficiencies in functional capacity of the tears and tear film typically manifest as a less-than-optimally moistened eye, more commonly referred to as some level of *dry eye*. Because anomalies of the tears and tear film can be caused by ocular surface problems or can cause problems with the surface of the eye, the term *ocular surface disease* is popular in describing tear- and tear film–related problems.[2]

The relevance of dry eye in clinical eye care is strong, with a 25% prevalence of at least one level of self-reported symptom of dry eye (by questionnaire survey) in patients presenting to optometric practices across Canada.[3] Dry eye symptoms are relatively common in the elderly population,[4] and, although women are thought to have more dry eye symptoms than men,[3,4] the association between dry eye and gender may not be as strong as once believed.[5]

We are making progress in expanding our knowledge base regarding dry eye conditions, but more basic and clinical research is needed for better understanding and treatment of the myriad of conditions and circumstances contributing to dry eye. This chapter is an effort to point out, with an eye firmly focused on clinical relevance, a portion of what is currently known about dry eye and its implications for contact lens wearers.

TEAR FLUID (AQUEOUS)

The tear fluid exists in the cul-de-sac, the tear meniscus, and the tear film. Tears exit from the anterior eye by absorption into the conjunctival capillaries, evaporation from the tear film, and drainage through the puncta and down the lacrimal canals. The basal tear turnover rate, expressed as a percent decrease of fluorescein concentration in the tear film per minute after instillation of fluorescein, is approximately 15% per minute.[6] The volume of the tears in the tear sac is approximately 10 μl, and the capacity of the sac is approximately 30 μl.[7] Systemic medications can have a deleterious effect on the aqueous production of the tears (Table 1-1).

PREOCULAR TEAR FILM

The preocular tear film has traditionally been described as three discrete, yet interactive, layers: the superficial meibomian oils, the aqueous liquid phase, and the innermost mucin glycoprotein layer.[8]

Goblet cells of the conjunctiva, the crypts of Henle, and the glands of Manz contribute the innermost mucin layer. The microvilli of the epithelia enhance the adsorption of the mucin to the ocular surface, and the mucin glycoprotein allows wetting of the surface cells of the cornea and conjunctiva by decreasing the surface tension of the tears, allowing for even spreading of a thin film across the ocular surface with the blink. The mucin also tends to capture and remove debris in the tear film and, in tears that are deficient in aqueous component, tends to develop mucus strands and filaments. The main lacrimal gland and the accessory lacrimal glands of Krause and Wolfring of the conjunctiva contribute the middle aqueous layer, constituting more than 90% of the thickness of the tear film. The main lacrimal gland contributes lysozyme, lactoferrin, metabolites, nutrients, and various immunoglobulins. The outermost lipid layer, the most discrete layer of the tears, is contributed by the meibomian glands that line the eyelid margins. The lipid layer of fatty acids, cholesterol esters, and phospholipids creates an optically smooth refracting surface, inhibits evaporation of the aqueous phase of the tears, and assists in keeping the tears in the tear meniscus from spilling over the lid margins. It is this layer of the tear film that is so readily assaulted by lid margin disease, such as blepharitis and meibomian gland dysfunction (MGD).

Acceptance of the three-layer model tempts one to view anomalies of the tears and tear film as deficiencies in one or more of these presumably discrete tear-film layers. A coacervate of mucin and aqueous and a highly integrated dynamic tear film, however, is more likely. This would limit the value of the dry eye mechanism theories that are based on the distinctly separate component layers view of the tear film. Techniques for viewing and evaluating the dynamic aspects of the outermost lipid layer of the tear film, because it is superficial and has optical and physical characteristics that make it relatively easy to view and evaluate, present hope for new understanding of the tear film's function and dysfunction.[9,10]

The regular blinking dynamics reconstitute the tear film after the interblink period and allow the film to thin and deteriorate again. The fluid within the very thin tear film across the anterior ocular surface is eventually drawn into the superior or inferior tear meniscus lining the upper and lower eyelid margins. During an extended interblink period, the superficial lipid layer eventually becomes disorganized and leads to breakup of the tear film. The mucin layer may be disrupted by contamination of the tear film coacervate by debris or by molecules of the lipid layer that make their way down into this layer of the tear film.

Anything that affects the production of the various component phases of the tears (i.e., lipid, aqueous, or mucin) as the building blocks for the tear film can have a deleterious effect on the tear film and its ability to preserve, protect, and nourish the ocular surface. In addition, if the dynamics of blinking, which continuously re-forms the tear film, are disrupted (e.g., by a decrease in blink rate, incomplete eyelid closure during the blinks, or irregularities in the eyelid anatomy), then the quality and completeness of the preocular tear film may be significantly compromised.

DIAGNOSTIC CHALLENGE OF TEAR AND TEAR FILM DEFICIENCIES

The diagnostic challenge of the dry eye and its causes is a widespread clinical problem. Establishing a valid and reliable set of clinical tests for diagnosis of dry eye is a formidable task, yet it is one that must be pursued because a dry eye is one of the most commonly self-diagnosed eye problems. The clinical challenge of diagnosing a dry eye is compounded in several ways. First, between the clearly normal (i.e., non–dry eye) and the clearly dry eye (i.e., severe keratoconjunctivitis sicca [KCS]) is the broad spectrum of what has been called the *marginally dry eye.*[2] Second, in addition to differences in the severity of dry eye, different types of dry eyes with different etiologies may also be present. For example, dry eyes may originate from deficiencies in the aqueous phase, mucin phase, or meibomian oil phase of the tear film, or from other causes such as lid anomalies and systemic conditions. Third, patients who complain of a dry eye do not necessarily have signs to confirm their symptoms,[11] and the idea of dryness may have been suggested to them by a previous doctor.[12] Occasionally, patients with frank signs of a dry eye do not report any ocular dryness or discomfort.

One of the more difficult considerations is an appropriate classification for the cases in which an isolated clinical test result or symptom indicates the possibility of dry eye, but the finding is inconsistent with other results. The diagnostic dilemma includes the following possibilities:

1. Dry eye symptoms with no clinical signs
2. Dry eye symptoms with minimal clinical signs
3. Dry eye symptoms with clinical signs
4. No dry eye symptoms but with clinical signs of dry eye
5. The wet eye as a sign of a dry eye
6. The marginal (i.e., periodic or occasional) dry eye

Obtaining an accurate profile of a dry eye by clinical testing has been largely unsuccessful owing to the dynamic nature of many dry eye conditions and the inherent shortcomings of the diagnostic tests and their administration. That the tears and tear film exist in an open system, unlike blood serum, for example, is a reminder that the moment-to-moment variability of the system also contributes to the difficulty in achieving reliable clinical measures. Describing and understanding the various types of dry eye so that predictably effective diagnosis and treatment of such problems can be achieved is another challenge. Aggravating conditions of this open system include low humidity, drafts, wind, smoke, air conditioning, atmospheric irritants, airline flights, and low tear production at night.

CATEGORIES AND CLASSIFICATIONS OF DRY EYE

Categories of the causes of dry eye generally have been tailored to the components of the tears and tear film, thought of as aqueous deficient, mucin deficient, lipid problems, lid surface problems, or epithelial defects. Although perhaps simplistic, this model serves as a useful approach for understanding the complex clinical diagnosis and treatment challenges presented by the various types of dry eyes and dryness symptoms.

If a series of clinical tests were available that allows for definitive diagnosis and leads to effective treatment of the particular type of dry eye condition, then this battery of tests would already be well known, generally accepted, and in common use. An important effort toward determining how dry eye conditions can better be understood, measured, and treated has begun with the publication of a National Eye Institute (NEI)/Industry Workshop on clinical trials in dry eyes.[13] This undertaking grew from a recognized need to provide clinical instruments for the conduct of epidemiologic studies and clinical trials of dry eyes. The three primary goals included development of a classification system for dry eyes, standardization of clinical tests used to diagnose dry eye states and assess treatment effects, and development of epidemiologic data concerning dry eyes. The workshop group's global definition of dry eye is "a disorder of the tear film due to tear deficiency or excessive tear evaporation which causes damage to the interpalpebral ocular surface and is associated with symptoms of ocular discomfort." The working group stated that most forms of dry eye exhibit the following features:

- Symptoms
- Interpalpebral surface damage
- Tear instability
- Tear hyperosmolarity

and that the following tests should be used to evaluate for the features:

- Validated questionnaire of symptoms
- Demonstration of ocular surface damage
- Demonstration of tear instability
- Demonstration of tear hyperosmolarity

According to the workshop group,[13] major classes of dry eye include tear-deficient dry eye and evaporative dry eye (EDE) (or *tear-sufficient dry eye*). Disorders in the tear-deficient dry eye group include Sjögren's syndrome tear deficiency, related to an underlying systemic condition, and non–Sjögren's tear deficiency. The non–Sjögren's tear deficiency stems from

1. Primary lacrimal gland deficiency;
2. Secondary lacrimal gland deficiency related to sarcoidosis, lymphoma, human immunodeficiency virus infection, xerophthalmia, or lacrimal gland ablation;
3. Reflex (neural) causes, such as sensory or motor deficiencies, from or to the lacrimal gland;
4. Obstructive lacrimal disease caused by such conditions as cicatrizing conjunctival disease, trachoma, cicatricial pemphigoid, erythema multiforme, and chemical and thermal burns.

These severe levels of dry eye and ocular surface disease are considered further in Chapter 10.

Disorders related to EDE include blepharitis, MGD, blink disorders, disorders of the lid aperture and lid/globe congruity, ocular surface disorder (e.g., elevated areas of the surface), other tear film disorders, and combined disorders.[13]

DIAGNOSTIC TESTS OF THE TEARS, TEAR FILM, AND OCULAR SURFACE

Taking the broad view, a reasonable—although not exhaustive—set of clinical tests may include the following:

1. Subjective impressions via patient history[14-16]
2. Tests of tears, such as:
   - Biomicroscopy, including evaluation of the tear meniscus,[7,17-20] tear film debris,[17,19,21] and mucus threads[17,19]
   - Schirmer's test[19]
   - Lacrimation kinetics[19,22,23]
   - Phenol cotton-thread test[24]
   - Tear osmolarity[2,7,19,21,25]
   - Total protein content[26,27]
   - Specific protein content[26,27]
   - Tear enzyme activity[26,27]
   - Lactoferrin immunoassay test[28]
   - Lactocard test[29]
3. Tests of the tear film
   - TBUT[7,9,17,30-33]
   - Tear evaporation rate[34,35]
4. Tests of the ocular surface
   - Vital staining with rose bengal[36-39]
   - Vital staining with sodium fluorescein[19,39]
   - Vital staining with lissamine green[13,40]
   - Impression cytology[41]
   - Tear cytology[42]

Patient History

Any screening questionnaire designed for broad clinical use must be valid, reliable, and economic in its design (i.e., in the number of questions and in the amount of time necessary to complete the questionnaire). McMonnies' Dry Eye Questionnaire is the best available screening tool for dry eye.[16] The questionnaire has been shown to have 98% sensitivity and 97% specificity in discriminating between persons with normal tear function and KCS patients[15] but incorporates a strong age bias against healthy females. The age and gender biases are misleading when attempts are made to identify healthy women older than 45 years. McMonnies and Ho[14] have reported that in a healthy population, women older than 45 years did not have an increased incidence of dry eye signs. Schein[5] found this as well in a group over the age of 65. In another age-related consideration, Whitcher[19] reported that senile changes in lacrimal gland function are probably not important causes of eye disorders. This was based on the observation that, despite atrophy of lacrimal tissue with advancing age, only 15% of patients older than 80 years have significantly decreased tear flow, and most have neither symptoms nor clinical signs that warrant the diagnosis of KCS.

An example of an expanded McMonnies' Dry Eye Questionnaire, with additional questions to increase its predictive and diagnostic value in clinical research, is offered in Appendix 1-1.

Tear Tests

Biomicroscopy Findings
Tear Viscosity   Viscosity of the tears and surface adhesion of the tear mucus are important in that they increase the retention of the tears as a tear film.[7] The tear viscosity can be evaluated by viewing the tear meniscus along the lower eyelid with low magnification and a parallelepiped beam of a biomicroscope.
Tear Meniscus   The tear meniscus can be evaluated with a biomicroscope for judging tear viscosity (Fig. 1-1). Measurement of the meniscus is difficult but can be facilitated by a measurement reticule in the eyepiece of the biomicroscope. The apparent height of the meniscus also depends on the position of gaze.[43] The average tear meniscus height in healthy subjects is 0.18 mm.[43] A helpful diagnostic sign in aqueous-deficient dry eye is the diminution of the tear meniscus (marked reduction in aqueous component of the tears),[19] and the size of the inferior lacrimal tear strip is reduced in moderate to severe KCS.[17] In spite of this, meniscus height is a poor test because many variables other than tear volume can affect meniscus size and shape.[18,20]

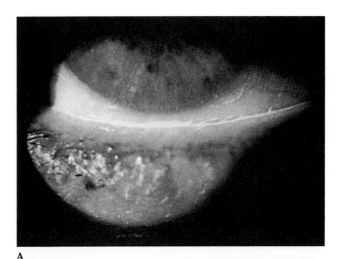

A

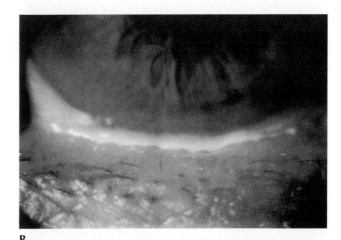

B

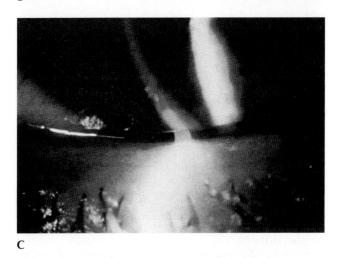

C

FIG. 1-1. *(A) A low tear meniscus height, as viewed with fluorescein and a biomicroscope (×16). (B) A low tear meniscus height as viewed with fluorescein and a biomicroscope (×30). Note the notched, irregular lid margin secondary in chronic blepharitis. (C) An average, normal tear meniscus height as viewed with fluorescein and a biomicroscope (×30).*

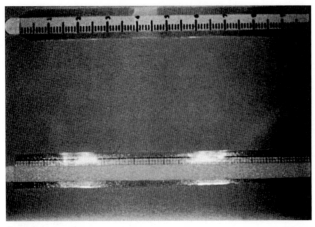

A

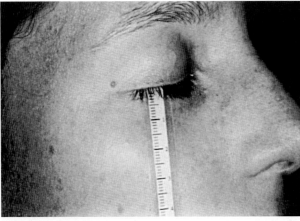

B

FIG. 1-2. *(A) Variations on lacrimation kinetics strips: top produced by Holly et al.[22,23]; bottom produced by Fullard.[26] (B) Lacrimation kinetics strip (after Holly[22,23]) in place under the lids. This strip reads 13 mm of wetting at 34 seconds along in the test.*

Tear Film Debris and Mucus Strands   The inferior lacrimal tear strip contains increased amounts of particulate matter and debris in moderate to severe KCS,[17,19] with particulate matter in the tear film correlating with dryness.[21] One of the earliest changes in dry eye is an increase in debris and mucus strands in the preocular tear film.[17,19]

Ocular Adnexa

Blepharitis   Blepharitis with KCS is caused by bacterial (staphylococcal) infection or is related to unknown factors associated with a dry eye.[17] The association of KCS with various types of blepharitis is significant.[44] Staphylococcal blepharitis, in particular, causes a variety of signs of ocular surface disease, including scaly exudate around eyelash bases, corneal staining, infiltrates from the exotoxins of the staphylococcal organisms, corneal ulcers, and phlyctenules. It can also cause significant disruption of tear film stability owing to lipase breakdown of lipids. This disruption allows resultant fatty acids to contaminate and destabilize the mucin layer of the tear film, leading to a lowered TBUT.

Meibomianitis   The lipid layer of the tear film is disrupted by alterations in the secretion of cholesterol esters, phospholipids, and fatty acids secondary to inflammation of the meibomian glands. MGD increases with age and causes significant disruption of tear film stability, which is reflected in a lowered TBUT (see Chapter 10).

Tear Flow Tests

Schirmer's Test   The Schirmer's test result is normal when the filter paper strip (5 × 35 mm) wets more than 15 mm in 5 minutes. Severe KCS is indicated when less than 5 mm of wetting is present, and mild to moderate KCS is indicated when 5–10 mm of wetting is present.[19] The Schirmer's I test is administered without anesthetic and the Schirmer's II test is essentially the Schirmer's I test administered with anesthetic.[19]

van Bijsterveld[36] proposed 5.5 mm of wetting as a cutoff for aqueous-deficient dry eye and suggested that this must be repeated three times on separate occasions.

Holly and colleagues[22,23] improved on the traditional Schirmer's test by using plastic-encased filter paper strips (Fig. 1-2) to eliminate the variable of tear evaporation from the strip during the test (when tear secretion comes to equilibrium with evaporation of tears off the strip, no further wetting is evident, even though tear secretion continues). This method also allows an assessment of the kinetics of lacrimation and can be performed using the same protocol as the traditional Schirmer's test to determine the tear flow. Cycles of lacrimal secretion can be identified and the weighted mean initial and final secretion rates can be determined, although this requires a relatively involved, nonroutine series of procedures for a clinical setting.

A disadvantage of the Schirmer's test, as well as of lacrimation kinetics testing, is that the interpretation and application of the test result are often questionable. An exception is when the patient has a dramatically dry eye; in such cases, the test result simply adds support to the diagnosis and management plan.

Phenol Red Thread Test   The phenol red thread test can be used for clinical assessment of tear flow. The crimped end of a 70 mm–long thread impregnated with phenol red dye is placed in the inferior conjunctival sac temporally for 15 seconds. The length of the thread wetted by the tears is indicated by a change from yellow to red because of the pH of the tears. Wetting lengths normally should be between 9 and 20 mm, with values less than 9 mm correlating with subjective symptoms of dryness.[24] This test is subject to the same constraints and limitations in interpretation and application as are the Schirmer's and lacrimation kinetics tests. It is commercially available as the Zone Quick phenol red thread tear test (distributed by Menicon, USA, Clovis, CA).

Osmolarity

The osmolarity of the tears is elevated in aqueous-deficient KCS dry eyes owing to the higher concentration of tear electrolytes dissolved in a relatively small amount of tear fluid (aqueous). The development of tear hyperosmolarity seems to precede rose bengal staining,[17] and osmolarity is elevated even after use of artificial tears.[19]

Farris et al.[45] proposed that tear osmolarity (312 mOsm/l cut-off) is a more sensitive test of the dry eye than rose bengal staining, basal tear volume, reflex Schirmer's test (3-mm wetting cut-off), and lysozyme in reflex tears. Gilbard[46] believes that the tear osmolarity test is better than the Schirmer's test, TBUT, and rose bengal staining for the diagnosis of KCS.

Although clinical measurement of tear osmolarity is not routinely performed in the practice setting, osmolarity levels may someday provide a clinical clue to effective dry eye diagnosis and management.[25,46]

Lactoferrin Immunoassay Testing

Measurement of the tear protein lactoferrin, produced by the lacrimal gland, is used to evaluate decreases in lacrimal gland output. Test kits known as *Lactoplate* are commercially available from Eagle Vision, Inc. (Memphis, TN) and require a filter paper moistened with tears to be placed on a test plate laden with antibodies to human tear lactoferrin. The test requires 3 days before a result can be read. The normal concentration in the tears is 1.42 mg/ml, and a value below 1 mg/ml is considered abnormal.

Tear Film Tests

Tear quality has traditionally been assessed by the staying power of the tear film, that is, its ability to remain as a complete, unbroken film over the anterior eye. An unstable tear film can lead to ocular surface damage that, in turn, can lead to a shortened TBUT and, therefore, a dry eye.

Tear Film Breakup Time

The traditional TBUT test involves the use of sodium fluorescein in the tear film and observation with the biomicroscope for the first randomly located discontinuity

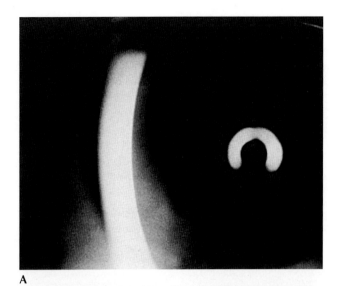

A

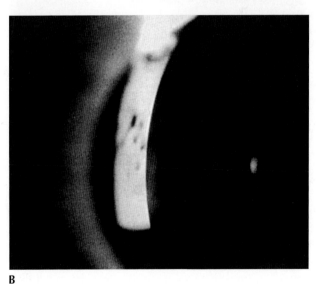

B

FIG. 1-3. *The traditional tear film breakup time.* **(A)** *Fluorescein instilled into the tear film.* **(B)** *Appearance of first nonstaining (black) spot or area indicating the tear film breakup time in seconds from the latest blink.*

in the tear film, as evidenced by a localized nonstaining (black) spot or area (Fig. 1-3). The appearance of the first nonstaining area indicates the breakup time in seconds from the latest blink. However, the instillation of fluorescein is invasive and should shorten the breakup time by lowering the surface tension of the tears and destabilizing the tear film. In addition, the amount of fluorescein instilled is important to the magnitude of these effects. A TBUT of less than 10 seconds implies an abnormal tear film and the likelihood of mucus deficiency,[30] but the

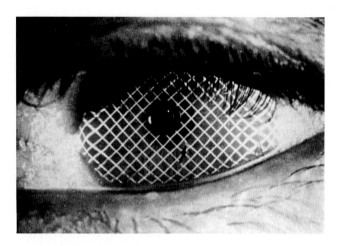

FIG. 1-4. *Reflected grid pattern image from the precorneal tear film of a healthy subject. The arrow shows distortion of the grid line with the beginning of discontinuity of the tear film. This indicates the noninvasive tear film breakup time of the tears from the latest blink. (Reprinted with permission from LS Mengher, AJ Bron, SR Tonge, DJ Gilbert: A non-invasive instrument for clinical assessment of the pre-corneal tear film stability. Curr Eye Res 4:1, 1985.)*

TBUT has been shown to be poorly reproducible in a given subject.[33]

Noninvasive Tear Breakup Time

A noninvasive technique for measurement of the TBUT has been developed that avoids the use of fluorescein.[30] This technique requires a grid pattern to be reflected from the tear film in a device called a *toposcope* or *xeroscope*, in which measurement of the noninvasive TBUT (NIBUT) commences immediately after the last complete blink (Fig. 1-4). Mengher et al.[30] reported the NIBUT values of healthy subjects to range from 4 to 214 seconds (mean, 41.5). They also reported, however, that the NIBUT range for the dry eye (KCS) was from 2 to 20 seconds (mean, 12.2), representing considerable overlap with the normal range. This type of NIBUT testing is not used in general clinical practice because of the need for special equipment.

In general, whether the traditional or the noninvasive TBUT test is used, cosmetics used on the eyelids, eyelid margins, and eyelashes may have deleterious effects on TBUT owing to contamination of the tear film.

Tear Thinning Time

Tear thinning time (TTT) is a noninvasive technique performed with a keratometer, in which the clinician notes the elapsed time after the blink to the first distortion of the keratometer mires.[47]

Tearscope

Another noninvasive tear film test is a technique to better evaluate the lipid layer of the tear film by observing the interference patterns created by the lipid layer and viewing the rupture of the lipid layer versus breakup of the entire tear film.[9] The commercially available Tearscope (Keeler Instruments, Inc., Broomall, PA) is used with a biomicroscope and is very user-friendly for clinical practice.

Tear Evaporation Rate   Tear evaporation rate has been found to be lowest on awakening, increasing in the first 2 hours of eye opening to a constant value for the rest of the day.[35] The explanation for this observation involves decreased tear production during sleep and an increased tear lipid layer (which would resist evaporation) on awakening.[35]

Ocular Surface Tests

Vital Staining with Rose Bengal

The use of rose bengal dye, an iodine derivative of fluorescein, to stain degenerating and devitalized epithelial cells on the anterior eye[36] was first used by Sjögren[37] to diagnose KCS and has been found by others to be a useful diagnostic tool.[39,42,48] Rose bengal is actually toxic to healthy epithelial cells if the cells are not adequately protected by the mucus layer of the tear film.[49] This may explain why some normal eyes stain minimally with rose bengal,[17] particularly in the area of application of the dye, and why staining increases when multiple drops are used or when the strength of the dye in solution is greater than 1%.[7] Characteristic rose bengal staining of exposed bulbar conjunctiva and cornea appears early in most patients with incipient dry eye.[17] Rose bengal also stains mucus and mucus threads.

A scoring system that can be used for rose bengal staining (after van Bijsterveld)[36] involves the external view of the patient's eye separated into three sections: the temporal third (bulbar conjunctiva), the central third (the cornea), and the nasal third (bulbar conjunctiva). The maximum score for each section is 3, allowing for a maximum score per eye of 9. Grade 0 indicates no staining, grade 1 is minimal scattered staining, grade 2 is moderate coalesced staining, and grade 3 is heavy coalesced staining over a large percentage of the area. Dividing the ocular surface into more areas for evaluation improves the sensitivity of any grading system.

Laroche and Campbell[50] proposed a 16-area grid for quantitative and location tracking of staining. The NEI/Industry Workshop group[13] proposed another grading system with three areas of temporal and nasal conjunctiva (six areas per eye), each graded 0–3 (Figs. 1-5

FIG. 1-5. *Conjunctival surface areas delineated for grading of rose bengal staining (after Lemp[13]). Each area is scored as grade 0–3. An eye's total score is the sum of scores from all areas of that eye.*

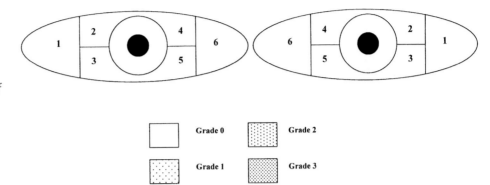

and 1-6). Their system excludes the cornea from the grading scheme.

Norn[39] considers rose bengal staining the most important diagnostic dry eye aid in practice. Combining rose bengal staining with the Schirmer's test was found to be no better than rose bengal alone in dry eye diagnosis.[36] Whitcher[19] agrees with Norn in believing that rose bengal staining is the most important diagnostic sign of KCS if KCS diagnosis is made when two of the three following abnormal results are present: (1) positive Schirmer's test, (2) positive rose bengal staining, and (3) reduced TBUT. Controversy still exists, however, concerning the value of rose bengal staining in the diagnosis of the patient with a dry eye. Rose bengal testing, tear prism height, and TBUT are all thought by Mackie and Seal[11] to be unreliable tests. Furthermore, Schein and colleagues[5] studied the signs and symptoms of dry eye in the elderly and found no correlation between symptoms (by questionnaire), Schirmer testing, and rose bengal staining.

Rose bengal dye can be instilled into the tear film by wetting a commercially available rose bengal–impregnated strip with one drop of saline and applying the strip to the tear film overlying the inferior bulbar conjunctiva. Among questions considered by the NEI/Industry Workshop group[13] were whether the strips or liquid rose bengal were better, and in what concentration and amount the dye should be used. One study concluded that the concentration of rose bengal delivered to the ocular surface by means of a wetted strip is relatively low and soak time/technique dependent, suggesting that results in clinical studies with rose bengal strip application may be different if controlled small-volume applications of 1% liquid rose bengal dye are used.[51] Consequently, small volumes of liquid dye may yield positive results while the strips may give a negative result, particularly in marginal or mild dry eye cases. The technique of using measured, small volumes of liquid rose bengal should give more sensitive and repeatable results than the dye-impregnated filter paper strips, and this protocol has been used in some dry eye research.[27]

Vital Staining with Lissamine Green

Lissamine green, an organic acid dye with a blue-green hue, is a relatively new entrant to the diagnostic armamentarium for dry eye. Lissamine green stains degener-

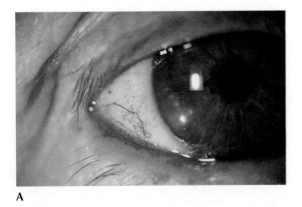
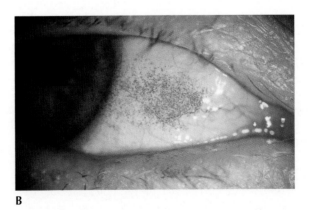

FIG. 1-6. *Examples of rose bengal conjunctival staining (16×) of (A) temporal and (B) nasal conjunctiva. Note a slight staining of the cornea as well.*

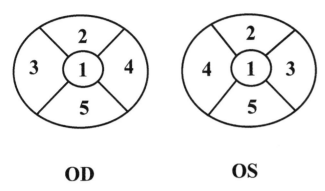

OD   OS

FIG. 1-7. *Corneal surface areas delineated for grading of sodium fluorescein staining. A standardized grading system of 0–3 is used for each of the five areas on each cornea (after Lemp [13]). (OD = right eye; OS = left eye.)*

ated cells and mucus[40] and has the advantage of not causing the stinging and discomfort associated with the use of rose bengal. It demonstrates the same staining pattern of ocular surface damage found with rose bengal, and the staining is easier to see than rose bengal because its color presents in contrast with the conjunctival blood vessels.

Lissamine green is commercially available in liquid form and in wettable, dye-impregnated filter strips. The preserved liquid form (15-ml bottle) of lissamine green (Dacryon Pharmaceuticals, Lubbock, TX) is marketed as an ophthalmic demulcent (artificial tear) for the temporary relief of burning and irritation caused by dryness of the eye. For use in clinical evaluation of the ocular surface, the drop is very generous, therefore, smaller, measured volumes of dye are recommended, as with liquid rose bengal. The ophthalmic filter-paper strips form of the lissamine green dye offers an advantage over rose bengal strips in that the dye releases much more readily with the addition of a drop of saline than does rose bengal.

Vital Staining with Sodium Fluorescein

Sodium fluorescein penetrates broken epithelial surfaces and diffuses through intercellular spaces without staining the cells,[50] easily demonstrating corneal epithelial breakdown secondary to dry eye conditions and other ocular surface disease states.[19]

The fluorescein dye is instilled into the tear film by wetting a commercially available fluorescein-impregnated ophthalmic strip with one drop of saline and applying the strip to the tear film overlying the inferior bulbar conjunctiva. Liquid fluorescein (2%) is available for topical use but offers no significant advantages over the strip form and, therefore, is rarely used. The NEI/Industry Workshop group[13] proposed a grading system for fluorescein staining (Fig. 1-7).

Impression Cytology

Conjunctival impression cytology allows the effects of tear deficiency on the ocular epithelium to be examined. A Millipore filter is pressed onto the conjunctiva and then removed. In the process, the filter paper pulls up epithelial cells, goblet cells, and mucus. The filter is fixed and stained, and the cells are inspected for their condition. This technique has a sensitivity of 100% and a specificity of 87% for a dry eye condition.[41] Squamous metaplasia is commonly encountered as the ocular surface disease caused by KCS. Although impression cytology traditionally has been done in laboratory and research settings, its clinical use is now becoming more feasible.

National Eye Institute/Industry Workshop Group Recommended Diagnostic Tests

The possible combinations of favorite or favored tear and tear film tests are numerous. In light of this, and after careful deliberation, the NEI/Industry Workshop group[13] offered their recommendations for diagnostic tests for dry eye. By following the recommendations of this group, researchers and clinicians should be better able to compare their results and experiences on a level playing field and work more in concert than they have in the past. The specifics of these recommendations are likely to be modified somewhat over time as new information comes to light.

TREATMENTS AND PROGNOSIS FOR COMMON DRY EYE

Treatment of dry eye and ocular surface disease conditions includes such approaches as conservation (e.g., tarsorrhaphy, punctal occlusion, humidifiers, and moisture chambers) and supplementation or replacement (e.g., artificial tears, ointments, and inserts). Many patients stabilize on a low-maintenance regimen of artificial tears and mucolytic agents.[52] Most patients using artificial tears develop a preference for a specific brand of drop (based on viscosity or initial comfort). A variety of artificial tears, preserved and nonpreserved, are available commercially. Patients who are sensitive to preservatives, who have allergies, or who are using the artificial tear products many times each day may do better with nonpreserved products. Albietz and Golding[53] recommended almost universally that preserved or nonpreserved artificial tears be instituted for mildly symptomatic dry eyes, and only nonpreserved tears be instituted for moderate and severe symptom conditions. Although appropriate as a part of most treatment plans, artificial tears are not recommended as a first-line treatment in conditions such as severe lipid anomaly (defer to lid hygiene and systemic antibiotics) or with severe allergic dry eye (recommending no contact lens wear; antihistamine, mast cell stabilizer, or both; and management of the underlying etiology).[53] Artificial tears are available in low-, moderate-, and high-viscosity choices, and ointments are also available for use during sleep. Most patients do not appreciate high-viscosity tear supplements for use during the day owing to the visual blurring that occurs with use.

Patients with a diagnosis of a questionably or marginally dry eye usually do not progress to severe dry eye,[21] and less than 1% of all dry eye patients suffer severe visual impairment.[54] Consideration of moderate to severe dry eye causes, diagnosis, and management is presented in Chapter 10.

CONTACT LENS–RELATED DRYNESS

It is an unnatural and significant challenge for the tear volume and tear film to support not only the anterior segment of the eye but also to support the surfaces and the bulk of a contact lens polymer. Dryness is a very commonly reported symptom of contact lens wearers, so much so that contact lens wear has been suggested as a provocative test for tear and tear film deficiency.[55] The sensation of dryness with contact lens wear, part of a *minimal sicca syndrome*, may result from loss of tears; a fast breakup of the tear film; or from physical interaction of the lens with the ocular tissues, lens dehydration, or rise in temperature because of vessel dilatation.[56] No clear-cut guidance exists concerning interpretation and application of the results of tear and tear film clinical tests in a predictable and repeatable fashion for symptoms of dryness related to contact lens wear. A variety of contributing factors have been identified, and approaches for management of contact lens–drying symptoms are reasonably well established.

The best way to avoid problems is to perform a thorough prefitting evaluation. Subjective input through appropriate case history or questionnaire[16] should be used to rule out absolute and relative contraindications to contact lens wear. Tests of the tears and tear film should then be performed. Problems associated with the frequency and completeness of the blink and with the general apposition of the eyelid to the globe can encourage dehydration with a hydrogel lens, peripheral corneal desiccation with a rigid gas-permeable lens, and exposure insult to the cornea and bulbar conjunctiva. Patients with keratopathy caused by exposure usually do not do well with hydrogel lens wear because the lens succumbs to the effects of exposure and consequent dehydration. Patients with

active blepharitis, ocular rosacea, or MGD should not wear contact lenses until the lid disease has been managed by conventional protocols, which include improved lid hygiene, lid scrubs, warm compresses, and sometimes systemic or topical antibiosis. For existing contact lens wearers with problems of discomfort and dryness, meibomian therapy can help them to become more comfortable. Twenty-one patients with contact lens intolerance (rigid gas permeable lens and hydrogel lens wearers) and some level of MGD experienced improved subjective comfort with contact lens wear and demonstrated increased TBUT after 2 weeks of daily eyelid scrubs and warm compresses.[57] The positive outcomes from eyelid hygiene for patients with dryness and discomfort, therefore, are emphasized and recommended as part of a general clinical approach in managing contact lens–related dryness symptoms, particularly with older patients. Clinicians should recommend against the use of commercially available eyelid hygiene (blepharitis) products while contact lenses are on the eye.

Tear Film Disruption and Evaporation

Contact lenses disrupt the tear film and actually enhance the evaporation of the tears[58] simply by the mechanical effects of their presence.[59] This effect of contact lens wear can transform a borderline dry eye to a symptomatic, contact lens–related dry eye.[35] Hydrogel lenses, because of the polymer's physical chemistry, have an imbibition pressure gradient much like that of the corneal stroma, in which a certain amount of water is held in balance within the body of the lens structure. The moisture within a hydrogel lens may be lost because of evaporation from the front surface of the lens, with moisture squeezed from the lens by the eyelids, or osmotic gradients.[60] The kinetics of the ocular environment require, as moisture is lost from the lens, moisture to be brought back into the lens polymer if it is available in the surrounding area (e.g., from the tears). Thus, if a hydrogel lens dries and requires moisture, it acts as a wick and pulls the moisture from the tear film. Study of diurnal variation in the human tear evaporation rate shows that the rate is lowest on awakening and increases within the first 2 hours to a fairly constant rate for the rest of the day, presumably because a thick, stable lipid layer inhibits evaporation in the early waking hours.[35] Drying symptoms late in the day for hydrogel lens wearers do not seem to be because of diurnal changes in tear evaporation but may be related to environmental changes or tear production changes throughout the day.[60]

Silicone elastomer lenses, which have no water content, allow water vapor to pass through the lens material. As moisture evaporates from the tear film on the anterior surface of the lens, an outward gradient of moisture movement occurs (pervaporation) from the tear pool behind the lens through the lens material to evaporate from the front lens surface.[61] Silicone elastomer lenses are commonly used as extended-wear devices in the management of pediatric aphakia. The difficulty with this feature of the silicone elastomer lens is that, if not fitted loosely enough, negative pressure can develop under the lens because of this movement of water vapor and can cause the lens to become immobile, which can be dangerous to the health of the eye.[61] Gas-permeable lenses, as well as hard lenses (polymethylmethacrylate [PMMA]), have essentially no water content (less than 1%) and, therefore, are relatively inert with regard to absorbing moisture from the tear film.

SPECIFIC CONTACT LENS–ASSOCIATED DRYNESS: VARIABLES AND TREATMENT

Corneal Hypoxia and Symptoms of Discomfort

Corneal hypoxia may be the source of drying symptoms because the cornea, after a number of hours, can cause some general, hypoxia-related nonspecific sensation and discomfort, and the patient may refer to this as dryness. Because of a lack of specific neural receptors for dryness in human tissue, the sensation of dryness must be a response to a multitude of nonspecific afferent neural inputs.[62]

Drying Symptoms at the Cellular Level

Impression cytology has enabled one to view, at the cellular level, the effects of soft contact lens wear in asymptomatic, clinical problem–free patients. Changes have been reported in the nuclear chromatin of conjunctival epithelial cells in successful, asymptomatic soft contact lens wearers, and these changes are the same as those seen in ocular surface disease (dry eye disorders, inflammation, and immunologic reactions).[63] The changes seen at the cellular level are signs of decreased metabolic activity and cellular dysfunction, and are thought to be caused by chronic mechanical irritation (rubbing) of the soft lens on the epithelial surface. Similar changes have been observed in squamous metaplasia in ocular surface diseases. The functional consequences of such intracellular changes in asymptomatic lens wearers may manifest at a clinical level after a longer time, presenting as a sensation of dryness secondary to the squamous metaplasia of the

epithelium. Perhaps this is why hydrogel lens drying symptoms are often not managed well with lens rewetting or lubricating drops for patients in whom a lack of moisture is not the problem and the true culprit is cellular change related to the mechanical effects of lens wear.

Rigid Gas-Permeable Lens Dryness

Rigid Gas-Permeable Polymers

A phenomenon seen with the refitting of the classic hard lens wearer into gas-permeable contact lenses is the development of drying symptoms, presumably because of the rehabilitation of the cornea, including a reawakening of corneal sensitivity. The cornea of a PMMA wearer is relatively numb secondary to the chronic swelling associated with the wearing of PMMA lenses. Many patients refitted from PMMA to gas-permeable lenses experience problems with increased awareness of the lenses as they are worn, and this is often interpreted as dryness, irritation, and scratchiness. This may be because of not only the awakening of the cornea with the more oxygen-transmissive gas-permeable materials but also, in part, to true differences in the lens polymer. The wettability of the surface of gas-permeable lenses has been a subject of debate. Certainly, the silicone added to the lens polymers, which is designed to encourage the transmission of oxygen through the lens material, does not enhance the wettability of the lens material. In fact, the silicone content tends to decrease lens surface wettability and to attract foreign material (e.g., lipids and proteins) to the lens surface. Such lens deposits can sometimes help wettability by encouraging a natural protective biofilm on the lens surfaces. The opposite can also be true: In some cases the deposits may alter lens wearability and wearing comfort, even to the point of setting up an ocular immunologic reaction to the deposits on the lens.

Another generation of lens materials is the family of fluorinated gas-permeable lenses. Addition of fluorine to the silicone acrylate lenses increases the solubility of oxygen within the lens material and decreases the surface tension of the lens, thereby increasing lens wettability. Drying symptoms and problems with wettability continue, however, with the fluorosilicone acrylate lenses.[64] Surface hazing caused by a drawing of the tear film away from the anterior lens surface toward either the inferior or superior tear prism, or both, is often clinically observed with the slit-lamp during the interblink period.[65] This type of lens surface hazing is a wettability problem that can sometimes cause a decrease in vision and lens-wearing comfort that may be described as dryness. The tear film over a rigid gas-permeable contact lens has been reported to be unstable,[66] and this may encourage evaporation of the tear film with ensuing drying symptoms; yet, for healthy, successful rigid gas-permeable lens patients, drier environments do not substantially reduce lens-wearing comfort.[67]

Gas-permeable lenses seem to allow better visual performance than hydrogel lenses when partial desiccation of the pre-lens tear film between extended, suppressed blinks is evaluated. They show small reductions (7%) in low-contrast visual acuity (mean loss of 0.3 lines), similar to the visual performance of patients wearing no contact lenses.[68] Hydrogel lenses, on the other hand, show a significant reduction of acuity (mean loss of 4.1 lines).[68]

Rigid Gas-Permeable–Related Peripheral Corneal Desiccation

Peripheral corneal desiccation, also known as *peripheral corneal drying, 3 and 9 o'clock staining*, and *4 and 8 o'clock staining*, occurs in approximately 80% of patients who wear gas-permeable lenses.[69] Signs of corneal drying include conjunctival hyperemia; punctate staining; corneal scarring and dellen; and symptoms that include itching, increased lens awareness, and dry eye sensation.[64,70] This phenomenon is thought to be caused by any of a number of contributory factors, including thinning of the tear film just beyond the lens edge (black line),[71] incomplete blinking,[64,70,72] unstable tear film or tear aqueous deficiency,[64,70,72,73] excessive lens edge thickness,[69] excessive edge lift,[72,74] insufficient edge lift,[70,74] inferior lens positioning,[64,74] and insufficient lens movement (lens stagnation).[74] Lens stagnation, particularly in an inferior position, keeps the peripheral corneal epithelial cells just beyond the lens edge from being washed and wiped with each blink. This leads to localized peripheral dry areas resembling a superficial punctate keratitis as seen with sodium fluorescein staining.

Peripheral corneal desiccation with rigid gas-permeable lens wear is often chronic, and can progress through stages as proposed by Henry and colleagues[73] (Table 1-2). The most advanced stage is now described as *vascularized limbal keratitis* (*VLK*). VLK has been described as a staged response to and a product of more severe peripheral corneal desiccation associated with gas-permeable contact lens wear[75] (Table 1-3). Management can range from no action to discontinuation of lens wear. Eye rewetting drops, lens lubricants, and antioxidant drops are recommended as part of a management protocol; however, changes in lens design and lens performance features are more likely to be effective in the management of this problem. Schnider[74] studied the effect of lens design of "known stainers" and concluded that large diameter lenses (10.2 and 9.6 mm) with moderate edge lifts (0.08 mm) outperformed lenses of small diameter (9.0 mm) with low edge lifts (0.04 mm), summarizing that peripheral corneal des-

TABLE 1-2. *Grading Scale for Peripheral Corneal Desiccation*

0 = Not present
1 = Diffuse punctate staining
2 = Mild density
3 = Moderate density
4 = Opacification/neovascularization

Source: Data from VH Henry, ES Bennett, JF Forrest: Clinical investigation of the Paraperm EW rigid gas-permeable contact lens. Am J Optom Physiol Opt 64:313, 1987.

iccation may be minimized by avoiding low-vertical centration, narrow or shallow tear pools under the peripheral curve system, erratic or insufficient lens movement, and smaller lens diameters.

Management of peripheral corneal desiccation includes changes in lens design (lens overall diameter, edge thickness, and edge lift), blinking exercises, use of artificial tears or lens lubricants, and—something that always works—refitting into a hydrogel lens.

Hydrogel Lens–Related Dryness

Environment, Dehydration, Lens Material, and Design

Many contact lens wearers are free of symptoms, have no need for rewetting drops, and wear their lenses happily. A significant number of lens wearers, however, have at least occasional or periodic symptoms of drying or discomfort. Others are burdened by constant discomfort, eventually becoming dropouts from contact lens wear. Many times, owing to lack of better information, we describe symptomatic lens-wearing patients as having a marginal dry eye. This is illustrated by a patient whose tear film does an adequate job of supporting the eye in its normal situation, even in the face of environmental challenges, such as low humidity and air drafts. When challenged with the need to support a contact lens as well, the

TABLE 1-3. *Classification of Vascularized Limbal Keratitis*

Stage I
  Hyperplasia (epithelial)
Stage II
  Inflammatory response
  Infiltration
  Conjunctival hyperemia
Stage III
  Vascularization
Stage IV
  Erosion

Source: Adapted from RM Grohe, KA Lebow: Vascularized limbal keratitis. Int Contact Lens Clin 16:197, 1989.

tear film may be pushed over the edge, and the patient develops a contact lens–induced dry eye. The patient may generally do well except for seasonal problems, flying in jet airplanes in which the air is very dry, or at high altitudes where the air is colder, dryer, and thinner. A survey of practitioners showed that 20% to 30% of hydrogel lens wearers experienced dry eye symptoms more often in dry than in humid environments when wearing their lenses.[76] Another significant environmental or ergonomic circumstance is use of a video display terminal, during which the patient may not blink fully or often enough and may be subjected to glare from the video display terminal screen and air drafts that dry out the tear film. Such situations may contribute to the marginal dry eye with contact lens wear. Counseling patients about their blinking skills and habits and encouraging them to blink fully and frequently help some patients. Regarding the internal (body) environment, Caffery has emphasized the importance of diet on tear function and, among other recommendations, has suggested increased water intake for generally improved body hydration.[77]

Hydrogel lenses lose water with wear,[78,79] and this can lead to changes in lens diameter, thickness, curvature, and oxygen transmissibility, thus affecting lens fit, vision, and wearing comfort. Patients who must reduce wearing time because of dry eye symptoms show normal tear meniscus height before lens wear but significantly reduced tear meniscus height after 4 hours of lens wear compared with a matched but symptom-free control group.[80] Therefore, pre-lens wear and prefitting tear meniscus height cannot predict which patients experience drying symptoms.

When hydrogel-wearing patients experience symptoms of drying with lens wear, the lens design, the material, and the water content are important factors. High–water content lenses (70% water), when made very thin (0.04-mm center thickness) to optimize oxygen transmission, cause significant fluorescein staining of the corneal epithelium.[81] The staining is worse in environments with low relative humidity and is not related to lens dehydration or degree of patient symptoms. The likely cause is that evaporation of moisture from the front surface of the lens pulls the tears from the post-lens space and the fluid from around and within the epithelial cells. Dehydration at the front surface of a hydrogel lens is more likely to penetrate through the cornea-lens interface with high–water content lenses than with low–water content lenses of the same thickness.[60] This may be why the staining reported by Orsborn and Zantos[81] occurred with thin, high–water content lenses. However, dehydration may vary not only with the water content but also with different lens materials of the same water content.[82]

Clinical impressions and opinions differ with regard to the best lens material and design for dry eye patients. The consensus seems to be that low to medium–water content lenses are best. Clinical studies by Finnemore (unpublished data) indicated that patients with drying symptoms preferred thicker lenses (0.12 mm) over thinner lenses (0.06 mm). Finnemore also found that marginal dry eye patients preferred prism-ballasted hydrogel lenses to thin or thick spheric lenses. This may be explained as the thicker, inferior portion of the lens protects the post-lens tears at the inferior cornea from depletion, especially with incomplete blinking. The aforementioned patient preferences are in concert with Orsborn and Zantos's finding that thicker, lower–water content lenses showed the least amount of corneal fluorescein staining.[81] Contrary to these findings, one published study found that 40% of patients wearing thick toric hydroxyethylmethacrylate lenses reported symptoms of dryness, whereas only 13% of patients wearing thinner spheric lenses reported dryness.[56] In a study of 10 marginally dry eye patients, a thinner, 58%–water content, spheric hydrogel lens was slightly preferred over the same lens material in a 33% thicker design; corneal staining was absent with the thinner lens, whereas it was present 37% of the time with the thicker lens.[83] Thus, traditional beliefs regarding lens water content and thickness remain open to question and further study.

Regarding choices of lens material, the U.S. Food and Drug Administration has allowed specific labeling for the hydrogel material omafilcon A, available as the Proclear line of contact lenses (Biocompatibles, Ltd., Tewksbury, MA), indicating that it may provide improved comfort for contact lens wearers who experience mild discomfort or symptoms related to dryness during lens wear. Through incorporation of the water-retaining polymer phosphorylcholine, this lens material combats dryness associated with the water loss of evaporative (non-Sjögren's) or aqueous tear deficiency. This lens material probably cannot help every patient, but the attainment of such U.S. Food and Drug Administration labeling is a first in the industry and is worthy of mention and consideration.

As clinical research continues toward development of even better hydrogel lens polymers for patients who have drying symptoms, it is wise to remember that rigid gas-permeable lenses are a good option because of their more inert nature relative to the tear pool and the tear film.

Lens Care Systems and Symptoms of Dryness

Lens care systems are important to the wearing comfort and ultimate lens-wearing success of contact lens patients. The components of a contact lens care system are themselves possible causes of dry eye symptoms, in addition to the lens material, lens design, lens fit, and the profile and stability of the patient's tear film. Lens care system components that are introduced to the tear film, even on a temporary basis, can be quite disruptive to the stability of the film. Product preservatives can exacerbate dry eye symptoms with lens wear,[84] and the possibility exists that surfactant agents in hydrogel lens multipurpose solutions can be inherently disruptive to the lipid layer of the tear film. Such effects should be short-lived because of the brief contact time. Any relationship between the surfactant and a longer-term discomfort reported to occur later in the wearing day undoubtedly would be weak.

Preservative-free care systems, such as thermal and hydrogen peroxide–based systems, for hydrogel lenses are a good alternative to so-called chemical disinfection systems. Gas-permeable lens wearers who change to a lens care system with a slightly different preservative may experience a difference in lens-wearing comfort. Often, the exact cause is not known, be it a particular care system component, concentration, or interaction with the patient's tear chemistry. It is simple enough, however, to try a different system. If the new care system works better, then one is often left not knowing the true source of the problem, but nevertheless successful in either suppressing or solving the difficulty.

Although not directly related to lens care, the use and type of facial and eye cosmetics should also be considered a potential contributor to tear and tear film difficulties. Contamination of the lens surface by cosmetics is the most direct challenge to wettability of the lens, and hypersensitivity (allergy) to the cosmetic ingredients is also a possibility. In both cases, some level of drying symptoms and lens intolerance is expected.

CONTACT LENSES FOR THERAPEUTIC USE

Severe cases of ocular surface disease, aqueous deficiency, or EDE can be treated with a hydrogel contact lens used as a bandage, offering protective and even therapeutic effects.[27] Such contact lenses are typically made of a collagen or hydrogel material and have a large diameter to cover the entire cornea; large scleral (haptic) lenses are also useful for eye protection in some cases. Therapeutic lenses are not used to correct refractive error, rather they are used to improve patient comfort, afford mechanical protection, promote healing, and maintain ocular surface hydration. Conditions treated with bandage contact lenses include, but are not limited to, recurrent corneal erosions, persistent epithelial defects, trichiasis, severe dry eye,

postphotorefractive keratectomy, and postphototherapeutic keratectomy.

Treatments, such as ocular lubricants, ointments, moisture chamber spectacles, and punctal occlusion, should be attempted before considering bandage contact lens therapy for the severe dry eye patient. If the patient's condition is so advanced, however, that lenses are worn as a bandage to protect the cornea from exposure to the air or to control corneal filaments and the discomfort associated with them, then lens wear may be considered.[85]

Because of the hydrophilic nature of hydrogel lenses, a dry ocular surface rarely, if ever, adequately supports the thirsty nature of the polymer of the soft lens. Consequently, the lenses dehydrate significantly on the eye and may deposit easily, and ocular infection potential may be increased. Lubricating drops for use with contact lenses may be used with lens wear to maintain lens hydration, but the positive effect is short-lived, requiring the very frequent instillation of drops to maintain lens-wearing comfort. Punctal occlusion may improve the retention of the patient's available tears on the ocular surface and maintain the hydration of the lens.

The choice of lens water content for dry eye patients is often debated. One view is that a higher–water content hydrogel lens should be worn because the lens has more water. Such a lens, however, has more moisture to lose and may be greatly affected by dehydration. Another view is that a lower–water content lens should be fitted and in a thicker lens design. This lens presents a greater barrier to lens dehydration and may be more comfortable for the patient. No clear direction exists on which is the best choice, and it may be highly patient dependent.

Because therapeutic lenses usually remain on the eye for an extended-wear basis, oxygen transmissibility should be maximized to minimize edema. Often, a middle–water content (approximately 50–60% water) disposable hydrogel lens not only may be a good choice for parameter and design considerations, but also may allow for frequent lens replacement at minimal cost.

For an in-depth discussion of the role of bandage therapeutic contact lenses, see Chapter 21.

COMMON TREATMENTS FOR CONTACT LENS–RELATED DRYNESS

Fluid Supplementation of the Tears

Many years ago, when hydrogel lenses were relatively new, no lens care systems included rewetting or lens lubricant drops. Dryness, scratching, and a gritty sensation late in the wearing time of a given day became common with so many hydrogel lens wearers that a market for lens rewetting drops developed, and such drops now are often included in hydrogel and gas-permeable lens care systems. The pre-lens tear film, however, does not seem to physically improve for longer than 5 minutes after instillation of either saline or on-eye lens lubricants.[86] Almost any rewetting drop affords some symptomatic relief, although more short term (10 minutes) than longer term.[87] Occlusion of the nasolacrimal drainage system extends the relief provided by these drops by extending retention time on the ocular surface.[88]

In addition to fluid-supplementing drops, eyelid massage is recommended for relief of symptoms of dryness with hydrogel lenses.[89] The lid massage is thought to use natural eye secretions to counteract lens or ocular surface changes associated with the symptoms of dryness. Soaking hydrogel lenses in the middle of a wearing day is also helpful. The midday lens soaking has two positive effects: rehydration of the lens, allowing a fresh start in a rewearing period, and a break for the eyes from lens wear, allowing the eyes to renew themselves for a return to lens wear later that day.

Nasolacrimal Punctal Occlusion

Nasolacrimal punctal occlusion is an easy procedure, which preserves the natural tears. Many clinicians believe that it can benefit many soft lens–wearing patients with symptoms of dryness. This is especially important for those who are diagnosed with borderline or marginally dry eye, and likely works best when the dryness symptoms stem from an aqueous tear deficiency. Dissolvable collagen plugs are typically used for a trial period to determine whether more permanent closure of the puncta is worthwhile. Although these benefits are widely held to be true, research calls this in question. A group of hydrogel lens–wearing patients with dryness symptoms had a single collagen plug placed in both canaliculi of one eye but were led to believe, through a sham procedure for the other eye, that they received this treatment in both eyes.[90] Results of clinical tests showed no difference between the treated and untreated eye, yet the patients indicated that the treated as well as the untreated eye had improvement in dryness symptoms. These results demonstrate a strong placebo effect and are a good example of the value of having controls in clinical studies. The results also cast doubt on the value of using the results of a trial with dissolvable punctal occlusion in establishing whether occlusion by nondissolvable plugs are productive.

Punctal occlusion with nondissolvable (silicone) punctal plugs may be more effective than that from collagen plugs because of the stability of the silicone material as well as the plug's dimensions. Silicone punctal plugs are inserted into the punctal opening, are visible, and may cause foreign-body sensation on occasion. Silicone intracanalicular plugs, however, are inserted down within the canaliculus, leave no outward evidence of their presence, and do not induce any sensation for the patient. Some newer designs of external punctal plugs have improved this situation by utilizing a more flush-fitting external cap.

A study with silicone punctal plugs showed a 72% improvement of drying symptoms in hydrogel lens wearers.[91] Intracanalicular plugs have been shown to improve drying symptoms and clinical signs for soft lens wearers.[88] Another benefit afforded from this type of lacrimal drainage occlusion is that the hydration effects of rewetting drops and artificial tears are enhanced.

More remains to be learned about the effects, desirable and undesirable, of punctal occlusion. The lacrimal gland proteins, lysozyme and lactoferrin, are elevated in the tears of patients after 1 week of punctal occlusion with nondissolvable plugs.[92] It is unknown whether this increased concentration of tear proteins leads to undesirable interactions with a contact lens or leads to an accumulation of denatured proteins under a lens, perhaps leading to inflammatory or infectious ocular events. In addition, the positive effects of nondissolvable plugs on hydrogel wearers' dryness symptoms may diminish over time,[88] which may be related to a decrease in basal tear production during punctal occlusion.[93] Tomlinson et al.[93] suggest that this may occur by some type of ocular surface homeostatic mechanism for downregulation of tear production. It is speculated that this homeostatic response is triggered by an increased tear volume or an increase in the concentration of a macromolecule in the tear film, secondary to occlusion of the puncta.

SUMMARY

The minimal sicca syndrome is a common complication of contact lens wear. Although some physiologic basis may exist for the observed symptoms and signs, minimal sicca is typically a consequence of water loss with hydrogel lenses, and a combination of polymer characteristics and lens design with rigid gas-permeable lenses. The practitioner should consider a variety of options that can be implemented in a conservative and methodic manner to alleviate the symptoms of contact lens–induced dryness.

Clinical management guidelines for drying symptoms with contact lens wear range from cessation of lens wear (rather extreme but 100% successful) to implementing any of a number of possible management options for the motivated patient.[94] These options include use of tear supplements and lubricants, blink training, avoidance of environmental challenges (e.g., smoke, drafts, and low humidity), decreasing lens-wearing time, increased frequency of lens cleaning and lens replacement, avoidance of contaminants (e.g., hand creams and cosmetics), and avoidance of diuretics (e.g., alcohol) and certain systemic medications. Other options include changes in lens design, lens materials, lens care system, and the use of punctal occlusion.

REFERENCES

1. Jordan A, Baum J: Basic tear flow: does it exist? Ophthalmology 87:920, 1980
2. Thoft RA: Relationship of the dry eye to ocular surface disease. Trans Ophthalmol Soc U K 104:452, 1985
3. Doughty MJ, Fonn D, Richter D, et al: A patient questionnaire approach to estimating the prevalence of dry eye symptoms in patients presenting to optometric practices across Canada. Optom Vis Sci 74(8):624, 1997
4. Bandun-Roche K, Munoz B, Tielsch JM, et al: Self-reported assessment of dry eye in a population-based setting. Invest Ophthalmol Vis Sci 38(12):2469, 1997
5. Schein OD, Tielsch JM, Munoz B, et al: Relation between signs and symptoms of dry eye in the elderly. Ophthalmol 104(9):1395, 1997
6. Kuppens EVMJ, Stolwijk TR, Keizer RJW, van Best JA: Basal tear turnover and topical timolol in glaucoma patients and healthy controls by fluorophotometry. Invest Ophthalmol Vis Sci 33:3442, 1992
7. Bron AJ: Duke-Elder lecture. Prospects for the dry eye. Trans Ophthalmol Soc U K 104:801, 1985
8. Holly FJ, Lemp MA: Tear physiology and dry eyes. Surv Ophthalmol 22:69, 1977
9. Guillon JP, Guillon M: Tear film examination of the contact lens patient. Contax 3:14, 1988
10. Doane MG: An instrument for in vivo tear film interferometry. Optom Vis Sci 66:383, 1989
11. Mackie IA, Seal DV: Confirmatory tests for the dry eye of Sjögren's syndrome. Scand J Rheumatol (suppl). 61:220, 1986
12. Mackie IA, Seal DV: Beta blockers, eye complaints, and tear secretion. Lancet 2:1027, 1977
13. Lemp MA: Report of the National Eye Institute/Industry Workshop on clinical trials in dry eyes. CLAO J 21(4):221, 1995
14. McMonnies CW, Ho A: Responses to a dry eye questionnaire from a normal population. J Am Optom Assoc 58:588, 1987
15. McMonnies CW, Ho A: Patient history in screening for dry eye conditions. J Am Optom Assoc 58:296, 1987
16. McMonnies CW: Key questions in a dry eye history. J Am Optom Assoc 57:512, 1986
17. Baum J: Clinical manifestations of dry eye states. Trans Ophthalmol Soc U K 104:415, 1985
18. Lamberts DW, Foster CS, Perry HD: Schirmer test after topical anesthesia and the tear meniscus height in normal eyes. Arch Ophthalmol 97:1082, 1979
19. Whitcher JP: Clinical diagnosis of the dry eye. Int Ophthalmol Clin 27:7, 1987
20. Scherz W, Doane MG, Dohlman CH: Tear volume in normal eyes and keratoconjunctivitis sicca. Graefes Arch Clin Exp Ophthalmol 192:141, 1974
21. Mackie IA, Seal DV: The questionably dry eye. Br J Ophthalmol 65:2, 1981
22. Holly FJ, Lamberts DW, Esquivel ED: Kinetics of capillary tear flow in the Schirmer strip. Curr Eye Res 2:57, 1983
23. Holly FJ, LauKaitis SJ, Esquivel ED: Kinetics of lacrimal secretion in normal human subjects. Curr Eye Res 3:897, 1984
24. Hamano H, Hori M, Hamano T, et al: A new method for measuring tears. CLAO J 9:281, 1983
25. Gilbard JP, Farris RL, Santamaria J: Osmolarity of tear microvolumes in keratoconjunctivitis sicca. Arch Ophthalmol 96:677, 1978
26. Fullard RJ, Snyder C: Protein levels in non-stimulated and stimulated tears of normal subjects. Invest Ophthalmol Vis Sci 31:1119, 1990
27. Snyder C, Fullard RJ: Clinical profiles of non-dry eye patients and correlations with tear protein levels. Int Ophthalmol 15:383, 1991
28. Jannsen PT, van Bjisterveld OP: A simple test for lacrimal gland function: a tear lactoferrin assay by radial immunodiffusion. Graefes Arch Clin Exp Ophthalmol 220:171, 1983
29. McCollum CJ, Foulks GN, Bodner B, et al: Rapid assay of lactoferrin in keratoconjunctivitis sicca. Cornea 13:505, 1994
30. Mengher LS, Bron AJ, Tonge SR, Gilbert DJ: A non-invasive instrument for clinical assessment of the pre-corneal tear film stability. Curr Eye Res 4:1, 1985
31. Mengher LS, Bron AJ, Tonge SR, Gilbert DJ: Effect of fluorescein instillation on the pre-corneal tear film stability. Curr Eye Res 4:9, 1985
32. Lang MA, Hamill JR: Factors affecting tear breakup time in normal eyes. Arch Ophthalmol 89:103, 1973
33. Vanley GT, Leopold IR, Gregg TH: Interpretation of tear film breakup. Arch Ophthalmol 95:445, 1977
34. Rolando M, Refojo MJ: Increased tear evaporation in eyes with keratoconjunctivitis sicca. Arch Ophthalmol 101:557, 1983
35. Tomlinson A, Cedarstaff TH: Diurnal variation in human tear evaporation. J Br Contact Lens Assoc 5:77, 1992
36. van Bijsterveld OP: Diagnostic tests in the sicca syndrome. Arch Ophthalmol 82:10, 1969
37. Sjögren H: Zur kenntnis der Keratoconjunctivitis sicca (Keratitis filiformis bei Hypofunktion der Tranendrusen). Acta Ophthalmol Scand (suppl). 2:S11:1, 1933
38. Shearn MA: Sjögren's syndrome. p. 43. In Major Problems in Medicine. Vol. 2. WB Saunders, Philadelphia, 1971
39. Norn MS: Rose bengal vital staining. Acta Ophthalmol (Copenh) 48:546, 1970
40. Norn MS: Lissamine green, vital staining of cornea and conjunctiva. Acta Ophthalmol (Copenh) 51:483, 1973

41. Nelson JD, Wright JC: Impression cytology of the ocular surface in keratoconjunctivitis sicca. p. 140. In Holly FJ, (ed): The Pre-Ocular Tear Film in Health, Disease, and Contact Lens Wear. Dry Eye Institute, Inc., Lubbock, TX, 1986

42. Norn MS: Dead, degenerated and living cells in conjunctival fluid and mucous thread. Acta Ophthalmol (Copenh) 47:1102, 1969

43. Port MJA, Asaria TS: The assessment of human tear volume. J Br Contact Lens Assoc 13:76, 1990

44. Bowman RW, Dougherty JM, McCulley JP: Chronic blepharitis and dry eyes. Int Ophthalmol Clin 27:27, 1987

45. Farris RL, Gilbard JP, Stuchell RN, Mandell ID: Diagnostic tests in keratoconjunctivitis sicca. CLAO J 9:23, 1983

46. Gilbard JP: Tear film osmolarity and keratoconjunctivitis sicca. CLAO J 11:243, 1985

47. Patel S, Murray D, McKenzie A, et al: Effect of fluorescein on the tear film breakup time and tear thinning time. Am J Optom Physiol Opt 62:188, 1985

48. Forster HW Jr: Rose bengal test in diagnosis of deficient tear formation. Arch Ophthalmol 45:419, 1951

49. Feenstra RPG, Tseng SCG: What is actually stained by rose bengal? Arch Ophthalmol 11:984, 1992

50. LaRoche RR, Campbell RC: Quantitative rose bengal staining technique for external ocular diseases. Ann Ophthalmol 20:274, 1988

51. Snyder C, Paugh J: Rose bengal dye concentration and volume delivered via dye-impregnated paper strips. Optom Vis Sci 75(5):339, 1998

52. Williamson J, Doig WM, Forrester JV, et al: Management of the dry eye in Sjögren's syndrome. Br J Ophthalmol 58:798, 1974

53. Albietz JM, Golding TR: Differential diagnosis and management of common dry eye subtypes. Clin Exp Optom 77(6):244, 1994

54. Wright P: Sjögren's syndrome. Its relationship with connective tissue disease and factors affecting visual prognosis. Trans Ophthalmol Soc U K 94:764, 1974

55. McMonnies C: Contact lens related tear deficiency. p. 584. In Harris MG, (ed): Contact Lenses and Ocular Disease: Problems in Optometry. Vol. 2. No. 4. JB Lippincott, Philadelphia, 1990

56. Brennan NA, Efron N: Symptomatology of HEMA contact lens wear. Optom Vis Sci 66:834, 1989

57. Paugh J, Knapp LL, Martinson JR, Hom MM: Meibomian therapy in problematic contact lens wear. Optom Vis Sci 67(11):803, 1998

58. Tomlinson A, Cedarstaff TH: Tear evaporation from the human eye: effects of contact lens wear. J Br Contact Lens Assoc 5:141, 1982

59. Guillon JP: Tear film structure and contact lenses. p. 914. In Holly FJ, (ed): The Pre-Ocular Tear Film in Health, Disease, and Contact Lens Wear. Dry Eye Institute, Lubbock, TX, 1986

60. Fatt I: A predictive model for dehydration of a hydrogel contact lens in the eye. J Br Contact Lens Assoc 12:15, 1989

61. ReFojo MF, Leong F: Water pervaporation through silicone rubber contact lenses: a possible cause of complications. Contact Intraocul Lens Med J 7:226, 1981

62. Brennan NA, Efron N: Vision and comfort problems with soft contact lenses. p. 221. In Harris MG, (ed): Special Contact Lens Procedures. Problems in Optometry. Vol. 2. No. 2. JB Lippincott, Philadelphia, 1990

63. Knop E, Brewitt H: Conjunctival cytology in asymptomatic wearers of soft contact lenses. Graefes Arch Clin Exp Ophthalmol 230:340, 1992

64. Grohe RM, Caroline PJ: RGP non-wetting lens syndrome. Contact Lens Spectrum 3:32, 1989

65. Grohe RM: Comparative surface hazing of silicone acrylate and fluorosilicone acrylate copolymer contact lenses. Poster presented at the Annual Meeting of the American Academy of Optometry. American Academy of Optometry, Toronto, Canada, 1986

66. Guillon M, Guillon JP, Mapstone V, Dwyer S: Rigid gas-permeable lenses in vivo wettability. J Br Contact Lens Assoc 6:24, 1989

67. Bickel PW, Barr JT: Rigid gas-permeable contact lenses in high and low humidity. J Am Opt Assoc 68(9):574, 1997

68. Timberlake GT, Doane MG, Bertera JH: Short-term, low-contrast visual acuity reduction associated with in vivo contact lens drying. Optom Vis Sci 69:755, 1992

69. Solomon J: Causes and treatments of peripheral corneal desiccation. Contact Lens Forum 11:30, 1986

70. Businger U, Treiber A, Flury C: The etiology and management of three and nine o'clock staining. Int Contact Lens Clin 16:136, 1989

71. Holly FJ: Tear film physiology in contact lens wear, part II. Contact lens tear film interactions. Am J Optom Physiol Opt 58:331, 1981

72. Jones DH, Bennett ES, Davis LJ: How to manage peripheral corneal desiccation. Contact Lens Spectrum 5:63, 1989

73. Henry VH, Bennett ES, Forrest JF: Clinical investigation of the Paraperm EW rigid gas-permeable contact lens. Am J Optom Physiol Opt 64:313, 1987

74. Schnider CM, Terry RL, Holden BA: Effect of lens design on peripheral corneal desiccation. J Am Opt Assoc 68(3):163, 1997

75. Grohe RM, Lebow KA: Vascularized limbal keratitis. Int Contact Lens Clin 16:197, 1989

76. Orsborn G, Robboy M: Hydrogel lenses and dry-eye symptoms. J Br Contact Lens Assoc 6:37, 1989

77. Caffery BE: Influence of diet on tear function. Optom Vis Sci 68:58; 1991

78. Andrasko G: Hydrogel dehydration in various environments. Int Contact Lens Clin 10:22, 1983

79. Brennan NA, Lowe R, Efron N, Harris MG: In vivo dehydration of disposable (ACUVUE) contact lenses. Optom Vis Sci 67:201, 1990

80. Orsborn GN, Zantos SG, Robboy M, et al: Evaluation of tear meniscus heights on marginal dry-eye soft lens wearers. Invest Ophthalmol Vis Sci (suppl). 30:501, 1989

81. Orsborn GN, Zantos SG: Corneal desiccation staining with thin high water content contact lenses. CLAO J 14:81, 1988

82. Brennan NA, Efron N: Hydrogel lens dehydration: a material-dependent phenomenon? Contact Lens Forum 12:28, 1987

83. Jurkus J, Gurkaynak D: Disposable lenses and the marginal dry eye patient. J Am Optom Assoc 65(11):756, 1994

84. Burstein N: The effects of topical drugs and preservatives on the tears and corneal epithelium in dry eye. Trans Ophthalmol Soc U K 104:402, 1985

85. John T, Mobilia EF, Kenyon KR: Therapeutic soft contact lenses. p. 887. In Ruben M, Guillon M, (ed): Contact Lens Practice. Chapman & Hall Medical, London, 1994

86. Golding TR, Efron N, Brennan FA: Soft lens lubricants and prelens tear film stability. Optom Vis Sci 67:461, 1990

87. Efron N, Golding TR, Brennan NA: The effect of soft lens lubricants on symptoms and lens dehydration. CLAO J 17:114, 1991

88. Slusser TG, Lowther GE: Effect of lacrimal drainage occlusion with nondissolvable intracanalicular plugs on hydrogel contact lens wear. Optom Vis Sci 75(5):330, 1998

89. Shuley V, Collins M: Lid massage and symptoms of dryness in soft contact lens wearers. Int Contact Lens Clin 19:121, 1992

90. Lowther GE, Semes L: Effect of absorbable intracanalicular collagen implants in hydrogel contact lens patients with the symptom of dryness. Int Contact Lens Clin 22(11,12):238, 1992

91. Giovagnoli D, Graham SJ: Inferior punctal occlusion with removable silicone punctal plugs in the treatment of dry-eye related contact lens discomfort. J Am Optom Assoc 63:481, 1992

92. Pearce EI, Tomlinson A, Craig JP, Lowther GE: Tear protein levels following punctal plugging. p. 669. In Sullivan DA, Dartt DA, Meneray MA, (ed): Lacrimal Gland, Tear Film, and Dry Eye Syndromes 2: Basic Science and Clinical Relevance. Plenum Press, New York, 1998

93. Tomlinson A, Craig JP, Lowther GE: The biophysical role in tear regulation. p. 371. In Sullivan DA, Dartt DA, Meneray MA, (ed): Lacrimal Gland, Tear Film, and Dry Eye Syndromes 2: Basic Science and Clinical Relevance. Plenum Press, New York, 1998

94. Lowther GE: Dryness, tears and contact lens wear. Butterworth–Heinemann, Boston, 1997

Appendix 1-1

Expanded Dry Eye Patient Questionnaire *

STUDY QUESTIONNAIRE

Please answer the following questions by checking the response most appropriate to you or by filling in the requested answer.

Currently wearing:
   No contact lenses, hard contact lenses, soft contact lenses

1. Do you ever experience any of the following symptoms? (Please check those that apply to you.):
    Soreness ❏   *Scratchiness* ❏   *Dryness* ❏   *Grittiness* ❏   *Burning* ❏

2. How often do you have these symptoms?
    Never ❏   *Sometimes* ❏   *Often* ❏   *Constantly* ❏

3. Have you ever had drops prescribed or other treatments for dry eyes?
    Yes ❏   *No* ❏   *Uncertain* ❏

4. Do you experience arthritis?
    Yes ❏   *No* ❏   *Uncertain* ❏

5. Do you experience thyroid abnormality?
    Yes ❏   *No* ❏   *Uncertain* ❏

6. Do you experience dryness of the nose, mouth, chest, or vagina?
    Never ❏   *Sometimes* ❏   *Often* ❏   *Constantly* ❏

7. Do you regard your eyes as being *unusually* sensitive to cigarette smoke, smog, air conditioning, central heating?
    Yes ❏   *No* ❏   *Sometimes* ❏

8. Do your eyes easily become very red and irritated when swimming in chlorinated freshwater?
    Not applicable ❏   *Yes* ❏   *No* ❏   *Sometimes* ❏

9. Do you take (please circle) antihistamine tablets or use antihistamine eyedrops, diuretics (water tablets), sleeping tablets, tranquilizers, oral contraceptives, medication for duodenal ulcer or digestive problems, or for high blood pressure?
    or other? (write in) _____

    _____

*Reprinted with permission from RJ Fullard, C Snyder: Expanded dry eye patient questionnaire.

10. Are your eyes dry and irritated the day after drinking alcohol?
Not applicable ❑   *Yes* ❑   *No* ❑   *Sometimes* ❑

11. Are you known to sleep with your eyes partially open?
Yes ❑   *No* ❑   *Sometimes* ❑

12. Do you have eye irritation as you wake from sleep?
Yes ❑   *No* ❑   *Sometimes* ❑

13. Do you wear eye makeup?
   - ❑   *Yes* (please fill in answers to all of this question)
   - ❑   *No* (please go directly to question 14 from here)
      a. Mascara: *Yes* ❑   *No* ❑
         If yes, do you apply a little or a moderate-to-heavy amount (please circle)?
         A little   Moderate to heavy
            do you apply it on the: _____ top lashes only?
                                    _____ top *and* bottom lashes?
      b. Eyeliner: *Yes* ❑   *No* ❑
         If yes, do you apply it on the: _____ top lid only?
                                          _____ top *and* bottom lid?
         If you apply it on the bottom lid, do you apply it above or below the lower eye lashes?
         Above ❑   *Below* ❑
      c. Eyeshadow: *Yes* ❑   *No* ❑
         If yes, do you apply a little or a moderate-to-heavy amount (please circle)?
         A little   Moderate to heavy
      d. Foundation: *Yes* ❑   *No* ❑
      e. Do you use hypoallergenic makeup? *Yes* ❑   *No* ❑

14. Do you have allergies that affect your eyes? *Yes* ❑   *No* ❑
   If yes, what are you allergic to? _____
      Is it seasonal? *Yes* ❑   *No* ❑
   Do you take medication for allergy? *Yes* ❑   *No* ❑
   If yes, is it in the form of shots, pills, or eyedrops? _____

15. Have you had any eye problems, including eye infections, abnormalities, and so forth?
Yes ❑   *No* ❑
   If yes, what _____,
      when _____,
      how was it treated _____,
      and, do you still have this eye condition? _____

16. Do you regularly use eyedrops or ointments of any kind? *Yes* ❑   *No* ❑
   If yes, what drops or ointments and why? _____

17. If you regularly take systemic (by mouth) medicine, do these medicines affect your eyes in any way?
Yes ❑   *No* ❑
   If yes, which medicine(s) and in what way(s)? _____

18. Do you use a computer regularly? *Yes* ❑   *No* ❑
   If yes, how many hours do you use a computer in an average day? _____
      If you have dry eye symptoms, do they occur just when using the computer?
Yes ❑   *No* ❑

(*Continues*)

19. Do you think you have a dry eye?
    - ❏ *Yes* (please go on to question 20)
    - ❏ *No* (you may stop here)

20. a. Are your dry eye symptoms worse in: the home / at work / elsewhere?
        Yes ❏   *No* ❏
    b. Is there anything in your home, work surroundings, or elsewhere, such as chemicals, fumes, or dust, that makes your eyes feel uncomfortable? *Yes* ❏   *No* ❏
        If yes, what is it and describe the feeling of discomfort that you experience: _____

21. a. If you have been diagnosed as having a dry eye,
        Who diagnosed this problem: _____ Optometrist
        _____ Ophthalmologist
        _____ Physician
        How long ago was this diagnosed? _____
        What treatment(s) were:
            Suggested? _____
            Prescribed? _____
    b. If a treatment was suggested or prescribed,
        Have you actually used this treatment? _____
        How often do you use this treatment? _____
        How long have you been using this treatment? _____
        Do you think the treatment helps your dry eye symptoms? _____
    c. Were you told that you could not wear contact lenses because of a dry eye?
        Yes ❏   *No* ❏

22. Are your dry eye symptoms worse in one eye? *Yes* ❏   *No* ❏
    If yes, which eye? *Right* ❏   *Left* ❏
    And why is it worse in this eye? _____

Thank you!

2

Corneal Edema

JOSEPH A. BONNANO

GRAND ROUNDS CASE REPORT

Subjective:
A 32-year-old woman, in good general health, who takes birth control pills. She has worn disposable extended-wear soft lenses for 2 years on a continuous 7-day-wear regimen. Lenses are removed after 1 week, with one night sleep without lenses. Despite advice to the contrary from her practitioner, she disinfects her lenses and uses them again for a second week before discarding.

Objective:
- Best corrected acuity: right eye (OD) 20/20, left eye (OS) 20/20, each eye (OU) (distance or near) with contact lenses or spectacles
- Biomicroscopy: grade 2 bulbar redness (see cornea and contact lens research unit [CCLRU] scale) and smooth palpebral conjunctival surface in area 2; grade 2 epithelial microcysts with mild staining OU (see Fig. 2-7)

Assessment:
Grade 2 epithelial microcysts secondary to long-term extended wear

Plan:
1. Discontinue extended wear. Revert to daily wear.
2. Continue use of disposable lenses, with lens replacement at 2-week intervals.
3. Follow up in 6 weeks; monitor number of microcysts.

Corneal edema secondary to the use of contact lenses is a well-documented and commonly observed clinical phenomenon. Many investigators have established the link between reduced oxygen delivery to the cornea (i.e., corneal hypoxia) and corneal edema. Hypoxia has also been implicated as the underlying cause of other complications, such as epithelial microcyst formation, superficial punctate staining, reduced corneal sensitivity, and neovascularization. Most of these problems, including corneal edema, can be either eliminated or significantly reduced by the use of oxygen-permeable soft or hard contact lenses that are removed on a daily basis.

Whereas oxygen-permeable soft and hard lenses can reduce the level of hypoxia, the oxygen transmissibility of commonly used extended-wear lenses is still insufficient to eliminate it altogether. Some rigid and silicone elastomer lenses (e.g., Silsoft, Bausch & Lomb, Inc., Rochester, NY) provide very high oxygen transmissibilities; however, other problems (e.g., lens adherence and lens coatings) prevent widespread acceptance. Continuous use of contact lenses extends the period of hypoxia to 24 hours, consequently eliminating the daily period of normoxic recovery. This gives the clinician a new set of more complex problems (e.g., contact lens acute red eye syndrome and corneal infection), bringing together effects of altered metabolism secondary to hypoxia, a stimulated immune system, and extended microbial resident times. Although significant corneal edema is present in users of extended-wear lenses, it should be stressed that, with proper lens selection, edema can be significantly reduced in daily-wear users.

Edema is an abnormal accumulation of water in body tissues. This chapter discusses the mechanisms by which water is accumulated in the cornea and how hypoxia stimulates this accumulation. To understand the mechanisms of edema, it is necessary to review some basic aspects of normal corneal physiology. What are the functions of the epithelium and endothelium? For what purpose is oxygen used? How does reduced oxygen delivery to the cornea alter cell function? Because the cornea is avascular, how does it get its oxygen? How can the hypoxic edema be prevented or reversed? This chapter provides the clinician with an understanding of the known etiologies of contact lens–induced corneal edema and relates these underlying mechanisms to the clinical picture. This chapter also presents basic guidelines for proper clinical management of hypoxic corneal edema.

SOME BASIC CORNEAL PHYSIOLOGY

Contact Lens Hypoxic Edema

In the 1950s, it became apparent that the epithelial haze and stromal edema observed after contact lens wear were caused by corneal hypoxia. Smelser and Ozanics[1] placed a tight-fitting goggle over the eye and perfused the goggle with 100% nitrogen gas in an attempt to displace the oxygen present in air. These authors found that the epithelial haze could be duplicated by removal of oxygen from the tears. Subsequent studies by Polse and Mandell[2] showed that polymethylmethacrylate (PMMA) contact lens–induced corneal swelling could be alleviated by exposing the lens-wearing eye to higher-than-normal levels of oxygen. Although this work is consistent with hypoxia as the cause of corneal edema, it also demonstrates that the oxygen must be getting to the cornea through the tears via tear pumping, because PMMA lenses are essentially impermeable to oxygen.

Much effort has been spent attempting to determine the minimal level of oxygen necessary to prevent corneal swelling. The rationale is that if a lens that delivered this critical amount of oxygen is designed, then metabolic interference to the cornea could be eliminated. Studies have indicated that approximately 7–10% oxygen is required to prevent edema, and possibly higher amounts in some individuals.[3] It is difficult to arrive at a precise number because of inherent individual subject variability and the limited sensitivity of the corneal thickness measurement. Seven percent oxygen is approximately the amount delivered by the palpebral conjunctiva to the corneal surface when the eyes are closed. If any amount of oxygen below this level is considered hypoxia, then all lenses, except possibly those made of a silicone elastomer, produce corneal hypoxia when the eyes are closed. Conversely, many of the rigid gas-permeable (RGP) lenses and hydrogel lenses worn with the eyes open satisfy the 7% or greater criterion.

Transparency and Hydration Control

Before considering the specific mechanisms by which hypoxia can lead to corneal edema, it is instructive to review how the cornea regulates its hydration and transparency. For example, to understand why the cornea becomes hazy and scatters light when it is edematous, it is necessary to understand how little light the normal cornea actually scatters.

The cornea provides the major refracting element for the eye and must be smooth, regular, and transparent. Light incident on the cornea can be either transmitted, absorbed, reflected, or scattered. During absorption, the energy of a photon is captured and usually reradiated as heat. Very little visible light is absorbed in the cornea; however, below 310 nm (i.e., in the ultraviolet spectrum) strong absorption occurs by corneal proteins—mainly collagen—and by cellular nucleic acids, DNA and RNA. High doses of ultraviolet light damage epithelial cells and cause severe keratopathy.

Light is reflected because of its interaction with particles larger than its wavelength that have an index of refraction different from the surrounding medium. Stromal keratocytes are large enough to reflect light. Because the keratocytes are located between the stromal lamellae, the reflected light enables an observer to see the fine lamellar appearance of the stroma when it is viewed with the slit-lamp using bright direct illumination. Relatively large differences in the refractive index also occur at the tear-epithelium and aqueous-endothelium interfaces and are, therefore, easily visualized in the slit lamp. Subcellular organelles, such as mitochondria, are larger than the wavelength of light and can reflect light traversing the epithelium, keratocytes, and endothelium. A high concentration of mitochondria is present in the endothelium. The endothelium, however, is very thin (5 μm), and therefore, very little net reflection occurs. The epithelium is relatively thick (50 μm) but contains very few mitochondria, again yielding little net reflection. Although the stromal keratocytes also contain mitochondria, these cells are relatively diffuse; therefore, the relative paucity of mitochondria is consistent with transparency. Because of the lack of mitochondria, the epithelium must rely heavily on glycolytic metabolism (not using oxygen) to generate cellular energy (see Oxygen Uses and Requirements section).

The collagen fibrils of the stroma are smaller than the wavelength of light and, therefore, contribute most of the small-particle light scatter in the cornea. Maurice[4] advanced the first hypothesis for corneal transparency. He argued that the orderly arrangement of the collagen fibrils acts as a perfect crystal lattice that yields destructive interference (i.e., elimination) of the scattered light. Hart and Farrell[5] later demonstrated that a perfect crystal lattice is not found in electron micrographs of the stroma and showed that a perfect lattice is not necessary for transparency. These authors found that the main requirement for destructive interference was that the local density of scatterers (collagen fibrils) must be uniform. For example, if the number of collagen fibrils is counted in a small volume of stroma and if the number of fibrils is the same in an adjacent area of equal volume, then destructive interference predominates. When the stroma becomes edematous, the collagen fibril distance increases, the density of fibrils becomes less uniform, and more light is scattered.[5,6] In the opaque sclera, the collagen fibrils have different diameters, and their density is not uniform. If the sclera is dried or becomes very thin (e.g., as in a staphyloma), the fibers are compressed into a smaller space. The variation in fiber density is thus decreased, and the sclera appears transparent. Given all these strategies to enhance transparency, the end result is that light transmission through the rabbit cornea is 80% at 400 nm and 98% at 700 nm.[6]

The corneal stroma is a gel-like substance that can absorb many times its weight in water. It is composed mainly of collagen fibrils (a protein) and a ground substance consisting of glycosaminoglycans and glycoproteins. The glycosaminoglycans are hydrophilic and absorb fluid like a gel. This is the basis for the negative fluid imbibition pressure of the stroma.[7] If the epithelium or endothelium is removed and the stroma is soaked in isotonic saline, it swells to many times its original thickness. Edematous stromas examined by electron microscopy show that the collagen fibril diameter has not changed; therefore, the water must be taken up into the ground substance. Conversely, a wide range of collagen fibril densities is seen, as well as lakes or separations between stromal lamellae.[8] These separations produce extensive light scatter. Furthermore, if the metabolic functions of the epithelium or endothelium are compromised, the cornea becomes edematous. Therefore, one of the functions of the corneal epithelium and endothelium is to maintain stromal hydration at a level low enough to minimize light scatter.

Stromal hydration is maintained by the passive barrier properties of the cell layers and by the active fluid pumping of these layers. The stromal imbibition pressure sucks water across the cell layers. The resistance of the cell layers acts to slow the leak of fluid into the stroma. The active fluid pump exactly offsets the leak to maintain a constant stromal hydration. *Active* implies the use of energy. Interference with energy production by the use of metabolic poisons[9] or by cooling the cornea[10] causes the cornea to become edematous. This active component, together with the stroma's passive tendency to imbibe water, is termed the *pump-leak hypothesis* for maintenance of corneal hydration[7] and is illustrated in Figure 2-1.

In general, epithelial cell layers pump ions from one side of the cells to the other, and water follows these ions by osmosis. These ion pumps are contained in the corneal epithelium and endothelium. However, the endothelium accounts for at least 90% of the total fluid pump[7,11]; therefore, damage to the endothelium caused by trauma (e.g., intraocular surgery) or disease (e.g., chronic high intraocular pressure or Fuchs' endothelial dystrophy) reduces the pump activity and leads to increased imbibition of water, corneal edema, light scatter, and poor vision. In contrast, the epithelium serves mainly as a barrier to the outside world. The epithelial resistance to water flow is about twice that of the endothelium.[12] To prevent infection, the epithelium constantly renews itself, shedding its superficial cells. Microbes attached to the superficial cells are thus washed away in the tears, not allowing a sufficient resident time for infection to occur. Therefore, contact lens wear, corneal disease, and trauma, all of which interfere with epithelial function, can increase the likelihood of corneal infection.

SOURCES OF OXYGEN

Because blood vessels and blood cells reflect light, the cornea must be avascular to maintain transparency. Nutrients, including oxygen and glucose, therefore, must be delivered to the cornea by diffusion. The nutrients may come from the tears, limbus, or aqueous humor. When the eyes are open, the tears equilibrate with the air and,

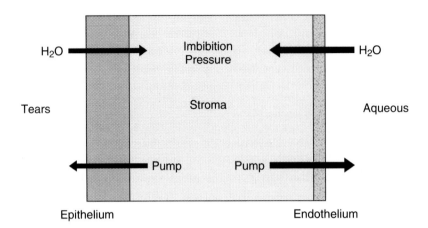

FIG. 2-1. *Pump-leak hypothesis: an anteroposterior cross section of the cornea. The imbibition pressure is the driving force for drawing water into the stroma. The rate at which water moves is determined by the resistance of the epithelium and endothelium. The total amount of water moving into the stroma is termed the leak. The relatively larger arrow for leak from aqueous to stroma compared with the arrow showing the leak from tears to stroma indicates that the resistance across the endothelium is approximately one-half that across the epithelium. This leak must be exactly counterbalanced by a pump mechanism for corneal hydration to remain at a steady state. The relatively large endothelial pump arrow indicates that at least 90% of the cornea's pumping is from this cell layer.*

thus, have an oxygen tension (P_{O_2}) equal to 155 mm Hg. In the closed eye, the tears receive oxygen by diffusion from the palpebral conjunctival blood vessels and the P_{O_2} is estimated to be 55 mm Hg.[13] As mentioned in the Contact Lens Hypoxic Edema section, a tight-fitting goggle over the eye perfused with pure nitrogen simulates the effects of contact lens wear[1] (e.g., corneal edema and epithelial haze), indicating that the tears are a primary source of oxygen to the cornea. The limbus provides oxygen only to the very periphery of the cornea.[7] The aqueous humor, however, supplies oxygen to the posterior cornea in the open eye and supplies close to one-half of the oxygen to the cornea in the closed eye.[13–15]

During contact lens wear, oxygen is delivered to the tears by (1) diffusion through the lens and (2) tear pumping around the lens. The oxygen permeability (Dk) of soft lenses is directly related to lens hydration.[16] In contrast, RGP lenses have little or no water content, and their Dk is determined by the chemical composition of the plastic. When no tear pumping takes place (e.g., during lens wear while sleeping), the precorneal oxygen tension can be determined from the lens oxygen transmissibility, Dk/t (in which oxygen transmissibility is inversely related to the lens thickness [L]).[17]

Lens movement and rocking cause fresh tears to be exchanged with tears under the contact lens. This is a significant source of tear oxygen in wearers of rigid lenses. Subjects who wear oxygen-impermeable PMMA lenses exhibit substantial stromal swelling within a few hours.

Polse and Mandell[2] showed that this swelling could be reduced by covering the eye with a goggle through which pure oxygen was passed, demonstrating the tear pumping component of oxygen delivery. Steady-state oxygen tension behind a PMMA lens is a function of the blink frequency, percent of tear exchange with each blink, and volume of the tear reservoir behind the lens.[18,19] When RGP lenses are compared with soft lenses having the same average Dk/t, the rigid lenses cause less corneal swelling.[20] This is because of the much-reduced tear reservoir and percent of tear exchange with soft lenses (1%)[21] relative to rigid lenses (10%).

OXYGEN USES AND REQUIREMENTS

Oxygen is used by all cells to generate the energy that maintains cell function and homeostasis. A great deal of energy is expended for precise maintenance of the ion concentration within the cell cytoplasm. All cells possess many copies of a membrane ion pump, which moves Na^+ out of the cell and K^+ into the cell. This pump is called the *Na^+/K^+ pump* or *Na^+/K^+ adenosine triphosphatase*, and its actions maintain a low Na^+ concentration and a high K^+ concentration within the cell relative to the extracellular space. These ion gradients are then used by other membrane proteins to transport ions for fluid movement (obviously important for the function of the corneal endothelium). They also regulate cell volume and cell pH (important in the regulation of metabolism and other functions) as well as uptake of glucose, amino acids, and other nutrients necessary for cell survival. The Na^+/K^+ pump needs energy to perform its function, and this energy is in the form of adenosine triphosphate (ATP).

In addition to their role in fluid transport, the corneal cell layers also act as a barrier. As mentioned in the Transparency and Hydration Control section, the cell layers resist water flow into the corneal stroma. The plasma membranes offer high resistance. The total resistance, however, is more often determined by the quality of the connections between cells. These connections form gaskets or seals between the cells to slow the movement of water across the cell layer. The seals are proteins called *tight junctions*. Without these seals, gaps through which fluid and ions could easily move would exist between the cells. The tight junctions are more extensive in the corneal epithelium (located in the superficial layer) than in the endothelium, which gives the epithelium approximately twice the resistance of the endothelium. The epithelium continuously renews itself, such that the tight junctions are lost concomitantly with the sloughing of superficial cells. Just before the old cells die, the cells immediately underneath them form new tight junctions so that the epithelial seal is never broken. This highly dynamic process requires synthesis of protein and RNA.[22] Furthermore, as old cells are lost, new cells arise in the basal cell layer via mitosis. All of these processes require ATP. An inadequate ATP supply to the epithelium can slow this renewal process, resulting in a thin fragile epithelium, which may be more susceptible to infection.

Understanding that the cells need ATP leads one to question how cells obtain it? ATP is produced by a series of complex metabolic pathways. Most ATP ultimately comes from the burning or metabolism of glucose. Glucose gets into the cells and enters the glycolytic pathway located in the cytoplasm. Each glucose molecule is converted to two pyruvate molecules, with a net production of two ATPs. The pyruvate can then enter mitochondria, where the citric acid cycle and oxidative phosphorylation pathways are located. The two pyruvates can then yield a net of 36 ATPs. These mitochondrial pathways, however, require the presence of oxygen. If oxygen is not present, the pyruvate is instead converted to lactate (Fig. 2-2A). Clearly, much more efficient energy production is achieved when oxygen is present.

When ATP is used, it is hydrolyzed to adenosine diphosphate (ADP) and a high-energy phosphate. The high-energy phosphate is transferred to the substrate, thus energizing it. The other by-product of this hydrolysis is a proton (hydrogen). Thus, ATP hydrolysis adds acid to the cytoplasm, which in turn could cause the intracellular pH to drop. The reverse of this hydrolysis occurs when

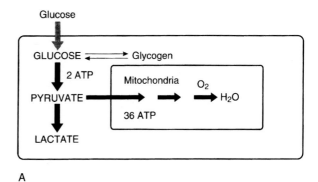

A

B

FIG. 2-2. *Glucose utilization and diffusion. (**A**) Adenosine triphosphate (ATP) production by utilization of glucose in glycolysis and oxidative pathways. Glucose enters cells, usually by facilitated diffusion, and is either stored as glycogen or utilized. Glycolysis metabolizes glucose to pyruvate and produces a net gain of two ATP molecules. If oxygen is available, some pyruvate can be further metabolized in the mitochondria to yield an additional 36 ATP molecules. Pyruvate not used in oxidative metabolism is converted to lactate, which must then be excreted from the cell. (**B**) Glucose uptake into the cornea. Almost all corneal glucose comes from the aqueous humor. Glucose is first taken up by the endothelial cells. Approximately one-third of it is metabolized and the remainder enters the stroma. In the stroma, approximately one-third of the glucose that entered the stroma is metabolized by the keratocytes. The remaining one-third enters the epithelium, where it is metabolized.*

ATP is made from ADP, phosphate, and an H^+ in the mitochondria. Therefore, if oxidative ATP production equals ATP consumption, zero net acid is produced, and cell pH is unaffected. If ATP consumption exceeds oxidative production, however, then a net production of acid is present, and the cell, tissue, or both may become acidotic. When tissues are made hypoxic, ATP production can drop, and tissue pH may drop as well.

The three components of the cornea, epithelium, stroma, and endothelium, consume oxygen at approximately equal rates.[23] Taking into account the much smaller cell volume of the endothelium, however, it has been shown that it consumes oxygen approximately six times more rapidly

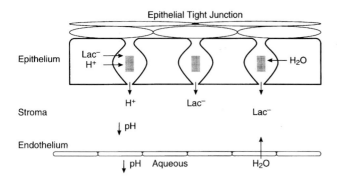

FIG. 2-3. *Cross section of the cornea showing the fate of lactate and H^+ produced by the epithelium. Lactate and H^+ diffuse from the cells to the extracellular space. Diffusion is limited anteriorly because of the tight junctions in the superficial epithelium, so all the lactate and H^+ diffuse into the stroma and out into the aqueous. Lactate accumulates between the epithelial cells and in the stroma as well. The higher lactate concentration osmotically draws fluid into these spaces. This leads to increased light scatter in the epithelium and causes the stroma to swell. The H^+ ions cause a drop in stromal and aqueous pH and may also change endothelial intracellular pH, which could have a small effect on pump function.*

than the epithelium. The epithelium has a relatively low density of mitochondria relative to the endothelium, so this finding is not surprising. The endothelium can generate ATP much more efficiently than the epithelium, even at the same oxygen tension. This may be important, because it does most of the fluid pumping. Even under normal oxygen conditions, at least 60% of the glucose consumed in the epithelium is converted to lactate, the remainder enters oxidative pathways[24]; therefore, the epithelium is normally a highly glycolytic tissue.

All of the glucose for the epithelium must come from the aqueous and not the tears, as the superficial cells are impermeable to glucose.[25] Again, the limbus probably provides glucose only to the very periphery of the cornea. Early attempts at refractive surgery using PMMA implants failed because the implants prevented glucose from diffusing to the anterior cornea, and the epithelium and stroma anterior to the implant soon degenerated.[26] As glucose is taken up by the endothelial cells, a small portion is used by these cells and is then transported to the stroma, where some is used by the keratocytes and the remainder feeds the epithelium. This process is shown schematically in Figure 2-2B.

What happens to all the lactate normally produced by the corneal epithelium? This lactate must be removed, because if the lactate concentration becomes high, glycolysis slows and even less ATP is produced. Lactate, like

glucose, is also impermeable to the superficial epithelium.[27] One study showed that lactate removal from corneal epithelial cells is facilitated by coupling to an H^+ via a specialized membrane protein called the *lactate-H^+ cotransporter*.[28] In this way, the epithelial cells can dispose of the two waste products, lactate and H^+. In essence, what is being removed is lactic acid. The lactate-H^+ cotransporter removes lactic acid from the cell, helping to regulate intracellular pH and preventing the inhibition of glycolysis.[29] The movement of lactate and H^+ ions out of the cornea is summarized in Figure 2-3.

When the cornea is made hypoxic (e.g., during contact lens wear), glycolytic metabolism is increased. A number of studies have shown that the cornea increases its consumption of glucose[24,30] and its production of lactate[27] and H^+[31] during hypoxia. As a consequence, stromal pH is reduced (Fig. 2-4).[31] In addition, aqueous pH is reduced,[32] which may have a negative impact on endothelial cells. If hypoxia is severe and of long duration (e.g., in the overwear syndrome), the epithelial cells cannot get glucose fast enough to make ATP, and the cells consequently die.[30]

During moderate hypoxia, cells undergo stress. This adversely affects many housekeeping functions, such as tight junction formation and mitosis. Evidence that this may occur in the cornea has been provided, for example, by studies showing decreased mitotic activity in corneal epithelium that has been made hypoxic.[33] This could make the epithelium more fragile and susceptible to infection, a condition more prevalent in wearers of contact lenses.

HYPOXIC EDEMA

Mechanisms

Epithelial Edema
Corneal edema can be classified as either epithelial edema or stromal edema. Generally, when one type is present, the other is likely to be present as well. During lens adaptation, mild amounts of edema can occur as the result of excess lacrimation. In the adapted lens wearer, however, epithelial edema is the most prominent sign of hypoxic stress. Because the requirement for the appearance of epithelial edema is moderately deep hypoxia for a few hours' duration, hypoxic stress can occur with either rigid or hydrogel lens wear. With rigid lenses, the clinical appearance is an epithelial haze in the area corresponding to the position of the lens (central circular clouding). It is best observed by indirect retroillumination or use of the sclerotic scatter technique in slit-lamp biomicroscopy. Central circular clouding is relatively easy to observe,

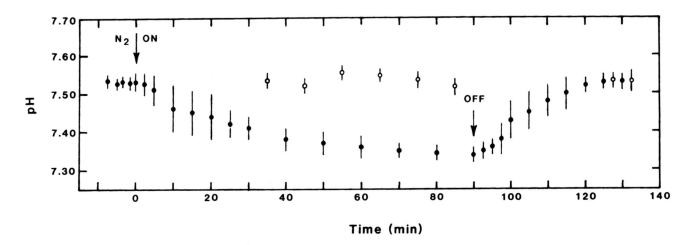

FIG. 2-4. *Application of the nitrogen goggle (i.e., anterior corneal hypoxia) leads to a decrease in stromal pH from 7.55 to 7.35 over 60–90 minutes. N_2 ON = nitrogen gas starting; OFF = goggle removed; open circles = control eye wearing a goggle with air being perfused. (Reprinted with permission from JA Bonanno, KA Polse: Corneal acidosis during contact lens wear: effects of hypoxia and CO_2. Invest Ophthalmol Vis Sci 28:1514, 1987. Copyright 1987, Association for Research in Vision and Ophthalmology.)*

because a clear demarcation exists between nonedematous peripheral cornea and edematous central cornea. Sufficient hypoxia for the formation of epithelial edema can occur in many instances of hydrogel lens use (e.g., low water content or thick plus lenses). The edema is spread over the entire cornea, however, which makes it more difficult to see. Nevertheless, the basic mechanism that causes edema is the same in both cases.

When the lenses are removed, patients may complain of hazy vision (sometimes called *Sattler's veil*) owing to increased light scatter within the epithelium. The hazy vision should disappear within 30–60 minutes. Rigid lens wearers who experience epithelial edema complain more often of spectacle blur. Because the edema can locally disrupt the normally smooth and regular surface of the epithelium, the corneal surface becomes distorted. Keratometry reveals increased curvature, and the mires often appear distorted. Refraction, therefore, tends to uncover increased minus correction. Because the edema is diffuse after hydrogel lens wear, distortion is less likely, and few, if any, refractive changes are observed. Epithelial edema and its associated effects can be minimized by reducing wearing time or increasing oxygen delivery to the cornea by refitting with a more oxygen-transmissible lens.

Epithelial edema is sometimes associated with superficial punctate staining, resulting in superficial punctate keratitis (SPK). This represents breaks in the epithelial surface that allow water to move into the epithelium and contribute to the light scatter. SPK is often not observed and is not necessary for the patient to experience Sattler's veil.[34,35]

Clinicians can observe epithelial edema resulting from the increased light scatter within the epithelium (Fig. 2-5). Patients, however, report seeing colored fringes around bright lights, the same symptom as in acute angle-closure glaucoma. In the 1950s, Finkelstein[34] demonstrated that Sattler's veil was caused by diffraction at the epithelium, leading to the projection of diffraction fringes onto the

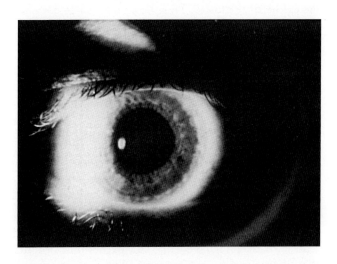

FIG. 2-5. *Epithelial edema and central corneal clouding seen in a polymethylmethacrylate lens wearer after 6 hours wearing time, using the sclerotic scatter technique. Note that the epithelial haze is confined to the central cornea where the lens was in place. The haze disappears within 10–20 minutes of removing the lens.*

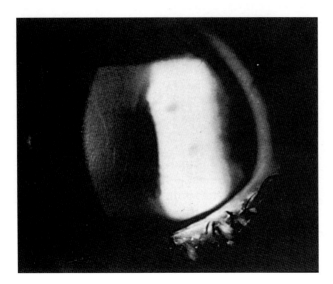

FIG. 2-6. *Corneal striae in a contact lens patient with significant stromal swelling.*

retina. What is the origin of the light scatter? By definition, areas within the epithelium of differing refractive index must be forming. Lambert and Klyce[35] showed that epithelial hypoxia in the rabbit cornea produced light scattering sites around the basal cells, which then acted as a large meshwork or diffraction grating. These authors hypothesized that water was accumulating between the basal cells.

Wilson and Fatt[36] showed that hypoxia does not affect the epithelial thickness. This shows that water does not accumulate in the epithelium and that epithelial light scatter must be caused by a redistribution of water. Lambert and Klyce[35] hypothesized that the increased lactate production during hypoxia causes lactate to accumulate between the basal cells. The lactate then begins to draw water out of the cells by osmosis. This leads to the formation of areas between cells that have a lower index of refraction relative to the cell cytoplasm, and light, therefore, scatters at the interface. Figure 2-3 shows this process schematically.

Stromal Edema and Corneal Striae

Contact lens–induced hypoxia causes the corneal stroma to swell, taking up water from the surrounding aqueous and tears. Unlike epithelial edema, stromal swelling of more than approximately 15% is needed to produce any significant light scatter.[7] This amount of swelling is rarely achieved with current modes of contact lens wear. The amount of swelling is inversely related to the amount of oxygen in the tears. As the oxygen tension increases, the amount of swelling decreases exponentially, making it difficult to determine the

exact level of oxygen required to prevent corneal swelling. A similar relationship holds true for stromal swelling as a function of the Dk/t of the contact lens worn,[37] which makes it difficult to determine exactly what lens transmissibility is needed to produce zero edema.

How does the swelling occur? To answer this question, one must examine the routes by which water moves in and out of the stroma. Outward movement of water is primarily caused by the endothelial pump, and reduced pump activity could, therefore, cause the stroma to swell. A reduction in the resistance of the cell layers (e.g., epithelial break) could cause the stroma to swell. Lastly, an increase in the imbibition pressure or osmotic activity of the stroma could cause stromal swelling. It seems apparent that swelling can occur in the absence of cellular breaks. For example, edema (8–10% swelling) produced with the nitrogen goggle technique usually does not lead to any noticeable breaks (i.e., staining) of the epithelium. Furthermore, acute corneal hypoxia of isolated, perfused rabbit corneas does not affect epithelial resistance.[27] The drop in stromal pH that occurs during lens wear could slow down the endothelial pump.[31] Recent in vitro experiments have shown, however, that decreases in pH within the physiologic range could not account for more than 3–4% swelling.[38] The increased lactate content in the stroma after hypoxia could osmotically result in swelling. Increases in stromal lactate were confirmed by Klyce[27] and by Klyce and Russel,[39] and the amount of lactate was sufficient to produce the observed water influx. Experimental alterations of the rate of lactate production during hypoxia gave results consistent with this lactate osmotic hypothesis.[40]

When the stroma swells, it swells into the eye (i.e., posteriorly), because the anterior collagen fibrils resist stretching. This can cause the posterior surface to buckle or fold in corneas that have swelled at least 6–7%.[41] Under direct illumination with the slit lamp, these folds (in the posterior stroma near Descemet's membrane) are seen as vertical lines or striae (Fig. 2-6). The density and number of striae increase in direct proportion to the amount of stromal swelling. Striae are relatively easy to observe and can be graded on a 0–3 scale, in which grade 0 indicates no striae, grade 1 indicates one or two faint lines, grade 2 indicates two to six lines, and grade 3 indicates many lines along with black folds. Corneal striae are most often observed in soft lens extended-wear patients, because the edema involves the entire cornea. Treatment is to reduce wearing time or refit with a more oxygen-transmissible lens, if possible.

Epithelial Microcysts

Contact lens extended wear is most often associated with the appearance of epithelial microcysts, first reported with soft lenses[42,43] and with RGP extended-wear lenses. The cysts are small (10–15 μm), transparent epithelial inclusions. Under the slit lamp, they can be observed with high magnification and bright direct and indirect retroillumination (Fig. 2-7). Beginning at the deeper layers of the epithelium, the cysts take at least 2–3 months to appear; subsequently, they seem to migrate anteriorly. When they reach the surface, they cause a break in the epithelium that stains with fluorescein. Documentation can be performed by counting or grading the microcysts. Because counting seems to be more difficult, a grading system based on the density and the presence or absence of epithelial staining has been recommended.[44] Grade 1 is a low density of microcysts with no staining, grade 2 is a moderate density with light staining, and grade 3 is high density of microcysts with punctate staining (Fig. 2-8).

Even when lenses are discontinued, microcysts persist for several weeks to months. A grade 2 or greater microcyst response should prompt a return to daily wear. Lens discontinuance is often not necessary. Remission of microcysts can occur with gas-permeable lenses on a daily-wear basis. The introduction of a break in continual hypoxia is essential for microcyst remission.

The appearance of microcysts can sometimes be confused with epithelial edema, and the condition is sometimes called *microcystic edema.* Although some degree of epithelial edema is likely to be present with microcysts, the two appear to be independent phenomena. Epithelial edema comes and goes in a matter of hours, whereas microcysts take months to develop. The persistence of cysts well past the normal epithelial turnover time indicates that the cysts are not tied to the normal migration of cells from basal to superficial layers. It is more likely that microcysts are associated with altered cell metabolism. Biopsies of microcysts suggest that they are composed of degenerated epithelial material.[45] Chronic hypoxia may alter the basal cell RNA/protein synthesizing machinery. The defect (whatever it is) may be passed on to daughter cells and perpetuated until it is somehow washed out.[46] The altered cell metabolism may be caused by the direct effects of hypoxia (i.e., reduced ATP levels) or possibly the indirect effects of the chronic hypoxic acidosis to which lens wearers are subjected.

Neovascularization

The new blood vessel growth into the cornea observed in wearers of contact lenses is often associated with significant levels of corneal edema.[46] Neovascularization was rare in PMMA wearers unless a significant degree of epithelial damage was present. Conversely, vessel growth was not uncommon with thick, daily-wear hydrogels. Clini-

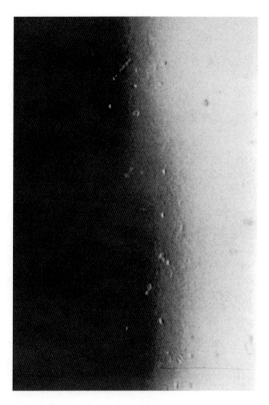

FIG. 2-7. *Epithelial microcysts secondary to contact lens–induced hypoxia.*

cians have clearly shown that hypoxia has some role in vessel formation, because the use of high Dk/t lenses can reduce vascularization considerably. Postsurgical lens wearers (e.g., penetrating keratoplasty and radial keratotomy) seem to be particularly susceptible to new vessel

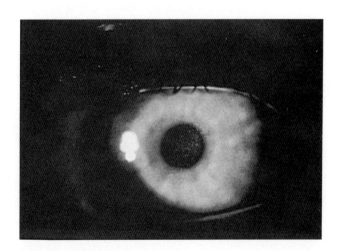

FIG. 2-8. *Example of superficial punctate keratitis in a patient with grade 3 microcysts.*

formation, especially when they are fitted with soft contact lenses. Therefore, an RGP lens is preferred for visual rehabilitation after surgery, if possible.

What is the stimulus to new blood vessel formation? Perilimbal stromal edema seems to be a prerequisite for vessel infiltration, which may explain why vascularization is relatively rare with rigid lenses and more common with hydrogels. Hypoxia alone cannot induce limbal vessels to grow. Other cellular distress signals derived from the epithelium and keratocytes are apparently required. These signals may then interact directly with limbal vascular endothelium or in conjunction with immune cells, or both, to provide all the necessary signals to stimulate growth.[47] Steroids and cyclo-oxygenase or lipo-oxygenase inhibitors interfere with immune metabolites and lessen the vessel response in experimental angiogenesis.[47] Furthermore, prostaglandins, promoters of vessel growth, are found in high concentrations after corneal injury.[48] Therefore, neovascularization can be slowed by steroids and nonsteroidal anti-inflammatory drugs; however, these drugs have many side effects. The best therapy for neovascularization is to discontinue lens wear. Refitting with a lens that allows substantially more oxygen transmission to the cornea, preferably a high Dk/t RGP lens that avoids mechanical damage, is preferred. A more detailed discussion of neovascularization appears in Chapter 4.

CLINICAL MANAGEMENT

Corneal edema can occur in response to the disruption of the normal physical barrier function, stromal ion balance, or ion transport systems of the corneal epithelium or endothelium. Typical contact lens–induced edema is caused by stimulation of glycolytic metabolism secondary to hypoxia. An increased corneal lactate content leads to the redistribution of water in the epithelium and osmotic accumulation of water in the stroma. Light scatter secondary to edema is confined to the epithelium, occurring in the stroma only in cases of pathologic edema (i.e., more than 15% swelling, as in Fuchs' endothelial dystrophy). Clinical evidence of hypoxia-induced edema is shown in patients who complain of transient hazy vision and spectacle blur, and presents with epithelial haze or corneal striae. These and other associated signs (e.g., epithelial microcysts, neovascularization, chronic SPK) should prompt discontinuation of lens wear. In more common, less severe cases, simply enhancing oxygen delivery to the cornea or shortening the wearing time (e.g., extended wear to daily wear) may ameliorate the problem. Because of the greater probability of infection when the epithelial barrier is broken, persistent epithelial defects should

prompt lens discontinuation until complete healing is achieved, at which time refitting or re-evaluation of wearing times can be considered.

Management of most contact lens–related corneal edema is relatively straightforward. From the patient's point of view, the most bothersome problem is typically spectacle blur. If the cornea is not being mechanically distorted by an improper fitting relationship, then the distortion has a hypoxic origin. Today, clinicians have much greater flexibility with the availability of a large range of high Dk RGP lenses. Refitting distorted corneas, which can result from long-term use of PMMA lenses, for example, can be done without discontinuing lens wear. Studies have shown that the corneal distortion from PMMA contact lens wear disappears in about 21 days after lens discontinuation.[49] When PMMA patients are fitted with RGP lenses without interruption of lens wear, the cornea also stabilizes after about 3 weeks.[49] Clearly, lens discontinuation is not needed. Once the 3-week period is complete, the lens fit should be re-evaluated. In most cases, it is possible to refract for glasses even if some small lens changes are indicated. If dramatic changes in corneal curvature are seen (e.g., greater than 1.5 diopters), it may be prudent to make the lens changes and wait another 2 weeks to ensure that the cornea has completely stabilized so that a proper spectacle correction can be given. From the outset, the patient should be made aware of the possible need for two sets of lenses and the need to wait before the correct spectacle prescription can be obtained. Demonstration of the extent of spectacle blur using trial lenses often helps to convince patients of the need for corneal rehabilitation. Explanation that the changes are caused by an altered physiology emphasizes to the patient that an RGP fit is indicated for the long-term health of the eye.

REFERENCES

1. Smelser GK, Ozanics V: Importance of oxygen for maintenance of the optical properties of the human cornea. Science 115:140, 1952
2. Polse KA, Mandell RB: Hyperbaric oxygen effect on edema. Am J Optom 48:197, 1971
3. Holden B, Sweeney D, Sanderson G: The minimum precorneal oxygen tension to avoid corneal edema. Invest Ophthalmol Vis Sci 25:476, 1984
4. Maurice DM: The structure and transparency of the cornea. J Physiol 136:263, 1957
5. Hart RW, Farrell RA: Light scattering in the cornea. J Opt Soc Am 59:766, 1969
6. Farrell RA, McCally RL, Tatham PER: Wavelength dependencies of light scattering in normal and cold swollen rab-

bit corneas and their structural implications. J Physiol 233:589, 1973

7. Maurice DM: The cornea and sclera. p. 1. In Davson H, (ed): The Eye. Vol. I. Academic Press, Orlando, 1984

8. Benedek GB: Theory of the transparency of the eye. Appl Opt 10:459, 1971

9. Dikstein S, Maurice DM: The metabolic basis to the fluid pump in the cornea. J Physiol 221:29, 1972

10. Davson H: The hydration of the cornea. Biochem J 59:24, 1955

11. Klyce SD: Enhancing fluid secretion by the corneal epithelium. Invest Ophthalmol Vis Sci 16:968, 1977

12. Mishima S, Hedbys B: The permeability of the corneal epithelium and endothelium to water. Exp Eye Res 6:10, 1967

13. Fatt I, Bieber MI: The steady-state distribution of oxygen and carbon dioxide in the in vivo cornea. I. The open eye in air and the closed eye. Exp Eye Res 7:103, 1968

14. Kwon M, Niimikoski J, Hunt TK: In vivo measurements of oxygen tension in the cornea, aqueous humor and anterior lens of the open eye. Invest Ophthalmol Vis Sci 11:108, 1972

15. Barr RE, Hennessey M, Murphy VG: Diffusion of oxygen at the endothelial surface of the rabbit cornea. J Physiol 270:1, 1977

16. Sarver MD, Baggett D, Harris MG, Louie K: Corneal edema with hydrogel lenses and eye closure. Am J Optom Physiol Opt 58:386, 1981

17. Fatt I, Bieber MI, Pye SD: Steady-state distribution of oxygen and carbon dioxide in the in vivo cornea of an eye covered by a gas permeable contact lens. Am J Optom Physiol Opt 46:3, 1969

18. Fatt I, Hill RM: Oxygen tension under a contact lens during blinking—a comparison of theory and experimental observation. Am J Optom 47:50, 1970

19. Fink BA, Carney LG, Hill RM: Rigid lens tear pump efficiency: effects of overall diameter/base curve combinations. Optom Vis Sci 68:309, 1991

20. Holden BA, Sweeney DF, LaHood D, Kenyon E: Corneal de-swelling following overnight wear of rigid and hydrogel contact lenses. Curr Eye Res 7:49, 1988

21. Polse KA: Tear flow under hydrogel lenses. Invest Ophthalmol Vis Sci 18:409, 1979

22. Wolosin JM: Regeneration of resistance and ion transport in rabbit corneal epithelium after induced surface cell exfoliation. J Membr Biol 104:45, 1988

23. Freeman RD: Oxygen consumption by the component layers of the cornea. J Physiol 225:15, 1972

24. Riley MV: Glucose and oxygen utilization by the rabbit cornea. Exp Eye Res 8:193, 1969

25. Hale PN, Maurice DM: Sugar transport across the corneal endothelium. Exp Eye Res 8:205, 1969

26. Knowles WF: Effects of intralamellar plastic membranes on corneal physiology. Am J Ophthalmol 51:1146, 1961

27. Klyce SD: Stromal lactate accumulation can account for corneal oedema osmotically following epithelia hypoxia in the rabbit. J Physiol 332:49, 1981

28. Bonanno JA: Lactate-proton cotransport in rabbit corneal epithelium. Curr Eye Res 9:707, 1990

29. Triverdi B, Danforth WH: Effect of pH on the kinetics of frog phosphofructokinase. J Biol Chem 241:4110, 1966

30. Uniacke CA, Hill RM: The depletion course of epithelial glycogen with corneal anoxia. Arch Ophthalmol 87:56, 1972

31. Bonanno JA, Polse KA: Corneal acidosis during contact lens wear: effects of hypoxia and CO_2. Invest Ophthalmol Vis Sci 28:1514, 1987

32. Thomas JV, Brimijoin MR, Neault TR, Brubaker RF: The fluorescent indicator pyranine is suitable for measuring stromal and corneal pH in vivo. Exp Eye Res 50:241, 1990

33. Hamano H, Hori M: Effect of contact lens wear on the mitoses of corneal epithelial cells: preliminary report. CLAO J 9:133, 1983

34. Finkelstein I: The biophysics of corneal scatter and diffraction of light induced by contact lenses. Arch Am Acad Optom 29:185, 1952

35. Lambert SR, Klyce SD: The origins of Sattler's veil. Am J Ophthalmol 91:51, 1981

36. Wilson G, Fatt I: Thickness of the corneal epithelium during anoxia. Am J Optom Physiol Opt 57:409, 1980

37. O'Neal MR, Polse KA, Sarver MD: Corneal response to rigid and hydrogel lenses during eye closure. Invest Ophthalmol Vis Sci 25:837, 1984

38. Huff JW: Contact lens–induced stromal acidosis and edema are dissociable in vitro. Invest Ophthalmol Vis Sci (suppl). 32:322, 1991

39. Klyce SD, Russel SR: Numerical solution of coupled transport equations applied to corneal hydration dynamics. J Physiol 292:107, 1979

40. Rohde MD, Huff JW: Contact lens–induced edema in vitro: amelioration by lactate dehydrogenase inhibitors. Curr Eye Res 5:751, 1986

41. Polse KA, Mandell R: Etiology of corneal striae accompanying hydrogel lens wear. Invest Ophthalmol Vis Sci 15:553, 1976

42. Humphreys JA, Larke JR, Parrish ST: Microepithelial cysts observed in extended contact lens wearing subjects. Br J Ophthalmol 64:888, 1980

43. Zantos SG: Cystic formations in the corneal epithelium during extended wear of contact lenses. Int Contact Lens Clin 10:128, 1983

44. Kenyon E, Polse KA, Seger RG: Influence of wearing schedule on extended wear complications. Ophthalmology 93:231, 1986

45. Lemp MA, Gold JB: The effects of extended-wear hydrophilic contact lenses on the corneal epithelium. Am J Ophthalmol 101:274, 1986

46. Holden BA: The Glenn A. Fry Award Lecture 1988: the ocular response to contact lens wear. Optom Vis Sci 66:717, 1989

47. Haynes WL, Proia AD, Klintworth GK: Effects of inhibitors of arachidonic acid metabolism on corneal neovascularization in the rat. Invest Ophthalmol Vis Sci 30:1588, 1989

48. Fruct J, Zauberman H: Topical indomethacin effect on neovascularization of the cornea and on prostaglandin E_2 levels. Br J Ophthalmol 68:656, 1984

49. Polse KA: Changes in corneal hydration after discontinuing contact lens wear. Am J Optom 49:511, 1972

3

Endothelial Complications

Jan P. G. Bergmanson

GRAND ROUNDS CASE REPORT

Subjective:
A 73-year-old woman with chief complaints of decreased vision and halos around lights. Medical history includes open heart surgery 1 year prior, high blood pressure under medication, and mild diabetes (diet controlled). Familial ocular history includes father, two sisters, and one brother with Fuchs' dystrophy (autosomal dominant transmission).

Objective:
- Best acuity with hyperopic correction: right eye (OD) $^{20}/_{100}$, left eye (OS) $^{20}/_{60}$ distance and near pupillary reflexes, extraocular muscles (EOMs), and peripheral vision normal each eye (OU)
- Biomicroscopy:
    Lens: bilateral cortical and nuclear cataracts, more advanced OD
    Cornea: bilateral Fuchs' dystrophy with well-developed guttae OU, and early corneal haze (see Figs. 3-17 and 3-18)
    Intraocular pressure (IOP): 10 mm Hg OU by applanation
    Fundus: healthy retinas, functional optic nerves

Assessment:
Acuity reduction owing to bilateral cataracts and, to some extent, from corneal haze of Fuchs' dystrophy. Dilemma from need to remove cataracts, which may aggravate the corneal condition.

Plan:
Consultation with anterior segment surgeon. Recommendation by surgeon: In view of compromised endothelium, a triple procedure would be required, consisting of extracapsular cataract extraction, intraocular lens implant, and a penetrating keratoplasty. (Phacoemulsification and intraocular lens implant require healthy corneal endothelium). Subsequent surgery was successful, and removed corneas were evaluated histopathologically.

Histopathology:
Complete endothelial coverage of posterior cornea, but at guttae, the cells were attenuated to the degree that only minimal cytoplasm separated anterior and posterior cell membranes. Whereas the normal young adult endothelium is 5 μm, the endothelial thickness at the guttae was only 0.24 μm, thus unable to allow presence of organelles. Posterior limiting lamina (PLL) was thickened across full width of cornea, with increased focal thickness points at the guttae. Posterior portion of the PLL was thickened and represents the abnormal collagen secretion by the endothelium that is the hallmark of Fuchs' dystrophy. The posterior displacement and stretching of endothelial

cells, especially at points of nodular thickening of the PLL, are responsible for depressed endothelial function, including corneal haze and symptom of halos around lights. As some endothelial insult occurs during lens phacoemulsification and the histopathologic evaluation reveals the compromised status of the endothelium, the wisdom of performing a triple procedure is confirmed (see Fig. 3-19).

Follow-up:
Postoperative follow-ups indicated successful surgery. At 3 months, corneas were clear OU, and aided visual acuities at distance were OD $^{20}/_{30}$, OS $^{20}/_{30}$. Prognosis is excellent for clear vision for the remainder of the patient's life.

The clinical evaluation of the corneal endothelium was first described in 1920 by Vogt,[1] who appears to have been the first to realize the possibilities and value of the specular reflection illumination technique for examining the cornea with a biomicroscope. Maurice[2] took this technique one step further and developed the endothelial specular microscope. These two important breakthroughs facilitated the study of the human corneal endothelium in the living eye for the purpose of clinical research and routine clinical anterior segment patient care.

Every contact lens patient should have the posterior cornea evaluated for two reasons. First, the patient may have or may develop an endothelial pathology that could interfere with or even preclude contact lens wear in any form. Such pathologies include, but are not limited to, Fuchs' dystrophy, congenital hereditary dystrophy, and keratic precipitates (KP). The practitioner must know the status of the endothelium before fitting the patient and should monitor this structure thereafter for changes in its status that may be related to contact lens wear.

Second, it is well established that the endothelium is a part of the overall corneal response to contact lens wear.[3–5] This overall response includes transient bleb changes[5] and the more lasting effect of polymegethism.[4,5] Given the delicate nature of the endothelial layer and its apparent inability to reproduce,[6] it seems prudent to be concerned with this layer in all contact lens wearers.

This chapter describes the contact lens–induced endothelial changes and discusses their clinical implications. Furthermore, endothelial disease and pseudoendothelial disease are described from the standpoint of differential diagnosis. The possible effect on the abnormality by lens choice and wearing schedule are also discussed. To discuss these fields in sufficient depth, it is paramount to consider first some of the fundamentals of endothelial morphology and function.

NORMAL ENDOTHELIUM

Embryology

The endothelium is present after 6 weeks of gestation.[7] Embryologically, it consists of two layers of mesenchymal cells originating from the perilimbic cell mass.[8,9] At birth, these two layers have been reduced to a monolayer of cells. During this transition from a two-layered to a one-layered structure, the cells change from an initial cuboidal configuration to a flat shape. The endothelium of the newborn consists of highly uniform cells that cover the posterior cornea and face the anterior chamber. Peripherally to the cornea, the endothelium modifies to form the trabecular meshwork. In the rabbit, however, the corneal endothelium continues uninterrupted across the meshwork all the way to the angle recess.[10]

After birth, the human endothelium is unable to reproduce, and therefore, dead cells are never replaced.[6] Instead, neighboring cells spread out to cover the space left by dead cells. The extreme uniformity of this corneal layer in the young is thus gradually lost during life. Aging, disease, and environmental factors can affect this uniformity, which is best studied clinically by observing the mosaic pattern formed by the cells.

Few of the apical tight junctions are formed at the time of birth.[11] The maturation of the endothelial tight junction in rabbits continues into young adulthood.[11] In some respects, the maturation of corneal endothelial tight junctions can be considered an incomplete process because these junctions never completely encircle the cells and, thus, make the endothelium a somewhat leaky fluid barrier.[11–14] Although these studies examined the development and structure of tight junctions in rabbits, good reason exists to believe that the discontinuity of such junctions is also present in the primate endothelium, which is known to be a permeable barrier.

The endothelium is a form of epithelium. Like all epithelia, it is associated with a basement membrane laid down by its own synthesis of the necessary material. The endothelial basement membrane is known as the PLL (older texts use the eponymous term *Descemet's membrane*). What makes the corneal endothelium unusual, however, is its productivity in secreting this material. At birth, the PLL is already one of the thickest basement membranes in the body (possibly challenged by the lens capsule), with a thickness of approximately 3 μm. The endothelium continues to add to the basement membrane at the astonishing rate of 1 μm per decade.[15] Therefore, in reaching, for example, the eighth decade, the PLL is approximately 10 μm or more and has established itself as the thickest basement membrane of the body.

Typically, descriptions of the cornea treat the endothelium and PLL as two separate structures. The PLL, however, is a part of the endothelium, as are all basement membranes, and that is the reason for discussing this structure in a chapter on the corneal endothelium (Fig. 3-1).

Gross Anatomy

The cornea is bathed in fluid, anteriorly in the tears and posteriorly in the aqueous. In this context, it is interesting that the bulk of the cornea is formed by stromal tissue, which is relatively dehydrated. As a consequence, the stroma continuously strives to absorb water, and this apparently passive activity explains the imbibition pressure exhibited by all normal corneas.[16] The dehydrated state of the stroma is necessary for corneal transparency, and when this normal hydration level is lost, edema ensues. Edema is the visible manifestation of loss of transparency. The stroma is lined by two cell layers, one anteriorly and the other posteriorly, to counter the undesirable effects of stromal imbibition pressure. Both layers have tight junctions between the cells to prevent uncontrolled intercellular leakage. Therefore, most of the fluid exchange occurs through the cells rather than between them. Current understanding of the endothelium suggests that its most vital physiologic role is control of fluid movements in and out of the cornea.

This functional concept is important to bear in mind when discussing the anatomy of the endothelium. Although the literature is not readily endowed with accounts on the structure of the endothelium, some good sources nevertheless exist and can be consulted for additional details.[8,17-20]

The corneal endothelium is formed by one layer of squamous cells measuring approximately 5 × 20 μm. In humans

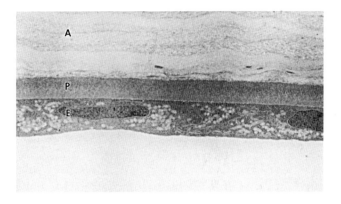

FIG. 3-1. *Low-magnification transverse section through the posterior cornea. Posterior stroma (A), posterior limiting lamina (P), and endothelium (E) are all present. The apical and basal sides of the endothelial cells have a parallel outline. Macaque mulatta monkey. (Transmission electron micrograph, ×2,500.)*

between 20 and 30 years of age, the density of this layer is 3,000–3,500 cells/mm,[2,21-23] which translates to a total number of cells of approximately 300,000–350,000. To perform its expected functional requirements in corneal hydration control, the endothelium must cover the complete posterior corneal surface. Only approximately 100,000 cells or less are needed to accomplish this. This means that a tremendous reserve is built into this layer. A significant cell loss can be accommodated by this layer without jeopardizing vision. Some safety margin is required because the endothelium does not exhibit mitotic activity after birth. In addition, over a lifetime, a number of factors negatively influence the overall population of endothelial cells (see Cell Density and Differential Diagnosis sections).

The apical side of the endothelial cells faces the aqueous, and the basal side closely lines the PLL. The cells are closely packed, leaving no intercellular spaces. The apical side of the endothelial cells follows a geometric mosaic, which is very uniform in the young eye. Most endothelial cells are hexagonal, but it is normal to observe five- and seven-sided cells, and occasionally even cells that do not fall into this group. Therefore, it is most correct to describe the endothelium as a layer of polygonal cells. This notion has also been put forward by other sources,[17,19,24,25] but older texts imprecisely describe the endothelium as being formed of hexagonal cells.

The posterior, apical surface of the cells is flat and smooth. The optical purpose of the cornea dictates this arrangement. The lack of surface irregularities is not absolute, however. Examination of this surface by scanning electron microscopy reveals microvilli that predominantly appear to mark the outline of the cell. The density of the endothelial microvilli, however, is far less

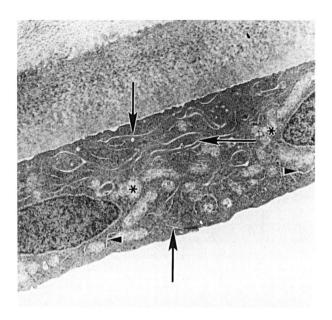

FIG. 3-2. *High magnification of the endothelium in transverse section. The cells contain many mitochondria (asterisks), most of which are adjacent to the nuclear poles. In addition, the cells are rich in rough endoplasmic reticulum (triangles). The lateral sides of cells show complex interdigitations (arrows). Macaque mulatta monkey. (Transmission electron micrograph, ×9,600.)*

than that found in the epithelium along the anterior surface of the cornea. An additional surface irregularity may be observed in the extreme periphery of the normal cornea.[26] These irregularities are bumps in the endothelial surface and are known as *Hassall-Henle warts*. Corneal guttae have a similar effect on this surface and are found, when present, across the entire cornea, including the central portion. Unlike Hassall-Henle warts, the guttae are not part of the normal picture (*gutta* is Latin for *drop*, whereas *guttata*, an adjective, is Latin for *droplike*. Although guttata is the term used frequently, the proper use of language when referring to an endothelial drop is gutta, and the plural form is guttae. Thus, this chapter uses the term *corneal gutta* and not *corneal guttata*).

The anterior or basal side of the endothelial cell is remarkably linear in outline. Only microscopic (less than 0.1 μm) pits are noted along the cell surface that lines its basement membrane (i.e., the PLL). Little or no difference is evident in the refractive indices between the endothelium and the PLL. Again, this highly organized arrangement promotes the transparency of the cornea. A possible legacy of the negligible variation in refractive indices of the endothelium and its basement membrane is the resultant difficulty in viewing the anterior side of the endothelial cells. In fact, the literature offers no account

or illustration of the wide-field mosaic formed by the basal side of these cells. In contrast, the mosaic formed by their apical sides has been studied extensively by specular endothelial microscopy and scanning electron microscopy. A few pioneering studies, however, have provided insight concerning the outline formed by the basal side of the endothelial cells.[12,27,28] Through these studies, it was learned that the anterior side is of a shape distinctly different from that of the posterior side. Many small overlapping processes along the posterior cellular outline produce an irregular cell contour. Ringvold et al.[27] correctly pointed out that the presence of tight junctions at the apical aspect of the cell leads to the uniform geometric mosaic of the posterior endothelial surface. No tight junctions exist along or near the basal side of the cells, and hence, the anterior surface mosaic appears to be dissimilar to its opposing side.

The lateral sides of the endothelial cells also have a more complex form. The outline of the lateral side follows an extensively invaginated course, but if its anterior and posterior extremes were linked together by a line, this line would be perpendicular to the plane of the cornea. Neighboring cells follow each other's lateral outline faithfully, leaving no intercellular spaces.

Three important points are made based on our knowledge of the endothelial cellular outline:

1. The complexity of the lateral sides does not permit the mosaic of the anterior surface to be as uniform as the posterior surface.
2. The invaginated lateral outline suggests that the cells are larger than space permits. This allows cells later in life to easily spread out to cover the gap left by lost cells (e.g., cells lost because of the decline in cell density that occurs as a function of age).
3. The two-dimensional images of the apical side as seen through the specular endothelial, and scanning electron microscopes do not enable us to predict the three-dimensional size or volume of these cells (such predictions are often made but are purely speculative).

Microanatomy

The endothelial cell contains a large nucleus, which in transverse section is round or somewhat oval, in longitudinal section is ellipsoid or sausage-shaped, and in flat section is kidney-shaped. In addition, endothelial cells possess a large number of mitochondria and have a high incidence of smooth and rough endoplasmic reticulum (Fig. 3-2). The high density of organelles in the endothelial cell suggests that these cells are very active metabolically. Indeed, their vital involvement in the normal hydration of the cornea received a great deal of attention from researchers, and this physiologic aspect of the endothelium is addressed in the Physiology section.

Cell junctions have three distinct but separate functions: fluid barrier, cell adhesion, and intercellular communications. To meet these functional requirements, different types of junctions evolved, and, when they occur close together, they are termed *junctional complexes*. As seen with other epithelia, the endothelial cells are linked together by these junctions and junctional complexes. These junctions are all located toward the apical side of the cell, and none are present near or on the basal side.

The zonula occludens (a tight junction) is perhaps the best-studied cell junction in the endothelium. The maturation of these junctions is slow and incomplete at birth.[11] The tight junction typically encircles the complete cell, but these junctions are discontinuous in the corneal endothelium, and as a functional consequence, they constitute an incomplete barrier to fluid movements.[11-14] This leakiness or permeability of the endothelium can be studied under in vivo conditions. In one study,[29] it was noted that endothelial permeability increased 23% between the ages of 5 and 79 years, but this age-related change was not associated with an increase in corneal thickness or endothelial pump rate. Corneas with enlarged endothelial cells show a decrease in endothelial permeability.[30,31] Consequently, it is likely that the increased endothelial permeability that appears to occur with age is not related to cell density but rather to other factors.

The zonula occludens is located along the lateral side and is the junction closest to the apical side. Sometimes, this junction is on the corner between the lateral and apical sides. The endothelial cell often projects on the apical side a small cytoplasmic flap over its neighbor. It is along this flap that the tight junction is most commonly found. This placement of the tight junctions is obviously strategically advantageous, considering their function (Fig. 3-3).

Anterior to the zonulae occludentes along the lateral wall, but still close to the apical side of the endothelium, are the gap junctions. Freeze-fracture studies have been particularly useful in observing the gap junctions, and in the corneal endothelium, these junctions form discontinuous linear arrays.[12-14] The gap junction provides the opportunity for intercellular exchanges and communications. To facilitate this interaction between neighboring cells, the opposing cell membranes have closed the intercellular space to less than 10 nm. This narrowing of the intercellular gap, however, does not form a barrier to fluid movements.

The endothelium does not have desmosomal contacts between cells. The desmosome, or macula adherens, is a

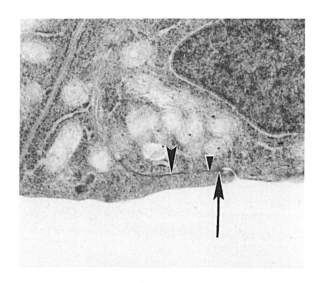

FIG. 3-3. *The apical aspect of the lateral sides of two neighboring endothelial cells shows a junctional complex consisting of a zonula occludens (arrow), an intermediate junction (triangle), and a gap junction (arrowhead). Macaque mulatta monkey. (Transmission electron micrograph, ×23,200.)*

very strong cell junction that not only helps the cells to attach to each other but also enables them to withstand significant physical forces. For instance, the corneal epithelium does not come apart even after the most vigorous rubbing of the eyes, and, to a great extent, this is probably because of the presence of many desmosomes. The endothelium is not an exposed structure and is unlikely to be subjected to such physical forces. Consequently, no need exists for desmosomal cell junctions. However, the cells must remain in their organized and relative positions throughout life, but neither tight junctions nor gap junctions are of any assistance in maintaining such intercellular adhesion. This is where intermediate junctions or *zonulae adherentes* enter the picture. *Intermediate junction* is the better name for two reasons, at least with regard to the corneal endothelium. The first reason is that the intermediate junction does not appear to encircle the cell completely, as is implied by the name *zonula* (*adherens*).[32] Second, this junction is always the intermediate junction in the endothelial junctional complex. It is found between the zonula occludens and the gap junction, and it maintains structural integrity by providing intercellular adhesion.

It is now understood how the endothelium preserves its integrity, but how does it remain attached to the overlying cornea? Unlike the case for the corneal epithelium, no hemidesmosomes are found along the basal side of the endothelial cells. The endothelial attachment to the over-

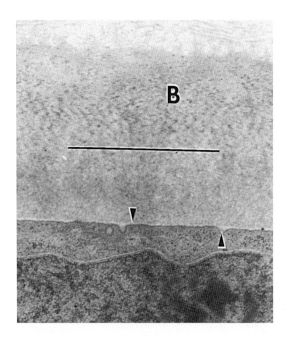

FIG. 3-4. *The posterior limiting lamina consists of an anterior banded region (B) and a posterior nonbanded region. The line marks the transitional zone between these two regions. Note the absence of hemidesmosomes along the apical endothelial side. Fine particles (triangles) are found in the space between the endothelium and the posterior limiting lamina. Macaque mulatta monkey. (Transmission electron micrograph, ×17,900.)*

lying cornea appears effective because cells remain attached throughout a lifetime. Furthermore, the normal endothelium cannot be forcibly detached from its basement membrane by, for instance, attempting to peel it off with the aid of a forceps. The mechanism of this surprisingly strong endothelial adhesion to the PLL has yet to be uncovered. The unsurpassed corneal endothelial basement membrane production may provide this strong linkage (Fig. 3-4).[32]

Physiology

The endothelium has two interlinked functions. First, in the interest of corneal transparency, the endothelial cells must also be transparent. Second, the endothelium participates in maintenance of the structural integrity of the cornea, which, indeed, is also essential to corneal transparency. In addition to these two functions, the endothelium forms the internal concave surface of the corneal lens. However, the refractive power of this surface is very small because of the slight change in refractive index between the cornea and the aqueous. Hence, the endothe-

lial contribution to the refractive power of the eye is negligible and does not constitute a meaningful function.

The transparency of the cornea is dependent on its thickness, and the thickness of an isolated cornea is related to its hydration.[33,34] However, the corneal stroma in situ is relatively dehydrated and, therefore, continuously strives to draw into it more water, a process called *imbibition*. To a degree, this is countered by the physical forces of the IOP and the barrier function of the endothelium. The endothelium has tight junctions that exhibit discontinuity[11-14] and, as a consequence, has been traditionally classified as a leaky fluid barrier.[29] In other words, the normal corneal stroma exerts a force to take up more water, and this force is incompletely checked by a barrier along its endothelial side. Therefore, the cornea would become slightly thicker (and less transparent) if it were not for the countering effect by another function that drives residual excess fluid out of the stroma and into the aqueous. The exact mechanism by which the fluid that leaked into the stroma is returned to the anterior chamber is still not universally agreed on and is still being studied.

Initially, Davson[35] demonstrated that a metabolic process maintains the normal corneal hydration and, as a result, normal corneal thickness. Later, Maurice[36] presented evidence indicating that the endothelium was the site of this metabolic activity and that this energy-requiring process was strong enough to counter the tendency for the stroma to swell.

Although this metabolic activity has often been termed the *endothelial fluid pump*, most authorities agree that it is not quite as simple as a straightforward water pump. It seems reasonable to postulate that a mechanism for maintaining the water balance in the stroma involves transportation of ions from the cornea into the anterior chamber. This movement of ions draws fluid with it. Initially, Na^+ was implicated, but later Hodson and Miller[37] suggested that the bicarbonate ion is the one actively transported into the anterior chamber. The validity of these hypotheses, however, has been challenged on the basis of methodologic errors.[38] Mechanisms in the cornea promote or maintain corneal hydration balance, but this deturgescence function has not been quantitatively associated with the transendothelial net fluid pump.[38-42] Doughty[38] postulates that the deturgescence activity is a constituent property of the stroma and that the endothelial contribution toward hydration control is to regulate the flow of bicarbonate from the aqueous into the stroma.

In the debate concerning the contribution of the bicarbonate ion to the transendothelial fluid pump, it is interesting to note that the net fluid pump activity in the presence of 35 mmol bicarbonate does not change at the low concentration of 2 mmol bicarbonate and 5% carbon dioxide, or in the nominal absence of bicarbonate and carbon dioxide.[40] The continuance of pumping activity in the absence of extracellular (exogenous) bicarbonate was also noted by Kuang et al.[43] These authors postulated that intracellular (endogenous) bicarbonate is the ion that drives the fluid pump. This hypothesis is based on the observation that high concentrations of acetazolamide (a carbonic anhydrase inhibitor) attenuated the pump activity in a bicarbonate-free medium. Conflicting evidence has been presented by Edelhauser et al.,[44] who found that carbonic anhydrase inhibitor did not produce significant corneal swelling in either rabbit or human. The study by Kuang et al.[43] assumes a cell-based carbonic anhydrase mechanism linking metabolic carbon dioxide to bicarbonate ion production. Because this relationship has never been proven and requires that all corneal metabolic carbon dioxide is used by the endothelium to produce bicarbonate, such a mechanism must be regarded as speculative.

It should be mentioned that the corneal epithelium and the IOP are contributors to the relatively dehydrated state of the corneal stroma. Their contributions, however, have not been fully assessed in comparison with that of the transendothelial flow. Studies have shown that the effect of IOP on corneal thickness is significant.[39,45] The IOP is, however, a passive mechanical force. The epithelium exerts its influence on corneal hydration in conjunction with a fluid barrier. Descriptions of these physiologic processes are offered by Maurice[46] and by Fatt and Weissman.[16] Furthermore, Doughty (M. J. Doughty, oral communication, January 1999) has found that the cornea without a scleral ring swells more than the cornea with a scleral ring. This suggests that stromal imbibition is also checked to some degree by the tissue surrounding the cornea. Many past corneal hydration (swelling) studies have been conducted on corneal buttons without the adjacent sclera attached.

An additional factor in the control of corneal hydration was proposed, suggesting that evaporation through the tears contributed as much as 80% to the corneal thinning after corneal swelling by 60 μm.[47] Other studies examining the effect of humidity (ranging from 0% to 100%) found that this presumed osmotically driven deswelling function is unaffected by humidity.[48,49] As a consequence, it is unlikely that evaporation from the precorneal tear film significantly contributes to corneal thinning after an episode of swelling, unless significant epitheliopathy is present.

Past literature often presented a rather simplistic view of the transendothelial pump and what drives it. The previously cited and often conflicting literature in this section should not provoke perturbation but should illuminate the complexity of normal corneal hydration. The issues

of where the pump is located, the exact nature of the endothelial contribution towards corneal deturgescence, and the exact nature of the involvement of the bicarbonate ion in this vital corneal process must await further research before a comfortable understanding of the mechanisms behind the corneal pump-leak hydration control is reached.

The ability of the cornea to recover its normal thickness after induced swelling, usually by means of a thick hydrogel lens, has been evaluated in several studies.[47,50,51] The initial rate of deswelling (deturgescence) by which the cornea returns to its normal thickness may decline as a function of age[50,52] and is adversely affected in Fuchs' dystrophy.[53,54] In these studies, the corneal thickness is monitored by optical pachometry, an excellent method for such measurements. This methodology, however, although excellent for the purpose of measurement, cannot reveal the physiologic process behind the corneal deswelling. The assumption that the deswelling function is a measurement of the endothelial functional ability, therefore, is speculative. Even if the presumption of a linkage between the deswelling function and the endothelium seems reasonable, the many other factors involved in corneal hydration control do not allow the conclusion that the speed with which the swollen cornea returns to its normal thickness is a measurement based solely on endothelial health and fluid pump function.

Anatomic observations of the endothelial cell demonstrate its high concentration of organelles. This is indeed highly suggestive of substantial metabolic activity, although the nature of this activity is not precisely defined. Nevertheless, to exert significant energetic activity, a high level of metabolism is necessary, and this requires a steady supply of metabolites. These metabolites are predominantly derived from the aqueous side. The aqueous delivers oxygen, glucose, protein, amino acids, and vitamins. Fatt and Weissman[16] offer a review of this aspect of endothelial physiology. Metabolic waste products are most likely to be returned to the aqueous. The perilimbal vasculature has not been shown to be of value as a supply route for metabolites to the endothelium, nor have the tears, although some authorities suggested that some of the atmospheric oxygen diffuses all the way to the endothelium. A number of studies contradict this notion, showing that all the endothelial oxygen supply is derived from the aqueous.[54-57]

Aging

The aging human endothelium exhibits distinct changes, some of which can be traced back to its inability to continue mitotic activity beyond birth. Consequently, when an endothelial cell is lost, it is not replaced through reproduction. When a cell disappears from the endothelial layer, the neighboring cells spread out to fill the gap. This response provokes a change in the endothelial mosaic, which is often studied clinically by specular endothelial microscopy. Because dead cells are not replaced, cell density naturally declines throughout life. Notable species differences exist in some of the characteristics of the endothelium. For example, it has been reported that the endothelial cells of the young rabbit can divide even after birth.[58] Another study showed that the cat endothelium does not suffer a significant decline in cell density with age.[59,60]

One study reported that human epidermal growth factor not only has beneficial effects on cell migration after wounding of the endothelium but also accelerates DNA synthesis in the aging cornea.[61] It is uncertain, however, whether increased DNA synthesis is necessarily a sign of nuclear or cell division. Another observation is that the human endothelium can contain multinuclear cells.[61–65] In general, however, most authorities seem to agree that human endothelial mitosis, amitotic division, and fusion occur only in response to trauma.

Cell Density

It is established that endothelial cell density declines with advancing age,[21,23,25,63,66,67] and that this decline in cell density also occurs in animals.[68] Table 3-1 illustrates the age-related loss of endothelial cells but also shows that considerable individual variations are already present at birth. The prevailing opinion is that an almost linear relationship exists between age and cell density.[21,67] Murphy et al.[67] stated that the direct link between age and cell density is "due to the loss of 0.56% cells per year from the endothelial layer." Some studies, however, reported a reduction in the rate of cell loss in the higher age groups,[22,23] whereas another study concluded that the cell density remained unaltered after the age of 50 years.[66] Age-related cell loss is accelerated by intraocular surgery, such as cataract surgery.[69] It was found that the annual decline in cell density was 2.5% in patients who had cataract extraction with or without an implant. This represents a fivefold increase in endothelial cell loss.

TABLE 3-1. *Cell Density as a Function of Age*

Age (yrs)	Cell density (cells/mm²)	Reference
Newborn–2	2,987–5,632	22, 63
20–30	3,000–3,500	21–23, 66
40–50	2,500–3,000	21–23, 66
≤80	2,000–2,500	21–23

The young endothelium has an enormous built-in reserve to sustain this steady decline in cell population over a lifetime. For most people, corneal edema never becomes a problem, even for those who live to become centenarians. In some cases, the cell density drops to the point at which the endothelium can no longer counter the swelling pressure to a sufficient degree, and these individuals develop chronic edema. Ultimately, such patients develop bullous keratopathy and corneal decompensation. To uphold a minimal level of physiologic function requires a density of approximately 1,000 cells/mm².[8,70] The limiting factor appears to be the minimal number of cells necessary to provide complete coverage of the posterior corneal surface.[8,70] The absolute limit for corneal coverage is somewhere between 400 and 700 cells/mm². Once the cell density is reduced to this level, corneal edema is a certain consequence.[8] That humans are born with approximately 400,000 endothelial cells and that this layer can uphold normal corneal hydration with as few as 100,000 cells (a 75% loss of the population) attest to the vast reserve built into this layer. These facts also demonstrate the remarkable ability of individual cells to spread out to cover the corneal surface left open by departing cells. The explanation for this ability of cells to stretch laterally must lie in their extensively invaginated lateral sides. These sides are longer than the endothelial thickness permits, and, consequently, room exists for straightening of the sides, enabling the cell to stretch in a lateral direction. A physical limit exists, however, to the cell's ability to straighten out its invaginated lateral sides, and that limit seems to have been reached when the cell count is reduced to 1,000 cells/mm² or perhaps as few as 400–700 cells/mm².

Cell Shape

The basic shape of the normal endothelial cell is described in the Gross Anatomy section. As the cell gets older, it changes from the pattern of the young human endothelial cell in a number of different ways, which have received different descriptive names that are often confused or misused (see Table 3-2 for correct definitions).

The specular microscope offers a unique view of the endothelium in the living eye, and this capability has been used in a large number of studies. The view obtained through this instrument shows the cellular mosaic formed by the interface between the apical endothelial surface and the aqueous humor. A body of literature developed over the years conclusively demonstrated that a number of changes in cell shape are associated with aging. In addition to overall cell loss, the endothelium shows increasing polymegethism, polymorphism, and polygonality as a function of aging.[23,29,70,71] These changes in cell shape because of aging occur regardless of contact lens wear. As discussed in the Polymegethism, Polygonality, and Polymorphism section, however, contact lens wear does mimic these changes in cellular form. It is of interest to note that the term *polymegethism* was first used to describe endothelial changes in a non–contact lens–wearing population.[72] The appearance of giant cells after trauma has been reported,[73] and thus, the endothelial trauma response may differ from the aging process of the endothelium. Atypically, large cells were also noted in a study in which the rabbit endothelium was challenged for 20 minutes with 15 mmol sodium lactate. This exposure led to a net increase in the fluid pump and the prompt manifestation of unusually large endothelial cells, which, it was postulated, were formed by cell fusion.[74] Potentially multinucleate cells were also observed by Jackson et al. in 1995.[73] The age-related decline in endothelial cell density is accelerated by intraocular surgery.[69] Endothelial cell loss caused by trauma leads to reorganization of the mosaic—that is, polymegethism, polymorphism, and polygonality—as occurs also in the aging cornea, but additional responses unique to the traumatized endothelium may also be present.

Cell Function

What are the functional consequences of the aging of the endothelium? If normal function is defined as a transparent, nonedematous cornea, then advancing age appears to have a negligible effect on a healthy individual. Endothelial coverage of the posterior cornea is a requirement for avoidance of edema, and this condition demands a cell density of approximately 1,000 cells/mm².[8,70] Corneas with no history of disease, trauma, or surgery rarely have cell counts below this threshold, and corneal edema, therefore, is not a common problem in the healthy but older eye.

Several studies have examined the speed at which a swollen cornea returns to its normal thickness. First, the cornea is challenged in a hypoxic stress test. The hypoxic stimulus is then removed, and the corneal thinning from its swollen state to its normal thickness is monitored with an optical pachometer. The time it takes for the cornea to recover its original thickness is a measure of the deswelling function of that cornea. With this technique, it has been shown that the older eye requires more time to return to normal.[50,54] It is not known, however, how much of the deswelling function is a measurement of the functional ability of the endothelial cell. The methodology used in such studies does not permit identification of the physiologic process being measured and the location of this activity.

An increase in endothelial permeability with age has been demonstrated.[29] This suggests that fluid leaks through

TABLE 3-2. *Terminology Relating to the Shape of the Endothelial Cell*

Term	Definition
Polymegethism	Variation in cell size
Polymorphism	Variation in cell shape
Pleomorphism	Variation in cell shape
Polygonal	Variation in number of sides forming the cell

the endothelial barrier more readily in the older person. However, if this is indeed the case, then the transendothelial pump compensates by becoming more efficient, because the cornea does not increase in thickness with age. The functional consequence of an increasingly permeable endothelium is uncertain.

The study of the aging corneal endothelium is a relatively new field, and our knowledge, therefore, is incomplete and often conflicting. Most of the literature on the subject focuses on cell density, which may be why this particular aging phenomenon is understood best. The functional consequence of other age-related changes in the endothelium, such as polymegethism, polymorphism, polygonality, and increased permeability, are far less well understood. None of these characteristics appears to constitute a hazard to the well-being of the endothelium or to provoke corneal edema. Table 3-3 summarizes the changes in the endothelium associated with aging.

POSTERIOR LIMITING LAMINA

The endothelium, like any other epithelium, has its own basement membrane. In the literature, this basement membrane, the PLL, is regarded as a separate corneal layer. It is an endothelial structure, however, and therefore, is included in this discussion.

The PLL has unique characteristics. As previously noted in the Embryology section, it is the thickest basement membrane found in the body. Also, over a lifetime, it exhibits the most dramatic thickening of any basement membrane. At birth, this basement membrane measures

TABLE 3-3. *Aging Endothelium*

Reduced cell density (cell loss)
Increased polymegethism
Increased pleomorphism
Increased polygonality
Increased permeability (?)
Reduced deswelling function (?)

? = proposed but not yet established functional changes.

approximately 3 μm, and in the eighth decade of life, it can reach a thickness of up to 17 μm.[15]

The adult PLL possesses an anterior and a posterior region. The anterior region is banded and remains at a constant thickness of 3 μm throughout life.[15] This portion is the only part present at birth, whereas the posterior nonbanded region becomes thicker as a function of age. The latter portion adds approximately 1 μm to the overall thickness of PLL for every decade of life[15] (see Fig. 3-4). The increased thickness can be explained only by continuous and vigorous basement membrane synthesis in the endothelial layer. No functional penalty seems to occur from this age-related change; on the contrary, the thickened basement membrane is expected to be more resistant in trauma and disease. Indeed, this structure is known for its resilience to insult; for example, in corneal melting caused by chronic inflammatory disease, the PLL is the last corneal structure to give way before perforation. In the literature, this last corneal stand is termed *descemetocele* and is clinically recognized as a forward bulging of the elastic PLL.

It is quite normal to find Hassall-Henle warts in the peripheral cornea of the adult. These warts are localized thickenings of the PLL.[26] As previously noted in the Gross Anatomy section, when these occur across the central cornea, they are known as *guttae*.

The epithelial basement membrane has a specific attachment apparatus for anchoring the epithelial cells and another for its own adhesion to the underlying stroma. None of these features appears to be replicated in the PLL. For example, no hemidesmosomes anchor the endothelial cells to the PLL, nor do reticular type VII collagen fibers issue from the stroma and fuse with this membrane, as is the case with the epithelial basement membrane.[75,76] The anterior adhesion of the PLL can be explained by the irregular outline of the interface, which allows some intermingling of the tissues. Posteriorly, it is more difficult to identify the anchoring of the endothelial cell to its basement membrane. The best explanation appears to lie in the phenomenal basement membrane production, which may work as an adhesive.[32] Whatever the answer to the mystery of endothelial adhesion, it is an effective mechanism because most unchallenged cells remain in their place throughout life.

ENDOTHELIUM IN CONTACT LENS WEAR

Clinical Observation Methods

The diameter of the endothelial cell is only between 0.01 and 0.03 mm. If we consider the minute size of the endothelial cells, their transparency, and that one must look through 90% of the corneal tissues to observe them, then it goes without saying that clinical examination of the endothelium is a challenge requiring excellent instrumentation and good clinical skills.

Because of these difficulties, it was not until 1920 that the clinical examination of the endothelium was first reported.[1] In this report, Vogt described the use of specular reflection to view the endothelium. In this technique, the light source is placed at an angle to the line of observation. Next to the bright reflex from the anterior corneal surface is the second, less-bright reflex, which is derived from the posterior corneal surface (i.e., the endothelial side). This less-bright reflex, sometimes referred to as the *second Purkinje image,* is a mirrorlike reflection of the light reflected from this surface. As can be expected, the laws of optics govern this reflex: The angle of reflection is equal to the angle of incidence. This is a good guideline to remember when the biomicroscope is set up for endothelial evaluation.

An angle of 60 to 70 degrees between the microscope and the light source is, for most occasions, ideal for specular microscopy of the endothelium. Most modern biomicroscopes of good quality have the necessary optical resolution and a halogen bulb for detailed evaluation of the endothelium. To study microscopic changes in this corneal layer, moderate to high magnification is usually required (30× to 60×). It should be remembered that the halogen bulb emits ultraviolet radiation and short-wavelength blue light, which may be hazardous to the patient during prolonged examination. In addition, the very bright light presented during endothelial examination tends to make patients somewhat uncomfortable. For these reasons, the examination period should be concise. Given the right equipment and experience, it should still be accurate.

The image seen by the observer reveals what is commonly called the *endothelial mosaic.* This mosaic is formed by the lateral border outline of the endothelial cells. Each individual cell contributes to the mosaic with its own outline. It is very important to understand that the cell outlines observed are derived from the interface between the cell and the aqueous of the anterior chamber. It is presumed that the change in refractive index is greater between the endothelium and the aqueous than between the endothelium and the PLL. Therefore, specular microscopy of the endothelium views the posterior or apical side of the cell. This is a two-dimensional image that, as a consequence, does not enable the observer to make assumptions about the three-dimensional shape or volume of the cell.

Specular microscopy is an excellent technique for viewing any irregularities along this surface. An irregularity (e.g., depression, elevation, or cell border) deflects light away from its normal path. The deflected light never reaches the eye of the observer, and areas that divert light, therefore, appear dark in specular microscopy. On the basis of these simple optical principles, the pioneers in this field were able to describe the in vivo appearance of a variety of endothelial entities. The first textbook on this subject, *Lehrbuch und Atlas der Spaltlampen Mikroskopie des lebenden Auges*, was published by Vogt in 1930.[77] Graves in 1924,[78] for example, offered an early account of Fuchs' dystrophy while also describing his clinical techniques. Holm in 1977[79] and Zantos and Holden in 1977[3] reported advanced photographic methods with the biomicroscope set up for specular microscopy. The latter researchers photographed the endothelium through the microscope eyepiece rather than through a split-beam arrangement.

Technologic advances allowed the development of a specular endothelial microscope. This instrument is designed for in vivo endothelial observations under high magnification, usually 50× to 200×,[21,80] and can be utilized for photography or video recordings.

The original specular endothelial microscope was developed by Maurice[2] in 1968 as a laboratory technique for in vitro studies. Later, such instruments became a valuable tool in eye banks, where it is important to screen potential donor corneas.[81]

In its current application, the specular endothelial microscope is used in conjunction with computerized morphometric methods to quantify the observation. The limitations of these instruments do not seem to be that the specular reflection represents only 0.02% of the light incident on that eye[82] but that the field of view is very narrow. This narrow field allows a detailed analysis of only a small number of cells; typically, a clinical sample involves 75–200 cells. Widening the slit leads to a vast increase in light scatter that blanches out details.

To overcome such obstacles, Maurice[83] in 1974 described a scanning mirror microscope, and this principle was utilized clinically by others.[84,85] This technique is commercially available as the Keeler-Konan widefield specular microscope. A drawback of this instrument is that it requires contact between the lens and the cornea. The modern endothelial camera does not demand corneal applanation and is, for that reason, noninvasive (Fig. 3-5).

Blebs

The early literature did not report an endothelial response to contact lens wear.[86] In clinical practice, the endothelium was surveyed for disease but was usually not evaluated for an adverse response in contact lens wearers. It was not until 1977 that Zantos and Holden[3] ended this

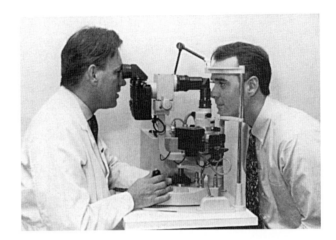

FIG. 3-5. *Clinical in vivo examination of the corneal endothelium. The most commonly used instrument for clinical evaluation of the endothelium is the specular endothelial microscope with a camera attachment. Illustrated here is the Nikon Non-Contact Endothelial camera. This instrument is noninvasive, as it does not touch the cornea.*

period of ignorance by describing the bleb response in the endothelium. The blebs can be seen in the biomicroscope when the familiar endothelial examination set-up for specular reflection is used. Because they represent irregularities in the endothelial layer, the blebs show up as dark areas, just as corneal guttae and Hassall-Henle warts do. The blebs appear approximately 10 minutes after the insertion of a rigid or soft contact lens and their numbers peak 10–20 minutes later.[3,87–89] The adapted contact lens wearer shows a lesser response than the unadapted wearer, thus pointing to an adaptive process. A unique feature of the bleb response is that it is transient even when the lens remains on the eye. Therefore, after peaking in incidence, the blebs begin to resolve, leaving an undisturbed mosaic. The cycle is completed in approximately 2 hours, but considerable individual variations exist (Fig. 3-6 and 3-7).

In 1985, Holden et al.[90] elegantly demonstrated that neither the contact lens itself nor the swelling that it often induces is the etiology of this transient endothelial response. The authors concluded that a hypoxia-provoked pH change in the acidic direction led to bleb formation, and that this response had no effect on corneal hydration control or endothelial barrier function. Although they linked a pH change only indirectly to the formation of blebs, a later study by Bonnano and Polse in 1987[91,92] confirmed that hypoxia leads to an acid pH shift in the stroma. A direct demonstration of bleb development caused by a pH change towards increased acidity has yet to be accomplished. The bleb phenomenon is also reported to result

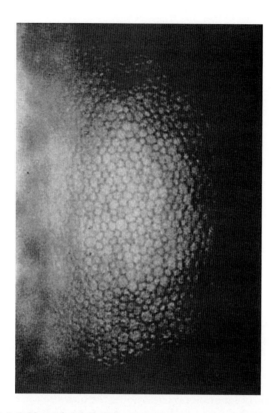

FIG. 3-6. *Normal endothelial mosaic in a non–contact lens–wearing eye. The endothelial cells are tightly packed, lacking intercellular spaces but maintaining a geometric mosaic. The normal endothelium is flat and free of vertical irregularities in the mosaic. (Courtesy of SG Zantos, Sydney, Australia.)*

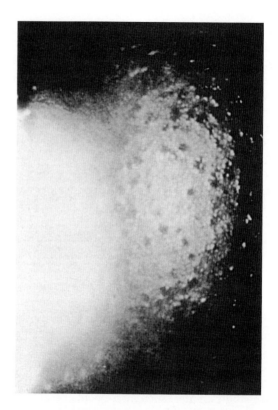

FIG. 3-7. *Endothelial mosaic in a contact lens–wearing eye. Approximately 20 minutes after the insertion of a standard thickness (0.1 mm) hydroxyethylmethacrylate contact lens, irregularities (blebs) are seen along the periphery of the cells and involve two or more cells. (Reprinted with permission from SG Zantos, BA Holden: Ocular changes associated with continuous wear of contact lenses. Aust J Optom 61:418, 1978.)*

from lid closure and from exposure to nitrogen and carbon dioxide.[90,93]

At the structural level, it is not known exactly what the endothelial blebs represent. A posterior bulging of the apical cell membrane has been reported in human corneas after hypoxic challenge.[94] One study suggested that intercellular edema may explain the bleb phenomenon.[95] In this latter study on human contact lens wearers, a randomly distributed pattern of fluid-filled pockets was described between cells. This histopathologic picture appears to correlate well with the clinical picture.

Endothelial Bedewing

The combination of chronic contact lens intolerance and active anterior segment inflammation has been reported to lead to endothelial bedewing.[96,97] Although the exact etiology of this entity is not known, the clinical picture

appears to be derived in part from the presence of inflammatory cells along the posterior corneal surface and also from a transient guttalike response in the endothelium. This gutta response may be a variant of the bleb response. This severe anterior segment response appears to be mainly associated with extended wear of possibly tight-fitting lenses.

Cell Density

It is well established that the cell density in the endothelium declines as a function of age.[21-23,66,98] A number of studies examined the question of whether contact lens wear leads to an acceleration of this decline. In 1982, Caldwell et al.[99] reported a reduced cell count among hard (polymethylmethacrylate [PMMA]) contact lens wearers and that this decrease went beyond the expected decline associated with age; however, the study lacked an adequate control group. Another study compared a group of long-term contact lens wearers (average of 10 years) with a control group and found that the mean cell density for the control group was 2,940 cells/mm², whereas the cell density in the lens-wearing group was 94 cells/mm² less.[100] Although the *p*-value was less than .05, the difference between the groups was 3.2%, which is a smaller number than the technology used was likely to detect (see Polymegethism, Polygonality, and Polymorphism section). In this study, all contact lens–wearing groups contained more subjects with a cell density in excess of 3,500 cells/mm² than the control group. The greatest discrepancy between these subgroups, in this respect, was between the PMMA wearers and the control group; therefore, the information from these two later studies is less dependable but, more important, has been contradicted by a number of well-controlled studies examining contact lens populations in this regard.[4,5,101–103] These latter studies used age-matched control groups for analyses of hard, rigid, soft, daily, and extended-wear groups. None of these studies demonstrated cell loss attributable to contact lens wear in any form. On the basis of available data, it is concluded that contact lens wear does not affect endothelial cell density.

Polymegethism, Polygonality, and Polymorphism

The triple Ps—polymegethism, polygonality, and polymorphism—were described and defined in the Aging section (see Table 3-2). These entities are all present in the aging endothelium and appear to be interlinked. The more pronounced the polymegethism, the more noticeable the polygonality and polymorphism are likely to be. In the contact lens wearer, polymegethism also shows a strong correlation to polygonality, but the relationship is not linear.[104] Because polymegethism, polygonality, and polymorphism are also associated with contact lens wear, it has led to fears that contact lens wear accelerates aging of the endothelium. In view of the inability of this corneal layer to regenerate, such a consequence would be most unwelcome. Therefore, this aspect of the endothelial response to contact lens wear deserves a thorough review. Almost all of the literature, however, is focused on polymegethism, and little has been said about polygonality and polymorphism.

The discovery of contact lens–induced polymegethism originated with Schoessler and Woloschak in 1982.[4] Subsequent studies have confirmed this important observation beyond doubt.[4,5,101–103] These studies have further demonstrated that the severity of the polymegethous response is closely linked to the degree of hypoxia gener-

ated by the lens itself and to the length of lens wear. The number of hours per day the lenses are worn and the number of months or years the lenses have been worn in a particular fashion determine the magnitude of the response. Here, again, the longer the wear, the greater the response. Therefore, PMMA wear and soft extended wear, being the most hypoxic wearing conditions, also produce the most polymegethism.[4,5,102,103] The physical presence of a contact lens on the eye appears to have little to do with this endothelial response because a highly gas-permeable lens, such as the silicon elastomer lens,[105] does not provoke a polymegethous response.[105–107] Indeed, these studies further strengthen the concept that the polymegethous response in contact lens wearers is strongly linked to reduced levels of oxygen along the anterior corneal surface (Figs. 3-8 and 3-9).

The link of this phenomenon to oxygen, or the lack thereof, may be indirect. Anterior hypoxia leads to corneal acidosis from inhibited carbon dioxide efflux,[92] and this change in the physical characteristics of the stroma may alter the corneal hydration control.[108] Clements[109] suggested that corneal acidosis is also a cause of polymegethism.

Polymegethism occurs with age and as a result of contact lens wear, but other causes of this phenomenon exist[60,110–113] (Figs. 3-10 and 3-11). Table 3-4 lists the other known causes. Fuchs' dystrophy, diabetes, and cystic fibrosis[110,111] are the only disease processes known to cause a polymegethous endothelial response. This list of diseases can be expected to lengthen with time as more is learned about the cornea and its pathologies.

The severity of the polymegethous response is quantified as the coefficient of variation (COV). This is an index derived by dividing the standard deviation of the cell areas observed by the arithmetic mean cell area of the total number of cells in the sample. Although the COV index is the most commonly used method for quantification of endothelial polymegethism, it is not without criticism.[19,114,115] The COV is usually calculated from micrographs taken with a specular endothelial microscope; as a consequence, it provides a size index only of the posterior side of the cell. In a simplistic view, the endothelial cell can be described as a brick-shaped structure. Using such an example, the specular micrograph gives information about one out of six sides (in the case of a brick). This is one of the limitations of the COV that often is not realized.

Other limitations of the COV index include the fact that the ratio is calculated from one cornea only and, for this reason, the obtained COV is only valid for that particular cornea; hence, its usefulness for comparisons with other eyes is limited. In addition, the COV does

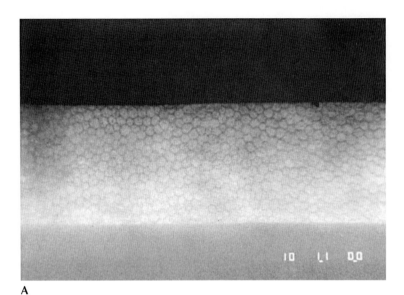

A

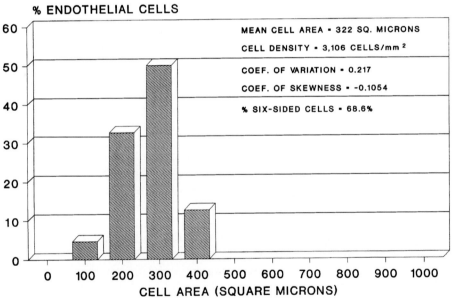

B

FIG. 3-8. *(A)* *Specular micrograph (Konan-Keeler) from a 21-year-old person with no history of contact lens wear. Note that this normal endothelium has many nonhexagonal cells. **(B)** Histogram with the distribution of endothelial cell areas calculated from Figure 3-8A. Other specifics for the endothelium are also listed. (Courtesy of JP Schoessler, Columbus, OH.)*

not tell whether cells are generally shifted toward larger or smaller surface areas. Both of these changes may occur without affecting the COV. In 1990, evaluation of these limitations of the COV led Doughty[114] to conclude that "the continued use of the COVs is thus not recommended."

The validity of the sample size for calculating the COV has also been questioned.[115] The typical clinical sample obtained by specular endothelial microscopy includes

75–200 cells, and the question is whether this small paracentral cell collection is representative of the endothelium in general. In 1989, Hirsch et al.[115] compared the COV from the smaller clinical type of sample with that derived from measuring the surface area of all the cells occupying the central 4 mm of the same cornea. The larger sample with endothelial cells from the central cornea included 2,800–5,300 cells. The results of these authors demonstrated that the smaller clinical sample is

FIG. 3-9. *(A) Specular micrograph (Konan-Keeler) from a 40-year-old person with 10 years of polymethylmethacrylate contact lens wear. Note the increase in pleomorphism and polymegethism compared with Figure 3-8A. (B) Histogram with the distribution of the endothelial cell areas calculated from (A). The endothelium of this person has approximately similar cell density and mean cell area to the one shown in Figure 3-8, but the coefficient of variation in the former is significantly larger than in the latter (see Fig. 3-8B). (Courtesy of JP Schoessler, Columbus, OH.)*

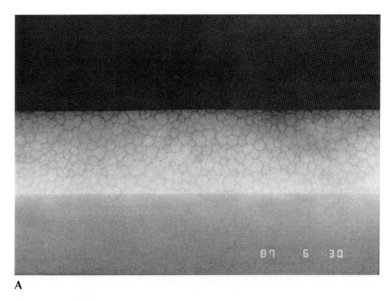

A

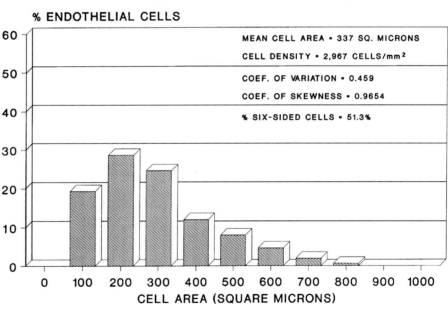

B

at least 10% off the mean cell size calculated from the cells in the central 4 mm of the cornea. Only the most uniform mosaic improved on that figure and obviously so, because in the extreme case in which all cells have an identical surface area, sampling a single cell is sufficient for obtaining a representative mean value. Conversely, the greater the polymegethism, the less representative or accurate the clinical sample. In 1993, Doughty et al.[116] also reached the conclusion that small

samples (e.g., 100 cells) yield unreliable COV estimates that, at best, may show ±4% reliability. They found, however, that cell density estimates based on small samples were more accurate.

Current technology does not permit cost-effective measurement of 3,000–5,000 cells to obtain an accurate COV. As a consequence, the COVs continue to be calculated as in the past, from a smaller and less representative sample. This is unfortunate but is more acceptable if it is

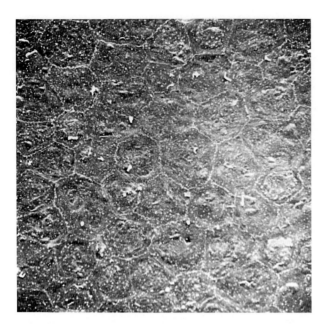

FIG. 3-10. *Polymegethous endothelium in a 66-year-old aphakic soft lens daily wearer who had worn such lenses for 8 years. Distinct variation in cell sizes is present. (Scanning electron micrograph, ×800.)*

acknowledged that the current methodology does not permit a greater accuracy than perhaps 10%; therefore, small changes in the COV of an individual may simply be the result of a variation in the sample rather than of an acute change in the endothelium.

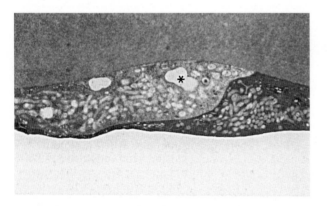

FIG. 3-11. *Polymegethous endothelium in an 82-year-old aphakic soft contact lens extended wearer who wore contact lenses for 25 years. Extreme cell overlapping is noted. Although cytoplasmic electron density varies, the cells contain normal organelles. Small intracellular spaces (asterisk) represent edema. (Transmission electron micrograph, ×9,000.) (Reprinted with permission from JPG Bergmanson: Histopathological analysis of corneal endothelial polymegethism. Cornea 11:133, 1992.)*

TABLE 3-4. *Causes of Polymegethism*

Cause	Associated cell loss
Age	Yes
Disease	Yes
Trauma	Yes
Surgery	Yes
Ultraviolet radiation	Yes
Contact lens wear	No

Endothelial Function in Contact Lens Wearers

Since contact lens wear was discovered to induce polymegethism of the endothelium, a great deal of interest has been focused on the possibility of the functional consequences of this change in cell shape. Almost two decades have passed since the original discovery by Schoessler and Woloschack,[4] and convincing evidence for any deficit in the functional ability of the endothelium has yet to be demonstrated. Nevertheless, a number of theories concerning functional changes in the polymegethous cornea have been put forward and are worthy of attention.

An early study evaluating physiologic changes in contact lens wearers compared 40 long-term contact lens wearers with 40 non–lens wearers.[117] This study found increased polymegethism in the contact lens–wearing group but found no difference between the two groups when corneal transparency, corneal thickness, and endothelial permeability were measured. Increased permeability of the endothelium, however, has been reported in contact lens wearers.[118,119] It was also noted in these studies that the endothelial pump rate had increased to compensate for the increase in endothelial permeability. No immediate physiologic consequences, therefore, seemed to arise from the change in endothelial permeability. The fact that the methodology used in studies measuring endothelial permeability has not been proven to actually measure such a characteristic and that data obtained from such methodology most likely does not represent the measurement of the presumed function deserves mention. In these studies, 15 drops of 0.25% fluorescein sodium/0.4% benoxinate hydrochloride were instilled over a 15-minute period. The toxicity of topical anesthetics is well known,[120–122] and because of the cytotoxicty of this drug, multiple applications are not recommended.[122] The contact lens wearer is more likely to have a compromised epithelium, and 15 drops of a topical anesthetic, therefore, is more likely to have a more profound effect on this individual.[123,124] In addition, the fluorescein was measured as it moved from the epithelium to the anterior chamber via the endothelium; however, the normal physiologic flow because of endothelial permeability is in the opposite direction through the endothelium (see Physiology section). We cannot assume without justification that these two fluid movements in opposite directions are the same.

Dutt et al.[119] noted that the cornea was thicker in the extended lens wearer, contradicting the findings by Carlson et al.,[117] who had found no difference in corneal thickness between contact lens wearers and non–lens wearers. In the former study, however, the thickness measurements were taken when the corneas of the contact lens wearers could not be expected to be completely returned to their normal thickness. In addition, the difference those authors found between the lens wearers and the control non–lens-wearing group was small, and the pachometer used may not have had the precision to discriminate the difference of 10 μm or less in thickness found between the two groups. Hence, no reliable study shows that the cornea is thicker in people who have worn contact lenses. Indeed, available evidence suggests that once the lenses are removed and after a recovery period with the eyes open, the cornea of a contact lens wearer is no thicker than that of someone who has no history of contact lens wear.[117] Holden et al.[102] found a 2.3% reduction in stromal thickness in long-term users of soft extended-wear lenses. In the extreme case, therefore, a small amount of stromal thinning may occur. In summary, available evidence indicates that contact lens wear does not affect normal corneal hydration.

The time it takes for the swollen cornea to regain its normal thickness has been used to describe corneal vigor. Recent studies have shown that this deswelling function decreases with age.[50,51] For example, O'Neal and Polse[50] stated that the recovery to normal corneal thickness takes 10% longer by the time an individual reaches age 65 years. As discussed in the Physiology section, the morphologic site of the deswelling function has not been located. It has often been assumed that this is an endothelial function, but that has not been proven. No convincing or statistically significant correlation was found when the effect of contact lens wear on the corneal ability to recover from hypoxia-induced swelling was examined. Again, a difference between age and contact lens wear with regard to recovery from hypoxic swelling is not surprising, even if the endothelium is concerned with this function. One reason for such difference is that the aging cornea undergoes a decrease in cell density, which has not been found to occur in contact lens wearers. One study measured the corneal swelling response in a group of contact lens wearers. It was found that the endothelial cell density was the only measure that correlated with corneal swelling,[125] whereas polymegethism and pleomorphism did not show such association. It seems most reasonable to conclude that no indication exists that a clinically meaningful and significant functional deficit is induced by contact lens wear.

Histopathology of the Endothelium in Contact Lens Wearers

Histopathologic examination of corneas from long-term human contact lens wearers revealed no significant degenerative cell changes.[95] The organelles of the endothelial cell were normal in all eyes. However, intercellular edema and alteration in cell shape were noted in the endothelium of the contact lens wearers. The most important change in shape was found along the lateral walls of cells, where the normally extensively interdigitated lateral sides had straightened out and had reoriented themselves obliquely from their normal orientation, which is perpendicular to the plane of the cornea. It was speculated that this alteration in cellular configuration was fluid driven. According to this theory, the intercellular edema unfolds the lateral interdigitations. Furthermore, the intercellular edema, which can reach significant proportions, may explain the endothelial bleb phenomenon.

The obliquely reoriented lateral sides of the endothelial cells led to the hypothesis (Fig. 3-12) that cells with a larger posterior surface area (as seen with the specular endothelial microscope) may have a smaller anterior surface area (not seen with the specular endothelial microscope). Consequently, cells may have similar volume or identical total size despite an apparent size variation as viewed by specular endothelial microscopy. A simple reorientation of cell shape must be viewed as a more benign response than if a cell becomes shriveled or enlarged. The prevailing concept that polymegethous endothelial cells randomly become larger or smaller is difficult to explain logically, because all initially uniform cells were subjected to the same stimulus: hypoxia. The question, therefore, should be the following: How can a uniform stimulus cause uniform cells to respond in a non-uniform fashion; that is, to swell and shrink? The proposed hypothesis[95] eliminates this troublesome question by stating that all cells maintain their normal volume. The reported lack of cell degenerative changes is supported by the fact that other studies found no statistically significant functional loss in the polymegethous endothelium.[53,117] The morphologic findings on the polymegethous endothelium clearly demonstrate that the two-dimensional view of the specular endothelial microscope does not permit extrapolation of the three-dimensional size or volume of cells.

Other Long-Term Changes and Responses

Do other negative consequences of contact lens–induced endothelial polymegethism exist? Two responses attributed to the effect of long-term contact lens wear have been proposed in the literature.

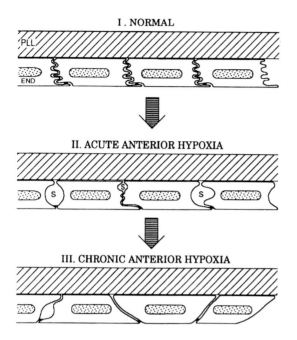

FIG. 3-12. *Schematic diagram illustrating a hypothesis on the formation of contact lens–induced endothelial polymegethism. (I) Normal endothelium with complex interdigitated lateral sides. (II) Acute anterior hypoxia causes cellular stress leading to intercellular edema (blebs?) and resultant straightening of lateral sides. (III) Chronic anterior hypoxia provokes an oblique reorientation of lateral sides. Thus, a cell with a large anterior surface may have a small posterior surface or vice versa. Consequently, cell volume is unchanged despite a variation in the posterior wall surface area of cells. The posterior wall is the cell side observed with the specular endothelial microscope. (Reprinted with permission from JPG Bergmanson: Histopathological analysis of corneal endothelial polymegethism. Cornea 11:133, 1992.)*

First, it has been postulated that endothelial polymegethism is more important than endothelial cell density in predicting the success of intraocular surgery.[72] A study found that pseudophakic bullous keratopathy was correlated with endothelial morphology rather than with cell density. A later study presented data contradicting this finding.[126] The study showed that the outcome of cataract surgery cannot be predicted on the basis of endothelial morphology. This may be a case in which the accused is innocent until proven guilty. More data is needed to resolve this issue. A cautious approach to interpreting the available data is recommended, and patients with polymegethism should not be told horror stories of what may happen if they need intraocular surgery.

The second proposed consequence of long-term contact lens wear has been termed the *corneal exhaustion syndrome*.[127-129] This syndrome is accompanied by signs, such as lens discomfort, lens intolerance, and periods of edema after 6–8 hours of lens wear. Distinct changes in the endothelial mosaic have also been described in these patients, and it has been suggested that these morphologic changes are responsible for the nontolerance to lenses.[129] According to these reports, PMMA and thick hydroxyethylmethacrylate lens wearers are most vulnerable to the corneal exhaustion syndrome, which manifests only after years of lens wear.[127-129] The existence of this entity affects large numbers of contact lens wearers who have worn such lenses for many years. It is also disturbing to the practitioner and the patient to know that endothelial damage eventually harms the cornea and prevents continued wear.

A closer look at the scant literature available on the corneal exhaustion syndrome reveals that the information is somewhat anecdotal and that no direct evidence exists, linking the endothelium to the loss of tolerance to low–oxygen permeability (Dk) contact lenses. This proposed syndrome does not affect everyone with polymegethism or every PMMA or hydroxyethylmethacrylate lens wearer. Other factors must be considered as the total or partial cause. Factors that provoke the corneal exhaustion syndrome may be exogenous or endogenous. For example, medication, ultraviolet radiation exposure, dry or simply drier eyes, hormonal changes, and allergies should all be considered potential causes that are just as likely as contact lens wear.

The older eye is not the same as the younger eye, nor are the tears the same, and this is unrelated to contact lens wear. In these cases, it may be that the older ocular system can no longer handle the stress or perform like the ocular system of the younger person. Contact lens problems and complications are more common in the older population. The underlying cause may be the aging of the cornea or the tear-forming apparatus, and, therefore, a lens that rests on the cornea with minimal stress is necessary, which usually requires a high-Dk rigid gas-permeable material.

Furthermore, social circumstances and the motivation to wear lenses are other factors that should not be underestimated. These are factors that change throughout life. What one gladly goes through or tries to achieve when young, often is not attempted when one gets older. The classic example of the effect that changing social circumstance has on contact lens wear is the married person's reversion to wearing spectacles. This is something all contact lens practitioners have observed, but it seems less common today, which attests to the great improvements in contact lenses.

No evidence exists to support the notion that the corneal exhaustion syndrome is caused by contact lens wear. If the syndrome exists, its cause is unknown and may be unrelated to an ocular structure or function. Sweeney[129] reported that three of her four reported cases of corneal exhaustion syndrome had significant endothelial pigment deposition, and this clinical entity is another factor that should be considered as a potential contributing cause. All cases described in this study were successfully refitted in higher-Dk material, which suggests that the syndrome is benign and can be successfully managed by classic approach of providing more oxygen to the cornea. This approach is what a responsible practitioner should do before the patient experiences difficulties.

Recovery

Great importance is placed on the reversibility of an induced change. Is polymegethism a reversible alteration in the endothelial morphology? Research indicates that a return to normal cell size does not occur quickly. In 1990, McLaughlin and Schoessler[130] found no significant change in the COV after 4 months when patients were switched from PMMA to an oxygen-permeable lens material, Itafocon A (Boston II, Bausch & Lomb, Inc., Rochester, NY). Switching from lower Dk/t (in which oxygen transmissibility is inversely related to the lens thickness [L]) lenses to higher Dk/t fluorocarbon lenses (Dk/t 70) did not improve previously induced morphologic changes during a 3-year period.[131] Furthermore, Holden et al.[132,133] have reported that after a 6-month abstinence from extended lens wear, no reduction in polymegethism occurred. Sibug et al.[134] found more encouraging results when long-term (15–32 years) contact lens wearers were followed for up to 5 years after cessation of lens wear. They found in this group a trend towards a reduction in COV, suggesting that, over a long period of time, polymegethism may be reversible.

As with many other aspects of endothelial polymegethism, further studies on the reversibility of contact lens–induced endothelial changes are awaiting. Available information suggests that the endothelium has at least some ability to recover its normal configuration, but that it occurs only over a prolonged period.

Management of Polymegethism, Polygonality, and Polymorphism

The fact that the contact lens effects the endothelium has been known for two decades and, perhaps not surprisingly, a number of questions are unanswered. A good deal of conflicting evidence exists on what endothelial polymegethism is and what it means. What should the practitioner do after diagnosing polymegethism? Table 3-5 summarizes the management options available. The alter-

TABLE 3-5. *Management Options for Endothelial Polymegethism*

Increase oxygen transmission
    Change material
    Increase water content
Reduce wearing time (extended wear → daily wear → less than full day)
Change fit (e.g., soft to rigid lenses or increase tear pump in a rigid lens fit by changing base curve, overall size, peripheral design)
Discontinue lens wear (suggested only when severe polymegethism occurs together with a disease process that threatens the corneal integrity)

natives generally are designed to increase the oxygen circulation to the cornea.

An increase in the COV in the endothelium indicates a change in the morphology. In the contact lens wearer, the stimulus for this change is a relative lack of oxygen, and the change occurs without cell degenerative changes or clinically significant functional deficits. Polymegethism in the contact lens wearer does not affect cell density, corneal thickness, or transparency. In the absence of known and truly degenerative changes in morphology and clinically significant functional losses, it seems reasonable to regard polymegethism as an adaptation to an altered environment rather than as a threat to corneal health. Further findings and results from future studies await, and one may indeed find that this concept requires modification.

Endothelial polymegethism in the contact lens wearer, however, is a sign of chronic hypoxic corneal stress, and hypoxia also affects the epithelium and the stroma. Common hypoxia-induced epithelial conditions include microcysts, microcystic edema, and thinning. In the stroma, lack of oxygen leads to edema (edematous corneal formations, central corneal clouding, and vertical striae). Hypoxia decreases the rate of epithelial mitosis, adhesion, and corneal sensitivity. Furthermore, it stimulates the growth of new vessels, leading to corneal vascularization in severe cases. The practitioner who cares for the cornea under hypoxic stress, however, has a variety of concerns. Perhaps the most severe potential complication of contact lens wear is ulceration of the cornea. Loss of vision and resulting keratoplasty are common consequences of corneal ulcers. The cornea challenged by severe hypoxic stress may develop a number of epithelial defects, and loss of integrity of the ocular surface barrier makes it vulnerable to microbial invasion. This is believed to be one reason why corneal ulcers are more prevalent among extended-wear patients than daily-wear patients.

Because the corneal ulcer starts in the epithelium, the immediate concern in cases of hypoxic stress is for the epithelium, not the endothelium. One should strive to provide the epithelium with the best possible environment, and when good epithelial health is achieved, a healthy endothelium results. The scientifically based understanding of the effects of contact lens wear on the corneal endothelium is that a benign alteration of cell shape occurs, with no known negative or positive consequences during a normal lifetime; however, this does not free the practitioner from the obligation to give the cornea of every contact lens patient a thorough and complete endothelial examination. This delicate cellular layer is sometimes compromised by disease that can affect the patient's ability to wear contact lenses; therefore, contact lens wear may be contraindicated. Furthermore, young contact lens patients, as well as non–contact lens wearers, may contract disease or develop degenerative corneal changes as they become older (see Endothelial Pathology section). Many of these anomalies can affect continued lens wear. Good reasons exist for continued endothelial evaluations in all patients.

DIFFERENTIAL DIAGNOSIS: POLYMEGETHISM, POLYGONALITY, AND POLYMORPHISM VERSUS ENDOTHELIAL PATHOLOGY

This chapter is not complete without a review of some of the more common or well-known endothelial disorders that may affect contact lens and non–lens wearers alike. Primary disease of the endothelium is normally divided into two categories: degeneration and dystrophy. Degeneration is an age-related process, whereas dystrophy is inherited. Age-related corneal degenerations usually do not manifest before age 50 years, whereas dystrophies are present in most cases by ages 20–30 years. Corneal dystrophies usually have an autosomal dominant inheritance, but three autosomal recessive dystrophies exist: macular dystrophy, congenital hereditary endothelial dystrophy (CHED) (infrequently), and posterior polymorphous dystrophy (PPD) (infrequently).[135] In addition, a number of other etiologies are associated with endothelial changes, including aging, contact lens wear, trauma, surgery, ultraviolet radiation, and pharmaceutical agents. Furthermore, endothelial changes may be secondary to disease processes, such as inflammation, diabetes, and glaucoma.

A number of abnormal corneal conditions manifest adjacent to the endothelium and, consequently, are difficult to distinguish clinically from true endothelial pathology. Such abnormalities—*pseudoendothelial* pathology—are included here because the clinician should always make

a differential diagnosis. The clinician, after making the diagnosis, should consider whether continued lens wear, or prescribing contact lenses in the case of a new patient, is appropriate. It is easy to say no to contact lens wear as soon as a problem occurs, but this decision does not serve our patients well if they want to wear contact lenses. Therefore, insightful understanding of the disease is paramount in this decision. Table 3-6 summarizes the differential diagnosis.

Cornea Farinata: Pseudoendothelial Pathology

The clinical manifestation of cornea farinata is characterized by many whitish-colored specks located in the most posterior extreme of the corneal stroma. The flour-like appearance of these small opacities gives this entity its name, which is derived from *farina*, the Latin word for *flour*. In most cases, the opacities are distributed across the entire cornea but may be more prominent centrally.

Cornea farinata is an age-related condition that is rarely reported to be inherited.[136,137] The condition is asymptomatic and usually affects both eyes. Visual acuity is good, which may be somewhat unexpected given its often dramatic presentation with the biomicroscope.

Cornea farinata is best evaluated with the biomicroscope, using direct focal illumination and red (choroidal) retroillumination. This condition may be confused primarily with corneal guttae and pre–Descemet's dystrophy. Specular reflection yields a normal mosaic, which distinguishes it from guttae. Differentiating farinata from pre–Descemet's dystrophy is more difficult; however, the often spindle-shaped appearance and more scattered distribution of the opacities in pre–Descemet's dystrophy, as opposed to the more spotlike shape and uniform corneal coverage of the farinata, are helpful clues in differential diagnosis. In pre–Descemet's dystrophy, some opacities are noted in the anterior third of the stroma, whereas in cornea farinata the opacities are strictly limited to the stroma adjacent to the PLL. In addition, if the patient is younger than 50 years of age, and especially if the patient is between 20 and 30 years of age, the opacities are likely a manifestation of pre–Descemet's dystrophy.

Histopathological similarities are apparent between cornea farinata and pre–Descemet's dystrophy, and differential diagnosis at the clinical level, therefore, is more difficult. In both of these disorders, lipofuscin deposits have been reported in keratocytes of the posterior stroma.[138] Lipofuscin is a degenerative pigment that aggregates in aging cells.

TABLE 3-6. *Differential Diagnosis: Endothelial versus Pseudoendothelial Pathology*

Pathology	True or Pseudo-endothelial Pathology	Disease Pattern	Age of Onset (yrs)	Most Common in Male vs. Female	Best Illumination for Observation	Specular Reflection	Contact Lens Wear
Fuchs' dystrophy	True	Inherited	50	Female	Specular reflection	Abnormal dark areas	Contraindicated, except in bullous keratopathy
Posterior polymorphous dystrophy	True	Inherited	Any age, sometimes congenital	No difference	Direct focal illumination, red retroillumination	Abnormal large dark area	Yes
Congenital hereditary endothelial dystrophy	True	Inherited	Congenital or sometimes before age 10	No difference	Direct focal illumination, diffuse illumination	Cannot be done because of stromal edema	Contraindicated
Iridocorneal endothelial syndrome	True	Nonfamilial	20–50	Female	Diffuse illumination, specular reflection	Beaten-metal appearance	Contraindicated
Pre–Descemet's dystrophy	Pseudo	Inherited (but not always)	30	Female	Direct focal illumination, retroillumination	Normal	Yes
Farinata	Pseudo	Degeneration	50(?)–70	No difference	Direct focal illumination, red retroillumination	Normal	Yes
Posterior mosaic shagreen	Pseudo	Degeneration	50(?)–70	No difference	Diffuse illumination	Normal	Yes
Keratic precipitates	True	Acquired	Any age	No difference	Direct focal illumination, retroillumination	Abnormal dark areas	Yes; monitor
Trauma or surgery	Deep trauma: true	Acquired	Any age	No difference	Direct focal illumination, specular reflection	Deep trauma: abnormal mosaic	Mostly yes; monitor

Cornea farinata has self-limiting morphologic characteristics and no known physiologic consequences. Hence, contact lens wear is not contraindicated.

Pre–Descemet's Dystrophy: Pseudoendothelial Pathology

Pre–Descemet's dystrophy is bilateral, more prevalent in females than in males, and may be inherited.[139] This condition does not affect vision. The patient is asymptomatic and often unaware of the affliction.

The close resemblance between pre–Descemet's dystrophy and cornea farinata, clinically and histopathologically, has led some authorities to regard these two disorders as variants of the same disease.[135,136] Other authorities, however, prefer to classify them as separate entities.[136] A good reason for this concept is that pre–Descemet's dystrophy appears relatively early, usually by the age of 30 years, whereas farinata normally manifests in the late 60s or early 70s. Subtle clinical differences exist as well.

Pre–Descemet's dystrophy (see Table 3-6), like cornea farinata, must be differentiated from corneal guttae; this is best accomplished by using specular reflection illumination for endothelial evaluation. Pre–Descemet's dystrophy should have a normal mosaic without dark areas. Narrowing the beam to an optical section reveals that the discrete opacities are primarily located deep in the stroma rather than in the endothelium. A few opacities may be

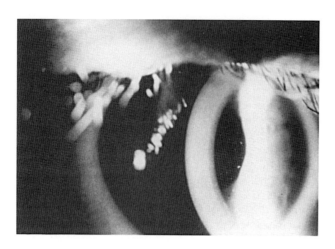

FIG. 3-13. *Pre–Descemet's dystrophy in a woman in her early 30s. The many small, scattered opacities are noted against the dark pupil by retroillumination.*

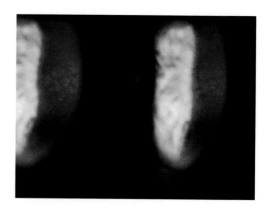

FIG. 3-14. *Posterior mosaic shagreen. The characteristic polygonally shaped cloudy areas with distinct borders occupy the central cornea. This clinical picture has sometimes been mistaken for central corneal clouding. (Courtesy of Professor Joel Silbert, Philadelphia, PA.)*

noted anteriorly in the stroma. Their distribution across the cornea may vary from patient to patient. As a consequence, the pre–Descemet's dystrophy may be recorded as annular when sparing the central cornea, or axial when found only in the central cornea.[139] Optical determination of the distribution of the opacities is done by red reflex retroillumination (Fig. 3-13).

In cornea farinata, the stromal densities appear more uniform, whereas pre–Descemet's dystrophy varies more in its clinical presentation. In the latter, the opacities have been classified as dendritic shaped, boomerang shaped, filiform shaped, comma shaped, circular, or linear.[139]

Histopathologic evaluation of this dystrophy demonstrated changes in the most posterior keratocytes.[138] The surrounding stromal tissue, together with the endothelium and the PLL, is normal. The keratocyte has a spindle shape, which correlates well with the common clinical picture of spindle-shaped opacities. Other shapes of the opacities may result when only a part of the cell is affected. The reported changes in the affected keratocyte include vacuolization and aggregation of lipofuscin.[138] As mentioned in the Cornea Farinata: Pseudoendothelial Pathology section, the presence of lipofuscin argues for a degenerative change rather than a dystrophic alteration. It has been suggested, however, that a primary genetic disorder predisposes the cells to the changes noted in pre–Descemet's dystrophy.

The self-limiting structural changes, together with the lack of known functional deficits in pre–Descemet's dystrophy, should permit contact lens wear without great concern.

Posterior Mosaic Shagreen: Pseudoendothelial Pathology

Posterior mosaic shagreen is sometimes referred to as *posterior crocodile shagreen* because the characteristic mosaic pattern resembles that of crocodile hide (Fig. 3-14). This is a degenerative stromal change about which relatively little is known. The practitioner should be familiar with this condition because it is sometimes confused with central corneal clouding in contact lens wearers. In differential diagnosis, the absence of Descemet's folds suggests mosaic shagreen, because these folds are almost always present in central corneal clouding. In contrast to corneal clouding, in which the stromal haze is relatively uniform in the affected area, posterior mosaic shagreen exhibit clear zones between areas of clouding. Symptomatology of halos around lights indicates central corneal clouding. Posterior mosaic shagreen should yield a normal endothelial mosaic on specular reflection.

The mosaic shagreen is bilateral and most dense centrally. Its characteristic polygonal pattern originates from the posterior stroma. An anterior variant, however, may be provoked by trauma or associated with band keratopathy.[136] The literature contains a histopathologic report on one case of posterior mosaic shagreen.[140] In this case, alterations were found in the normal arrangement of collagen lamellae. Some lamellae in the posterior stroma oriented perpendicular to the plane of the cornea, and other lamellae displayed a sawtooth outline. Furthermore, a change in the banding interval was noted in some patches of collagen fibers.

Posterior mosaic shagreen is not associated with symptomatology of any kind and appears inconsequential to the patient. Therefore, this condition should present no obstacle to normal contact lens wear.

Posterior Polymorphous Dystrophy: Endothelial Pathology

Patients with PPD are almost always asymptomatic. The condition usually follows an autosomal dominant inheritance pattern, but infrequent cases of autosomal recessive inheritance have been reported.[141] PPD is usually a bilateral anomaly but may occasionally be manifest on only one side. The age of onset may vary widely, although this is difficult to determine in a subtle, asymptomatic disease. PPD may be present at birth.

The clinical presentation is asymmetric and exhibits a great deal of variation. Typically, larger and/or smaller hazy, grayish-white vesicular and blisterlike lesions, together with so-called stretched cellophane sheets, are noted in general examination of the cornea (Fig. 3-15). The exact location of these features is at the PLL and the endothelial level. Specular endothelial reflection does not reveal guttae as in Fuchs' dystrophy. The mosaic shows polymorphous cells with indistinct borders. In red retroillumination, the blisterlike lesions are refractile and of the same brilliance as the surrounding tissue.

Electron microscopy of PPD has demonstrated that the disease is of endothelial origin and that a spillover to the PLL occurs.[136,142,143] These reports on the PPD cornea have demonstrated epithelial-like behavior by the endothelial cell, which may develop many microvilli, desmosomes, and keratin. In addition, the endothelium can become multilayered instead of the normal monolayered configuration. The PLL shows increased but uneven thickness in PPD.[136,142,143] This is perhaps not surprising in view of elevated endothelial activity. The membrane is often distinctly laminar. Areas with coarse granular substance may be seen, and other zones may contain collagen fibers with 100-nm banding.

PPD seems to be a self-limiting disease, and treatment is rarely needed. In a few cases, however, uncontrolled edema has been reported, requiring penetrating keratoplasty. Therefore, contact lenses can usually be worn by patients with PPD, but close monitoring is recommended at first. Interestingly, it was reported that PPD may sometimes coexist with keratoconus.[144] Consequently, the practitioner in such a case faces a unique challenge.

Fuchs' Dystrophy: Endothelial Pathology

Fuchs' dystrophy is inherited in an autosomal dominant manner. It is a bilateral condition that may exhibit some

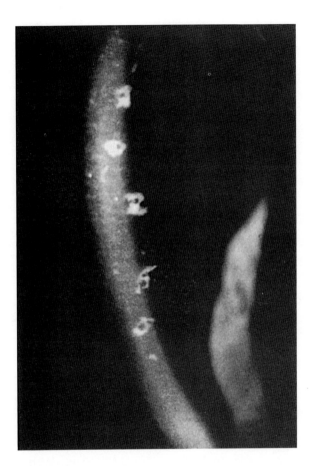

FIG. 3-15. *Posterior polymorphous dystrophy. This patient has the characteristic discrete posterior opacities, together with blisterlike areas, usually associated with posterior polymorphous dystrophy. (Courtesy of Professor Joel Silbert, Philadelphia, PA.)*

asymmetry. Fuchs' dystrophy is more common in women than in men. The disease starts with the formation of asymptomatic guttae, which are clear, small vesicular endothelial secretions projecting into the potential space between the endothelium and the PLL (Fig. 3-16). These guttae are common in patients older than 40 years, but in a small proportion of patients the anomaly continues to develop, eventually constituting a full-blown Fuchs' dystrophy. This is an unpredictable development, and in the early stages it requires clinical skill to determine whether it is Fuchs' dystrophy. The basic criterion for calling this condition *Fuchs' dystrophy* rather than *corneal guttae* is the presence of corneal edema (Figs. 3-17, 3-18, and 3-19). When the endothelial integrity has been compromised to a point at which its function is sufficiently inhibited for corneal edema to develop, it is termed *Fuchs' dystrophy*. It is at this time or sometime afterwards that

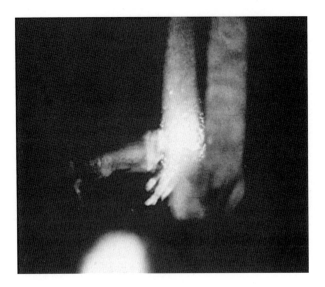

FIG. 3-16. *Corneal guttae. This patient is in her early 50s and has distinct guttae formations across both corneas. No clinical signs of corneal edema are present.*

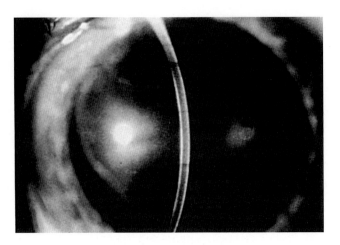

FIG. 3-18. *Fuchs' dystrophy. The same patient as in Figure 3-17. The narrow corneal section reveals the refractile nature of the endothelial secretion that forms the guttae. In contrast, the endothelium of the normal cornea scatters less light than the epithelium. (Courtesy of Drs. J Goosey and J Snyder, Houston, TX.)*

the patient becomes symptomatic. As the stromal edema progresses, fluid eventually exerts pressure on the epithelium where most nerve terminals are located, and the patient becomes aware of the condition. In advanced stages, severe pain is experienced when epithelial fluid–filled bullae have formed.

The practitioner should determine whether a patient is a suitable candidate for contact lens wear. If the patient has guttae with pre-existing stromal edema, he or she should avoid contact lens wear. In the more subtle cases, it is best to look for fine vertical striae. These are the

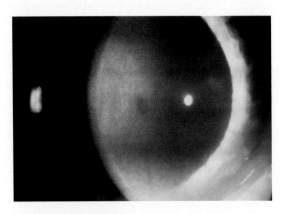

FIG. 3-17. *Fuchs' dystrophy. The history of this patient is presented in the Grand Rounds Case Report. This biomicroscope view utilizing a broad beam reveals some central corneal haziness. (Courtesy of Drs. J Goosey and J Snyder, Houston, TX.)*

first clinical manifestations of stromal edema and represent 5–8% corneal swelling. Pachometry can also be used to establish the presence of increased corneal thickness, but this reading has limited usefulness unless an earlier reading exists with which to compare it. Guttae without stromal edema should not preclude a patient as a candidate for contact lens wear. It would be wise in such circumstances to choose a more oxygen-permeable material and a conservative wearing schedule. Such patients also require more frequent monitoring. It has been pointed out that the deswelling of the cornea takes longer in Fuchs' dystrophy.[52] It should be noted, however, that bandage contact lenses are often helpful in the treatment of patients when painful epithelial bullae become manifest (Figs. 3-20 and 3-21).

Over the gutta, the endothelial cell is often thinned to the point where no space is available for organelles (see Fig. 3-19) and, therefore, at these points, little or no pump action can occur. This observation led to the hypothesis that the most important endothelial function is to provide a complete coverage of the posterior corneal surface.[145] As the disease progresses from simple guttae to epithelial bullae via stromal edema, the eventual outcome is corneal decompensation, necessitating a penetrating keratoplasty. Histopathologically, the guttae formations are collagenous secretions probably derived from abnormal endothelial cells. In fact, the abnormal secretion, probably incomplete basement membrane material, is distributed over the entire PLL and is known as the *posterior*

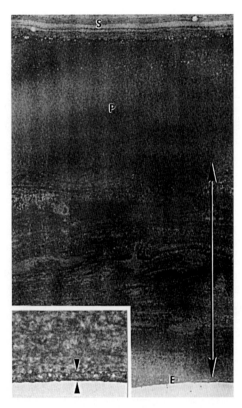

FIG. 3-19. *Histopathologic preparation of the cornea from the Grand Rounds Case Report. The transverse section through a corneal guttae illustrates the enormous buildup of abnormal basement membrane material (here indicated with a line with an arrowhead at each extreme) located between the endothelium (E) and the posterior limiting lamina (P). At this point, the endothelium has become extremely thinned (0.24 μm), while the stroma (S) is normal. (Transmission electron micrograph, ×1,700) (Inset). High magnification of extreme endothelial thinning, leaving little or no room for organelles. Presumably, the only function provided by the endothelium at this point is simple coverage. The two triangles indicate endothelial thickness. (Transmission electron micrograph, ×7,600.)*

collagenous layer.[145] As the disease progresses, cells gradually exhibit a more abnormal and degenerative appearance. Because no give exists in the tissue anterior to the secretions, their effect is to deflect the endothelial cell in a posterior direction. In this way, the endothelial cell is pushed out of the plane of view in specular microscopy. Hence, dark areas can be seen, which at one time were mistakenly believed to be holes in the endothelium. Perhaps this physical distortion of the cell contributes to the loss of function of this layer in Fuchs' dystrophy. Cell loss and polymorphism are associated with Fuchs' dystrophy. The cells may become attenuated over the guttae, and they develop more microvilli.[143]

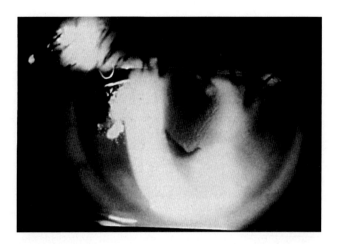

FIG. 3-20. *The end stage of Fuchs' dystrophy is known as bullous keratopathy, which is manifested here as an area with a so-called ground glass effect by retroillumination against the dark pupil. This appearance is caused by subepithelial buildup of fluid. (Courtesy of Dr. William Jones, Albuquerque, NM.)*

Congenital Hereditary Endothelial Dystrophy: Endothelial Pathology

CHED is usually inherited in an autosomal dominant pattern but may also occur in autosomal recessive form.[136] The recessive form is present at birth, whereas the dominantly inherited variant appears within a few years after birth.

This condition is caused by a degeneration of the endothelium that commences in fetal life. However, the anterior banded portion of the PLL is normal in CHED, suggesting that the endothelial cell develops normally until

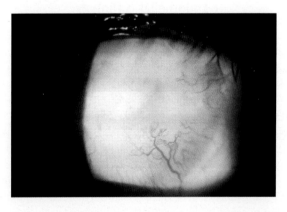

FIG. 3-21. *Full-blown bullous keratopathy leads to opacification and often to vascularization of the cornea, as in this aphakic patient. (Courtesy of Dr. William Jones, Albuquerque, NM.)*

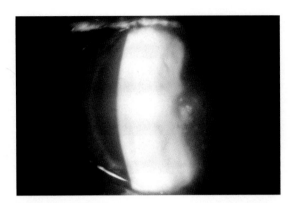

FIG. 3-22. *A herpes simplex keratitis triggered a uveitis with the resultant formation of keratic precipitates, or mutton-fat precipitates. In retroillumination, the keratic precipitates appear as discrete grayish spots in the lower one-third to one-half of the cornea. (Courtesy of Dr. William Jones, Albuquerque, NM.)*

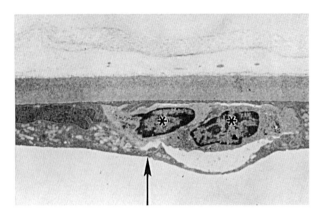

FIG. 3-23. *Histopathologic preparation of keratic precipitates consisting of two white blood cells (asterisks). They have become entrapped within the endothelium in the potential space between two neighboring endothelial cells. This space is sealed from the anterior chamber by a zonula occludens (arrow). Macaque mulatta monkey. (Transmission electron micrograph, ×3,000.)*

the fifth fetal month. Thereafter, aberrant basement membrane material is noted in the PLL.

Clinically, CHED is distinguished by bilateral, generalized stromal edema. The stroma is thickened two- or threefold. The typical absence of symptoms is probably because of the observation that epithelial bullae are not seen in these patients.[135] Raised IOP and corneal vascularization are not associated with CHED.

Progression of the disease leads to the need for keratoplasty. However, penetrating keratoplasty in young children is more difficult and seems to yield a shorter span of corneal clarity before decompensation recurs. Contact lenses are not a realistic consideration for these unfortunate patients.

Iridocorneal Endothelial Syndrome (Chandler's Syndrome): Endothelial Pathology

The iridocorneal endothelial syndrome (ICE) is a unilateral nonfamilial disorder that becomes manifest between ages 20 and 50 years.[135,136] In ICE, abnormal endothelial cells start to proliferate peripherally across the trabecular meshwork and onto the iris. Clinically, this results in elevated IOP, peripheral anterior synechiae, and iris defects. The progressing endothelial cells may be seen as a fine white sheet over the iris. These cells may cause atrophy and distortion of the delicate iris tissue.

Observation of the endothelium reveals a so-called beaten metal appearance. The mosaic is abnormal, with apparent polymorphism, polymegethism, and reduced cell density.[136]

Although stromal and epithelial edema may develop,[136] the immediate problem is the significantly raised IOP, which responds poorly to medications and, therefore, routinely requires surgical intervention to preserve vision.

As a consequence, patients with ICE are poor candidates for contact lenses.

Keratic Precipitates

KP represent an acquired disorder that is mostly derived from inflammatory cells released into the aqueous during an anterior uveitis. These cells become adherent to the posterior cornea. Other material known to adhere to the posterior endothelial surface includes noninflammatory cells, pigmented or nonpigmented, that arrive as a result of trauma or aging.[136,146,147] Occasionally, these deposits may consist of erythrocytes or precipitates from neoplasms.[136,146]

The KP are characteristically distributed over the inferior one-third of the cornea in a triangular pattern, with the apex of the triangle toward 12 o'clock (Fig. 3-22). Convection currents in the anterior chamber dictate this pattern of deposition. Although KP can be observed in most biomicroscopic illuminations, the most dramatic way to observe these features is through retroillumination against the dark pupil. This reveals the soft, milky-white appearance of the keratic deposits. Specular microscopy may be helpful in differentiating KP from guttae. The dark empty areas seen in guttae are not observed in KP.

Only patients with an active anterior uveitis are symptomatic, reporting a constant dull pain; however, the practitioner usually observes a quiet eye when noting KP. In the quiet eye, KP is the only telltale sign of what once happened.

Histopathologic examination of corneas with KP has demonstrated that, instead of being simply adherent to the posterior endothelial surface, the KP actually have become entrapped intercellularly (Fig. 3-23).[20] Initially, however, the inflammatory cell must adhere to the endothelial surface before it can gain entry to the potential intercellular space between the lateral sides of these cells. This seems to be accomplished by an intercellular adhesion molecule.[148]

In general, the existence of KP in the endothelium of the quiet eye should not preclude the wearing or fitting of contact lenses. Closer monitoring of the patient is advisable. The practitioner should remember that pigment dispersion glaucoma is associated with KP, and more frequent follow-ups are often recommended for this reason.

Acknowledgments

I am very grateful to Professor Barry Weissman, who offered his expertise and constructive critique during the preparation of this manuscript. Mrs. Yvonne Blocker made a valuable contribution with her technical assistance on the tissue and photographic work. I would also like to thank Dr. John Goosey for the corneal button I evaluated for the Grand Rounds Case. Illustrations used in this chapter are acknowledged with gratitude and were generously provided by Drs. John Goosey, William Jones, John Schoessler, Joel Silbert, Barry Weissman, and Steve Zantos.

REFERENCES

1. Mayer DJ: Clinical Wide-Field Specular Microscopy. Balliere-Tindall, London, 1984
2. Maurice DM: Cellular membrane activity in the corneal endothelium of the intact eye. Experientia 24:1094, 1968
3. Zantos SD, Holden BA: Transient endothelial changes soon after wearing soft contact lenses. Am J Optom Physiol Opt 54:856, 1977
4. Schoessler JP, Woloschak MJ: Corneal endothelium in veteran PMMA contact lens wearers. Int Contact Lens Clin 8:19, 1981
5. Schoessler JP: Corneal endothelial polymegethism associated with extended wear. Int Contact Lens Clin 10:144, 1983
6. Kaufman HE, Capella JA, Robbins JE: Human corneal endothelium. Am J Ophthalmol 61:835, 1966
7. Hay ED: Development of the vertebrate cornea. Int Rev Cytol 61:263, 1980
8. Klyce SD, Beuerman RW: Structure and function of the cornea. p. 3. In Kaufman HE, Barron BA, McDonald MB, Waltman SR (eds): The Cornea. Churchill Livingstone, New York, 1988
9. Ozanios V, Jakobiec FA: Prenatal development of the eye and its adnexa. p. 1. In Tasman W, Jaeger EA (eds): Duane's Foundations of Clinical Ophthalmology. Vol. 1. JB Lippincott, Philadelphia, 1991
10. Bergmanson JPG: The anatomy of the rabbit aqueous outflow pathway. Acta Ophthalmol 63:493, 1985
11. Stiemke MM, McCartney MD, Cantu-Grouch D et al: Maturation of the corneal endothelial tight junction. Invest Ophthalmol 32:2757, 1991
12. Hirsch M, Renard G, Faure JP et al: Study of the ultrastructure of the rabbit corneal endothelium by freeze-fracture technique. Apical and lateral junctions. Exp Eye Res 25:277, 1977
13. Kreutziger GO: Lateral membrane morphology and gap junction structure in rabbit corneal endothelium. Exp Eye Res 23:285, 1976
14. McLaughlin BJ, Caldwell RB, Sasaki Y, et al: Freeze-fracture quantitative comparison of rabbit corneal epithelial and endothelial membranes. Curr Eye Res 4:951, 1985
15. Johnson DH, Bourne WM, Campbell RJ: The ultrastructure of Descemet's membrane. I. Changes with age in normal corneas. Arch Ophthalmol 100:1942, 1982
16. Fatt I, Weissman BA: Physiology of the Eye. An Introduction to the Vegetative Functions. 2nd ed. Butterworth–Heinemann, Boston, 1992
17. Hogan MJ, Alvarado JA, Weddel JE: Histology of the Human Eye: An Atlas and Textbook. WB Saunders, Philadelphia, 1971
18. Kuwabara T: Current concepts in anatomy and histology of the cornea. Contact Intraocul Lens Med J 4:101, 1978
19. Doughty MJ: Toward a quantitative analysis of corneal endothelial cell morphology: a review of techniques and their application. Optom Vis Sci 66:626, 1989
20. Bergmanson JPG, Weissman BA: Hypoxic changes in the corneal endothelium. p. 37. In Tomlinson A (ed): Complications of Contact Lens Wear. Mosby-Yearbook, St. Louis, 1992
21. Bourne WM, Kaufman HE: Specular microscopy of human corneal endothelium in vivo. Am J Ophthalmol 81:319, 1976
22. Bigar F: Specular microscopy of the corneal endothelium: optical solutions and clinical results. Dev Ophthalmol 6:1, 1982
23. Yee RW, Matsuda M, Schultz RO, et al: Changes in the normal corneal endothelial cellular pattern as a function of age. Curr Eye Res 4:671, 1985
24. Waring GO: Corneal structure and pathophysiology. p. 3. In Liebowitz HM, (ed): Corneal Disorders: Clinical Diagnosis and Management. WB Saunders, Philadelphia, 1984
25. Duke-Elder S, Wybar KC: The Anatomy of the Visual System. Vol. II. In Duke-Elder S (ed): System of Ophthalmology. Henry Kimpton, London, 1961
26. Svedbergh B, Bill A: Scanning electron microscopic studies of the corneal endothelium in man and monkeys. Acta Ophthalmol 50:321, 1972
27. Ringvold A, Davanger M, Gronvold-Osen E: On the spatial organization of the corneal endothelium. Acta Ophthalmol 62:911, 1984
28. Sherrard ES, Ng YL: The other side of the corneal endothelium. Cornea 9:48, 1990
29. Carlson KH, Bourne WM, McLaren JW et al: Variations in human corneal endothelial cell morphology and permeability to fluorescein with age. Exp Eye Res 47:27, 1988
30. Bourne WM, Brubaker RF: Decreased endothelial permeability in transplanted corneas. Am J Ophthalmol 96:362, 1983

31. Bourne WM, Nelson LR, Buller CR, et al: Long-term observation of morphologic and functional features of cat corneal endothelium after wounding. Invest Ophthalmol Vis Sci 35:891, 1994

32. Bergmanson JPG, Zhang X: Endothelial adhesion—morphological considerations. Opt Vis Sci (suppl.) 69:134, 1992

33. Maurice DM: The structure and transparency of the cornea. J Physiol 136:26, 1957

34. Maurice DM: The cornea and the sclera. In Davson H (ed): The Eye. Vol. 1. Academic Press, Orlando, FL, 1969

35. Davson H: The hydration of the cornea. Biochem J 59:24, 1955

36. Maurice DM: The location of the fluid pump in the cornea. J Physiol 221:43, 1972

37. Hodson S, Miller F: The bicarbonate ion pump in the endothelium which regulates the hydration of rabbit cornea. J Physiol 263:563, 1976

38. Doughty MJ: Evidence for a direct effect of bicarbonate on the rabbit corneal stroma. Optom Vis Sci 68:687, 1991

39. Doughty MJ: New observations on bicarbonate—pH effects on thickness changes of rabbit corneas under silicone oil in vitro. Am J Physiol Optom 62:879, 1985

40. Doughty MJ, Maurice D: Bicarbonate sensitivity of rabbit corneal endothelium fluid pump in vitro. Invest Ophthalmol Vis Sci 29:216, 1988

41. Doughty MJ: Side effects of bicarbonate on rabbit corneal endothelium in vitro. Clin Exp Optom 70:168, 1987

42. Doughty MJ: Physiologic state of the rabbit cornea follow 4C moist chamber storage. Exp Eye Res 49:807, 1989

43. Kuang K, Xu M, Koniarek JP, et al: Effects of ambient bicarbonate, phosphate and carbonic anhydrase inhibitors on fluid transport across rabbit corneal endothelium. Exp Eye Res 50:487, 1990

44. Edelhauser HF, Williams KK, Holley GP, et al: The effect of sulfonamide carbonic anhydrase inhibitors on the physiological function of the rabbit and human endothelium. Invest Ophthalmol Vis Sci 33:1402, 1992

45. Anseth A, Dohlman CH: Influence of the intraocular pressure on hydration of the corneal stroma. Acta Ophthalmol 35:85, 1957

46. Maurice DM: The cornea and sclera. p. 1. In Davson H (ed): The Eye. 3rd Ed. Vol. 16. Vegetative Physiology and Biochemistry. Academic Press, Orlando, FL, 1984

47. O'Neal MR, Polse KA: In vivo assessment of mechanisms controlling corneal hydration. Invest Ophthalmol Vis Sci 26:849, 1985

48. Cohen SR, Polse KA, Brand RJ, et al: Humidity effects on corneal hydration. Invest Ophthalmol Vis Sci 31:1282, 1990

49. Bourassa S, Benjamin WJ, Boltz RL: Effect of humidity on the deswelling function of the human cornea. Curr Eye Res 10:493, 1991

50. O'Neal MR, Polse KA: Decreased endothelial pump function with aging. Invest Ophthalmol Vis Sci 27:457, 1986

51. Polse KA, Brand RJ, Vastine DW, et al: Clinical assessment of corneal hydration control in Fuch's dystrophy. Optom Vis Sci 68:831, 1991

52. Polse KA, Brand RJ, Mandell R, et al: Age differences in corneal hydration control. Invest Ophthalmol Vis Sci 30:392, 1989

53. Mandell RB, Polse KA, Brand RJ, et al: Corneal hydration control in Fuch's dystrophy. Invest Ophthalmol Vis Sci 30:845, 1989

54. Polse KA, Brand RJ, Cohen SR: Hypoxic effects on corneal morphology and function. Invest Ophthalmol Vis Sci 31:1542, 1990

55. Riley MV: Glucose and oxygen utilization by the rabbit cornea. Exp Eye Res 8:193, 1969

56. Fatt I, Freeman RD, Lin D: Oxygen tension distributions in the cornea: a reexamination. Exp Eye Res 18:357, 1974

57. Weissman BA, Fatt I, Rasson J: Diffusion of oxygen in human corneas in vivo. Invest Ophthalmol Vis Sci 20:123, 1981

58. Oh JO: Changes with age in the corneal endothelium of normal rabbits. Acta Ophthalmol 41:568, 1963

59. Chan-Ling T, Curini J: Changes in corneal endothelial morphology in cats as a function of age. Curr Eye Res 7:387, 1988

60. Ling T, Vannas A, Holden BA: Long-term changes in corneal endothelial morphology following wounding in the cat. Invest Ophthalmol Vis Sci 29:1407, 1988

61. Hoppenreijs VPT, Pels E, Vrensen GFJM: Effects of human epidermal growth factor on endothelial wound healing of human corneas. Invest Ophthalmol Vis Sci 33:1946, 1992

62. Nartey IN, Sherrard ES: Amitosis in human donor corneal endothelium—a serendipity? Br J Ophthalmol 74:63, 1990

63. Speedwell L, Novakovic P, Sherrard ES, et al: The infant corneal endothelium. Arch Ophthalmol 106:771, 1988

64. Neubauer L, Laing RA, Leibowitz HM, et al: Coalescence of endothelial cells in the traumatized cornea. I. Experimental observations in cryopreserved tissue. Arch Ophthalmol 101:1787, 1983

65. Neubauer L, Baratz RS, Laing RA, et al: Coalescence of endothelial cells in the traumatized cornea. III. Correlation between specular and scanning electron microscopy. Arch Ophthalmol 102:921, 1984

66. Wilson RS, Roper-Hall MJ: Effect of age on the endothelial cell count in the normal eye. Br J Ophthalmol 66:513, 1982

67. Murphy C, Alvarado J, Juster R, et al: Prenatal and postnatal cellularity of the human corneal endothelium. A quantitative histologic study. Invest Ophthalmol Vis Sci 25:312, 1984

68. Doughty MJ. The cornea and corneal endothelium in the aged rabbit. Optom Vis Sci, 71:809, 1994.

69. Bourne WM, Nelson LR, Hodge DO. Continued endothelial loss ten years after lens implantation. Ophthalmology 101:1014, 1994.

70. Rao GN, Waldron WR, Aquavella JV: Morphology of graft endothelium and donor age. Br J Ophthalmol 64:523, 1980

71. Suda T: Mosaic pattern changes in human corneal endothelium with age. Jpn J Ophthalmol 28:331, 1984

72. Rao GN, Aquavella JV, Goldberg SH, et al: Pseudophakic bullous keratopathy: relationship to pre-operative corneal endothelial status. Ophthalmology 91:1135, 1984

73. Jackson AJ, Gardiner T, Archer DB. Morphometric analysis of corneal endothelial giant cells in normal and traumatized corneas. Ophthal Physiol Opt 15:305, 1995

74. Doughty MJ, Nguyen KT. Rapid morphological reorganization of the rabbit corneal endothelium after acute exposure to sodium lactate in vitro. Ophthalmic Res 27:80, 1995

75. Gibson IK, Spurr-Michaud SJ, Tisdale AS: Anchoring fibrils form a complex network in human and rabbit cornea. Invest Ophthalmol Vis Sci 28:212, 1987

76. Bergmanson JPG: Corneal epithelium. p. 3. In Bennett ES, Weissman BA (eds): Clinical Contact Lens Practice. JB Lippincott, Philadelphia, 1991

77. Vogt A: Lehrbuch und Atlas der Spaltlampen Microskopie des lebenden Auges. Springer, Berlin, 1930

78. Graves B: A bilateral chronic affection of the endothelial face of the cornea of elderly persons, with an account of the technical and clinical principles of its slit-lamp observation. Br J Ophthalmol 8:502, 1924

79. Holm O: High magnification photography of the anterior segment of the human eye. Acta Ophthalmol 56:475, 1977

80. Laing RA, Sandstrom MM, Leibowitz HM: In vivo photomicrography of the corneal endothelium. Arch Ophthalmol 93:143, 1975

81. Hoefle FB, Maurice DM, Sibley RC: Human corneal donor material: a method of examination before keratoplasty. Arch Ophthalmol 84:741, 1970

82. Laing RA, Sandstrom MM, Leibowitz HM: Clinical specular microscopy. I. Optical principles. Arch Ophthalmol 97:1714, 1979

83. Maurice DM: A scanning slit optical microscope. Invest Ophthalmol 13:1033, 1974

84. Koester CJ, Roberts CW, Donn A, Hoefle FB: Wide-field specular microscopy. Clinical and research applications. Ophthalmology 87:849, 1980

85. Hirst LW, Aver C, Abbey H, et al: Quantitative analysis of wide-field endothelial specular photomicrographs. Am J Ophthalmol 97:488, 1984

86. Obrig T: Contact Lenses. Chilton, Philadelphia, 1942

87. Barr J, Schoessler J: Corneal endothelial response to rigid contact lenses. Am J Optom Physiol Opt 57:267, 1980

88. Vannas A, Makitie J, Sulonen J, et al: Contact lens induced transient changes in corneal endothelium. Acta Ophthalmol 59:552, 1981

89. Schoessler JP, Woloschak MJ, Mauger TF: Transient endothelial changes produced by hydrophilic lenses. Am J Optom Physiol Opt 59:764, 1982

90. Holden BA, Williams L, Zantos S: Etiology of transient endothelial changes in the human cornea. Invest Ophthalmol Vis Sci 26:1489, 1985

91. Bonanno JA, Polse KA: Measurement of in vivo human corneal stromal pH: open and closed eyes. Invest Ophthalmol Vis Sci 28:522, 1987

92. Bonanno JA, Polse KA: Corneal acidosis during contact lens wear: effects of hypoxia and CO_2. Invest Ophthalmol Vis Sci 28:1514, 1987

93. Khodadoust A, Hirst L: Diurnal variation in corneal endothelial morphology. Ophthalmology 91:1125, 1984

94. Vannas A, Holden B, Makitie J: The ultrastructure of contact lens induced changes. Acta Ophthalmol 62:320, 1984

95. Bergmanson JPG: Histopathological analysis of corneal endothelial polymegethism. Cornea 11:133, 1992

96. McMonnies CW, Zantos SD: Endothelial bedewing of the cornea in association with contact lens wear. Br J Ophthalmol 63:478, 1979

97. Zantos SD, Holden BA: Guttate endothelial changes with anterior eye inflammation. Br J Ophthalmol 65:101, 1981

98. Laing RA, Sandstrom M, Berrospi A, et al: Changes in corneal endothelium as a function of age. Exp Eye Res 22:587, 1976

99. Caldwell DR, Kastle PR, Dabezies OH, et al: The effect of long-term hard lens wear on the endothelium. Contact Intraocul Lens Med J 8:87, 1982

100. Setala K, Vasara K, Vesti E, Ruusuvaara P: Effects of long-term contact lens wear on the corneal endothelium. Acta Ophthalmol Scand 76:299, 1998

101. Hirst LW, Aver C, Cohn J, et al: Specular microscopy of hard lens wearers. Ophthalmology 91:1147, 1984

102. Holden BA, Sweeney DF, Vannas A, et al: Effects of long-term extended contact lens wear on the human cornea. Invest Ophthalmol Vis Sci 26:1489, 1985

103. MacRae SM, Matsuda M, Shellans S, et al: The effects of hard and soft contact lenses on the corneal endothelium. Am J Ophthalmol 102:50, 1986

104. Doughty MJ, Fonn D: Pleomorphism and endothelial cell size in normal and polymegethous human corneal endothelium. International Contact Lens Clinic 20:116, 1993

105. Weissman BA, Fatt I, Phan C: Polarographic oxygen permeability measurement of silicon elastomer contact lens material. J Am Optom Assoc 63:187, 1992

106. Schoessler JP, Barr JT, Fresen DR: Corneal endothelial observations of silicon elastomer contact lens wearers. Int Contact Lens Clin 11:337, 1984

107. Carlson KH, Ilstrup DM, Bourne WM, et al: Effect of silicon elastomer contact lens wear on endothelial morphology in aphakic eyes. Cornea 9:45, 1990

108. Cohen SR, Polse KA, Brand RJ, et al: Stromal acidosis affects corneal hydration control. Invest Ophthalmol Vis Sci 33:134, 1992

109. Clements LD: Corneal acidosis, blebs and endothelial polymegethism. Contact Lens Forum 15:39, 1990

110. Burns RR, Bourne WM, Brubaker RF: Endothelial function in patients with cornea guttatae. Invest Ophthalmol Vis Sci 20:77, 1981

111. Lass JH, Spurney RV, Dutt RM, et al: A morphologic and fluorophotometric analysis of the corneal endothelium in Type I diabetes mellitus and cystic fibrosis. Am J Ophthalmol 100:783, 1985

112. Bergmanson JPG, Pitts DG, Chu L: The efficacy of a UV-blocking soft contact lens in protecting cornea against UV radiation. Acta Ophthalmology 65:279, 1987

113. Good GW, Schoessler JP: Chronic solar radiation exposure and endothelial polymegethism. Curr Eye Res 7:157, 1988

114. Doughty MJ: The ambiguous coefficient of variation: polymegethism of the corneal endothelium and central corneal thickness. Int Contact Lens Clin 17:240, 1990

115. Hirsch LW, Yamauchi K, Enger C, et al: Quantitative analysis of wide-field specular microscopy. II. Precision of sampling from the central corneal endothelium. Invest Ophthalmol Vis Sci 30:1972, 1989

116. Doughty MJ, Fonn D, Nguyen KT. Assessment of the reliability of calculations of the coefficient of variation for normal and polymegethous human corneal endothelium. Optom Vis Sci 70:759, 1993

117. Carlson KH, Bourne WM, Brubaker RF: Effect of long-term contact lens wear on corneal endothelial cell morphology and function. Invest Ophthalmol Vis Sci 29:185, 1988

118. Lass JH, Dutt RM, Spurney RV, et al: Morphologic and fluorophotometric analysis of the corneal endothelium in long-term hard and soft contact lens wearers. CLAO J 14:105, 1988

119. Dutt RM, Stocker EG, Wolff CH, et al: A morphologic and fluorophotometric analysis of the corneal endothelium in long-term extended wear soft contact lens wearers. CLAO J 15:121, 1989

120. Brewitt H, Bonatz E, Honegger H: Morphological changes in the endothelium after application of topical anesthetic ointments. Ophthalmologica 180:198, 1980

121. Burstein NL: Corneal cytotoxicity of topically applied drugs, vehicles, and preservatives. Surv Ophthalmol 25:15, 1980

122. Bartlett JD, Jaanus SD: Local anesthetics. In Bartlett JD, Jaanus SD (eds): Clinical Ocular Pharmacology. 2nd ed. Butterworth, Boston, 1989

123. Bergmanson JPG: Histopathological analysis of the corneal epithelium after contact lens wear. J Am Optom Assoc 58:812, 1987

124. Bergmanson JPG: Contact lens-induced epithelial pathology. p. 13. In Bennett ES, Weissman BA (eds): Clinical Contact Lens Practice. JB Lippincott, Philadelphia, 1991

125. Erickson P, Doughty MJ, Comstock TL, Cullen AP: Endothelial cell density and contact lens-induced corneal swelling. Cornea 17:152, 1998

126. Bates AK, Cheng H: Bullous keratopathy: a study of endothelial cell morphology in patients undergoing cataract surgery. Br J Ophthalmol 72:409, 1988

127. Holden BA: Suffocating the cornea with PMMA. Contact Lens Spectrum 4:69, 1989

128. Holden BA, Sweeney DF: Corneal exhaustion syndrome (CES) in long-term contact lens wearers: a consequence of contact lens-induced polymegethism? Am J Physiol Opt 65:95P, 1988

129. Sweeney DF: Corneal exhaustion syndrome with long-term wear of contact lenses. Optom Vis Sci 69:601, 1992

130. McLaughlin R, Schoessler J: Corneal endothelial response to refitting polymethyl methacrylate wearers with rigid gas-permeable lenses. Optom Vis Sci 67:346, 1990

131. Bourne WM, Holtan SB, Hodge DO: Morphologic changes in corneal endothelial cells during 3 years of fluorocarbon contact lens wear. Cornea 18:29, 1999

132. Holden BA, Sweeney DF, Vannas A, et al: Contact lens induced endothelial polymegethism. Invest Ophthalmol Vis Sci (suppl.) 26:275, 1985

133. Holden BA, Williams L, Sweeney DF, et al: The endothelial response to contact lens wear. CLAO J 12:150, 1986

134. Sibug ME, Datiles MB, Kashima K, et al: Specular microscopy studies on the corneal endothelium after cessation of contact lens wear. Cornea 10:395, 1991

135. Waring GO, Rodrigues MM, Laibson PR: Corneal dystrophies. p. 57. In Liebowitz HM (ed): Corneal Disorders: Clinical Diagnosis and Management. WB Saunders, Philadelphia, 1984

136. Arffa RC: Grayson's Diseases of the Cornea. 3rd ed. Mosby-Yearbook, St. Louis, 1991

137. Sugar A: Corneal and conjunctival degenerations. p. 441. In Kaufman HE, Barron BA, McDonald MB, Waltman SR (eds): The Cornea. Churchill Livingstone, New York, 1988

138. Curran RE, Kenyon KR, Green WR: Pre-Descemet's membrane corneal dystrophy. Am J Ophthalmol 77:711, 1974

139. Grayson M, Wilbrandt H: Pre-Descemet's dystrophy. Am J Ophthalmol 64:276, 1967

140. Krachmer JH, Dubord PJ, Rodrigues MM, Mannis MJ: Corneal posterior crocodile shagreen and polymorphic amyloid degeneration. A histopathologic study. Arch Ophthalmol 101:54, 1983

141. Waring GO, Bourne WM, Edelhauser HF, Kenyon KR: The corneal endothelium. Normal and pathological structure and function. Ophthalmology 89:531, 1982

142. Boruchoff SA, Kuwabara T: Electron microscopy of posterior polymorphous degeneration. Am J Ophthalmol 72:879, 1971

143. Miller CA, Krachmer JH: Endothelial dystrophies. p. 425. In Kaufman HE, Barron BA, McDonald MB, Waltman SR (eds): The Cornea. Churchill Livingstone, New York, 1988

144. Weissman BA, Ehrlich M, Levenson JE, et al: Four cases of keratoconus and posterior polymorphous dystrophy. Optom Vis Sci 68:243, 1987

145. Bergmanson JPG, Sheldon TM, Goosey JD: Fuchs' endothelial dystrophy: a fresh look at an aging disease. Ophthalmic and Physiological Optics. 19:210, 1999

146. Duke-Elder S, Leigh AG: Diseases of the outer eye. Vol. VIII. Part 2. System of Ophthalmology. CV Mosby, St. Louis, 1965

147. Catania LJ: Primary care of the anterior segment. Appleton & Lange, East Norwalk, CT, 1988

148. Elner VM, Elner SG, Pavilack MA, et al: Intercellular adhesion molecule-1 in human corneal endothelium. Modulation and function. Am J Pathol 138:525, 1991

4

Noninfectious Corneal Staining

Larry J. Davis and Kenneth A. Lebow

GRAND ROUNDS CASE REPORT

Subjective:

A 27-year-old woman presented with complaints of discomfort and reduced wearing time with her 2-year-old rigid, gas-permeable (RGP) contact lenses. The patient had no contact lens history before these lenses. She used Allergan Wet-N-Soak care system (Allergan, Irvine, CA), with weekly use of an enzyme cleaner. The patient was in good health, took no medications, and denied allergies. Familial ocular and medical histories were unremarkable.

Objective:

- Best acuity with lenses: right eye (OD) $^{20}/_{20}$ J-1 @ 16 in, left eye (OS) $^{20}/_{20}$ J-1 @ 16 in
- Postwear keratometry: OD 42.50 @ $^{180}/_{43.00}$ @ 90, OS 42.25 @ $^{180}/_{43.00}$ @ 90
- Manifest refraction: OD –8.00 = –0.50 × 180, OS –7.50 = –0.75 × 180

Lens Observations:

High-riding lenses, with lower edge of lenses 2 mm below the pupil. Inferior arcuate staining with fluorescein each eye (OU) corresponding to area just outside of inferior lens edge. Fluorescein pattern aligned centrally and superiorly, but excessive inferior edge lift.

Lens Verification:

	OD	OS
Base curve	8.04 mm	8.08 mm
Diameter	9.4 mm	9.4 mm
Optic zone diameter	7.8 mm	7.8 mm
Back vertex power	–7.00 D	–6.50 D
Center thickness	0.14 mm	0.14 mm
Edge	Single cut	Single cut (nonlenticularized)

Assessment:

The arcuate punctate staining corresponded to the region below the inferior lens edges. The high-riding lenses were excessively lifted by the upper lids and moved only during the blink. The thick lens edges and relatively flat peripheral curves, thus, were malpositioned, riding over a steeper area of the cornea just 2 mm below the pupil. Extreme lid gap was created by the thick lens edges, which prevented the lids from rubbing mucin over the lower portion of the cornea, leading to the development of arcuate punctate staining OU. The etiology of this staining, seen with high-riding, high-minus lenses, is not unlike the corneal staining that forms at the 3 and 9 o'clock positions in patients wearing more optimally centered RGP lenses.

Plan:
The lenses were remade in essentially the same parameters, except that a myolenticular (plus-edge lenticular) design was used. This design reduced the lens mass overall and allowed for a thin edge (0.12-mm edge thickness) that was heavily tapered. The upper lids subsequently "squeezed" against a thin edge, pushing the lens back to a more centered position. A fluoropolymer with a Dk of 30 was used.

Follow-up:
The patient was reexamined on several occasions after dispensing of the new lenses and was enjoying all-day wearing time and good comfort. Biomicroscopy revealed resolution of the inferior arcuate staining.

The corneal epithelium functions to provide a smooth ocular surface, which demonstrates good optical properties. It also forms a vital barrier to superficial particulate matter and potential infectious organisms. The corneal epithelium consists of five or six cell layers having three major cell types, including from posterior to anterior:

1. Basal cell layer
2. A wing cell layer (which is overlain by a thin layer of flattened cells, two to three cells thick)
3. The most anterior layer, which contains many microvilli that extend into the tear layer and function to promote vital interactions between the hydrophobic corneal epithelium and mucous tear components[1]

Thus, disruptions of any layer of the corneal epithelium or tears that overlie this tissue may result in compromised integrity of the epithelium. This chapter describes various clinical techniques used to evaluate corneal epithelial integrity. Representative clinical presentations of epithelial compromise associated with contact lenses that manifest as corneal and conjunctival staining are also described.

VITAL DYES AS INDICATORS OF CORNEAL INTEGRITY

Although large epithelial defects are often detected during routine slit-lamp biomicroscopy, others may go unnoticed until the clinician applies one of several corneal stains. Various vital dyes have been used to observe compromised epithelium and disruptions of cell structure. A vital dye is considered to stain living cells without affecting their integrity.[2] Although sodium fluorescein[3] is the sub-

stance most often used for this purpose, other dyes, such as rose bengal, fluorexon,[4] lissamine green,[5] tetrazolium-alcian blue mixture,[6,7] trypan blue,[8] methylene blue, and bromothymol blue have been investigated. Fluorexon is a high-molecular-weight fluorescein derivative primarily used with soft lenses to eliminate lens discoloration.[9] It has few predictive properties for evaluation of fitting relationships and determination of the ability to wear a contact lens.[10] Alcian blue is a copper-containing dye that selectively stains mucus and connective tissue.[11] Bromothymol blue is a hydrogen ion indicator that appears yellow in acid media and blue in alkaline;[12] it can be used to judge the relative pH of the tear film but, in general, has weak properties.[13] Although all these vital dyes are available to evaluate corneal integrity, their frequency of clinical application is very low. Because fluorescein and rose bengal are the best-suited dyes currently available for clinical practice, the majority of our discussion is limited to these.

Sodium Fluorescein

Sodium fluorescein itself is relatively insoluble in water; therefore, the sodium salt is used for clinical practice.[2] It is available for topical use in the eye as a 2% solution or as impregnated filter paper strips.[14] Fluorescein promotes bacterial growth; therefore, the filter paper strips are usually preferred.[15] In the event that a solution is necessary, a low-volume sterile unit dose is preferred.

A fundamental property of fluorescent substances is that they absorb light at specific wavelengths and emit this absorbed energy at longer wavelengths. Fluorescein has a maximal absorption spectrum at 460 to 490 nm, with a maximal emission spectrum at 520 nm.[16] The observed intensity of fluorescence may be affected by several fac-

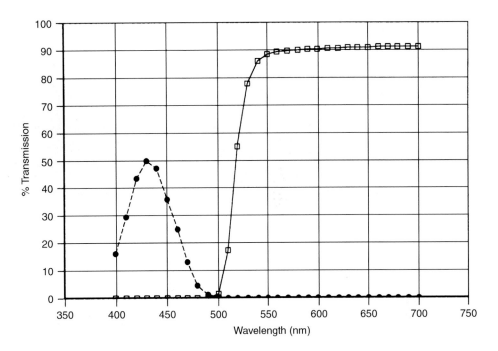

FIG. 4-1. *Transmission characteristics of barrier filters (square, Wratten No. 12; circle, Wratten No. 47B, Kodak Corp., Rochester, NY).*

tors. Intensity increases with the concentration of fluorescein until it is sufficiently high to result in attenuation, also known as *quenching* of fluorescence.[16,17] Therefore, patients who have a low tear volume are often observed to exhibit a less intense tear fluorescence despite repeated applications of fluorescein. It is often helpful to apply a drop of artificial tears to reduce the fluorescein concentration, thereby enhancing the observed fluorescence. Extrinsic contaminants, such as protein and heavy metals, or halogens, such as chloride, may also result in attenuation of fluorescence.[18] Fluorescence increases with the thickness of the tear layer until the concentration reaches the point at which quenching begins.[18] The observed intensity may also be enhanced via barrier filters placed in the illumination and observation system.[19-22] The excitation filter should have a maximal transmission between 400 and 500 nm, approaching zero above 500 nm, as is observed with the Wratten No. 47B (Kodak Corp., Rochester, NY) filter. Furthermore, the introduction of a yellow Wratten No. 12 or equivalent filter into the observation system, which absorbs all wavelengths below 500 nm and provides for maximal transmission at approximately 530 nm, further enhances the observed fluorescence (Fig. 4-1). These wavelengths correspond to the maximal emission peak of fluorescein under most clinical conditions. Enhancing the visualization of fluorescein aids the practitioner in evaluating subtle degrees of staining as well as in analyzing the fit of a contact lens (Figs. 4-2 and 4-3). Proper use of filters enables the practitioner to distinguish subtle varia-

tions in tear film thickness and incipient superficial punctate keratitis (SPK).[23] Fluorescence increases with increasing pH until quenching begins at a pH of approximately 8.[18,23]

It is generally believed that fluorescein is not absorbed by or adsorbed to cells. Rather, it diffuses into areas with loose cellular attachments, where a disruption of cell-cell junctions occurs.[24] Some investigators have reported fluorescein staining of cells under special conditions, although it is usually not observed clinically.[25,26] Often, it diffuses through the corneal stroma and may result in *pseudo-flare* in the anterior chamber. Fluorescein is also widely used to observe the tear layer thickness under con-

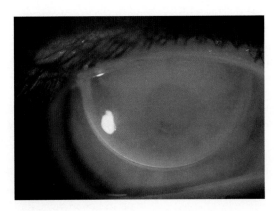

FIG. 4-2. *Fluorescein evaluation of contact lens fit observed without yellow excitation filter.*

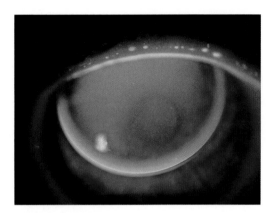

FIG. 4-3. *Fluorescein evaluation of contact lens fit observed with yellow excitation filter.*

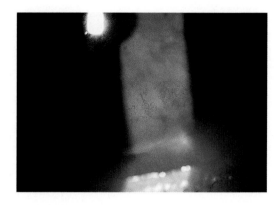

FIG. 4-4. *Rose bengal staining in keratoconjunctivitis sicca.*

tact lenses to achieve a desired fitting relationship.[27,28] Tear layer stability is observed through tear breakup time. A normal tear film shows uniform fluorescence with biomicroscopy until breaks or holes, which look like dark spots within the tear layer, are observed in the tear film. Any disruption of the tear layer thickness may result in a dark area observed (negative staining), as is seen after rigid lens adherence or in basement membrane corneal dystrophies.

Fluorescein, with a molecular weight of 376, is smaller than the calculated theoretical pore size of hydrogel lenses. Therefore, it is absorbed by soft hydrogel contact lenses and permanently adheres to the material, giving a yellow-orange tint to the lens. Fluorexon, on the other hand, is a high-molecular-weight (710) derivative of fluorescein. Because it is larger than the pore size of hydrogel lenses, fluorexon does not enter the lens and can be easily rinsed from the lens.[9,29] Despite these potential advantages, it has not gained wide clinical use because of its reduced fluorescent properties compared to sodium fluorescein.[30] Furthermore, a high degree of stinging and patient discomfort has been observed with the use of this product.

Often, the initial application of fluorescein does not show staining, particularly in asymptomatic non–contact lens wearers. The intensity of stain increases with time.[31] *Sequential corneal staining* may be a more sensitive technique predictive of epithelial complications with contact lens wear.[32] It is performed by repeated application of nonpreserved fluorescein dye over a period of minutes, followed by observation of staining. This phenomenon is thought to indicate a defective adhesive matrix of the epithelial cells, which predisposes the epithelium to break down in the event of lens trauma.[33] Variations of this technique have been used to investigate changes over a period of 30 days, and diurnal variance has been reported.[33-36] A positive sequential result may be associated with contact lens intolerance and

a propensity for dry eye and surface disease. The significance of patient variation with sequential corneal staining has yet to be determined, although cytotoxic effects of sodium fluorescein cannot be ruled out.[37]

Rose Bengal

The second most often used vital dye for clinical practice is rose bengal. It is adsorbed to and absorbed by compromised epithelial cells and mucus.[38] Rose bengal is available as a 1% ophthalmic solution and as impregnated filter paper strips.[14] Some investigators have suggested that even healthy epithelial cells may absorb rose bengal if the superficial mucin layer is removed.[25] Therefore, epithelial staining by rose bengal is often used to investigate dry eye and surface disease conditions (Fig. 4-4). The resulting amount of rose bengal staining is highly influenced by the concentration of the dye. It has been shown that a 10% solution causes a marked increase in uptake of the dye compared to a 1% concentration.[38]

It is thought that the 1% solution is better than filter strips for maximal penetration of the corneal epithelium. Small defects often go undetected unless the solution is used.[39] Rose bengal diffuses through the corneal stroma at a much lower rate than fluorescein does. Feenstra and Tseng[25] showed that tears probably have a blocking effect on dye uptake by healthy epithelial cells. Therefore, epithelial staining by rose bengal often demonstrates a tear deficiency as the primary defect, with epithelial compromise being only a secondary result. Rose bengal also demonstrates antiviral properties;[40] therefore, it should not be used before performing viral cultures. Rose bengal is known to produce phototoxic effects in the presence of light. The increased stain observed with higher concentrations of dye may, in part, result from these effects (Table 4-1).

TABLE 4-1. *Summary of Differences between Fluorescein and Rose Bengal Staining*

	Fluorescein	*Rose Bengal*
Experimental data		
Staining of healthy cells[a]	No	Yes
Intrinsic toxicity	No	Yes
Phototoxicity	No	Yes
Increased staining in dead cells	Yes	Yes[b]
Staining blockable by tear components	No	Yes[b]
Stromal diffusion	Rapid	Limited
Clinical extrapolation		
Staining promoted by:	Disruption of cell-cell junctions	Insufficient protection of preocular tear film[c]

[a]Staining is defined by stainability detected by clinical means (i.e., by the naked eye or under a biomicroscope using blue light).
[b]Even for dead or degenerated cells, the rose bengal staining can still be blocked by tear components.
[c]Insufficient protection can come from either decreased tear components or abnormal epithelial cells.
Source: Reprinted with permission from RPG Feenstra, SCG Tseng: Comparison of fluorescein and rose bengal staining. Ophthalmology 99:605, 1992.

CLASSIFICATION OF CORNEAL STAINING

Corneal staining occurs in a wide spectrum of shapes, locations, and intensities. It is the most frequently observed

TABLE 4-2. *Classification of Corneal Staining**

Categories	*Type*	*Severity*
Arcuate abrasions	Punctate stains	Superficial stains
Punctate abrasions	Diffuse stains	Moderate stains
Superficial abrasions	Line stains	Deep stains
Deep epithelial abrasions	Dimple stains	
Linear abrasions		
Limbal abrasions		
Superficial conjunctival abrasions		

*See JR Larke: Contact lens and the epithelium. p. 42. In JR Larke (ed): The Eye in Contact Lens Wear. Butterworth, London, 1985.

complication of contact lens wear. Few reports of the incidence of contact lens–associated corneal staining exist, and no standardized techniques exist for description and measurement of corneal staining. The threshold of detection varies with instrumentation and observation techniques, therefore, devising a classification system to include all clinical presentations is difficult. A classification scheme based on those by previous authors that divides staining into seven categories by appearance was proposed; these are further divided into four categories by type and severity (Table 4-2).[41] Figure 4-5 shows an alternative system for the evaluation and grading of corneal staining proposed by Begley et al.[42,43]

FIG. 4-5. *A representative corneal staining grading system. The cornea is divided into five zones. The number of stains in each section is then counted or estimated. (C = central; I = inferior; N = nasal; S = superior; T = temporal.) (Reprinted with permission from CG Begley, B Weirich, J Benak, NA Pence: Effects of rigid gas permeable contact lens solutions on the human corneal epithelium. Optom Vis Sci 69:347, 1992.)*

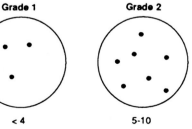
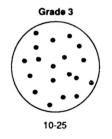
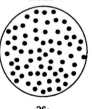

Grade 1   < 4

Grade 2   5-10

Grade 3   10-25

Grade 4   26+ (Difficult to count)

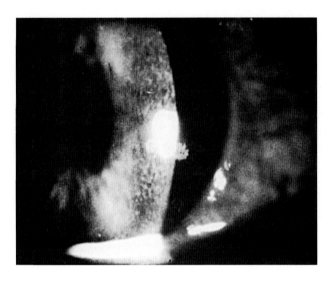

FIG. 4-6. *Peripheral subepithelial infiltration associated with subtle overlying epithelial staining.*

Because the clinical appearance of quite different causes of corneal staining may look similar, we group corneal staining according to the probable mechanism of the various causes. A discussion of the first four mechanisms follows. Infectious causes are discussed in other chapters.

Etiologies

The causes of corneal staining are as follows:

- Drying
- Mechanical
- Toxic or allergic
- Physiologic
- Infectious

In discussing corneal staining, most authors provide descriptive information as well as probable causes. It is necessary to consider the patient history when attempting to determine the definitive cause of epithelial defects. Similarly, it is important to evaluate epithelial integrity via biomicroscopy at all follow-up visits because it has been reported that the incidence of staining in the hydrogel lens–wearing population alone occurs in 33% to more than 60% of patients.[43–45]

Drying

Superficial Punctate Keratitis

A general term for diffuse corneal staining, *SPK* refers to small, dotlike epithelial changes that fill with fluorescein

when epithelial cells are damaged or missing. SPK is initially described as a localized, diffuse epithelial disturbance appearing as grayish white clouding in areas of isolated, discrete punctate corneal staining.[46] Lesions that initially appear as either fine or coarse ultimately coalesce, eroding the epithelium and predisposing the cornea to potentially more serious complications. A more detailed differentiation of SPK is based on the morphologic appearance of staining and includes superficial punctate epithelial erosions (SPEE), superficial punctate epithelial keratitis, and combined epithelial and subepithelial punctate keratitis.[47]

SPEEs appear as fine, slightly depressed spots that are invisible without fluorescein and are believed to represent areas of focalized epithelial disruption.[48,49] They are a nonspecific response to injury and are frequently found in staphylococcal blepharoconjunctivitis, keratitis sicca, exposure keratitis, and toxicity reactions.[47] Superficial punctate epithelial keratitis presents as small, grayish white opacities in the epithelium and is differentiated from SPEE by not staining with fluorescein. These lesions represent accumulations of epithelial cells surrounded by an inflammatory cell infiltrate[50] and are found in many clinical conditions, including microcystic edema associated with extended wear of hydrogel lenses.[51] They may ultimately rupture on the epithelial surface and appear subsequently as epithelial erosions. Combined epithelial and subepithelial punctate keratitis is usually associated with adenovirus infections of the cornea[51] and inclusion conjunctivitis.[52]

Areas of peripheral or midperipheral subepithelial infiltration associated with subtle overlying epithelial staining or drying may occur with hydrogel contact lenses as a result of tight lens syndrome (contact lens–induced acute red-eye syndrome),[53] preservative reactions,[54] or peripheral corneal edema[55] (Fig. 4-6). SPK has many causes, including desiccation, mechanical injury (foreign body or dehydration), preservative-induced allergic reactions, lens deposits, hypoxia, and infection. Because these other complications are discussed elsewhere, it is important to consider the diffuse pattern of SPK resulting from dehydration-induced corneal desiccation. These central diffuse punctate lesions stain with fluorescein and are also visible as grayish white lesions with white light. This condition is frequently observed with high-water ultrathin lens designs. It is thought to result from full-thickness dehydration and is directly related to water content and thickness (Fig. 4-7).[56,57] Corneal desiccation staining has been associated with a rapidly destabilizing pre-lens tear film and a thinning lipid layer. It can be exacerbated in the presence of low humidity, as occurs with forced-air heat or in arid environments. Incomplete blinking can also cause this form of SPK, as can the presence of a bor-

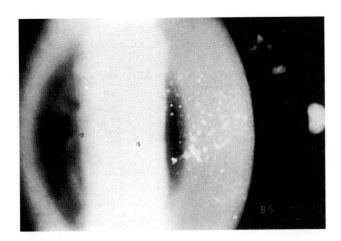

FIG. 4-7. *Superficial punctate keratitis associated with dehydration of high-water-content ultrathin lens. (Courtesy of Dr. Steve Zantos.)*

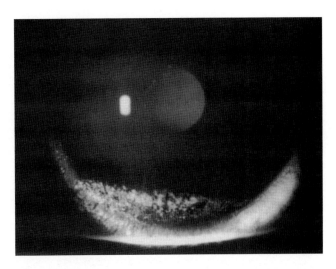

FIG. 4-8. *Superficial punctate keratitis associated with contact lens–associated keratitis sicca.*

derline dry-eye condition. It can typically be diagnosed initially via steepening of the base curve radius and resultant decrease in lens movement with the blink. Changing to a thicker lens with a lower water content usually reduces this problem, especially if adequate movement is present with the blink. It may be necessary to supplement this management option with a 10-minute saline soak during the middle of the day to rehydrate the lens. Lubricating drops are of little value unless instilled frequently throughout the day.

Contact Lens–Associated Keratitis Sicca

Although the term implies an infectious or inflammatory etiology, *contact lens–associated keratitis sicca* is most often associated with a deficiency in the quantity or quality of tears. It may cause mild to moderate SPK, particularly in the inferior one-half of the cornea, which is usually most exposed (Fig. 4-8). Patients may experience symptoms of burning, stinging, or dryness. The condition is most common in women and in patients in their third through fifth decades. Environmental factors may exacerbate it, including low humidity, wind, ventilated areas, smoke, dust, or other particulate matter. Various medications, such as antihistamines, decongestants, diuretics, and birth control pills, may contribute. The diuretic effect of alcohol consumption should also be considered. Usually, patients are asymptomatic and the clinical signs are absent without lens wear, which assists in differentiating contact lens–associated dry eye from true pathologic dry eye. Contact lens–associated keratitis sicca can be considered to result from borderline dry eye. Soft contact lens wear has been shown to result in an increase in

the tear evaporation rate.[58] Therefore, contact lens wear may stress a tear layer that has a tendency to provide borderline moisture and stability. A change to a thicker soft lens may enhance comfort by providing a larger reservoir for tears with reduced lens dehydration.[59] Medium-water lenses, which show a lower absolute percentage of drying than do high-water lenses, may provide further relief.[60-62] *Silicone sicca* is reported to occur in patients who are refitted from polymethylmethacrylate (PMMA) lenses into a silicone-acrylate, rigid, gas-permeable material.[63] In the event that the patient is a RGP lens wearer, a change to a polymer that contains fluorine may enhance comfort. See Chapter 1 for additional information on these conditions.

Lagophthalmos and Other Eyelid or Blinking Abnormalities

Incomplete closure of the palpebral aperture is often associated with drying and SPK of the inferior one-half of the cornea. Acceleration of the tear evaporation rate from exposure, with improper renewal of the pre-lens tear film, promotes local drying. Lens coating and soiling may promote further irritation. Frequent tear supplements are often indicated. These patients may also benefit from more frequent enzymatic treatment.

Peripheral Corneal Staining

Peripheral corneal staining (PCS) is an inflammatory process primarily limited to the cornea. The term describes the morphologic changes in corneal appearance represented by a broad group of epithelial alterations without implying a specific etiology or clinical course.[64] Although

TABLE 4-3. *Differential Diagnosis of Peripheral Corneal Staining Patterns Based on Corneal Location*

Inferior Cornea	Superior Cornea	Peripheral Cornea
Staphylococcal blepharitis	Superior limbic keratoconjunctivitis	Pterygium
Acne rosacea	Giant papillary conjunctivitis	Vascularized limbal keratitis
Exposure keratitis	Vernal catarrh	Elevated limbal mass
Entropion	Inclusion conjunctivitis	Conjunctival lesions
—	Molluscum contagiosum	Marginal furrow or gutter dystrophy
—	Trachoma	Terrien's marginal dystrophy
—	—	Peripheral corneal ischemia

SPK associated with contact lens wear is generally attributed to desiccation[47,65] and an unstable tear film,[66] practitioners should be aware that *desiccation* refers only to the process of corneal drying, whereas *staining* involves the actual visualization of the sequelae of desiccation with sodium fluorescein.[67] Although clinically these terms are used somewhat interchangeably, subtle differences exist in their meaning. Corneal desiccation is only one of several factors related to PCS (Table 4-3). Several classifications of PCS among RGP-wearing patients have been proposed based on the severity of staining, patient symptomatology, and associated loss of corneal transparency (Table 4-4).[68–71]

It appears that PCS secondary to contact lens wear is a progressive process directly related to lens wearing time.[72] As PCS progresses, several important objective signs and subjective patient symptoms develop. During the early stages of PCS, localized dustlike areas of epithelial staining appear along the horizontal axis of the peripheral cornea. This is frequently referred to as *3 and 9 o'clock staining* (Fig. 4-9). At this stage, the patient is frequently asymptomatic and rarely reports any complications with the lenses. Initially, no intervention is required, but as the amount of staining and coalescence enlarges, observation and documentation, along with lubricating drops and blink training, are helpful remedial procedures.[73] Mod-

TABLE 4-4. *Comparative Classification of Peripheral Corneal Staining Based on Severity of Staining, Patient Symptoms, and Loss of Corneal Transparency*

Grade	Henry, Bennett, and Forrest[68]	Andrasko[69]	Schnider[71]	Lebow[70]
0	Not present	No staining < 10 widely scattered spots	Absence of staining Cornea wets well *No intervention*	No staining No patient symptoms
1	Diffuse punctuate staining	Extremely light staining 10–50 spots Not coalesced	Diffuse light staining No coalescence *No intervention*	Microscopic superficial punctate keratopathy No significant symptoms
2	Mild density	Light staining > 50 spots Not coalesced	Light coalescence Absence of penetration *Observe*	Superficial punctate keratopathy Subjective burning
3	Moderate density	Light-to-moderate staining Partial and incomplete coalescence	Marked coalescence Some deep penetration *Modify fit* Redesign the lens *Adjust wearing schedule*	Coalesced superficial limbal punctate keratopathy *Reduce wearing time* Conjunctival hyperemia
4	Opacification Neovascularization	Moderate coalesced staining Coalescence over a large area	Complete coalescence Loss of epithelium *Remove lenses*	Abraded limbal keratopathy Dellen, scarring, invasive vasculature Intolerance to lens wear
5	—	Heavy staining Completely coalesced No thinning, dellen, or ulcer	—	—
6	—	Heavy staining Associated limbal pathology Thinning, dellen, or scarring	—	—

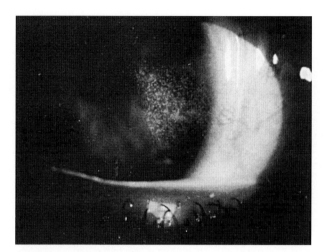

FIG. 4-9. *Mild 3 and 9 o'clock peripheral corneal staining, showing isolated micropunctate epithelial keratopathy.*

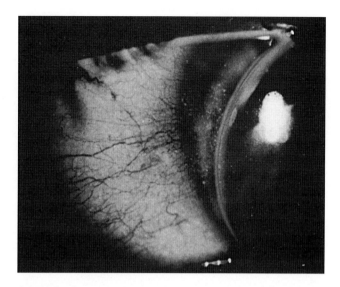

FIG. 4-11. *Severe 3 and 9 o'clock peripheral corneal staining, showing opacification of tissue.*

erate corneal staining is represented by an increase in the density of the staining pattern, evolving into diffuse, coalesced areas of staining (Fig. 4-10). With increased physiologic involvement, patients often complain of conjunctival hyperemia, burning, itching that increases with wearing time and persists after lens removal, increased lens awareness, dry eyes, and reduced wearing time.[66,73] At this stage of corneal involvement, practitioners should modify the fit of the existing lens, completely redesign the lens using a different fitting philosophy, or reduce the patient's wearing time.[74] Ultimately, advanced PCS is characterized by opacification of the stained areas (Fig. 4-11), collateral invasive vascularization and, in severe

cases, corneal thinning, erosion, or ulceration. If patients persist in wearing lenses with this degree of staining, they are often oblivious to their ocular problem and are generally negligent in following instructions about the care of their lenses. Lenses should be discontinued immediately and wearing time not resumed until the condition completely heals.

Etiology of Peripheral Corneal Staining with Rigid Gas-Permeable Lenses PCS associated with contact lens wear has long been attributed to corneal desiccation, especially as a result of disruption to the mucous layer of the precorneal tear film.[75,76] It may also be associated with an accumulation of connective tissue in the conjunctiva similar to pinguecula.[77-79] One theory suggests that shearing forces caused by viscous drag may be at work in some patients.[80] Environmental irritants, such as wind, ultraviolet exposure, low humidity, and noxious vapors, as well as hypersensitivity or toxic reactions to contact lens solutions, preservatives, and topical ocular medications, may also produce PCS (Table 4-5).

Inappropriate contact lens designs may mechanically exacerbate marginally dry eyes and physically induce PCS in otherwise healthy eyes. This may occur when the prelens tear film is disrupted, the flow of the post-lens tear film is reduced, or the mucous layer of the cornea is disturbed.[81] Two types of mucins are believed to exist in the tears: an invisible mucin that dissolves in the tears[72] and a visible form that represents degraded mucin and is of lesser benefit in promoting wetting of the ocular surface.[82] In contact lens wear with an abnormal mucin layer,

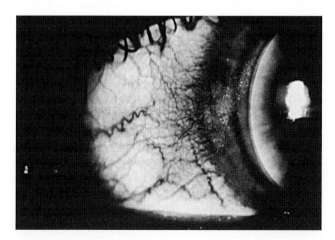

FIG. 4-10. *Moderate 3 and 9 o'clock peripheral corneal staining, showing increased density and coalescence of the epithelial keratopathy.*

TABLE 4-5. *Types of Peripheral Corneal Staining Induced by Rigid Gas-Permeable Lenses, Characteristics, and Therapeutic Recommendations*

Type of Staining	Characteristics	Therapy
Peripheral curve indenture	Negative staining Nonmoving lens Tear film break	Heavy blend P/C Flatten P/C Ocular lubrication
Patch staining	Away from lens edge Lid gap (thick edge)	C/N taper lens edge Reduce optic zone diameter
	Systemic medications	Ocular lubrication
Juxtapositional staining	Adjacent to lens edge Sharp demarcation line of staining Low edge-lift profile	Flatter P/C Wider P/C Smaller overall lens diameter

C/N = heavy cone tool tapering; P/C = peripheral curve.

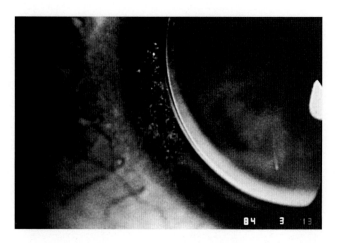

FIG. 4-12. *Black line formation or negative tear meniscus around the circumference of a contact lens associated with excessive edge lift of the peripheral curve system. (Courtesy of Dr. William Benjamin.)*

excessive degradation of tear mucins and decreased tear film wetting of the corneal surface may lead to excessive mucin debris and increased corneal staining.[83]

A variety of contact lens design factors should be considered in the evaluation of PCS (Table 4-6). Several distinct groupings of interrelated contact lens factors that should be evaluated by the practitioner are sagittal depth relationship (overall lens diameter, optic zone diameter, and base curve); peripheral curve systems and lens edge (edge profile, thickness, contour, and lift); lens centration characteristics; blinking; wearing time; and contact lens material (Figs. 4-12–4-15). Thus, PCS associated with rigid lenses probably has a multifactorial mechanism. It has been observed to occur along the flattest corneal meridian in

TABLE 4-6. *Contact Lens Factors Associated with Peripheral Corneal Staining*

Overall lens diameter
Optic zone diameter
Peripheral curve system
   Edge profile
   Edge thickness
   Edge contour
   Edge lift
Lens centration
Lens material
   Lens wettability
   Silicone acrylate
   Fluorosilicone acrylate
Wearing time
   Daily wear
   Extended wear
Negative tear meniscus
Blink inhibition

some patients.[84] Furthermore, rigid designs with large diameter and moderate edge lift have been shown to be associated with less PCS than are designs with small diameter and low edge lift.[85] Therefore, adequate peripheral edge clearance is recommended, particularly along the flattest corneal meridian in eyes having with-the-rule astigmatism.

Peripheral Corneal Staining with Hydrogel Lenses
Peripheral corneal or 3 and 9 o'clock staining occurs primarily with PMMA and RGP contact lenses. Hydrogel contact lenses can also induce PCS despite their inherent better wettability.[86] However, PCS with hydrogel lenses is less severe and is seen less frequently than with RGP lenses.[87,88] As with rigid lenses, the ultimate success of hydrogel lens wear depends on adequate mucin coating of the cornea as well as complete blinking to rewet the lens surface.[89] Staining with hydrogel lenses is usually not described as a cumulative process, such as that which occurs with RGP lenses. As with rigid lenses, however, characteristic staining patterns exist that point the practitioner to specific causes of peripheral staining with hydrogel lenses. Staining with hydrogels may be characterized as diffuse (as a result of hypoxia or trapped debris under a tight lens) or inferior (caused by improper blinking[90] or lens dehydration[91]). More frequently, hydrogel lens materials, especially when worn for extended periods, may lead to diffuse corneal punctate staining secondary to hypoxia and accumulation of metabolic wastes.[92,93]

Hypoxia-induced SPK with hydrogel materials is presumed to result from premature desquamation of stressed superficial epithelial cells, which leave microscopic gaps on the corneal surface where fluorescein may accumulate.[94]

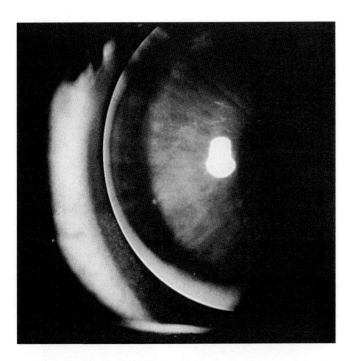

FIG. 4-13. *Excessive edge lift secondary to too flat a peripheral curve system.*

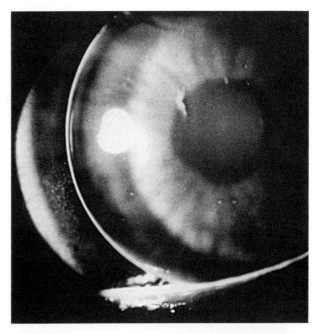

FIG. 4-15. *Low edge lift secondary to too steep a peripheral curve system.*

Chahine and Weissman describe prolonged use of extended-wear soft contact lenses as etiologic factors associated with pannus formation and peripheral furrow stain[95] (Fig. 4-16).

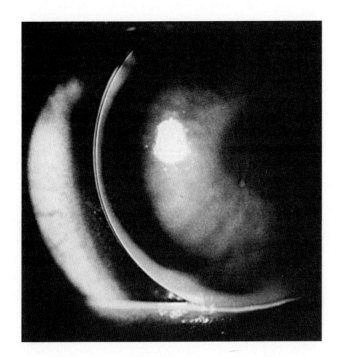

FIG. 4-14. *Ideal or moderate edge lift.*

The authors implicate hypoxia as the primary cause because high-minus lens powers were worn. Resolution was complete after refitting with rigid contact lenses.[95]

Epithelial pits have also been reported on the corneal surface with extended wear of hydrogel lenses, but these do not actively stain and should be differentiated from true corneal staining.[96] Hydrogel wearers also have more conjunctival staining than non–lens wearing controls.[97] As with RGP lenses, hydrogel-induced PCS is multifactorial in nature (Table 4-7).

Vascularized Limbal Keratitis

Vascularized limbal keratitis (VLK) is a rare but progressive aggregate of signs and symptoms associated with primarily large-diameter, low edge-lift lens designs worn for RGP extended wear. It is manifest by significant corneal inflammation and invasive vascularization but, unlike contact lens–induced pseudopterygium, is reversible and nonscarring. Initially, epithelial chafing with various degrees of microscopic SPK causes an epithelial heaping of hyperplastic corneal or limbal epithelium, or both. These changes are caused by desiccation and the fluid dynamics associated with low edge-lift peripheral curve designs that disturb the tear film meniscus. An inflammatory or immunologically mediated component is demonstrated by the presence of conjunctival hyperemia and corneal infiltration. Ultimately, a vascular leash ema-

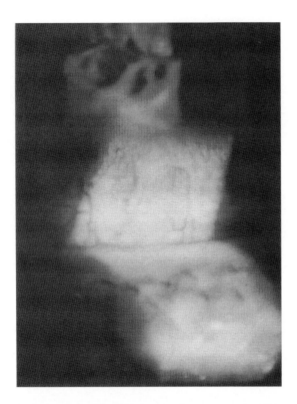

FIG. 4-16. *Limbal epithelial hypertrophy associated with large hydrogel contact lenses. (Courtesy of Dr. Joel Silbert.)*

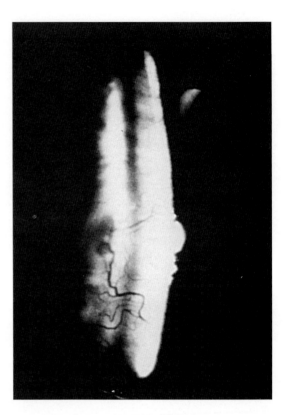

FIG. 4-17. *Vascularized limbal keratitis, demonstrating invasive vascularization and raised hyperplastic epithelial heaping. (Courtesy of Drs. R. Grohe and K. Lebow.)*

nating from the conjunctiva and across the edematous limbus leads to the raised epithelial mass with superficial and deep invasive vascularization. Finally, there may be erosion of the elevated hyperplastic epithelium with significant ocular staining and hyperemia (Fig. 4-17).[98]

Immunologic Basis of Vascularized Limbal Keratitis
The significance of the corneal limbus and its physiologic response to PCS is clearly demonstrated by VLK. The limbus delineates a unique portion of cornea that exhibits many anatomic, physiologic, and immunologic factors that differentiate this tissue from the central cornea and conjunctiva-sclera complex. Although the cornea has been described as *immunologically privileged* owing to the absence of

TABLE 4-7. *Possible Causes of Peripheral Corneal Staining with Hydrogel Contact Lenses*

Lens dehydration
Lens-induced hypoxia
Damaged contact lenses
Edge defects
Trapped retrolental debris
Keratitis from solutions
Corneal exposure and inadequate blinking

blood vessels and immunoreactive cells, the peripheral cornea marks a transitional buffer from the highly reactive conjunctival tissue. However, the physical proximity of the limbus to the conjunctiva, peripheral vascular plexus, and lymphatic system establishes unique characteristics that may predispose diseases affecting the limbus to allergic and immunologic mechanisms.[99] The presence of many mast cells within limbal tissue provides a pathway for the release of potent vasoactive substances that dilate conjunctival blood vessels, produce peripheral corneal or conjunctival edema, and attract inflammatory cells, especially eosinophils.[100] Increased awareness and itching associated with chronic PCS may indicate a contact lens–induced disruption of the stability of limbal mast cells. Moreover, the greater concentration of Langerhans' cells in the peripheral cornea represents a significant factor in the development of ocular hypersensitivity and the development of peripheral corneal infiltration and ulceration.[100,101] Although greater concentrations of immunoglobulin M (IgM) and C-1 complement are also located in the peripheral cornea, this can be attributed to the physical size of these molecules and their inability to diffuse from the limbal vascular plexus

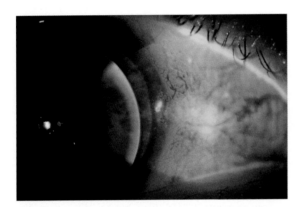

FIG. 4-18. *Active vascularized limbal keratitis, demonstrating significant invasive vascularization, raised hyperplastic limbal-epithelial mass, and acute hyperemia with pingueculitis before lubrication therapy. (Courtesy of Drs. R. Grohe and K. Lebow.)*

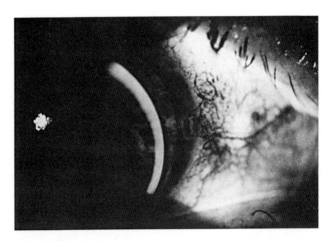

FIG. 4-19. *Reduced elevation of limbal-epithelial mass and staining after 1 week of ocular lubrication and decongestant supplements, with no alteration in wearing time or lens design. (Courtesy of Drs. R. Grohe and K. Lebow.)*

into the central cornea.[102,103] However, because IgM is the most effective agglutinant and cytolytic immunoglobulin, and C-1 complement is an integral factor in immune system stimulation, the unequal distribution of IgM and C-1 complement serves to protect the peripheral cornea more than the central tissue.[104] Chronic irritation to these systems from long-term PCS may trigger the development of more severe peripheral corneal complications.

The role of corneal edema in inducing contact lens–related inflammation is extremely difficult to establish.[105] However, the demonstration that corneal stem cells are primarily located in the limbus suggests an anatomic vulnerability of the limbus to large, mechanically impinging RGP lens diameters.[106] Moreover, studies with rabbit eyes have demonstrated that abnormal corneal epithelial healing can occur when partial limbal deficiency exists.[107] Adverse effects on the conjunctival goblet cells and mucus production occur once the corneal epithelium in the limbal area is compromised.[108] Because limbal stem cells are viewed as a primary source for the differentiation and proliferation of the corneal epithelium, any sustained insult to the limbus could compromise the cornea's ability to heal.[109-111] Disruption of the precorneal tear film induces PCS that deteriorates corneal and conjunctival surfaces even further, ultimately destabilizing the tear film and resulting in progressive exacerbation of the problem.[112]

Management of Vascularized Limbal Keratitis Treatment of VLK is specifically directed toward lens design deficiencies rather than incompatibility of lens material with the ocular surface. Initial design modifications include flatter and wider peripheral curve widths to reduce epithelial chafing, smaller overall lens diameters to eliminate mechanical impingement into the limbal sulcus, and concomitant use of ocular lubricants, decongestants, and antioxidants

to facilitate corneal wetting. Application of lubricants, decongestants, and antioxidative drops in isolation of lens design modifications may also cause VLK regression. Initially, the vasoconstrictive effect of ocular decongestants reduces vascular engorgement and limits the permeability of the vessels, thus reducing the involvement of VLK (Figs. 4-18 and 4-19). Further use of antioxidative lubrication without changes in wearing time or lens modification may reverse VLK in isolated situations (Fig. 4-20). However, as

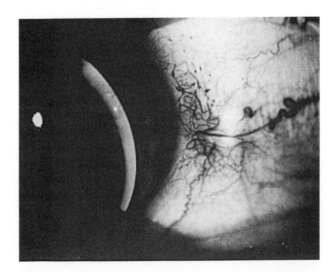

FIG. 4-20. *Elimination of raised limbal-epithelial mass, vascular leash, and conjunctival staining after 1 month of antioxidative drops, with no alteration in wearing time or lens design. (Courtesy of Drs. R. Grohe and K. Lebow.)*

CASE REPORT 1

Subjective:
A 40-year-old man presents with symptoms of dry and uncomfortable rigid lenses, increasing redness of eyes with contact lens wear, and a raised white spot visible on the cornea OS. He had a 10-year history of RGP lenses, with occasional periods of extended wear for several days' duration. Medical and familial ocular history are unremarkable.

Objective:
Visual acuities: OD $^{20}/_{15}$ with plano over-refraction (OR)
OS $^{20}/_{20}^-$ with OR of PL = -1.00×170 ($^{20}/_{15}$)
Biomicroscopy: Grade 3+ conjunctival, corneal, and limbal punctate staining; raised, hyperplastic limbal epithelial mass immediately adjacent to nasal limbus that stains with fluorescein (OS); superficial and deep invasive vascular leash emanating from the limbus to the hyperplastic tissue.
Lens evaluation: Interpalpebral lens design, with alignment patterns by fluorescein assessment OU; low edge-lift peripheral curve configuration, lenses centered, with 1- to 2-mm movement with the blink; lenses heavily coated with debris and lacquered mucoid deposits; poor surface wetting and moderate surface scratching.
Ophthalmoscopy: Unremarkable OU
Refraction: Low myopia OU

Assessment:
VLK, OS. Invasive corneal vascularization, PCS, peripheral corneal edema.

Plan:
1. Temporarily discontinue contact lens wear.
2. Institute ocular lubrication.
   a. Use an ocular decongestant for hyperemia.
   b. Use antioxidative or wetting agent for lubrication.
3. Redesign contact lens fit for OS.
   a. Smaller overall diameter.
   b. Flatter peripheral curve radius.
   c. Wider peripheral curve width.
4. Eliminate extended wear of contact lenses; use hypertonic saline for corneal edema.

---

the condition progresses, exhibiting greater staining, inflammation, invasive vascular proliferation, and erosion, temporary lens discontinuation is required until regression of the condition occurs. Refitting with RGP contact lenses that present a flatter lens-to-cornea relationship helps to avoid recurrence.[98] However, the creation of excessive edge-lift profiles with shallower sagittal depth fitting relationships may disturb the marginal tear meniscus and reestablish a mechanism for the development of PCS.[113]

Lens Decentration
Rigid Lenses Rigid lens decentration can result in many problems, including reduced or fluctuating vision, lens awareness, corneal distortion, and corneal desiccation. The desiccation, or 3 and 9 o'clock staining, is often the result of an inferiorly decentered lens, which can compromise the quality of the blink (Fig. 4-21).[67] Similarly, when a lens is decentered, poor corneal alignment is present, resulting in harsh regions of bearing adjacent to areas of excessive clearance. This fitting relationship can result in several diopters of corneal curvature change, often observed in the midperiphery and, therefore, not diagnosed with keratometry.[114,115]

The most common form, with the greatest problems, is inferior decentration. Patients may complain of lens awareness, dryness, and flare. Several lens design changes are beneficial in managing decentration. The selection of a lid attachment edge design often solves the problem. In addition, the use of a lenticular design is recommended when applicable. For example, a minus

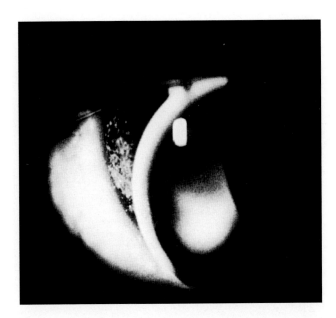

FIG. 4-21. *Corneal desiccation staining adjacent to an inferiorly positioned rigid gas-permeable lens.*

for the management of RGP-induced decentration is provided in Figure 4-22.

Hydrogel Lenses   As a result of the large overall diameter and improved manufacturing methods, hydrogel lens decentration resulting in corneal exposure is rare. When exposure is present, corneal desiccation staining may result in this region. Often, this takes the form of an arcuate stain, which appears to be a result of mechanical trauma by the lens edge.[117] This problem is typically managed quite easily by selecting either a large-diameter lens or an ultrathin design that may drape the cornea in a more well-centered position.

Mechanical Staining

Rigid Lenses

An arcuate or foreign-body abrasion can result from an unfinished lens edge. The softer RGP materials available today are more difficult to manufacture with a consistent smooth edge. Careful manufacture and verification are necessary to prevent sharp, abraded, or chipped edges, any of which may result in patient symptoms ranging from lens awareness to pain. The greater the edge defect, the more likely the resulting corneal abrasion is to be deep and more widespread. This problem can be avoided by careful verification of the lens edge with a comparator (reticule magnifier) or similar instrument. Unless the lens is chipped, a simple edge polish eliminates patient symptoms. If it is a frequent problem, the laboratory should be made aware of this quality-control problem.

lenticular edge is recommended for all plus and low-minus (less than 1.50 diopter [D]) lens powers, and a plus lenticular edge is recommended for all high-minus (greater than 6 D) lens powers. If possible, reducing center thickness by a minimum of 0.04 mm reduces mass by 25% or more, therefore increasing the possibility of greater lifting action by the upper lid.[116] A nomogram

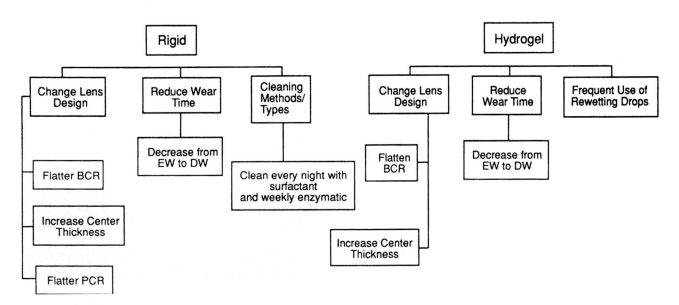

FIG. 4-22. *Management nomogram for rigid and hydrogel lens adherence. (BCR = base curve radius; DW = daily wear; EW = extended wear; PCR = peripheral curve radius.)*

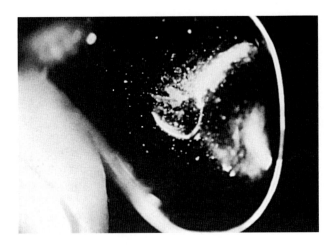

FIG. 4-23. *A small central tear in a hydrogel lens.*

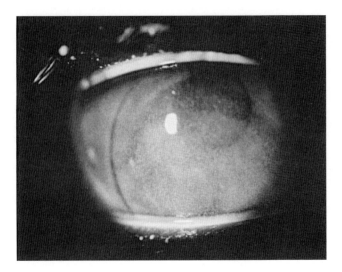

FIG. 4-24. *A negative area of staining can be observed, resulting from a lens with unblended peripheral curve junctions.*

Hydrogel Lenses

Hydrogel lens defects or tears may be small and difficult to detect (Fig. 4-23). However, when the defect is small, the patient typically has symptoms of discomfort and lens awareness. In this case, it is important to inspect the lens with the biomicroscope centrally and circumferentially because edge defects can be subtle. It is advantageous to observe the lens, off the eye, placed in the plane of the patient's eye with the biomicroscope. If the lens tear is central, foreign-body staining corresponding to the tear is often observed. It is rarely severe enough for antibiotic therapy, and simply replacing the lens accompanied by patient re-education on proper care and handling is sufficient. Discontinuation of lens wear is not necessary if staining is not present; however, the patient must be advised of the presence and implications of the tear. Similarly, if an edge tear or nick is present and the patient is asymptomatic, this is rarely a problem because corneal insult seldom results. Nevertheless, lens replacement is advised.

Arcuate Staining Unrelated to Decentration

Rigid Lens An arcuate stain, commonly observed with rigid lens wearers, can be seen in the midperipheral region of the superior cornea.[118] Although it can result from a steep base curve radius, a large optical zone diameter, or inadequate lens movement with the blink, it most often results from inadequately blended peripheral curve junctions. An arcuate negative stain is observed in a depression overlying an intact epithelium (Figs. 4-24 and 4-25). Blending this junction should resolve the staining.

Hydrogel Lens Arcuate staining in the midperipheral cornea just below the pupil is reported to occur with soft lenses of various designs, water content, and fitting rela-

tionships (Fig. 4-26).[119] It is often associated with a loose-fitting soft lens made from the crofilcon material.[120] The unusual rigidity of this unique lens polymer is considered a factor in the irritation. Patients are typically asymptomatic except in severe cases. A similar staining pattern has been observed in some patients wearing extended-wear disposable contact lenses.[121] The problem can be managed by either selecting a steeper base curve radius, changing to another hydrogel lens material, or reducing wearing time.

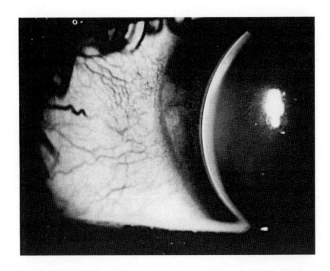

FIG. 4-25. *Midperipheral corneal staining associated with an inadequately blended junction between optic zone and the peripheral curve.*

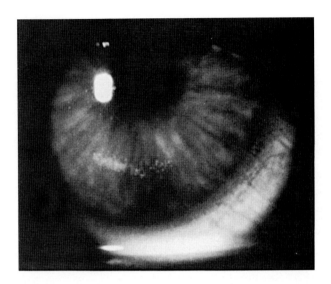

FIG. 4-26. *The so-called smile arcuate staining induced by a loose-fitting crofilcon lens.*

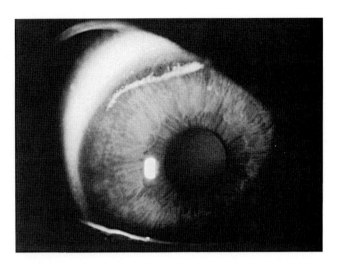

FIG. 4-27. *Epithelial splitting.*

Epithelial Splitting

Epithelial splitting is characterized by a horizontal lesion, usually adjacent to the superior limbus resulting from hydrogel lens wear.[122] The lesions appear as diffuse, scattered punctate dots, aligned in a linear or arcuate fashion in the superior cornea, under the upper lid (Fig. 4-27).[123]

As the coalescence of the staining progresses, the lesions can be viewed in white light as a line or arc. Because of its location and the fact that practitioners do not use fluorescein routinely for evaluation of the corneal integrity of hydrogel lens wearers at follow-up visits, this is often undiagnosed in its early phases when the patient is asymptomatic. As the condition progresses, however, the patient complains of lens awareness, burning, itching, and redness. With discontinuation of lens wear, these lesions heal in anywhere from a few days to a few weeks. The causative mechanisms appear to represent a combination of mechanical and hypoxic effects.[124] The causative factors may include tightening of lens fittings through tear hypertonicity, localized drying associated with the upper lid tear meniscus, overall lens dehydration, poor edge design, or giant papillary conjunctivitis.[118,125] As with dehydration-induced SPK, the presence of tight-fitting hydrogel lenses, with either low or high water content, can result in epithelial splitting. It is important to refit such patients into new lenses, preferably with a planned replacement or disposable lens material. If this condition continues to occur, refitting into RGP lens material is indicated.

Foreign-Body Tracking

Trapped debris under a contact often results in epithelial compromise with superficial staining. It appears as arcuate or linear tracks in the area of the trapped particle (Fig. 4-28). It may persist for several minutes to hours. The severity depends on the amount of lens excursion with a blink. Therefore, when it occurs in rigid lens wearers, it is usually more dramatic, and patients tend to be more symptomatic. However, long-term sequelae are rare.

CASE REPORT 2

A patient new to contact lens wear was dispensed RGP lenses and advised to gradually increase wearing time. The patient indicated that the lenses were quite uncomfortable from the moment of insertion. Tearing persisted longer than average, approximately 20 minutes. The patient was advised that the lenses should gradually feel better with each passing day. However, he returned in 1 week complaining that the comfort was not improving and that he was unable to wear the lenses for more than 4 hours. With biomicroscopy, an arcuate area of staining was observed surrounded by diffuse staining. No staining was observed after discontinuing contact lens wear for 24 hours and, after polishing the edge, comfort and ocular health were good.

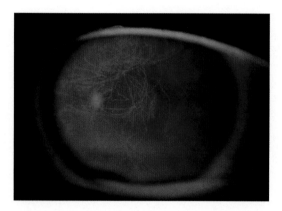

FIG. 4-28. *Foreign-body staining in a patient wearing rigid lenses.*

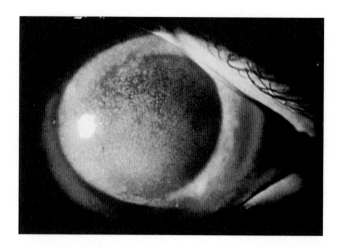

FIG. 4-29. *A thimerosal hypersensitivity reaction. (Courtesy of Patrick J. Caroline.)*

Solution- or Care-Induced Staining

Solution Toxicities or Allergies

All preservatives for antimicrobial use in contact lens solutions are potentially toxic. The tissue damage that may result from this toxicity is influenced by exposure time and concentration.[124] Therefore, a balance must be reached between safety and efficacy of these agents, such that the desired organisms are eradicated with no resulting subjective symptoms of redness, itching, photophobia, and conjunctival edema, or clinical signs, such as conjunctival hyperemia and diffuse corneal staining. A more immediate hypersensitivity reaction (not toxic) is a more common response to contact lens preservative use. In a delayed hypersensitivity reaction, the chemicals act as haptens, which require combination with a tissue protein to initiate an allergic response.[126] This not only results in diffuse staining but dendriform lesions, infiltrates, and neovascularization are possible. This type of reaction is most likely to occur in patients who present with an atopic history of general hypersensitivity to a variety of antigens.

Several preservatives are in current use. Those that have been used for many years include thimerosal, chlorhexidine, and benzalkonium chloride (BAK). All three preservatives can induce a cell-mediated hypersensitivity reaction, although this is less likely to occur with BAK-preserved solutions.[127]

Thimerosal   Thimerosal is an organic mercury compound whose use has been declining in recent years. An incidence of 6.6–8.0% hypersensitivity to thimerosal has been reported, with accompanying infection, edema, and diffuse corneal staining (Fig. 4-29).[127] Often, a reaction occurs in individuals who have been previously exposed and sensitized to mercurial compounds (i.e., merthiolate, mercurochrome). Contact lens–induced superior limbic keratitis has been associated with soiled lenses and solution preservatives, particularly thimerosal. It is charac-

terized by redness, foreign-body sensation, and decreased visual acuity. Typical signs include superior bulbar injection, superior limbal epithelial irregularity, and pannus, with superior subepithelial corneal opacification and neovascularization. The superior cornea and conjunctiva typically show fluorescein and rose bengal staining (Fig. 4-30). Refitting with fresh lenses along with elimination of thimerosal in the care system is indicated once resolution occurs, typically in 7 to 21 days.

Chlorhexidine   Chlorhexidine digluconate has bactericidal properties. Although rarely a cause of allergic reactions in rigid lens solutions, chlorhexidine tends to bind strongly and reversibly to the backbone of many hydrogel polymers; notably, binding to lysozyme occurs over time and a delayed hypersensitivity reaction can result.[128]

Benzalkonium Chloride   BAK, used in many rigid lens solutions, although compatible with PMMA and fluorinated lens materials appears to bind to the surface of silicone-acrylate lenses to reach toxic concentrations.[129] Tear-film destabilization and a diffuse SPK form of staining can occur.

Polyaminopropyl Biguanide   Studies by Begley et al.[42,130] have demonstrated a high incidence of toxicity to the epithelium with the use of the preservative polyaminopropyl biguanide (PAPB) in rigid lens solutions (Fig. 4-31). Although PAPB is relatively nontoxic in soft lens solutions, under the trade name Dymed (Bausch & Lomb, Rochester, NY), it is present at a concentration of 30–50 times greater in rigid lens solutions.

When compared with solutions preserved with BAK and chlorhexidine, corneas exposed to PAPB demonstrate significantly more fluorescein staining. Any patient expe-

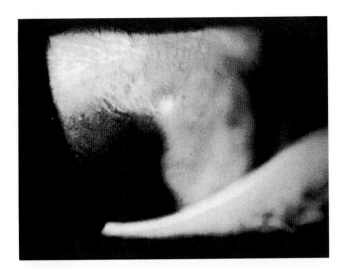

FIG. 4-30. *Contact lens–induced superior limbic keratitis.*

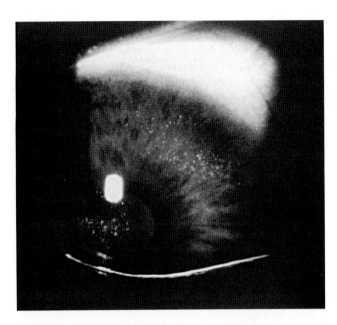

FIG. 4-31. *Corneal staining associated with a reaction to a rigid lens solution preserved with polyaminopropyl biguanide. (Courtesy of Dr. Joseph Vehige.)*

riencing itching, burning, and redness after application of a wetting solution should be provided with a care system that contains a different preservative, especially if this is confirmed by the presence of diffuse epithelial staining.

See Chapter 8 for an in-depth discussion of complications associated with solution toxicity and sensitivity.

Poor Patient Compliance

Poor patient compliance can result in chemical reactions similar to those described earlier (i.e., redness, burning, diffuse staining). Improper neutralization of hydrogen peroxide can result in a generalized epitheliopathy (Fig. 4-32). Chemical staining that may have been induced by accidental exposure of the cornea to a surfactant cleaner applied inappropriately to a rigid or soft lens can be very severe and painful.[117] This could be the result of either mistakenly using the cleaner as a wetting drop or improperly rinsing the cleaner off of the lens. In addition, the use of an inappropriate preservative with a given lens material (e.g., a BAK-preserved solution, which rapidly binds to hydrogel lenses) results in a similar reaction. The incidence of these problems can be minimized by a comprehensive four-step education process. This should include verbal instruction on care and handling, a supplemental written booklet, observation of a videotape on lens care, and (most important) reinforcement of care instructions by questioning the patient about lens care product use at all follow-up evaluations.

If the patient does not adequately clean the contact lenses, diffuse corneal staining can result because of debris accumulation on the back surface of the lens (Fig. 4-33).[117] The need for regular, thorough cleaning of the lens, sup-

plemented by weekly enzyme use, should be emphasized to these patients.

Physiologic Complications as a Source of Staining

Overwear Syndrome
Long-term wear of PMMA or low-Dk RGP lenses can result in what is termed *overwear syndrome* or *corneal*

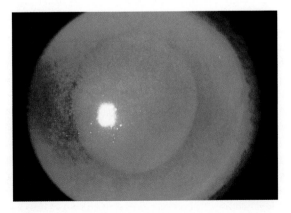

FIG. 4-32. *Epitheliopathy induced by improper neutralization of hydrogen peroxide. (Courtesy of Dr. Joseph Shovlin.)*

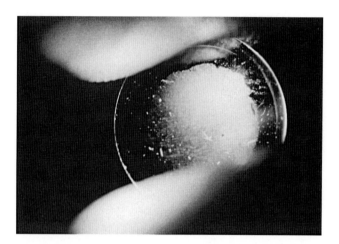

FIG. 4-33. *Inadequate cleaning of a rigid gas-permeable lens, resulting in deposits on the posterior surface.*

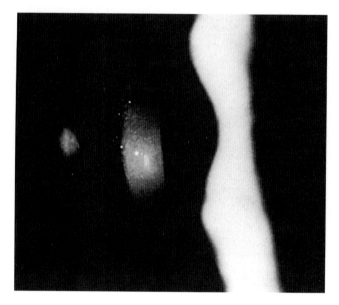

FIG. 4-34. *Central corneal abrasion resulting from overwear of a polymethylmethacrylate lens.*

warpage syndrome. Because these materials do not meet the cornea's oxygen demand for daily wear, a hypoxic condition is present. Therefore, the epithelium is prevented from reproducing at a rate necessary to match the sloughing off of dead cells.[131] Hypoxia is often manifested clinically by edema (present in 98% of PMMA wearers) and scattered epithelial erosion, which is sometimes termed *corneal stippling.*[132] Moderate-to-severe central corneal clouding or edema precedes the epithelial cell disruption and resultant staining. When this condition exists, the possibility of corneal abrasion is high if the patient wears the rigid lenses for longer than recommended by the practitioner. Typically, the patient either sleeps with the lenses on or, after replacement of a lost lens, increases wearing time at a greater rate than recommended. After lens removal, return of corneal sensitivity occurs in approximately 2 to 3 hours and the patient experiences extreme pain if overwear abrasion is present. In addition to acute ocular discomfort, symptoms include photophobia, tearing, reduced visual acuity, foreign-body sensation, and lens intolerance.[117] Using biomicroscopy, an epithelial abrasion is observed (Fig. 4-34).

In the absence of infection, management of this condition is primarily supportive. Patients should avoid sun and other sources of bright light. Lubricating drops or broad-spectrum antibiotic drops may be used every 4–6 hours. If severe photophobia is present, a bandage soft contact lens can be used. Antibiotic drops should be used four to six times per day until re-epithelialization occurs. Pressure patching should be avoided because it has been associated with subsequent corneal ulceration in the contact lens wearer.[133] Lens wear may resume 1–2 days after complete re-epithelialization or after symptoms cease. The wearing time should be increased gradually, begin-

ning with 4 hours the first day and increasing by 2 hours each day. The patient should continue to be monitored because chronic hypoxia can result in polymegethism and compromised endothelial function, resulting in greater risk of abrasion. Rather than resuming wear with the same material, the recommended management alternative for overwear syndrome case is refitting into a higher oxygen-permeable rigid lens material. A material with a Dk between 25 and 50 is recommended; this provides enough oxygen for successful daily wear but minimizes the incidence of warping- and dryness-related problems, which are common with PMMA wearers who are refitted into a superpermeable lens material.[63,134]

Rigid Lens Adherence
Rigid lens adherence to the cornea is a commonly observed complication of extended-wear lenses, seen in 40–50% of individuals immediately on awakening. Most adherent lenses, however, begin to move shortly after the eye opens and blinking commences. The cause of this adherence is believed to be thinning of the post-lens tear film as a result of eyelid pressure during sleep.[135] While the lens is adherent, tear circulation is absent behind the lens, allowing debris and contaminated mucus to remain trapped behind the lens. In addition, it is possible that a steep fitting relationship can cause adherence owing to the large tear volume between the lens and cornea.[136] Lens adherence can also occur with daily wear of RGP lenses owing to such factors as lens decentration (an adherent lens is almost always decentered, result-

---

CASE REPORT 3

A patient wakes up with extreme pain, and the practitioner on call is informed of the problem. Once in the office, the patient complains of pain, light sensitivity, and a foreign-body sensation in her left eye. She has worn Polycon I (Wesley-Jessen, Inc., Chicago, IL) lenses for 8 years, preceded by 15 years of PMMA wear. She has noticed that it is difficult to wear the lenses all day without experiencing some lens awareness in the evening. The previous night, she accidentally fell asleep for a few hours with the lenses on and then, realizing her mistake, removed the lenses immediately on awakening, returned to bed, and woke up in pain a few hours later. Her unaided visual acuity is OS $20/400$ (improves to $20/30$ with pinhole) and OD $20/100$ (improves to $20/30$ with pinhole). With slit-lamp examination, a dense epithelial abrasion is observed OS and diffuse stippling is observed OD.

This patient has experienced *overwear corneal abrasion* with excessive corneal edema, resulting from chronic hypoxia induced by a combination of PMMA and very low oxygen–permeable RGP lens wear. The presence of diffuse corneal staining in the right eye also indicates that eventually a similar complication may develop in that eye. The patient is instructed to rest indoors for the next 24 hours. Gentamicin drops are prescribed every 4–6 hours OU. She is told to discontinue contact lens wear until the abrasion has completely healed. Because she has no spectacle prescription, she is allowed to continue wearing her right contact lens. At the 24-hour visit, most of the re-epithelialization process has occurred, and only diffuse staining is present. She continues gentamicin solution four times daily, supplemented by ointment at bedtime until her next visit 3 days later. Her cornea is clear at the next visit, and she is provided with "loaner" RGP lenses to gradually build up wearing time until the refit visit 1 week later. All medications are discontinued, and she is refitted into Fluoroperm 30 (Paragon Vision Sciences, Mesa, AZ) lenses and allowed to gradually achieve all-day wear. To further illustrate to her the importance of wearing a higher oxygen-permeable lens material, she is shown photographs of such hypoxia-related complications as central corneal edema, epithelial abrasion, and corneal distortion.

ing in a large region of tear pooling adjacent to localized bearing), an unusual corneal topography (some patients are *binders*, in which practically every rigid lens adheres), an excessively steep fitting relationship, and a noncompliant patient who does not clean the lenses properly, resulting in trapped deposits forming a mucuslike glue.

In most cases, the patient is asymptomatic. The lenses show an absence of movement with biomicroscopy. On removal, an indentation ring is present where the lens edge indented the precorneal tear film (Fig. 4-35). In addi-

tion, an arcuate staining pattern is present slightly inward from the indentation ring, representing the region of trapped debris (Fig. 4-36).

Management of rigid lens adherence depends on the cause. A patient who uses extended-wear lenses may benefit by going to a daily-wear schedule. A daily-wear patient with mucoprotein deposits on the posterior surface should

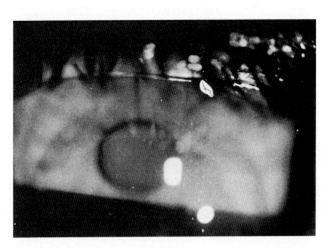

FIG. 4-35. *An indentation ring present after removal of a rigid gas-permeable lens.*

FIG. 4-36. *Diffuse corneal staining resulting from trapped debris under an adherent lens.*

benefit from re-education about proper and regular cleaning of the lenses. Lens parameter changes, such as flattening of the base curve radius, increasing center thickness, or flattening the peripheral curve (to allow more peripheral tear exchange), often solve the problem. In some cases, refitting into a hydrogel lens is indicated if the patient is a persistent binder.

Hydrogel Lens Adherence

Tight-fitting hydrogel lenses can cause various forms of corneal staining (i.e., epithelial splitting, desiccation). The so-called furrow staining is a variation of limbal epithelial hypertrophy in which the hydrogel lens is believed to act as a tight bandage, preventing normal sloughing of

the epithelium.[95,117] Furrow staining is a form of corneal staining, however, because it persists after irrigation. Scleral indentation staining can also be observed (Fig. 4-37).

Inferior desiccation staining may also result. Diffuse SPK may also be present with the extended-wear patient because hydrogel lenses may tighten during overnight wear, with lens adherence still occurring long after awakening, resulting in prolonged entrapment of contaminants between lens and cornea (Fig. 4-38).

The patient is typically asymptomatic unless the adherence is so great that, on forcibly removing the lens, the epithelium is damaged. In addition, an acute red-eye reaction or the so-called tight lens syndrome can occur. The patient is typically awakened by severe unilateral pain

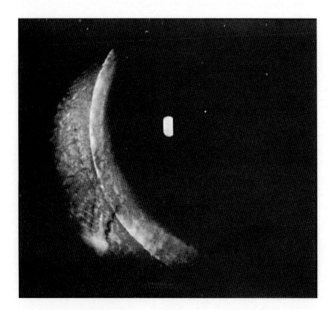

FIG. 4-37. *Indentation of the sclera associated with a tight-fitting hydrogel lens.*

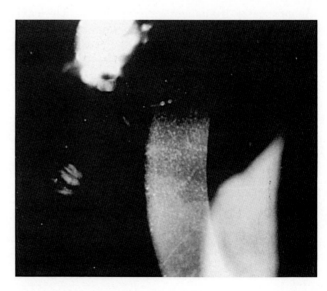

FIG. 4-38. *Superficial punctate keratitis in an aphakic patient using extended-wear lenses.*

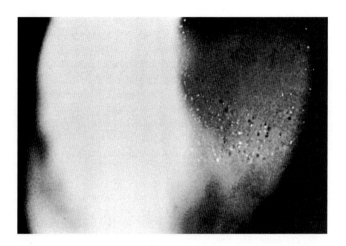

FIG. 4-39. *Superficial punctate keratitis associated with epithelial microcysts. (Reprinted with permission from SG Zantos: Cystic formations in the corneal epithelium during extended wear of contact lenses. Int Contact Lens Clin 10:128, 1983.)*

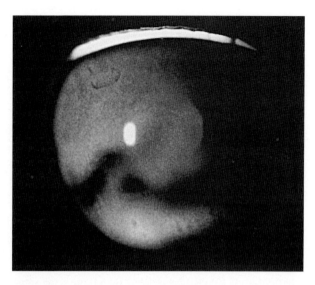

FIG. 4-40. *A region of negative staining associated with an epithelial basement membrane abnormality.*

with redness, tearing, and photophobia.[137] Conjunctival hyperemia, subepithelial infiltrates, and, on lens removal, epithelial staining corresponding to the pattern of trapped debris may be noted.

See Chapter 6 for an in-depth discussion of contact lens–induced acute red-eye syndrome and inflammatory tight lens complications.

Epithelial Microcysts

A long-term complication of extended wear most often reported with soft lenses is epithelial microcysts. They appear as translucent fine opacities that show reversed illumination with an indirect slit beam.[138,139] They are considered to result from hypoxia and represent abnormal cell debris that develops in the basal cell layer of the epithelium.[140] As these microcysts move to the surface during the desquamation process, SPK often results (Fig. 4-39).[138] The severity of microcysts and staining is reported to increase after discontinuation of overnight wear.[141] Patients often experience a foreign-body sensation once lenses are removed. It is a self-limited condition that resolves over 1–3 months after cessation of overnight wear.

Epithelial Basement Membrane Abnormalities

Any of the corneal diseases associated with epithelial basement membrane dystrophy may lead to interruption of the smooth ocular tear film. Reduplication of the basement membrane creates a localized area of elevated epithelium. This can be observed as *negative staining* after application of fluorescein. Distinct patterns of tear breakup

are observed in the affected areas (Fig. 4-40). These conditions are associated with recurrent erosions and true fluorescein staining. Patients typically experience a moderate-to-severe foreign-body sensation during the morning hours soon after awakening. The presence of significant basement membrane disease is a relative contraindication for rigid contact lens wear.

REFERENCES

1. Hogan MT, Alvarado JA, Weddell JE: Histology of the Human Eye. p. 55. Saunders, London, 1971
2. Norn MS: Vital staining of cornea and conjunctiva. Acta Ophthalmol Scand 50(suppl.):1, 1972
3. Norn MS: Vital staining of external eye of rabbit by fluorescein, rose bengal, tetrazolium and alcian blue. Acta Ophthalmol Scand 58:454, 1980
4. Norn MS: Side-effects of vital staining with tetrazolium-alcian blue. Acta Ophthalmol Scand 51:159, 1973
5. Norn MS: Lissamine green vital staining of cornea and conjunctiva. Acta Ophthalmol Scand 51:483, 1973
6. Norn MS: Flourexon vital staining of cornea and conjunctiva. Acta Ophthalmol Scand 51:670, 1973
7. Norn MS: Tetrazolium-alcian blue mixture vital staining of cornea and conjunctiva. Acta Ophthalmol Scand 50:277, 1972
8. Norn MS: Trypan blue vital staining of cornea and conjunctiva. Acta Ophthalmol Scand 45:380, 1967
9. Refojo MF, Korb DR, Silverman HI: Clinical evaluation of a new fluorescent dye for hydrogel lenses. J Am Optom Assoc 43:321, 1972

10. Mandell RB: Basic principles of hydrogel lenses. p. 517. In Mandell RB: Contact Lens Practice. Thomas, Springfield, IL, 1988

11. Lupelli L: A review of lacrimal function tests in relation to contact lens practice: Part II. Contact Lens J 16:3, 1988

12. Larke JR: Contact lens wear and the epithelium. p. 88. In Larke JR (ed): The Eye in Contact Lens Wear. Butterworths, London, 1985

13. Norn MS: Bromothymol blue. Acta Ophthalmol Scand 46:231, 1968

14. Lippincott JB: Ophthalmic drug facts. Facts & Comparison, Inc., St. Louis, 1989

15. Vaughan DG: The contamination of fluorescein solutions with special reference to *Pseudomonas aeruginosa*. Am J Ophthalmol 39:55, 1955

16. Maurice DM: The use of fluorescein in ophthalmic research. Invest Ophthalmol Vis Sci 6:464, 1967

17. Rollefson GK, Dodgen HW: The dependence of intensity of fluorescence on the composition of a fluorescing solution. J Chem Phys 12:107, 1944

18. Langham M, Wyber KC: Fluorophotometric apparatus for the objective determination of fluorescence in the anterior chamber of the living eye. Br J Ophthalmol 38:52, 1954

19. Romanchuk KO: Fluorescein: Physico-chemical factors affecting its fluorescence. Surv Ophthalmol 26:269, 1982

20. Poster M: An important new development. Int Cont Lens Clin 4:41, 1977

21. Courtney RC, Lee JM: Predicting ocular intolerance of a contact lens solution by use of a filter system enhancing fluorescein staining detection. Int Cont Lens Clin 9:302, 1982

22. Cox I, Fonn D: Interference filters to eliminate the surface reflex and improve contrast during fluorescein photography. Int Cont Lens Clin 18:178, 1991

23. Rozwadowski M: Effect of pH on the fluorescence of fluorescein solutions. Acta Physiol Pol 20:1005, 1961

24. Norn MS: Micropunctate fluorescein vital staining of the cornea. Acta Ophthalmol Scand 48:108, 1970

25. Feenstra RPG, Tseng SCG: Comparison of fluorescein and rose bengal staining. Ophthalmology 99:605, 1992

26. Wilson G, Ren H, Laurent J: Corneal epithelial fluorescein staining. J Am Optom Assoc 66:435, 1995

27. Brungardt TF: Fluorescein patterns: they are accurate and they can be mastered. J Am Optom Assoc 32:73, 1961

28. Davis LJ, Bennett ES: Observation of the base curve fitting relationship with UV absorbing rigid contact lenses. Contact Lens Spectrum 4:49, 1989

29. Holly FJ, Lamberts DW: Adsorption of high molecular weight fluorescein by polymacon hydrogel contact lenses. Contact Intraoc Lens Med J 5:160, 1979

30. Mosse P, Scott V: What use is large molecular fluorescein in soft contact lens fitting? Optician 171(suppl.):15, 1976

31. Hickey TE, Beck GL, Botta JA. Optimum fluorescein staining time in ocular irritation studies. Toxicol Appl Pharmacol 26:571, 1973

32. Korb DR, Herman JP: Corneal staining subsequent to sequential fluorescein instillations. J Am Optom Assoc 50:316, 1979

33. Kame RT, Hayashida JR: Lens evaluation procedures and problem solving. In: Bennett ES, Weissman BA (eds): Clinical Contact Lens Practice. Lippincott, London, 1991

34. Korb DR, Herman JP: Corneal staining subsequent to sequential fluorescein instillations. J Am Optom Assoc 50:361, 1979

35. Caffery BE, Josephson JE: Corneal staining after sequential instillations of fluorescein over 30 days. Optom Vis Sci 68:467, 1991

36. Josephson JE, Caffery BE: Corneal staining characteristics after sequential instillations of fluorescein. Optom Vis Sci 69:570, 1992

37. Thomas ML, Szeto VR, Gan CM, Polse KA: Sequential staining: the effects of sodium fluorescein, osmolarity, and pH on human corneal epithelium. Optom Vis Sci 74:207, 1997

38. Norn MS: Rose bengal vital staining: staining of cornea and conjunctiva by 10% rose bengal compared with 1%. Acta Ophthalmol Scand 48:546, 1970

39. Snyder C, Paugh JR: Rose bengal dye concentration and volume delivered via dye-impregnated paper strips. Optom Vis Sci 75:339, 1998

40. Roat MI, Romanowski E, Araullo-Cruz T, Gordon J: The antiviral effects of rose bengal and fluorescein. Arch Ophthalmol 105:415, 1987

41. Larke JR: Contact lens wear and the epithelium. p. 92. In Larke JR (ed): The Eye in Contact Lens Wear. Butterworth, London, 1985

42. Begley CG, Weirich B, Benak J, Pence NA: Effects of rigid gas permeable contact lens solutions on the human corneal epithelium. Optom Vis Sci 69:347, 1992

43. Begley CG, Barr JT, Edrington TB, et al: Characteristics of corneal staining in hydrogel contact lens wearers. Optom Vis Sci 73:193, 1996

44. Guillon JP, Guillon M, Malgouyres S: Corneal desiccation staining with hydrogel lenses: tear film and contact lens factors. Ophthalmic Physiol Opt 10:343, 1990

45. Bennett ES, Morgan BW, Henry VA, Stulc S: The incidence of corneal staining in hydrogel lens wearers. (in press)

46. DeDonato LM, Barresi BJ: Cornea. p. 331. In Barresi BJ (ed): Ocular Assessment. Butterworth, Boston, 1984

47. Lemp MA, Holly FJ: Recent advances in ocular surface chemistry. Am J Optom Arch Am Acad Optom 49:669, 1970

48. Jones BR: The differential diagnosis of punctate keratitis. Trans Ophthalmol Soc UK 80:665, 1960

49. Pfister RR, Burstein N: The effects of ophthalmic drugs, vehicles, and preservatives on corneal epithelium. Invest Ophthalmol 15:246, 1976

50. Coster DJ: Superficial keratitis. In Duane TD (ed): Clinical Ophthalmology. Harper & Row, Philadelphia, 1981

51. Jawetz E, Thygeson P, Hanna L, et al: The etiology of epidemic keratoconjunctivitis. Am J Ophthalmol 43:79, 1957

52. Stenson S: Adult inclusion conjunctivitis. Arch Ophthalmol 99:605, 1981

53. Mertz G, Holden B: Clinical implications of extended wear research. Can J Optom 43:201, 1981

54. Mondino J, Groden LR: Conjunctival hyperemia and corneal infiltrates with chemically disinfected soft lenses. Arch Ophthalmol 26:337, 1982

55. Bonanno JA, Polse KA: Central and peripheral corneal swelling accompanying soft lens extended wear. Am J Optom Physiol Opt 62:74, 1985

56. Orsborn GN, Zantos SG: Corneal desiccation staining with thin high water content contact lenses. CLAO J 14:81, 1988

57. Little SA, Bruce AS: Role of the post-lens tear film in the mechanism of inferior arcuate staining with ultrathin hydrogel lenses. CLAO J 21:175, 1995

58. Cederstaff TH, Tomlinson A: A comparison study of tear evaporation rates and water content of soft contact lenses. Am J Optom Physiol Opt 60:167, 1983

59. Zantos S, Orsborn G, Walter M: Studies on corneal staining with thin hydrogel contact lenses. J Br Contact Lens Assoc 9:61, 1986

60. Andrasko C, Schoessler JP: The effect of humidity on the dehydration of soft contact lenses on the eye. Int Contact Lens Clin 7:21, 1980

61. Fatt I, Chaston J: The effect of temperature on refractive index, water content, and central thickness of hydrogel contact lenses. Int Contact Lens Clin 7:250, 1980

62. Mirejovsky D, Patel AS, Young G: Water properties of hydrogel contact lens materials: a possible predictive model for corneal desiccation staining. Biomaterials 14:1080, 1993

63. Grohe RM, Caroline PJ: Surface deposits on contact lenses. p. 1. In Bennett ES, Weissman BA (eds): Clinical Contact Lens Practice. Lippincott, Philadelphia, 1991

64. Petit TH, Meyer KT: The differential diagnosis of superficial punctate keratitis. Int Ophthalmol Clin 24:79, 1984

65. Norn MS: Vital staining of the cornea and conjunctiva. Acta Ophthalmol Scand 40:389, 1962

66. Businger U, Treiber A, Flury C: The etiology and management of three and nine o'clock staining. Int Contact Lens Clin 16:136, 1989

67. Henry VA, Bennett ES, Forrest JF: Clinical investigation of the Paraperm EW rigid gas-permeable contact lens. Am J Optom Physiol Opt 64:313, 1987

68. Henry VA, Bennett ES, Forrest JF: Clinical investigation of Paraperm EW rigid gas-permeable contact lens. Am J Optom Physiol Opt 64:313, 1987

69. Andrasko G: Peripheral corneal staining: incidence and time course. Contact Lens Spectrum 5:59, 1990

70. Lebow KA: Three and nine o'clock staining. Contact Lens Update 8:1, 1989

71. Schnider CM: Rigid gas permeable extended wear. Contact Lens Spectrum 5:101, 1990

72. Jenkins MS, Brown SI, Lempert SL, et al: Ocular rosacea. Am J Ophthalmol 88:618, 1979

73. Waring GO: Acne rosacea. Dermatological disorders. p. 147. In Fraunfelder FT, Roy FH (eds): Current Ocular Therapy. Saunders, Philadelphia, 1980

74. Jones DH, Bennett ES, Davis LJ: How to manage peripheral corneal desiccation. Contact Lens Spectrum 4:63, 1989

75. Holly FJ: Tear film physiology and contact lens wear: I. Pertinent aspects of tear film physiology. Am J Optom Physiol Opt 58:324, 1981

76. Holly FJ: Tear film physiology and contact lens wear: II. Contact lens–tear interaction. Am J Optom Physiol Opt 58:331, 1981

77. Schnider CM, Bennett ES, Grohe RM: Rigid extended wear. p. 10. In Bennett ES, Weissman BA (eds): Clinical Contact Lens Practice. Lippincott, London, 1991

78. Jones DH, Bennett ES, Davis LJ: How to manage peripheral corneal desiccation. Contact Lens Spectrum 4:63, 1989

79. Finnemore V: Common factors in contact lens failure. Am J Optom Arch Am Acad Optom 50:50, 1973

80. Bell GR: A new theory on 3 and 9 o'clock staining. Contact Lens Spectrum 12:44, 1997

81. Friend J, Kiorpes T, Thoft RA: Conjunctival goblet cell frequency after alkali injury is not accurately reflected by aqueous tear mucin content. Invest Ophthalmol Vis Sci 24:612, 1983

82. Adams AD: The morphology of human mucus. Arch Ophthalmol 97:730, 1979

83. Farris RL: Contact lens wear in the management of the dry eye. Int Ophthalmol Clin 27:54, 1987

84. Buch JR, Fogt N, Barr JT: Peripheral corneal staining and scarring with rigid gas permeable contact lenses: a case report. Int Contact Lens Clin 23:183, 1996

85. Schnider CM, Terry RL, Holden BA: Effect of lens design on peripheral corneal desiccation. J Am Optom Assoc 68:163, 1997

86. Spinell MR: Staining. p. 165. In: A Clinical Guide to Soft Contact Lenses. Chilton, Radnor, PA, 1979

87. Terry R, Schnider C, Holden BA: Maximizing success with rigid gas permeable extended wear lenses. Int Contact Lens Clin 16:169, 1989

88. Fonn D, Holden BA: Rigid gas permeable vs. hydrogel contact lenses for extended wear. Am J Optom Physiol Opt 65:168, 1988

89. Feldman GL: Hydrocurve soft contact lens wear. In Harstein J (ed): Extended Wear Contact Lenses for Aphakia and Myopia. Mosby, St Louis, 1982

90. Mandell RB: Anatomy and physiology of the cornea. p. 67. In: Contact Lens Practice. 4th ed. Thomas, Springfield, IL, 1988

91. Andrasko G, Schoessler JP: The effect of humidity on the dehydration of soft contact lenses on the eye. Int Contact Lens Clin 7:210, 1980

92. Lebow KA, Plishka K: Ocular changes associated with extended-wear contact lenses. Int Contact Lens Clin 7:11, 1980

93. Zantos SG, Holden BA: Ocular changes associated with continuous wear of contact lenses. Aust J Optom 61:418, 1978

94. Bonanno JA, Polse KA: Hypoxic changes in the corneal epithelium and stroma. p. 27. In Tomlinson A (ed): Com-

plications of Contact Lens Wear. Mosby–Year Book, St Louis, 1992

95. Chahine T, Weissman BA: Peripheral corneal furrow staining: a sign to discontinue hydrogel contact lens use? Int Contact Lens Clin 23:229, 1996

96. Bourassa S, Benjamin WJ: Transient corneal surface "microdeposits" and associated epithelial surface pits occurring with gel contact lens extended wear. Int Contact Lens Clin 15:338, 1988

97. Lakkis C, Brennan NA: Bulbar conjunctival fluorescein staining in hydrogel contact lens wearers. CLAO J 22:189, 1996

98. Grohe RM, Lebow KA: Vascularized limbal keratitis. Int Contact Lens Clin 16:197, 1989

99. Mondino BJ: Experimental aspects and models of peripheral corneal disease. Int Ophthalmol Clin 26:4, 1986

100. Silberberg-Sinakin I, Baer RL, Thorbecke GJ: Langerhans cells: a review of their nature with emphasis on their immunological function. Prog Allerg 24:268, 1978

101. Gillette TE, Chandler JW, Greiner JV: Langerhans cells of the ocular surface. Ophthalmology 89:700, 1982

102. Mondino BJ, Brady KJ: Distribution of hemolytic complement activity in the normal cornea. Arch Ophthalmol 99:1430, 1981

103. Allansmith MR, McCellan BH: Immunoglobulins in the human cornea. Am J Ophthalmol 80:123, 1975

104. Mondino BJ: Inflammatory diseases of the peripheral cornea. Ophthalmology 95:4, 1988

105. Efron N: Review: Is contact lens-induced corneal oedema inflammatory? Aust J Optom 68:167, 1985

106. Lavker RM, Cotsarelis G, Dong G, et al: Limbal location of corneal epithelial stem cells. In Cavanagh HD (ed): The Cornea: Transactions of the World Congress on the Cornea III. Raven, New York, 1988

107. Chen JJY, Tseng SCG: Corneal epithelial wound healing in partial limbal deficiency. Presented at the Annual Meeting of the Association for Research in Vision and Ophthalmology, Sarasota, FL, April 1989

108. Lemp MA: General measures in management of the dry eye. Int Ophthalmol Clin 27:36, 1987

109. Kinoshita S, Friend J, Throft RA: Ocular surface epithelial regeneration and disease. Int Ophthalmol Clin 24:169, 1984

110. Throft RA: The role of the limbus in ocular surface maintenance and repair. Acta Ophthalmol Scand 67(suppl. 192):91, 1989

111. Tseng SCG: Topical tretinoin treatment for dry-eye disorders. Int Ophthalmol Clin 27:47, 1987

112. Doughty MJ: The pathophysiology of dry eye. Practical Optom 2:28, 1991

113. Stewart CE: Blinking and corneal lenses. Am J Optom Arch Am Acad Optom 61:418, 1966

114. Wilson SE, Lin DTC, Klyce SD, et al: Topographic changes in contact lens-induced corneal warpage. Ophthalmology 97:734, 1990

115. Rohler S, Bennett ES, Davis LJ, et al: The short-term effect of RGP parameter changes on corneal topography. (in press)

116. Hill RM, Brezinski SD: The center thickness factor. Contact Lens Spectrum 2:52, 1987

117. Mandell RB: Hydrogel lenses: symptomatology and aftercare. p. 620. In Mandell RB (ed): Contact Lens Practice. 4th Ed. Thomas, Springfield, IL, 1988

118. Dougal J: Abrasions secondary to contact lens wear. p. 123. In Tomlinson A (ed): Complications of Contact Lens Wear. Mosby–Year Book, St. Louis, 1992

119. Zadnik K, Mutti DO: Inferior arcuate corneal staining in soft contact lens wearers. Int Contact Lens Clin 12:110, 1985

120. Dittoe RJ: Corneal smile staining. Contact Lens Spectrum 3:49, 1988

121. Watanabe K, Hamano H: The typical pattern of superficial punctate keratopathy in wearers of extended wear disposable contact lenses. CLAO J 23:134, 1997

122. McMonnies CW: After-care symptoms, signs and management. p. 714. In Phillips AJ, Stone J (eds): Contact Lenses. 3rd ed. Butterworth, London, 1989

123. Josephson JE: A corneal irritation uniquely produced by hydrogel lathed lenses and its resolution. J Am Optom Assoc 49:869, 1978

124. Schnider CM. Keratitis. p. 105. In Tomlinson A (ed): Complications of Contact Lens Wear. Mosby–Year Book, St. Louis, 1992

125. Gasson A: Soft (hydrogel) lens fitting. p. 382. In Phillips AJ, Stone J (eds): Contact lenses. 3rd ed. Butterworth, London, 1989

126. Cai F, Backman H, Baines M: Thimerosal: an ophthalmic preservative which acts as a hapten to elicit specific antibodies and cell mediated immunity. Curr Eye Res 7:341, 1988

127. Larke J: Preserved soft lens storage solutions. p. 170. In Larke J (ed): The eye in contact lens wear. Butterworth, London, 1985

128. Refojo MF: Reversible binding of chlorhexidine gluconate to hydrogel contact lenses. Contact Intraocular Lens Med J 2:47, 1976

129. Sterling JL, Hecht AS: BAK-induced chemical keratitis. Contact Lens Spectrum 3:62, 1988

130. Begley CG, Waggoner PJ, Hafner GS, et al: Effect of rigid gas permeable contact lens wetting solutions on the rabbit corneal epithelium. Optom Vis Sci 68:189, 1991

131. Bergmanson JPG: Corneal epithelial mitosis. Contacto 25:19, 1981

132. Finnemore VM, Korb JE: Corneal edema with polymethylmethacrylate versus gas-permeable rigid polymer contact lenses of identical design. J Am Optom Assoc 51:271, 1980

133. Bergmanson JPG: Contact-lens-induced epithelial pathology. p. 1. In Bennett ES, Weissman BA (eds): Clinical contact lens practice. Lippincott, Philadelphia, 1991

134. Bennett ES, Tomlinson A, Mirowitz MC, et al: A comparison of overnight swelling and lens performance in RGP extended wear. CLAO J 14:94, 1988

135. Swarbrick HA, Holden BA: Rigid gas-permeable lens adherence: a patient-dependent phenomenon. Optom Vis Sci 66:269, 1989

136. Bennett ES, Grohe RM: How to solve stuck lens syndrome. Rev Optom 124:51, 1987

137. Holden BA, Swarbrick HA: Extended wear: physiologic considerations. p. 1. In Bennett ES, Weissman BA (eds): Clinical Contact Lens Practice. Lippincott, Philadelphia, 1991

138. Zantos SG: Cystic formations in the corneal epithelium during extended wear of contact lenses. Int Contact Lens Clin 10:128, 1983

139. Zantos SG: Corneal infiltrates, debris, and microcysts. J Am Optom Assoc 55:196, 1984

140. Tripathi R, Bron A: Cystic disorders of the corneal epithelium II. Pathogenesis. Br J Ophthalmol 57:376, 1973

141. Holden BA, Sweeney D, Vannas A, et al: Effect of long term extended contact lens wear on the human cornea. Invest Ophthalmol Vis Sci 26:1489, 1985

5

Corneal Vascularization

Joshua E. Josephson and Barbara E. Caffery

GRAND ROUNDS CASE REPORT

Subjective:
A 24-year-old woman presented for routine checkup. Wears Cibasoft (CIBA Vision, Duluth, GA) hydrogel lenses (tefilcon, 37.5% water) 15 hours per day. Uses daily surfactant, biweekly enzyme cleaning, and a disinfection solution preserved with a quaternary ammonium compound and thimerosal. The patient has no visual symptoms but reports that her eyes have become redder in the past year.

Objective:
- Best corrected acuity with contact lenses: distance right eye (OD) $^{20}/_{20}$, left eye (OS) $^{20}/_{20}$; near (16 in) OD J-1+, OS J-1+.
- Lens centration, movement, and lag are excellent.
- Lens condition: slight hazy gray film over anterior lens surfaces.
- Biomicroscopy: After 6 hours of wear, no staining or corneal striae exists. However, vascularization of 0.7-mm penetration in inferior quadrants and 0.5-mm penetration in superior quadrants each eye (OU) (over baseline) is noted.
- Grade 2 bulbar conjunctival injection exists; lid eversion reveals a smooth tarsal mucosa without papillae, but with pronounced hyperemia (grade 4, CCLRU scale).

Assessment:
Protein deposits on aging lenses. Corneal vascularization OU secondary to prolonged use of chemical lens care system.

Plan:
1. Discard lenses and replace with fresh lens product. Replacement lenses recommended.
2. Reduce average daily wearing time to 12 hours per day until hyperemia recedes.
3. Switch to preservative-free hydrogen peroxide disinfection system, and avoid exposure to solutions containing thimerosal or quaternary ammonium compounds.
4. Perform clinical assessments every 3 months over next 12 months to monitor vascularization.

Corneal vascularization in contact lens wearers is a noteworthy event that requires careful management. It is a particularly common change in the cornea of contact lens wearers. The normal cornea is typically avascular except for a 1-mm area adjacent to the limbus, in which small superficial capillaries (marginal arcades) are found.[1] These arcades originate from the episcleral branches of the anterior ciliary artery. The growth of blood vessels into the cornea is a sequela of corneal insult from hypoxic, allergic, toxic, or immune causes.

CLINICAL IMPORTANCE OF CORNEAL VASCULARIZATION

Vascular penetration of the cornea as a complication of contact lens wear can serve as a warning sign of corneal distress. When observed in its earliest and mildest stage, it is typically associated with a subtle and often prolonged corneal or limbal insult. In its more advanced stages, if it penetrates the pupillary region, vascularization can be a sight-threatening complication, especially when associated with lipid deposits and fibrous opacification of the surrounding tissues. Furthermore, the presence of vessels extending into the cornea that are associated with the healing process of a focal site of inflammation puts the cornea at risk. This is true because lymphatic changes that accompany vascularization make that area a more reactive site, which may be irritated by the normal biochemical events in the cornea.[2] For example, microbial corneal ulcers associated with contact lens wear often result in corneal vascularization.[3] After the ulcer resolves from the progressive stage to the healing stage, blood vessels begin to form. Vessels grow toward the ulcer. When the healing is completed, the vessels usually empty of red blood cells and constrict. They remain as ghost vessels unless further insult occurs.

Corneal neovascularization may be a serious complication for patients who require a future penetrating keratoplasty because there may be a significant risk of failure from allograft rejection.[4] Corneal vascularization secondary to contact lens wear may, in the extreme, require a corneal graft.[5]

PREVALENCE OF CORNEAL VASCULARIZATION AND NEOVASCULARIZATION

One of the great difficulties in interpreting the statistical prevalence of corneal vascularization in contact lens wear relates to vague and inconsistent standards for description and definition of vascularization. In general, the most complete record of the prevalence of vascularization is associated with extended-wear contact lenses. The prevalence of vascularization associated with daily wear has been only sparsely documented.

The prevalence of corneal vascularization reported among wearers of daily-wear rigid lens is extremely low. Dixon[6] observed only one case of neovascularization in a consecutive series of 3,000 patients (0.03%). Studies of extended-wear rigid lenses after 12 months of use have made no mention of abnormal corneal vascularization.[7,8] The limbal vascular response of cosmetic daily wearers of rigid contact lenses was compared with that of nonwearers and was found to be indistinguishable from that of nonwearers.[9] However, corneal vascularization associated with rigid lens wear has been associated with prolonged epithelial breakdown in the limbal region, manifested by such conditions as dellen[6,10-13] and chronic corneal epithelial desiccation associated with 3 to 9 o'clock staining.[14] When this peripheral desiccation (sometimes also associated with bulbar conjunctival desiccation) is sustained over a long period, corneal vascularization is possible in the affected area.[10,15-20]

The reported incidence of neovascularization in hydrogel lens wearers ranges from 0.2 to 33.9%.[21-34] The reported incidence of corneal vascularization in patients fitted with therapeutic hydrogel lenses also varies significantly, from 2.88% to 35%.[35,36]

In a retrospective study of 246 consecutive hydrogel contact lens–wearing patients fitted with daily- and extended-wear contact lenses, corneal vascularization was the most common aftercare problem encountered (Fig. 5-1). This patient group, however, consisted of private outpatients observed at a hospital cornea service and did not represent the larger population of primarily cosmetic wearers of rigid and hydrogel lenses. Twenty-nine percent of cases seen presented with corneal vascularization; 47% of these patients were wearing extended-wear contact lenses and 16% were wearing daily-wear lenses. Only 10% of the cases presented with vascularization greater than 1 mm of penetration; 39 patients presented with less than 1 mm of vascularization. Significantly, 21 of those 39 patients had aphakia, and nine were aphakic graft patients. Furthermore, of this same patient group, 77% used extended-wear contact lenses. According to the study, aphakic patients who wore lenses on an extended-wear basis developed neovascularization four times more often than did daily-wear lens users with aphakia.[37]

A more interesting and practical investigation for the clinician was the result of a retrospective analysis of two patient groups.[34] One group consisted of 827 soft contact lens wearers. The second group consisted of 900 nonwearers.

Both groups were examined for corneal vascularization by biomicroscopy. The prevalence of corneal vascularization in the soft lens group was 33.9% compared with 2% in the nonwearer group. In the soft contact lens group, 98.6% of the vascularization was located in the superficial stroma. Vascular penetration into the cornea did not exceed 4.5 mm in either the contact lens or nonwearer group. There was no significant correlation between age and gender. The total daily wearing time and the total length of time for which contact lenses had been worn were significantly related to the observed frequency of corneal vascularization in the contact lens–wearing group. In the contact lens–wearing group, 96.8% of the vascular responses did not exceed 1.5 mm. The incidence of corneal vascularization was significantly greater in contact lens–wearing patients with refractive errors in excess of –4.00 diopter (D). Contact lens wearers who wore their lenses in excess of 12 hours per day but who did not sleep in their lenses had a higher prevalence of corneal vascularization than did those who wore their extended-wear soft contact lenses on an extended-wear basis. Corneal vascularization increased over the first 3 years of soft contact lens wear, at which time the prevalence remained constant.[34]

TERMINOLOGY

The terms *vascularization* and *neovascularization* have acquired ambiguity from their use by some authors who seem to use the two terms to describe the same phenomenon.

- *Vascularization* is the formation and extension of vascular capillaries within and into any avascular cornea.[38–40]
- *Neovascularization* is the formation of new vascular capillaries from pre-existing capillaries and their extension into a previously vascularized cornea.[38,39] The vascular response at this stage is essentially irreversible (even if the stimulus is removed, ghost vessels remain).[40,41]
- *Limbal hyperemia* (limbal injection, limbal engorgement, vascular engorgement) can be defined as increased blood flow into the limbal arcades resulting in distention of the limbal blood vessels.[38,40]
- *Vessel penetration* is the apparent ingrowth of vessels, typically toward the corneal apex, measured from an arbitrary reference point at the corneal scleral junction.[38]
- *Vasoproliferation* is an increase in the number of vessels[38,39] with a corresponding degree of fibrous response.[40]

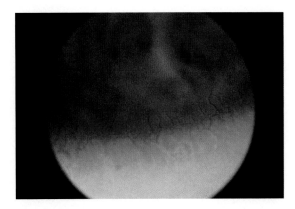

FIG. 5-1. *Corneal vascularization secondary to hydrogel lens extended wear.*

- *Fibrovascular pannus* is the specific clinical presentation of vascularization and connective tissue deposition beneath the epithelium.[38,40]

Pannus is typically found in the superior or inferior limbal region. The term *micropannus* is used when the extent of vessel penetration is less than 2 mm from the limbus.[42] Pannus is infrequently seen in contact lens wearers, but when present, it is typically associated with superior limbic keratoconjunctivitis.[43] A very narrow form of micropannus is also rarely observed in rigid lens wearers.[20] The term *pannus* associated with contact lens wear was used in a single reference, where it was not defined by the authors. The term may have been misused because the vascularization that the authors described was superficial and the authors did not describe any fibrovascular changes, merely vascular ones in the context of blood column regression.[44] Furthermore, the papers that the authors cited in association with their references to pannus did not use that terminology to describe the superficial vascularization.

A careful review of the literature indicates that clinicians and authors using the term *vascular regression* typically refer to the loss of the blood column in the capillaries observed in the cornea with vascularization or neovascularization.[44,45] The emptied vessel is referred to as a *ghost vessel*. Ghost vessels are often observed when the conditions that caused vascularization are no longer present.

STAGES OF CONTACT LENS–INDUCED VASCULAR CHANGE

Stages[40] of contact lens–induced vascular change include the following:

- Stage 1, limbal hyperemia
- Stage 2, vascularization
- Stage 3, neovascularization
- Stage 4, vasoproliferation

CLINICAL PRESENTATION OF NEOVASCULARIZATION

In its earliest phase, corneal vascularization is characterized by engorgement of the limbal plexus followed by the development of sprouts, spikes, or bulbs projecting from the normal limbal arcades. Newly formed vessels then invade the cornea.[46] The vascular invasion may be localized or extended around the limbus.

Vascular invasion may occur at various depths, usually invading at the level of the pathologic process. Thus, the depth at which the vessel appears is a clinically observed clue to the insult involved. Vascularization is observed as superficial, interstitial, or deep.

Superficial Vascularization

Superficial vascularization is the most common type seen as a complication of contact lens wear.[1,47] The initial invasion of superficial vessels derives from the small capillaries (marginal arcades) in the limbal region and originates from the episcleral branches of the anterior ciliary artery. The vessels may have a relatively straight, sharp loop at the digital end. The arterial and venous portions may lie close together, giving the appearance of a single vessel when viewed under low magnification.[48]

Stromal (Interstitial and Deep) Vascularization

Contact lenses have been known to produce vascularization at all levels of the stroma.[47] Vessels emerge sharply from the limbus, typically in the midstroma, and appear to be rather straight with virtually no branching if they do not penetrate more than 1.5 mm past the limbal transition zone. With increased penetration, small buds or small vessel anastomoses may be observed. The increased branching as the stromal vessel penetrates deeper into the cornea is thought to result from a loss of compactness of the more central corneal tissues.[48] Stromal corneal vascularization secondary to contact lens wear has been reported in cosmetic contact lens wearers, but it is typically a benign peripheral disease not associated with significant loss of visual acuity.[49–51] However, occasional reports exist of deep corneal vascularization associated

with lipid deposition and marked central scarring, resulting in decreased vision.[52] Therefore, deep stromal vessels are potentially more serious.[1,9] Deep vascularization is rarely seen except as an end result of interstitial keratitis, usually of syphilitic origin.[50,52]

Differentiation between Stromal Vessels and Superficial Vessels

Superficial vascularization can be differentiated from deep vascularization. Typically, superficial vessels are more tortuous, irregular, and arborescent than deep vessels.[53] Deep vessels end abruptly at the limbal region, whereas superficial vessels are seen to be continuous with the small capillaries or limbal arcades. On occasion, a midstromal vessel appears to enter the cornea with a nerve fiber. This finding may not have a pathologic origin, although such vessels may fill with blood in response to various forms of irritation. Blood vessels located deeper in the cornea tend to be darker and much straighter than superficial vessels.

METHODS OF EXAMINATION

The optimal method for observing filled or partially filled vessels in the cornea is initial use of moderately high magnification and direct focal illumination, followed by high-intensity indirect or marginal retroillumination. Ghost vessels are best observed with the biomicroscope by indirect retroillumination. A green (red-free) filter aids in increasing the visibility of the blood-filled vessels. They can be differentiated from nerve fibers by their apparent transparency when viewed by indirect illumination, whereas nerve fibers look more opaque.

METHODS OF DOCUMENTATION

The best practical method for accurate documentation of the degree of vessel penetration is the use of a calibrated eyepiece reticule for the slit lamp.[9] Alternative methods include photographic or videotaped documentation, which may allow for better precision from visit to visit. Stevenson and Chawla,[40] adapting the method of Meyer,[54] recommend using a COHU 4712 CCD (Cohn, Inc., San Diego, CA) video camera, which achieves a peak light sensitivity at 520 nm. This system should be adapted to a slit lamp with a halogen light source filtered by a 500- to 580-nm pass interference band filter (Schott Glas, Mainz, Germany). Stevenson and Chawla reported that this method allows close examination of the configuration of the limbal vessels, particularly the arrangement of loops and the flow of blood in vessels. In vivo measurement of corneal angiogenesis has also been recorded by video image capture and processed by computerized image analysis.[55] This method of recording and analysis is faster and perhaps more precise than other sources.

The normal limbus is an area rather than a point.[56] Vascularization should be measured from a point at which the translucent region of the conjunctiva and subconjunctival tissue ends and clear (translucent) cornea begins. The point at which the measurement begins is called the *transition zone*. The limbal transition zone may vary in appearance. In some individuals, no translucent region exists and the clear cornea extends right to the opaque sclera.[9] Vessel penetration past the limit of the visible iris of more than 1 mm can be a useful criterion for identifying the condition as corneal vascularization.[39,57]

Because of the variations within the transition zone, it is critical that the area of new vessel growth be considered only from the beginning of the clear zone.[39] The ability to distinguish the transition zone somewhat depends on the degree of pigmentation of the corneal region in heavily pigmented individuals or by the loss of peripheral corneal transparency seen in some individuals. At the superior limbus, a zone of vascularized transitional conjunctiva and subconjunctival tissue is often present. This tissue covers the transparent corneal stroma and has been described as a *conjunctival wedge*.[53] The overlying conjunctival tissue is translucent rather than transparent because the conjunctival epithelium is thicker and less regular than the transparent corneal epithelium. The variable width of the translucent region of overlying conjunctival tissue corresponds to variation in location of the limit of Bowman's membrane, from which full corneal transparency is established. This feature may vary 0–2.5 mm from the limit of opaque sclera or visible iris.[58]

Vessels should be documented by the following:

1. *Location*: Vessels can be located at the limbus by considering the limbus part of an arc of a circle or, alternatively, by considering the limbus as a clock and the vessel location by positions of the clock. One can also describe their position by quadrant (e.g., inferotemporal, inferonasal, superotemporal, or superonasal).
2. *Depth*
   a. Superficial vessels can be seen to be continuous with the conjunctival vessels. Superficial vessels are tortuous and irregular.
   b. Deep stromal vessels appear straight and can be seen emerging from the sclera into the transparent stroma.

TABLE 5-1. *Grading Scale for Contact Lens–Induced Corneal Vascularization*

Grade*	Description
1	Vessels that penetrate into the cornea past the limbal transition zone that do not exceed: 0.4 mm with daily-wear rigid lenses 0.6 mm with daily-wear hydrogel lenses 1.4 mm with extended-wear hydrogel lenses
2	Vessel penetration into the cornea exceeding grade 1 and extending as far as (not entering) the pupil area (as judged with the consulting room lights on)
3	Vessel penetration into the pupillary area (as judged with the consulting room lights on)

*The severity grade number should be followed by the suffix *S* if the vascularization is superficial or the suffix *D* if the vascularization is deep (stromal).
Source: Adapted from N Efron: Vascular response of the cornea to contact lens wear. J Am Optom Assoc 58:841, 1987.

3. *Degree of penetration* into the cornea is best measured by the use of a calibrated slit-lamp reticule eyepiece and can be recorded by video or slit-lamp photomicroscopy.
4. *Severity* is assessed by how much the vessel penetrates toward the central cornea and by vessel depth. The greater the depth of the vessels or the greater the penetration toward the corneal apex (or both), the more severe the condition of vascularization.

Efron[38] has developed a grading scale for contact lens–induced corneal vascularization. Table 5-1 presents a summary of Efron's grading system.

CLINICAL APPROACH TO MANAGEMENT OF VASCULARIZATION

One must recognize the early and subtle signs of vascularization and neovascularization and make prompt changes that lead to remission. A careful preliminary examination of the limbal region of the prospective contact lens patient should be completed so that vascularization observed after contact lens fitting is not incorrectly attributed to contact lens–induced changes. Particular care must be given to the detection of ghost vessels because they may refill during contact lens wear. The etiology of ghost vessels in the cornea must be elucidated by careful review of the patient's health history and history of contact lens wear, and managed by either careful monitoring or intervention. Ghost vessels have been known to

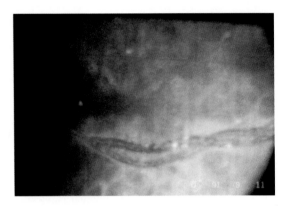

FIG. 5-2. *The spike phase of new vessel growth at the terminal end of the vessel (far left). Photographed by confocal scanning slit microscopy. (Courtesy of Dr. James D. Auren, New York, NY.)*

regress in animals.[2,59–61] However, long-standing ghost vessels have been observed in rabbit corneas.[10] McMonnies et al.[9] proposed that regression of blood vessels may or may not occur, depending on some critical point in vessel formation. If the critical point is passed, the fully established vessel regresses and remains as a ghost vessel; only the blood column regresses. If the critical point in the development is not reached, however, the relatively mature vessels may become obliterated.[39]

All follow-up examinations of contact lens–wearing patients should include a careful examination of the limbal vessels throughout the entire corneal circumference. Documentation by photography or diagrams can serve as a baseline for future comparisons.

Practitioners must be alert for signs of active growth or red blood cell filling of vessels, especially when the vessels are very near the acceptable limit of penetration. Signal observations are the maximal filling of the terminal capillaries and the presence of new vessel spikes surrounded by exudate[39] (Fig. 5-2). At the vessel penetration limit, if blood vessel growth appears active, discontinuation of all contact lens wear must be seriously considered. Chronic injection of the limbal capillaries should be regarded as an indication of reduced contact lens tolerance[48] or reduced tolerance to the solutions used in the care of contact lenses.[62]

If the limbal vasculature is engorged in a hydrogel lens wearer at the initial follow-up examination and the patient is using a preserved storage solution, the patient should change to an oxidation disinfection system (such as one that uses hydrogen peroxide) combined with a preservative-free sterile saline solution for the final stage of soaking.[9,62] If the hydrogel lens–wearing patient is already using a preservative-free system, refit the lens with a design

that increases movement during blinking or eye motion. Although it is now well known that blink-induced tear exchange is minimal, some slight exchange might be responsible for reducing the entrapment of metabolic by-products and cell debris over a day (or, in the case of extended wear, overnight). Lens motion can usually be increased by fitting lenses with a flatter base curve or by using a smaller diameter, or both.

Patients using extended-wear lenses should be refitted with a lens that transmits more oxygen. If blink-induced lens movement can be increased by changing the contact lens parameters without compromising lens fit or comfort, this may also help to remedy factors that may stimulate hyperemia or vessel growth. If the results are not satisfactory, the patient's wearing pattern must be changed from extended wear to daily wear.[48,63]

Patients who wear lenses on a daily-wear basis, who are already wearing an optimally fitted lens, and who are also using an optimal solution disinfection system should be refitted with a lens that transmits more oxygen.[63] If this approach is unsuccessful, the patients should wear their final optimal lens design and material combination with their wearing time reduced by at least 3 hours from their previous average daily wearing time.

In certain situations in which the contact lens wearer is using a preservative-free care system and is wearing a lens that is highly permeable to oxygen, the patient may present with neovascularization. In this situation, oxygen may not play a role in the vascularizing process, and one must suspect some mechanical element of low-level trauma.[64] Additionally, it is our impression that a hypothetical and possibly rare cause of vascularization may be the cumulative effect of chronic exposure of the hydrogel lens–wearing patient to toxic environmental vapors. Should the vapors be absorbed by the lens and gradually and continuously eluted onto the ocular surface under the lens, the toxic substance may stimulate vessel growth, indirectly or directly. If the environmental stimulus cannot be removed or if wearing contact lenses is preferred, refitting with rigid lenses should resolve this situation because rigid lenses do not absorb and elute chemical fumes.

If progressing vascularization in hydrogel lens wearers cannot be arrested by any means, a rigid contact lens may be physiologically acceptable, provided that it is physically tolerable. Because rigid lenses do not cover the peripheral cornea or the limbal region, more oxygen is available to the peripheral corneal regions. Therefore, taking into account the statistics mentioned earlier in the Prevalence of Corneal Vascularization and Neovascularization section, the rigid lens presents a much lower risk for corneal vascularization.

Rigid lens wearers who have had chronic limbal irritation and who present with vascular changes must be refitted with a slightly different design to minimize the causative factors of vascularization. Ideally, oxygen-permeable rigid lenses should be fitted in a central or slightly superior central position. During the interblink interval, the lens should not tend to drop into the lower limbal region and rest there. Furthermore, on blinking, upper lid–induced lens motion toward the lower limbal region must not cause traumatic compression of the inferior cornea, inferior limbus, or bulbar conjunctiva. When these adverse fitting characteristics are present, they can be improved and the problem resolved by designing a lens with an adequately flat base curve or by flattening the peripheral curve. Rigid lens wearers fitted with an optimal lens who have persistent vascular changes should discontinue contact lens wear. For rigid lens wearers who have never worn hydrogel lenses, it may be possible to refit with a hydrogel lens and, thus, resolve the tendency toward vascular engorgement. With rigid lenses, it is particularly important to carefully monitor and resolve any form of limbal irritation that presents as desiccation (manifested by mild dry spots), 3 to 9 o'clock staining, or dellen.

WHAT IS ACCEPTABLE VASCULARIZATION IN HYDROGEL LENS WEARERS?

It is inevitable that vessels will grow to some extent into the cornea in some contact lens wearers. Based on the U.S. Food and Drug Administration criteria for significant vascularization, vascular penetration of less than 1 mm may be considered clinically acceptable for safe contact lens wear. Vessel growth typically stops at a point approximately 1 mm in from the limbus because the corneal structure changes at this point. The fibers become more closely packed and, thus, act as a barrier to further penetration. Therefore, this is as far as vascularization should be permitted in elective contact lens wear.

Ruben[65] suggests that a noninflammatory 1- to 2-mm micropannus is consistent with the normal eye that is well compromised. In contrast, an inflammatory micropannus can have a cellular or even granular appearance, which can throw an entire sector of the cornea into a vascular pattern (indicating a poorly compromised eye).

Efron[38] has recommended that vessel penetration of up to 1.4 mm in patients using extended-wear hydrogel lens is acceptable, but vessel penetration should not exceed 0.6 mm with daily-wear soft lenses and 0.4 mm with daily-wear rigid lenses. He recommends that when vessel penetration exceeds 1 mm, caution is required and action should be taken to change the lens design or material or the solution. Furthermore, Efron suggests that when ves-

sels begin to encroach on the pupillary area, even if the situation is resolvable, contact lens wear should be discontinued because of the risk of vision loss if the vessels continue to penetrate into the pupillary region.

ETIOLOGY OF CONTACT LENS–INDUCED VASCULARIZATION

The ophthalmic literature presents several proposed causes of corneal vascularization. The current belief is that multiple factors usually contribute to stimulate the process of vascularization or neovascularization in contact lens wear. Notwithstanding the causative factors, vascular endothelial growth factors (VEGF),[66] a family of growth factors involved in the process of regulating neovascularization, have been shown to be present in the normal human corneal epithelium.[67] The appearance of VEGF in the corneal epithelium may have a possible role in the regulation of corneal vascularization associated with contact lens wear.

Contact Lens Factor

Chronic limbal hyperemia has been reported to be common among contact lens wearers.[9,15] McMonnies and colleagues[9] observed and measured the mean extent of stimulated capillary filling beyond the translucent zone of the conjunctival overlay of the transparent stroma. These authors found 0.12 mm in nonwearers, 0.25 mm in rigid lens wearers, and 0.4 mm in hydrogel lens wearers. Therefore, hydrogel lens wear presents the greatest risk. The chronic dilation of limbal vessels associated with hydrogel contact lens wear may be a precursor to new vessel growth.[9,62] Lens wearers examined by fluorescein angiography presented a greater proliferation of limbal loops with many interconnections, and, as a result, a haze or leakage of fluorescein was often observed within the limbal region.[40] Passive hyperemia caused by a tight-fitting soft contact lens or a decentered rigid lens that impinges on the limbal conjunctiva may cause venous compression and, ultimately, localized corneal vascularization.[68] In addition, a tight-fitting hydrogel lens may cause restricted venous drainage, thus, resulting in lactic acid accumulation in the corneal periphery, which is a possible stimulus to corneal vascularization.[64,69]

Lens Design Factor

The cross-sectional design of a negative-power hydrogel contact lens affects the thickness and oxygen transmissibility of the portion of lens that covers the limbal region. The increasing thickness that occurs toward the lens periphery, especially in high-powered lenses, may be of particular concern.[70]

Hypoxia Factor

The earliest reports of corneal vascularization associated with contact lens wear suggested corneal edema as the primary cause.[68] It was later suggested that corneal edema in itself was not a stimulating factor.[71] Some research has considered the oxygen factor more significant.

Hypoxia in hydrogel lens wear has been associated with increased lactic acid production,[72] edema and reduced compactness of the corneal tissues,[68,73] peripheral stromal softening, breakdown of ground substance,[74] and corneal pannus.[44] The results of earlier research indicated that loss of tissue compactness was not in itself a sufficient stimulus for corneal neovascularization and that other factors, combined with loss of tissue compactness sustained over some period, play a role.[75]

Contact lens–induced hypoxic stress has been shown to stimulate the endogenous formation of two biologically active metabolites in rabbit models. In rabbits, these metabolites are at least partially responsible for marked conjunctival inflammation characterized by corneal neovascularization.[76] This may also be true in humans. It has been suggested that contact lens–induced hypoxic stress could either directly or indirectly cause prolonged half-time of VEGF normally present in corneal epithelium, triggering or even initiating neovascularization.[67]

In a 3-year prospective investigation of high school–aged subjects, the population was randomly selected for spectacle wear or hydrogel lens wear. After 18 months of use, there was a statistically significant difference between the two populations with respect to edema and neovascularization.[61]

Conjunctival hyperemia may prove to be an important marker of corneal health, and limbal hyperemia may be a precursor to corneal neovascularization.[16] Low-Dk hydrogel lenses were found to produce a marked increase in limbal hyperemia compared to no lens or when an experimental high-Dk hydrogel was worn.[77] This observation was confirmed in a randomized double-blind study[11] with controls using high-Dk (140 × 10^{-11}) hydrogel lenses compared with low-Dk hydrogel lenses.[78] Dilation of limbal and conjunctival vessels resulting from contact lens hypoxia could be caused by the release of metabolites from hypoxic epithelial cells into the preocular tear film. The endogenous formation of

these metabolites is stimulated only after prolonged contact lens wear.[76]

Hypoxia and Inflammatory Response Factors

Despite evidence implicating hypoxia in corneal vascularization, a larger body of information points to an intimate relationship between the inflammatory response and the growth of blood vessels into the cornea.[79–81] Inflammatory stimuli or processes may be the primary mechanisms in corneal vascularization.[63,67,76,82–88]

Current theories suggest that inflammatory mediators are produced as a result of the altered metabolic state of the hypoxic ocular tissues, secondary to contact lens wear. Biological changes in the corneal epithelium after contact lens wear include glycogen depletion and altered adenosine triphosphate levels.[17]

In patients with extended-wear contact lenses, vascularization has been associated with an inflammatory response secondary to the chronic entrapment of mucus and exfoliated corneal epithelial cells between the lens and the eye.[89] This is consistent with reports of the effects of by-products of stressed corneal metabolism and lysed exfoliated epithelial cells held at the limbal region, in daily wearing of contact lenses, as a possible stimulus of vessel growth.[90–92] A corneal epithelial factor stimulated by inflammatory cells has also been suggested as a possible stimulus of vessel growth.[93]

Lactic acid is a metabolic by-product of corneal stress and has been implicated as an angiogenic factor.[75,90–92,94] Furthermore, lactic acid and hypoxia cause macrophages to release angiogenic factors that stimulate angiogenic activity.[95]

Other Inflammation-Related Factors

Stimulated lymphocytes that are present in an infiltrate near the limbal region can also stimulate blood vessel growth into the cornea.[60,96] The plasminogen activator–plasmin system seems to be involved in the pathologic progress of vascularization.[97] An abundance of plasmin disturbs the normal balance of the plasminogen activator–plasmin system.[98] Plasmin has been found in the tear film associated with use of daily-wear and extended-wear soft contact lenses.[99] However, only a minimal amount of plasmin was associated with the wearing of oxygen-permeable rigid contact lenses. The occurrence of plasmin in the tear film was associated with increased severity of corneal vascularization.[99] Daily-wear soft contact lens wearers had approximately 20% less plasmin in their tears than did those using extended-wear soft contact lenses. This may be one of the factors that makes extended-wear contact lens patients more prone to vascularization than are daily-wear contact lens patients. It is noteworthy that plasmin was also found in the preocular tear film of oxygen-permeable rigid contact lens wearers. However, the concentration of plasmin in the tears of these patients was not significantly different from the concentration of plasmin in the tears of a control group consisting of 50 healthy non–lens-wearing eyes.[99]

Although inflammatory processes have been mentioned as a primary mechanism in corneal vascularization, some contact lens–wearing patients who present with corneal inflammation do not develop vascularization. McMonnies[48] has speculated that it is possible for a small but significant amount of vasostimulating substances to be produced in an area that is too remote for an adequate concentration to reach the limbal vessels and promote new vessel growth. This speculation is further substantiated by the familiar observation of central corneal infiltrates in hydrogel lens wearers without associated vascularization.[100]

Trauma

Trauma has also been suggested as a possible cause of corneal vascularization.[10,16-18] Trauma often occurs as a result of sustained minor epithelial damage with hydrogel, silicone, or rigid lens wear. The epithelial damage may be associated with the production of vasostimulating factors. Vascularization has also been associated with the release of enzymes resulting from mechanical or peripheral injury to the epithelium.[38,101] Mechanical irritation of the cornea may contribute to contact lens–induced pathophysiologic changes.[76]

Contact Lens Solutions

The extrinsic effects of solution preservatives have also been associated with neovascularization in contact lens wear.[9,48,62,99] The toxic effects of some disinfecting agents in contact lens solutions[102,103] that are presented to the corneal epithelium or are eluted from a hydrogel lens into the preocular tear film might contribute to plasmin occurrence in the tears[99] and subsequent corneal vascularization (Fig. 5-3).

Coated-Lens Factor

It has been observed that coated or dirty lenses may be associated with limbal hyperemia. If this condition does

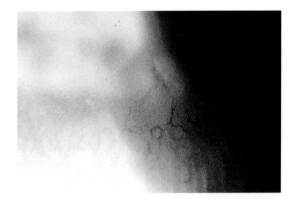

FIG. 5-3. *Corneal vascularization secondary to a reaction from solution preservatives. This figure illustrates the active phase of vessel growth. (Reprinted with permission from CW McMonnies: Contact lens induced corneal vascularization. Int Cont Lens Clin 10:12, 1983, with permission from Elsevier Science.)*

not resolve, the hyperemia becomes chronic and may be associated with corneal vascularization.

Rigid Contact Lens Wear as a Stimulus of Vascularization

The vascular response of an eye properly fitted with a hard lens is indistinguishable from that of an eye that does not wear a contact lens.[9] Chronic epithelial irritation, however, such as corneal epithelial desiccation associated with 3 to 9 o'clock staining, along with the frequently associated adjacent bulbar conjunctival desiccation, can produce chronic vasodilation.[14] If this epithelial trauma is sustained over a long period, corneal vascularization is possible in the affected area.[10,15-19]

An extreme form of desiccation that can occur in the limbal region may give rise to dellen. Dellen present as areas of extreme corneal thinning caused by local dehydration, often caused by an adjacent raised mass (e.g., a pterygium or large pinguecula), or occasionally from a thick contact lens edge. If present for a long period, dellen can cause corneal vascularization in the affected area in a rigid lens wearer.[6,10-13]

The passive hyperemia caused by a decentered rigid lens, even though it impinges on the limbal conjunctiva, results in venous compression and engorgement of the limbal vessels in the immediate area.[104]

Influence of Individual Susceptibility

McMonnies et al.[48] suggested a hypothesis of individual susceptibility to vascularization in contact lens wearers, particularly in those with chronic limbal injection. The critical combination of factors that leads to vascularization in some contact lens–wearing patients is not known.

It is possible that the predominance of anaerobic metabolism and inadequate venous flow,[105] combined with the loss of corneal compactness, may predispose certain patients toward vascularization. This may also be factored in with increased edema or collagenase production caused by epithelial damage or the presence of inflammatory cells in the limbal region. Lysed, exfoliated cells retained against the cornea by a contact lens, contact lens–induced trauma to the bulbar conjunctiva, and venous compression[64] may produce the chemical stimuli necessary for vascularization. All these cofactors may be present in contact lens wearers.

Patients with certain related systemic or ocular conditions, such as acne rosacea, trachoma, or keratitis, already have a compromised ocular environment and may be predisposed to neovascularization as a result of contact lens wear. Furthermore, patients with diabetes or renal disease are also at increased risk.

SUMMARY

Corneal vascularization is a relatively common complication in hydrogel lens wearers but an infrequent complication in rigid lens wearers. It is typically the result of corneal insult or inflammation. Vascularization should be considered a warning of long-standing and chronic stress to corneal physiology. The guidelines provided here help the contact lens fitter to anticipate and prevent this complication, and enable the fitter to manage the condition to prevent any significant exacerbation.

REFERENCES

1. Arentsen JJ: Corneal vascularization in contact lens wearers. In Cohen EJ (ed): Contact Lenses and External Disease. Int Ophthalmol Clin 26:15, 1986
2. Klintworth GK, Burger PC: Neovascularization of the cornea: current concepts of its pathogenesis. In Foulks GN (ed): Noninfectious Inflammation of the Anterior Segment. Int Ophthalmol Clin 23:27, 1983
3. Schein OD, Ormerod, LD, Barraquer E: Microbiology of contact lens related keratitis. Cornea 8:281, 1989
4. Khodadoust AA: The allograft rejection reaction: the leading cause of late failure of clinical corneal grafts. p. 151. In Jones BR (ed): Corneal Graft Failure. Elsevier, Amsterdam, 1973
5. Ghafoor SY, MacEwan CG: Contact lens induced keratopathy. Emirates Med J 5:60, 1987
6. Dixon JM: Corneal vascularization and corneal contact lenses: the clinical picture. Trans Am Ophthalmol Soc 65:333, 1967
7. Kamiya C: Cosmetic extended wear of oxygen permeable hard contact lenses: one year follow-up. J Am Optom Assoc 57:182, 1986
8. Levy B: Rigid gas-permeable lenses for extended wear—a one-year clinical evaluation. Am J Optom Physiol Opt 62:889, 1985
9. McMonnies CW, Chapman-Davies A, Holden BA: The vascular response to contact lens wear. Am J Optom Physiol Opt 59:795, 1982
10. Zauberman H, Michaelson IC, Bergman F, Maurice DM: Stimulation of neovascularization of the cornea by biogenic amines. Exp Eye Res 8:77, 1969
11. Mandelbaum J: Corneal vascularization in aphakic eyes following the use of contact lenses. Arch Ophthalmol 71:633, 1964
12. Ullen RL: Corneal vascularization in the wearing of contact lenses. Precision Cosmet Digest. Precision Cosmet Company, Minneapolis 3(1):1, 3(10):1, 1963
13. Goldberg JB: Biomicroscopy for Contact Lens Practice. Professional Press, Chicago, 1971
14. Stain GA, Brightbill FS, Holm P, Laux D: The development of pseudopterygia in hard contact lens wearers. Cont Intraoc Lens Med J 7:1, 1981
15. Larke JR, Humphreys JA, Holmes R: Apparent corneal neovascularization in soft lens wearers. J Br Cont Lens Assoc 4:105, 1981
16. Collin HB: Limbal vascularization response prior to corneal vascularization. Exp Eye Res 16:443, 1973
17. Thoft R, Friend J: Biochemical aspects of contact lens wear. Am J Ophthalmol 80:139, 1975
18. Henkind P: Ocular neovascularization. Am J Ophthalmol 85:287, 1978
19. Rochels R: Tierexperimentelle Untersuchungen zur Rolle von Entzundungsmediatoren bei der hornhaut Neovaskulariaation. Doc Ophthalmol 57:215, 1984
20. Lebow KA, Grohe RM: Vascularized limbal keratitis. Int Cont Lens Clin 16:197, 1989
21. Roth HW: The etiology of ocular irritation in soft lens wearers: distribution in a large clinical sample. Cont Intraoc Lens Med J 4:38, 1978
22. Maguen E, Nesburn AB, Verity SM, et al: Myopic extended wear contact lenses in 100 patients. A retrospective study. Cont Lens Assoc Ophthalmol J 10:335, 1984
23. Spoor TC, Hartel W, Winn P, et al: Complications of continuous-wear soft contact lenses in a nonreferral population. Arch Ophthalmol 102:1312, 1984
24. Stark WJ, Martin NF: Extended wear contact lenses for myopic correction. Arch Ophthalmol 99:1963, 1981
25. The Hydrocurve Extended Wear Study, 1977–1983: Report presented to Health Protection Branch, Canada, 1983
26. Athanassiadia P, Ruben M: The continuous wear of contact lenses. Ophthalmic Optician May 26:390, 1979
27. Slatt BJ, Stein H: Extended wear soft contact lenses in preservative. Int Cont Lens Clin Sept/Oct:35, 1977

28. Solomon OD, Sholiton D, Slonim C, Lamping K: Bausch & Lomb "O" lenses for extended wear. Cont Lens Assoc Ophthalmol J 9:137, 1983

29. Schonder A, Conklin T, Angelini E: Clinical evaluation of extended wear lidofilcon B contact lenses with aphakia. Am J Ophthalmol 14:222, 1982

30. Stark W, Krucher G, Covan C, et al: Extended wear contact lenses and intraocular lenses for aphakic correction. Am J Ophthalmol 88:11, 1979

31. Binder P: Myopic extended wear with Hydrocurve II soft contact lenses. Ophthalmology 60:578, 1983

32. Hill JF, Anderson FL, Johnson TK, et al: Eighteen-month clinical experience with extended wear silicone contact lenses on 400 patients. Am J Optom Physiol Opt 60:578, 1983

33. Sak J, Schlanger J: Complications of aphakic extended wear contact lenses encountered during a seven year period on 100 eyes. CLAO J 9:241, 1983

34. Jantzi JD, Jackson WE, Smith KM: Corneal vascularization in a group of soft contact lens wearers: prevalence, magnitude, type and related factors. Can J Optom 49:174, 1987

35. Dohlman CH, Boruchoff MD, Mobilia EF: Complications in use of soft contact lenses and corneal disease. Arch Ophthalmol 90:367, 1973

36. Schecter DR, Emery JM, Soper JW: Corneal vascularization in therapeutic soft lens wear. Cont Intraoc Lens Med J 1:141, 1975

37. Cunha MC, Thomassen TS, Cohen EJ, et al: Complications associated with contact lens use. CLAO J 13:107, 1987

38. Efron N: Vascular response of the cornea to contact lens wear. J Am Optom Assoc 58:836, 1987

39. McMonnies CW: Corneal vascularization. In Bennett E, Weissman B (eds): Clinical Contact Lens Practice. Lippincott, Philadelphia, 1991

40. Stevenson RWW, Chawla JC: Vascular response of limbus to contact lens wear. J Br Cont Lens Assoc 16:19, 1993

41. Becker MD, Kruse FE, Joussen AM, et al: In vivo fluorescence microscopy of corneal neovascularization. Graefes Arch Clin Exp Ophthalmol 236:390, 1998.

42. Grayson M: Diseases of the Cornea. 2nd ed. Mosby, St. Louis, 1983

43. Sendele DD, Kenyon KR, Mobilia EF, et al: Superior limbic keratoconjunctivitis in contact lens wearers. Ophthalmology 90:616, 1983

44. Chan W-K, Weissman BA: Corneal pannus associated with contact lens wear. Am J Ophthalmol 121:540, 1996

45. Tan DTH, Pullam KW, Buckley RJ: Medical applications of scleral contact lenses, 2: gas permeable scleral contact lenses. Cornea 14:130, 1995

46. Iomata H, Smelser GK, Pollack FM: Corneal vascularization in experimental uveitis and graft rejection. Invest Ophthalmol Vis Sci 10: 840, 1971

47. Ruben M: Corneal vascularization. In Miller D, White PF (eds): Complications of Contact Lenses. Int Ophthalmol Clin 21:27, 1981

48. McMonnies CW: Contact lens induced corneal vascularization. Int Cont Lens Clin 10:12, 1983

49. Weinberg RJ: Deep corneal vascularization caused by aphakic soft contact lens wear. Am J Ophthalmol 83:121, 1987

50. Nivankari VS, Karesh J, Lakhanpal V, et al: Deep stromal vascularization associated with cosmetic, daily wear contact lenses. Arch Ophthalmol 101:46, 1983

51. Braude LS, Sugan J: Circinate-pattern interstitial keratopathy in daily wear soft contact lens wearers. Arch Ophthalmol 103:1662, 1985

52. Rozenman Y, Donnenfeld ED, Cohen EJ, et al: Contact lens–related deep stromal neovascularization. Am J Ophthalmol 107:27, 1989

53. Duke-Elder S, Leigh AG: Diseases of the outer eye. p. 676. In Duke-Elder S (ed): System of Ophthalmology. Vol. 8. Henry Kimpton, London, 1977

54. Meyer PAR: The circulation of the human limbus. Eye 3:121, 1989

55. Conrad TJ, Chandler DB, Corless JM, Klintworth GK: In vivo measurement of corneal angiogenesis with video data acquisition and computerized image analysis. Lab Invest 70:426, 1994

56. Van Buskirk EM: The anatomy of the limbus. Eye 3:101, 1989

57. Allansmith M: Neovascularization—how much and how far? J Am Optom Assoc 55:199, 1984

58. Wolff E: Anatomy of the Eye and Orbit. HK Lewis, London, 1958

59. Ausprunk DH, Falterman K, Folkman J: The sequence of effects in the regression of corneal capillaries. Lab Invest 38:284, 1978

60. Madigan MC, Penfold PL, Holden BA, et al: Ultrastructural features of contact lens-induced deep corneal neovascularization. Clin Exp Optom (poster abstract) 72:207, 1989

61. Madigan MC, Holden BA, Billson FA: Ultrastructural features of contact lens induced deep corneal neovascularization and associated stromal leucocytes. Cornea 9:144, 1990

62. McMonnies CW, Chapman-Davies A: Assessment of conjunctival hyperemia in contact lens wearers. Part II. Am J Optom Physiol Opt 64:251, 1987

63. Cooper CA, Bergamini MVW, Leopold IH: Use of flurbiprofen to inhibit corneal neovascularization. Arch Ophthalmol 98:1102, 1980

64. Josephson JE, Caffery BE: Case report: progressive corneal vascularization associated with extended wear of a silicone elastomer contact lens. Am J Optom Physiol Opt 64:958, 1987

65. Ruben M: Picture tests and contact lenses. Optician 6:23, 1990

66. Ferrara N, Houck KA, Jakeman LB, et al: The vascular endothelium growth factor family of polypeptides. J Cell Biochem 47:211, 1991

67. Van Setten GB: Vascular endothelial growth factor (VEGF) in normal human corneal epithelium: detection and physiological importance. Acta Ophthalmol Scand 75:649, 1997

68. Campbell FW, Michaelson IC: Blood vessel formation in the cornea. Br J Ophthalmol 3:248, 1949

69. McMonnies CW: Risk factors in the etiology of contact lens induced corneal vascularization. Int Contact Lens Clin 5:286, 1982

70. Fatt I, Weissman BA, Ruben CM: Areal differences in oxygen supply wearing an optically powered hydrogel contact lens. CLAO J 19:226, 1993.

71. Cogan DG: Vascularization of the cornea. Arch Ophthalmol 41:406, 1949

72. Hamano H, Hori M, Kawabe H, et al: Effects of contact lens wear on mitosis of corneal epithelium and lactate content, in aqueous humor of rabbit. Jpn J Ophthalmol 27:457, 1983

73. Thoft RA, Friend J, Murphy HS: Ocular surface epithelium and corneal vascularization in rabbits: the role of wounding. Invest Ophthalmol Vis Sci 18:85, 1979

74. Holden BA, Sweeney DF, Vannas A, et al: The effects of long-term extended contact lens wear on a human cornea. Invest Ophthalmol Vis Sci 26:1489, 1985

75. Ashton N, Cook C: Mechanism of corneal vascularization. Br J Ophthalmol 37:193, 1953

76. Davis KL, Conners MS, Dunn MW, et al: Induction of corneal epithelial cytochrome P450 arachidonate metabolism for contact lens wear. Invest Ophthalmol Vis Sci 33:291, 1992

77. Papas EB, Vadjilc CM, Austen R, Holden BA: High oxygen transmissibility soft contact lenses do not induce limbal hyperemia. Curr Eye Res 16:942, 1997

78. Du Toit R, Simpson TL, Fonn D, Chalmers R: Recovery from hyperemia after overnight wear of hydrogel lenses. Poster no. 1560; Association of Research and Vision in Ophthalmology. Ft. Lauderdale, FL, 1998

79. Duffin RM, Weissman BA, Glasser DB, Pettit RM: Flurbiprofen in the treatment of corneal neovascularization induced by contact lenses. Am J Ophthalmol 93:607, 1982

80. Klintworth GK: Neovascularization of the cornea: an overview. p. 327. In BenEzra D, Ryan SJ, Glaser B, et al. (eds): Ocular Circulation and Neovascularization. Martinus Nijhoff/Dr W Junk, Dordrecht, 1987

81. Fromer CH, Klintworth GK: An evaluation of the role of leukocytes in the pathogenesis of experimentally induced corneal vascularization: I. Comparison of experimental models of corneal vascularization. Am J Pathol 79:537, 1975

82. Klintworth GK: The hamster cheek pouch. Am J Pathol 73:691, 1973

83. Robin J, Regis-Pacheco L, Kash R, Schanzlin D: The histopathology of corneal vascularization. Arch Ophthalmol 103:284, 1985

84. BenEzra D: Neovasculogenesis: triggering factors in possible mechanisms. Surv Ophthalmol 98:1102, 1980

85. Inomata H, Smelser GK, Polack FM: Corneal vascularization in experimental uveitis and graft rejection. Invest Ophthalmol Vis Sci 10:840, 1971

86. Fromer CH, Klintworth GK: An evaluation of the role of leukocytes in the pathogenesis of experimentally induced corneal vascularization: III. Studies related to the vaso-proliferative capability of polymorphonuclear leukocytes and lymphocytes. Am J Pathol 82:157, 1976

87. BenEzra D: Mediators of immunological reactions: function as inducers of neovascularization. Metabol Ophthalmol 2:339, 1978

88. Howard WH, Lee MD, Klintworth GK: An evaluation of spontaneously developing corneal angiogenesis in nude (nu/nu) and hairless (hr/hr) mice (abstract). Invest Ophthalmol Vis Sci 33:777, 1992

89. Mertz GW, Holden BA: Clinical implications of extended wear research. Can J Optom July(suppl.):203, 1981

90. Imre G: The role of increased lactic acid concentration in neovascularization. Acta Morphol Hung 32:97, 1984

91. Levene R, Shapiro A, Baum J: Experimental corneal vascularization. Arch Ophthalmol 70:242, 1963

92. Morley N, McCullock C: Corneal lactate and pyridine, nucleotides with contact lenses. Arch Ophthalmol 66:379, 1961

93. Vannas A, DeDonato LM: Corneal vascularization in hydrogel contact lens wearers. J Am Optom Assoc 52:235, 1981

94. Imre G: The mechanism of corneal vascularization. Acta Morphol Acad Sci Hung Tomus 14:99, 1966

95. Jensen DR, Hunt TK, Scheuenstuhl H, et al: Effect of lactate, pyruvate, and pH on secretion of angiogenesis and mitogenesis factors by macrophages. Lab Invest 54:574, 1986

96. Epstein RJ, Stulting RD, Hendricks RL, et al: Corneal vascularization: pathogenesis and inhibition. Cornea 6:250, 1987

97. Berman M, Withrop S, Ausprunk D, et al: Plasminogen activator (urokinase) causes vascularization of the cornea. Invest Ophthalmol Vis Sci 22:191, 1982

98. Berman M, Kenyon K, Hayashi K, et al: The pathogeneses of epithelial defects and stromal ulceration. p. 35. In Cavanagh D (ed): The Cornea. Transactions of the World Congress on the Cornea III. Raven, New York, 1988

99. VanSetten GB, Tervo T, Andersson R, et al: Plasmin and epidermal growth factor in the tear fluid of contact-lens wearers. Effect of wearing different types of contact lenses and association with clinical findings. Ophthal Res 22:333, 1990

100. Josephson JE, Caffery BE: Infiltrative keratitis in hydrogel lens wear. Int Cont Lens Clin 6:223, 1979

101. Sholley MM, Grimbone MA, Coltran RS: The effect of leucocyte depletion on corneal neovascularization. Lab Invest 38:32, 1978

102. Rai Mehta M, Kumar Dada V, Mohan M: Epitheliotoxicity of contact lens solutions: an experimental study using scanning electron microscopy. p. 840. Consilium Ophalmologicum Proc XXV, Int Congr Ophthalmol, Rome, 1986 in Acta XXV. Kugler and Ghendini, Amsterdam, 1987

103. Paugh JR, Brennan NA, Efron N: Ocular response to hydrogen peroxide. Am J Optom Physiol Opt 65:91, 1988

104. Mosquera JM, Voss EH, Moguilner MH: Corneal angiography and contact lenses. Int Cont Lens Clin 1:94, 1974

105. Ashton N: Neovascularization in ocular disease. Trans Ophthalmol Soc U K 81:145, 1961

II

Inflammation, Allergy, and Toxicity

6

Inflammatory Responses in Contact Lens Wear

Joel A. Silbert

GRAND ROUNDS CASE REPORT

Subjective:
A 19-year-old man presents with a history of wearing extended-wear disposable lenses for the past 5 years. He reports an acute episode of pain and foreign-body sensation in the left eye (OS) occurring the night before that was severe enough to have awakened him from sleep. On self-inspection of his eye, there was pronounced redness and extreme light sensitivity. Attempts at lens removal are difficult, and he had to add saline over a 5-minute period to loosen the lens and allow removal. He has not used any new lens care products and takes no medications.

   Examination in the practitioner's office the following morning shows a hyperemic eye. Persistent photophobia exists, which makes examination difficult.

Objective:
- Best corrected acuity with spectacles: right eye (OD) $20/20$, OS $20/30$, each eye (OU) $20/20$.
- Pinhole acuity OS is $20/25$.
- Equal ocular movements (EOMs) are full; pupillary reflexes are patent (no afferent defect).
- Biomicroscopy: corneas show no central staining, but subepithelial infiltrates exist OS only in the central 6-mm zone. The anterior chamber shows grade 1 cells but no flare.
- Tonometry: 13 mm Hg OD, 11 OS (Goldmann applanation).
- Ophthalmoscopy: Unremarkable.

Assessment:
Corneal inflammatory episode secondary to contact lens–induced acute red-eye (CLARE) syndrome. Corneal infiltrates are probably secondary to presence of gram-negative bacteria adherent to extended-wear soft lenses. Tight lens syndrome. Because no corneal staining overlies the infiltrates, the acute reaction, thus, is inflammatory but is not a corneal ulcer.

Plan:
1. No contact lens wear until corneal inflammation resolves. Patient does have a spectacle prescription.
2. As patient had been wearing lenses on an extended-wear basis, the risk of pseudomonal presence is high. Thus, rather than just discontinuing lens wear and monitoring the patient, a 2-day course of antibiotic ther-

apy is initiated, with good coverage for gram-negative organisms (ciprofloxacin ophthalmic solution, 1 drop OS four times daily). Also, patient given 1 drop homatropine 5% OS for the anterior uveitis, with topical steroids held in abeyance. See patient the next day.

3. The following day, the eye is less red, and photophobia is greatly reduced. No foreign-body sensation exists. No corneal staining exists, but infiltrates are still present. A mild topical steroid is prescribed to reduce the inflammatory effects (fluorometholone 1 drop OS three times a day) with a tapering of dosage over the next 2 days. Antibiotic dosage is reduced to twice a day and is to be discontinued within 2 days.

4. Follow-up visit in 2 days shows total resolution of inflammatory episode, with acuity of 20/20 in each eye, absence of infiltrates, and no photophobia. Contact lens wear may resume within 1 week, but only on a daily-wear basis. Reassess lens movement under conditions of daily-wear use; if inadequate, refit with looser lens.

Inflammation is a complex biological process that occurs in response to tissue damage. Tissue damage may come about from endogenous as well as exogenous factors, such as mechanical injuries (e.g., corneal abrasions), chemical burns (e.g., hydrogen peroxide burn of the cornea), infection by microbial agents, and hypersensitivity reactions. Although inherently protective in its role against injury and infection, inflammation may at times limit or diminish functions of the affected tissue while the offending agent is being attacked or while damaged tissue is beginning its repair. This is particularly true of hypersensitivity reactions. For contact lens wearers, inflammation is typically associated with corneal abrasions, infections, and acute red-eye syndrome, or it may come about from a variety of toxic and allergenic causes.

Because the potential list of inflammatory causes of a contact lens–induced red eye is relatively large, the clinician must take a detailed and methodical history to help narrow the field. A thorough examination of the eyes and adnexa, combined with inspection of the patient's lenses, should enable a differential diagnosis and, more important, a tentative diagnosis. This is not always a straightforward task, however, because many inflammatory stimuli may express themselves in only a limited number of signs and symptoms. Although good observational skills are essential, the clinician must also be a good listener and must exercise sound clinical intuition.

The four classic signs of inflammation contributed by Celsus almost 2,000 years ago still exquisitely and succinctly describe the inflammatory process:

- *Rubor, or redness.* This response is commonly encountered in contact lens practice in the form of increased conjunctival or perilimbal injection, dilatation of palpebral conjunctival vessels, or lid hyperemia.
- *Tumor, or swelling.* Some examples of tissue swelling include edema that may present as tissue exudation, corneal thickening, conjunctival chemosis, blepharoedema, papillary hypertrophy, and even granulation tissue seen in a chalazion.
- *Calor, or heat.* Increased tissue warmth accompanies inflammatory processes, especially in infections.
- *Dolor, or pain.* Discomfort and pain are caused by vascular dilatation and secondary nerve ending compression by surrounding edematous tissue, by corneal epithelial compromise, and by the release of inflammatory mediators at the site of insult. More than any other sign or symptom, pain or discomfort alerts the patient that something is not right and, thus, also serves as a subjective protective mechanism. Deeper pain associated with true photophobia may be a warning of more severe inflammation, as seen in anterior uveitis or in microbial keratitis.

The four cardinal signs of inflammation were later elaborated with the addition of a fifth sign, that of *functio laesa,* or loss of function. This is commonly observed in many aspects of inflammatory reactions and is primarily caused by nerve fiber involvement and tissue edema.[1]

INFLAMMATORY RESPONSE

Inflammation represents a complex sequence of events that occurs in injured or compromised tissues. Very shortly after injury, the inflammatory process is initiated by the activation of acute-phase proteins. In the case of microbial insult, C-reactive protein binds to the membrane of microbes and triggers the complement system cascade. This cascade stimulates special cells whose function is phagocytosis (i.e., ingestion and destruction) and ultimate lysis of the microbial organism.[2] Most cells involved in the phagocytic response are polymorphonuclear leukocytes (i.e., white blood cells), which respond within 30–60 minutes. If the cause of the inflammatory response persists beyond this period, mononuclear macrophages and lymphocytes infiltrate the region to bolster the phagocytic response. This is an example of *innate* or *natural immunity* present in the body, which serves to provide nonspecific protection against substances or microbes that are threatening or injurious.

An inflammatory response is likely to involve the *acquired immune system* when the host tissue has had prior exposure to an inflammatory agent. Repeated exposure to antigens provokes a rapidly expanding defensive response, which can be noncellular or cellular. When noncellular, the defense mechanisms involve plasma components, antibodies, and the complement cascade. When cellular, acquired immunity depends on the presence of macrophages and T lymphocytes.[3]

In addition to the supplementation of the phagocytic response, macrophages further add to the inflammatory defense system by presenting the foreign antigen of the invading substance or microbe to the lymphocytes. This brings into play the acquired immune system, which responds specifically to the foreign antigen by producing antibodies and then triggering the complement cascade.

An inflammatory response is considered *toxic* when the host tissue has had no prior exposure to an inflammatory agent. A local inflammatory reaction without much tissue damage caused by the toxic agent is known as a *nonnecrotizing* response and is exemplified by reactions to solution preservatives. *Necrotizing* inflammatory responses, in contrast, produce considerable tissue damage and are exemplified by corneal perforations or melting, observed with released enzymes and toxins in pseudomonal corneal ulcers.[4]

The intensity of an inflammatory response depends on the structure and nature of the inflammatory stimulus, the degree of prior exposure and, to some extent, on the characteristics of the host tissue. Immunologic responses often exceed normal levels and may give rise to hypersensitivity or allergic reactions, in which a full-blown reaction may follow the reintroduction of a very small stimulus. Quantity and contact time of the stimulus also influence the severity of the inflammatory response.

MECHANISMS OF INFLAMMATION: OVERVIEW

Many events occur during acute inflammatory episodes. The primary mechanisms of inflammation are summarized in this section. For a more detailed treatment of these topics, consult a current text in immunology.

Increased Vascular Permeability

Inflammatory swelling is present in almost all cases of acute inflammation and represents increased accumulation of tissue fluid during the early hours or days of an inflammatory event. This swelling is distinct from another type of swelling that may occur when inflammation persists for some time: the formation of hyperplastic connective tissue. Both can contribute to the tumor or swelling response of inflammation. The former is best illustrated by the focal blepharoedema of a newly formed hordeolum or stye. The latter is exemplified by a stye that has poorly drained, leading to granulation tissue and the formation of a chalazion (i.e., a firm nodule that walls off and contains the spread of inflammation). The focus here, however, is more on the events that take place during early acute inflammation, in which fluids escape from capillaries and produce tissue edema.

As a response to injury, inflammation may cause leakage from vessels from mechanical causes in which vessels are directly damaged (e.g., in a skin cut). Of greater interest, particularly in contact lens–related ocular inflammation, are the events leading to vascular leakage that are not caused by direct injury. In this case, chemical mediators released from damaged tissue stimulate uninjured venules in the area around the site of injury. This, in turn, causes vessels to leak as a result of loosened tight junctions between capillary endothelial cells. These events occur when mast cells are ruptured during allergic, traumatic, and inflammatory events, releasing large numbers of histamine granules. As mast cells are typically located near venules, their degranulation causes initial vasodilation and subsequent increases in capillary permeability. Plasma and proteins leak from the venules, causing tissue swelling. This is further compounded by additional leakage of neutrophils, lymphocytes, and macrophages into the site of the damaged tissue.[3]

In addition to histamine, other mediators increase vascular permeability and are released from basophils, mast cells, macrophages, polymorphonuclear leukocytes, and

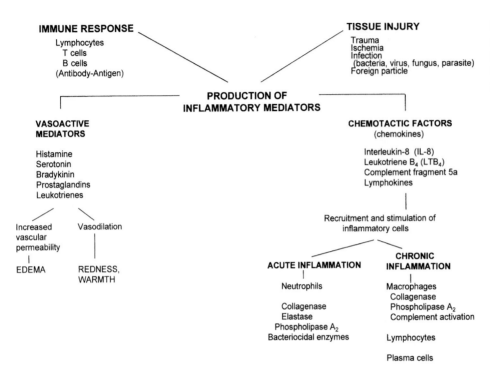

FIG. 6-1. *An overview of the consequences of the production of inflammatory mediators in the immune response to tissue injury. (Courtesy of Dr. Joan Wing.)*

platelets. These include prostaglandins, bradykinins, leukokinins, kallikrein, globulin permeability factor,[4] and platelet-activating factors (PAFs). PAFs are capable of increasing vascular permeability by inducing neutrophil migration and the formation of prostaglandin precursors.[5]

Early vascular leakage of the histamine model appears to occur when mediators trigger the endothelial cells of venules to contract, pulling away from each other and, thus, creating gaps for fluid and protein exudation.[6] As the inflamed tissue swells because of increased vascular permeability, the characteristics of the exudate can vary. For example, serous or watery exudate has few cells, is similar to blood serum, and is typical of mild vascular insult. Assuming a properly functioning immune system, the lack of cells suggests the lack of bacterial stimuli. Exudate containing cells is puslike, contains many neutrophils, and is typical of inflammation triggered by bacterial infection. Hemorrhagic exudate is a result of pronounced damage to capillaries, whereas fibrinous exudate is found more typically on surfaces such as the pleura or pericardium[7] or on the palpebral conjunctiva.

Figure 6-1 presents an overview of the consequences of the production of inflammatory mediators.

Leukocyte Infiltration and Chemotaxis

Leukocytes originate from the blood, initially sticking to the walls of the blood vessels. They then chemo-tactically move in the direction of an inflammatory stimulus. This might, for example, be movement toward a bacterial focus or toward the site of a chemical burn. Having arrived at the site of the insult, the leukocyte's function is to phagocytose or digest the offending agent.

Bacteria and damaged tissue release chemotactic factors that alter the endothelial lining of venules, leading first to sticking and then exiting of large numbers of leukocytes, which squeeze out of the venular wall between closely apposed endothelial cells. Although histamine-type mediators may create actual gaps between cells, it is clear that leukocytes do not require such gaps for this emigration process, or *diapedesis.*[7]

In the early stages of inflammation induced by a bacterial stimulus, a high percentage of neutrophils emigrate into the inflammatory site, followed later by an infusion of monocytes (mononuclear phagocytes), which can remain at the site for days. *Chemotaxins* are substances that cause phagocytic cells to migrate from regions of low concentration to regions of higher concentration. When the complement cascade is activated after an inflammatory stimulus, the chemotaxin C5a is released, which chemically attracts phagocytic neutrophils. In addition, a monocyte chemotactic factor may also be released by neutrophils.[7]

How leukocytes sense directionality in their chemotactic response is a complex topic still under active study. With-

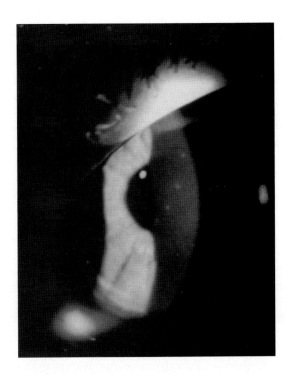

FIG. 6-2. *Subepithelial corneal infiltrates.*

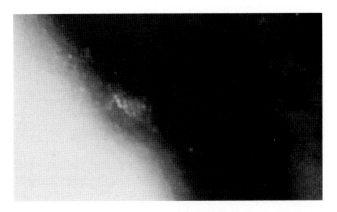

FIG. 6-3. *Epithelial infiltrate located near the limbus, observed with marginal retroillumination. (Reprinted with permission from JE Josephson, S Zantos, BE Caffery, et al: Differentiation of corneal complications observed in contact lens wearers. J Am Optom Assoc 59:679, 1988.)*

out chemotaxis, the body's ability to respond rapidly and accurately to the source of an infection is sorely limited.

Phagocytosis

The primary functions of neutrophils and mononuclear phagocytes are digestion and destruction of bacteria and damaged cells. Neutrophils contain granules composed of lysosomal enzymes, peroxidase, and the antibacterial proteins lysozyme and lactoferrin. The mononuclear phagocytes can be thought of as monocytes when in the blood and macrophages when the cells are in tissues. They contain granules composed of acid hydrolases as well as pinocytic vesicles.[7]

For bacteria to be ingested, their surfaces must first become coated with serum factors or *opsonins* before they can attach to a phagocyte. These include immunoglobulin G (IgG) antibodies specific to the particle surfaces, as well as opsonic fragments of the C3 or third component of the serum complement system (see Complement Cascade section). Once opsonized, the bacteria can be attached to the phagocyte because this cell has receptors for antibody molecules and the opsonized C3 fragments. It is not well understood how phagocytes know when to destroy a damaged or worn-out host cell (i.e., self).[7]

The opsonized foreign particle is captured in the cell in a phagocytic vacuole. Bacteria are killed by a combination of factors, including lysosomal degranulation, leading to discharge of hydrolytic enzymes into the vacuole; acid pH inside the vacuole; and release of lysozyme, lactoferrin, peroxide, superoxide radicals, and other destructive agents into the vacuole. Among these, it appears that peroxide is the neutrophil's primary antimicrobial agent. The cell protects itself against the effects of free peroxide by the presence of catalase in its cytoplasm.[8,9]

CORNEAL INFILTRATION

Corneal infiltrates represent aggregated neutrophils, macrophages, and lymphocytes, which migrate chemotactically to the site of the inflamed host tissue. In the cornea, they may localize in the epithelium, but more commonly, they localize in the subepithelium and stroma (Fig. 6-2). They migrate along nonvascular corneal lamellae from their source at the limbal vasculature (Fig. 6-3).[10] The limbus is the site of initial leukocyte migration and is rich in mast cells and capillaries. It thus serves as a site of deposition for circulating immune complexes and is clinically viewed as the source of a number of peripheral corneal disease entities.[11]

Leukocytes can also arrive externally at the site of corneal inflammation via chemotactic substances in the tears, coming from limbal transudation or from the conjunctival lymphatic system.[12] Corneal infiltrates may also be induced by the presence of viruses,[13] by inflammatory stimuli from contact lens solution preservatives, and by bacterial exotoxins and endotoxins.[14]

The clinical description of corneal infiltrates and their management is discussed later in the Clinical Signs of Contact Lens–Related Inflammation section.

INFLAMMATORY MEDIATORS

The inflammatory response involves changes in the caliber of blood vessels and increased movement and functions of cells. The communication necessary to trigger these events requires nerve stimulation but mostly occurs via chemical mediators or messengers. These can originate outside of the body (*exogenous*) or can come from within (*endogenous*).

Exogenous Mediators

Neutrophils and macrophages are key components of the phagocytic process of foreign organism removal. Bacterial products are representative of exogenous or external mediators of the inflammatory response, which can cause increases in vascular permeability and chemotaxis of leukocytes. Of greater importance, however, are the endogenous mediators of inflammation.

Endogenous Mediators in the Plasma

Three endogenous mediator systems exist in the plasma, all of which are interrelated: the complement cascade, the kinin system, and the clotting mechanism.

Complement Cascade

Complement is a group of serum proteins that activate each other in an orderly and serial fashion to ultimately cause the lysis of cells or microbes. These proteins are synthesized in the liver by tissue macrophages, blood monocytes, and epithelial cells of the intestinal tract. They are inactive when released into the serum but become activated during the complement cascade. The complement system plays a critical role in inflammatory reactions in the plasma. The binding of specific antibodies to foreign antigen triggers the *classic complement system* in the plasma (Fig. 6-4). After an antigen-antibody complex binds to a cell surface, a series of cascading and amplifying enzymatic reactions involving the activation of nine major plasma protein components (designated C1 through C9) is brought into action,[15] in which the following events transpire:

- Chemotactic attraction of phagocytic leukocytes to the site of inflammation
- Adherence of microbes to these cells

- Potentiation of mast cell degranulation by anaphylatoxins (C3a, C5a), which releases histamine and heparin
- Vasodilation with increased cell membrane permeability (caused by histamine) leading to local edema (edema fluid contains more antibodies and components of complement, thus, further amplifying the reaction)
- Cell membrane attack and damage leading to disturbances in osmotic equilibrium and cell lysis
- Activation of serotonin, PAFs, leukotrienes, and prostaglandins

The classic complement system is also chemotactic for eosinophils, which aid in the elimination of foreign substances or organisms that are too large to be ingested by neutrophils and macrophages. If microbial, this process destroys cell membranes by proteolytic action.[3] In addition, complement can interact with the clotting system, producing plasmin and collagenase. Inhibitors closely regulate the activity of the complement system so that adverse reactions are prevented.

An *alternative complement pathway* that does not require antigen-antibody complexes for activation has been found in which serum is triggered by cell walls of some bacteria and yeasts, lipopolysaccharides, IgA aggregates, cobra venom, and endotoxins from the cell walls of gram-negative bacteria, further exacerbating the inflammatory response.[15]

Kinin System

The kinin system is activated after tissue injury, leading to inflammation. It is triggered by activation of the clotting mechanism (Hageman factor), which produces a protease known as *kallikrein*. This series of cascading events in the fibrinolytic system ultimately produces a number of kinin peptides (bradykinin being the best known). Bradykinin causes slow contraction of certain smooth muscles, increases vascular permeability by way of contraction of vascular endothelial cells, and is responsible for much of the pain associated with inflammation.[2,7]

Clotting System

During clotting, the action of thrombin releases fibrinopeptides from fibrinogen molecules. This can lead to neutrophil chemotaxis and increased vascular permeability. The breakdown of fibrin by plasmin can also serve as a chemotactic trigger for neutrophils.[7]

Endogenous Mediators in the Tissues

Histamine and Anaphylactic Hypersensitivity

Although immunity serves to provide protection, it can sometimes produce results that are so exaggerated that

FIG. 6-4. *The complement cascade: classic and alternate pathways.*

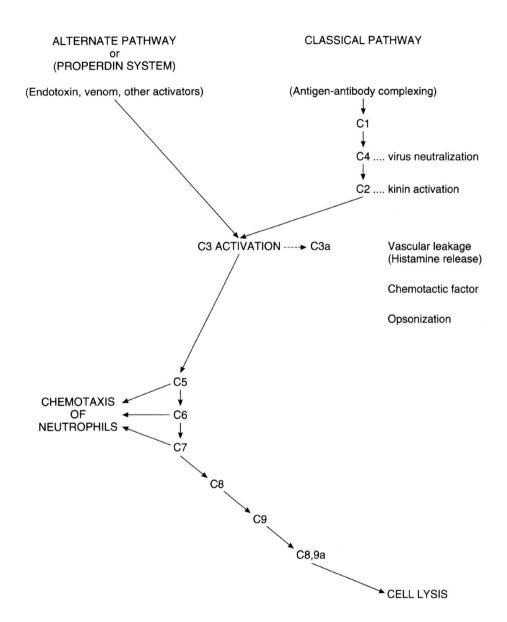

ALTERNATE PATHWAY
or
(PROPERDIN SYSTEM)

(Endotoxin, venom, other activators)

CLASSICAL PATHWAY

(Antigen-antibody complexing)

C1

C4 .... virus neutralization

C2 .... kinin activation

C3 ACTIVATION ----▶ C3a

Vascular leakage
(Histamine release)

Chemotactic factor

Opsonization

C5

CHEMOTAXIS
OF
NEUTROPHILS

C6

C7

C8

C9

C8,9a

CELL LYSIS

they may damage the host tissue. This is seen in *hypersensitivity* or *allergic* reactions. Four categories of hypersensitivity reactions exist: anaphylactic, cytotoxic, immune complex, and delayed-type hypersensitivity.[2,16]

Type I, or anaphylactic (immediate hypersensitivity), reactions are mediated by IgE antibodies, as well as by histamine, PAF, and serotonin. The contact lens patient who develops a sudden allergic reaction to the application of a new cosmetic product or contact lens solution and the patient who develops immediate allergic conjunctivitis to plant pollens are examples of a type I immediate hypersensitivity reaction. In the eye, such histamine-triggering reactions may lead to hyperemia,

chemosis, and itching, and in the adnexa, urticaria (hives) and angioneurotic edema.[17] A systemic example of type I hypersensitivity occurs when a sensitive patient is reexposed to an antibiotic (e.g., penicillin or sulfa), leading to skin rash, bronchospasm, laryngeal edema, and shock. Among contact lens wearers, a reaction known as *contact lens–induced papillary conjunctivitis*, or *giant papillary conjunctivitis*, involves elements of a type I IgE-mediated hypersensitivity reaction, as well as a type IV delayed sensitivity reaction (Figs. 6-5 and 6-6).[18]

Histamine is a vasoactive amine found within the granules of mast cells and basophils (as well as in platelets and in the intestinal tract). Mast cells are found in loose

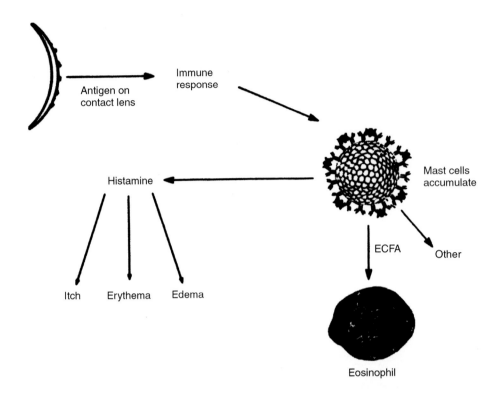

FIG. 6-5. *Type I allergic component in contact lens–induced papillary conjunctivitis. (ECFA = eosinophilic chemotactic factor of anaphylaxis.) (Courtesy of Fisons Pharmaceuticals, Loughborough, England.)*

connective tissue. The cornea and iris have no mast cells, but in contrast, the blood vessel–rich conjunctiva has many.[19] Approximately 50 million mast cells exist in the ocular tissue and adnexa of one human eye.[20] However, mast cells are normally found in the conjunctival substantia propria, not in the epithelium.[3] Therefore, it is not surprising that the conjunctiva is a prime location for ocular inflammation and anaphylactic reactions common to mast cell degranulation. Mast cells also contain

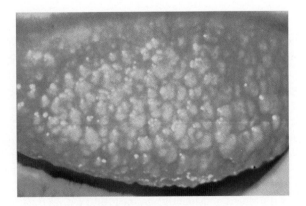

FIG. 6-6. *Giant papillary conjunctivitis. (Courtesy of Fisons Pharmaceuticals, Loughborough, England.)*

heparin (an anticoagulant), serotonin, enzymes, and chemotactic factors for eosinophils, lymphocytes, and neutrophils.[3] In hypersensitivity or allergic states, in which a patient already sensitized to an antigen is reexposed to the same antigen, the offending antigen stimulates an exaggerated inflammatory response by binding to two adjacent IgE molecules on the surface of mast cells (Fig. 6-7). The immediate response is an *anaphylactic reaction* occurring within seconds or minutes after reexposure, in which the mast cells degranulate and secrete mediators. These include preformed mediators already present in the mast cells, such as histamine and eosinophil chemotactic factor of anaphylaxis as well as newly synthesized mediators after allergen exposure. These longer-acting inflammatory substances include slow-reacting substance of anaphylaxis (SRS-A), PAF, and secondarily, the prostaglandins (Fig. 6-8).[2]

Type II, or cytotoxic (complement-dependent), reactions are mediated by antibodies of IgG and IgM, which activate the complement system, resulting in the destruction of cells.

Type III, or immune complex, reactions occur when IgG and IgM antigen-antibody complexes accumulate and activate the complement system. These large complexes result in the release of vasoactive mediators, chemotactic substances, and cytotoxins, which cause exaggerated

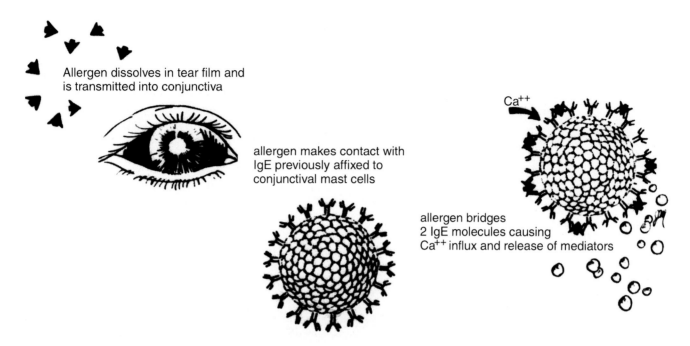

FIG. 6-7. *Mechanism of type I immediate hypersensitivity reactions (ocular allergic reactions) or immunoglobulin IgE–mediated anaphylaxis. (Courtesy of Fisons Pharmaceuticals, Loughborough, England.)*

inflammatory reactions and cell destruction. Neither type II nor type III reactions play a significant role in contact lens–related allergic reactions.

Type IV, or delayed-type hypersensitivity (cell-mediated immunity), reactions are mediated by T cells rather than by antibodies. The T cells release lymphokines, which activate macrophages, causing tissue damage. These delayed-onset reactions occur 1–2 days after presentation

of the antigen (or allergen). The most well-known example of a type IV reaction is the delayed skin reaction occurring after intradermal injection of tuberculin. Among contact lens wearers, a type IV immunologically mediated reaction is likely involved in the development of giant papillary conjunctivitis. Gebhardt and Hamano[21] have postulated that self-proteins may become denatured and adsorbed onto contact lens surfaces, resulting in T cells

FIG. 6-8. *Release of inflammatory mediators in type I ocular allergic reactions. (Courtesy of Fisons Pharmaceuticals, Loughborough, England.)*

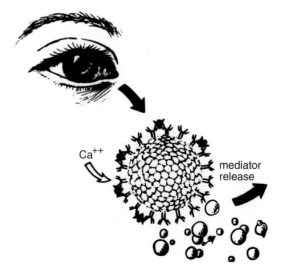

Histamine

- redness and itching

Eosinophil Chemotactic Factor

- attracts eosinophils

Neutrophil Chemotactic Factor

- attracts neutrophils

Other Mediators that Contribute to Inflammation

- leukotrienes
- prostaglandins
- platelet activating factor

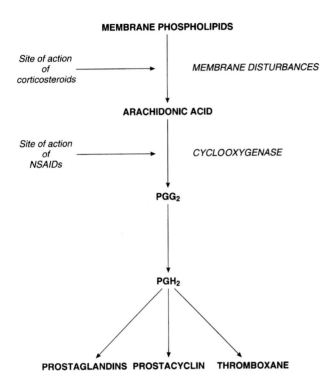

FIG. 6-9. *Schematic showing cyclooxygenase conversion of arachidonic acid into precursors, leading to the formation of prostaglandins. Note the sites of interference by corticosteroids and nonsteroidal anti-inflammatory drugs (NSAIDs). (PGG2 = prostaglandin G; PGH2 = prostaglandin H.)*

reacting to them as non-self. In addition, exogenous substances depositing on contact lens surfaces act as antigens or haptens that may bind to self-protein on corneal or conjunctival epithelial cell membranes. This process activates T cells, triggers the secretion of mediators, and leads to an antigen-antibody response.

Slow-Reacting Substance of Anaphylaxis

SRS-A is a set of peptides that is coupled to an arachidonic acid metabolite. Together, they are known as *leukotrienes*.[2] Whereas histamine produces more rapid and transient effects, SRS-A produces a slow and sustained contraction of smooth muscle. This is particularly evident in the narrowing and obstruction of bronchiolar passageways during a systemic allergic reaction and in asthma.[22,23]

Prostaglandins

Prostaglandins, a complex group of fatty acids, are released from a variety of tissues in response to primarily mechanical inflammatory stimuli. They are synthesized at the local site of tissue inflammation as a result of cell mem-

brane disturbances during mast cell stimulation, and they release arachidonic acid.[4]

Arachidonic acid can be oxygenated by lipoxygenase to produce leukotrienes, or by cyclooxygenase, which produces prostaglandins and thromboxanes. Cyclooxygenase, present in all ocular tissues, has the highest levels concentrated in the conjunctiva (Fig. 6-9).[24] This is not surprising, given the large numbers of mast cells present in this tissue. Cyclooxygenase is also present in moderate levels in the iris and ciliary body, with the lowest ocular levels in the retina and cornea.[4]

Mechanical irritation is the primary stimulus for release of prostaglandins into the anterior chamber as mediators of ocular inflammation. The eye's inflammatory response provoked by the release of prostaglandins includes pupillary miosis, hyperemia, production of cells and protein in the anterior chamber, and subsequent elevation of intraocular pressure.[25,26]

In addition, prostaglandins have been reported to produce the following inflammatory effects[18]:

- Increased vessel permeability (probably related to histamine release from mast cells)
- Chemotactic activity (neutrophils)
- Fever (when injected intravenously)
- Pain (headache; triggering of pain receptors)

Although prostaglandins may be involved in furthering an inflammatory reaction, it is known that they can also inhibit certain inflammatory processes, particularly those caused by release of SRS-A from mast cells in type I hypersensitivity reactions. In this case, prostaglandin activity inhibits the release of SRS-A, which is an important consideration in the management of asthmatic patients.[22]

Neutrophilic Lysosomal Products

Many substances that act as mediators also come into play in inflamed tissues as the result of breakdown of neutrophilic lysosomes. These include cationic proteins, acid proteases, and neutral proteases. The latter are important in that they are responsible for breakdown of tissue in a variety of disease states (e.g., tissue abscesses and arthritis).[7]

Although this chapter touches only the surface of what is known about endogenous inflammatory mediators, a summary of their general effects follows:

- Increased permeability and vascular leakage is caused primarily by histamine, bradykinin, and the prostaglandins
- White blood cell infiltration is mostly triggered by the chemotactic effects of the complement cascade
- Tissue damage is caused primarily by neutrophilic lysosomal breakdown

With so many cascading processes occurring during inflammation, one might wonder why inflammatory reactions are generally self-limiting and why an acute process ever comes to an end. The answer, although highly complex and beyond the scope of this chapter, revolves around the depletion of unstable enzymes, exhaustion of substrate, lymphatic cleansing, cell regeneration and repair as part of wound healing, and tissue modification observed in chronic inflammatory states in which an irritant persists.

It is also clear that inflammation is designed to eliminate foreign agents from the body (especially microbial ones) and to rid the body of damaged tissue, whether from infection or injury. Although it is an inherently protective process, inflammation may be insufficient to deal with the offending onslaught, leading to chronic inflammation, or it may cause physical deformity or immobility (e.g., in rheumatoid arthritis). Therefore, pharmacologic intervention is often necessary to mitigate many of the deleterious effects of the inflammatory process.

PHARMACOLOGIC INTERVENTION IN INFLAMMATION

Pharmacologic agents have proven to be highly successful in mitigating many of the undesirable aspects of the inflammatory response. For example, the nonsteroidal anti-inflammatory drugs (NSAIDs), such as aspirin, indomethacin, and indoxole, can inhibit cyclooxygenase, thus interfering with the production of arachidonic acid and its end products, the prostaglandins.[27] Corticosteroids can also disrupt the production of arachidonic acid by acting on mast cell membrane phospholipids, thus inhibiting prostaglandins.[28]

Although beneficial from a systemic standpoint, aspirin and other salicylates have not found use for controlling inflammation directly within the eye. However, newer NSAIDs have been under development for the control of ocular inflammation, without the significant side effects and ocular complications that accompany the use of corticosteroids (e.g., elevated intraocular pressure, microbial supra-infection, and posterior subcapsular cataract). The use of indomethacin-like drugs to suppress prostaglandin formation and resulting inflammation during the early manipulative stages of ocular surgery, such as in cataract extraction and penetrating keratoplasty, has been very promising.[29] Topical ocular NSAIDs are coming into wider use, not just for postoperative care but also for the management of seasonal allergic itching, for inflammation when steroids are contraindicated, and for the control of pain in corneal abrasions and keratorefractive surgery.

Corticosteroids are the most widely used agents in the treatment of ocular inflammation because of their nonspecific anti-inflammatory properties.[30] *Nonspecific* means that the inhibition of the inflammatory response occurs regardless of whether the etiology stems from infectious, allergic, or traumatic sources. The benefits of corticosteroid therapy[31] arise from their ability to do the following:

- Reduce permeability of blood vessels and the formation of cellular exudates
- Inhibit white blood cell migration
- Inhibit vasoactive mediators
- Inhibit prostaglandin, leukotriene, and thromboxane formation
- Inhibit fibroblast activity
- Inhibit immune reactions

It is important to remember that despite their ability to suppress inflammation, corticosteroids do not treat the actual cause of the inflammatory stimulus. For example, in infectious etiology of inflammation, an antibiotic is required to treat the actual cause, although conservative use of corticosteroids may, at times, be indicated to reduce the sequelae of the inflammatory response. Furthermore, conservative use of steroids is also indicated because their immunosuppressive action can facilitate bacterial, viral, or even fungal supra-infection.[32] Practitioners must closely monitor intraocular pressure when corticosteroids are prescribed because about one-third of the population is genetically predisposed to intraocular pressure elevation with strong topical steroids (*steroid responders*).[31]

Practitioners wishing to use a topical corticosteroid in the presence of contact lens–related immediate hypersensitivity reactions may elect to use the newer soft steroids. Topical steroids, such as *lotoprednol*, are effective in suppressing the signs and symptoms of ocular allergy with much less reason for concern about the more serious side effects of corticosteroid therapy. Other palliative measures to treat acute allergic or anaphylactic reactions include ocular decongestants (topical vasoconstrictors), antihistamines (topical and oral), and cold compresses.

Topical nonsteroidal mast cell stabilizers are effective in suppressing the immediate and long-term effects of type I IgE-mediated hypersensitivity reactions. Cromolyn sodium inhibits mast cell degranulation in the presence of an allergen, thus inhibiting the release of preformed and newly synthesized endogenous mediators.[33] This is also true of lodoxamide, a newer and somewhat more potent topical ophthalmic mast cell stabilizer. These agents have found wide acceptance by practitioners in the treatment of symptoms of hay fever conjunctivitis, vernal conjunctivitis, atopic keratoconjunctivitis, and, in contact lens wearers,

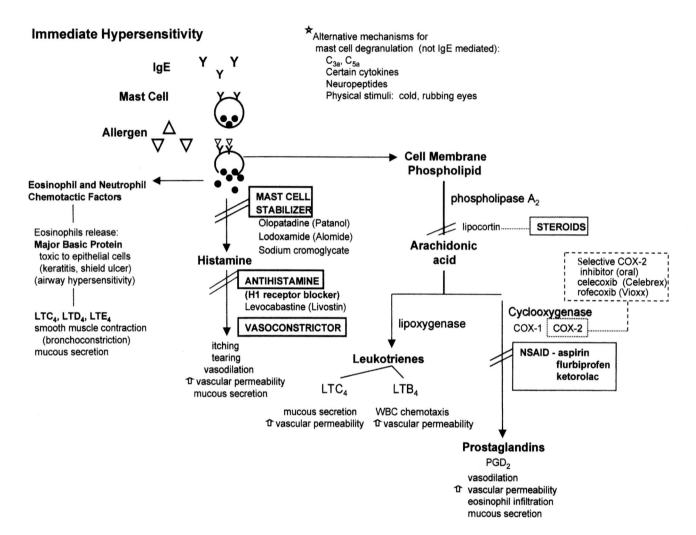

FIG. 6-10. *Overview of sequence of events in immediate hypersensitivity reactions, including levels of inhibitory action of pharmacological agents. (COX-1 = cyclooxygenase-1; COX-2 = cyclooxygenase-2; IgE = immunoglobulin E; LTB$_4$ = leukotriene B; LTC$_4$ = leukotriene C; LTD$_4$ = leukotriene D; LTE$_4$ = leukotriene E; NSAID = nonsteroidal anti-inflammatory drug; PGD$_2$ = prostaglandin D; WBC = white blood cell.) (Courtesy of Dr. Joan Wing.)*

giant papillary conjunctivitis. Figure 6-10 provides an overview of the sequence of events in immediate hypersensitivity reactions as well as the level of inhibition of various pharmacologic agents.

CLINICAL SIGNS OF CONTACT LENS–RELATED INFLAMMATION

Corneal Infiltrates

For the most part, contact lens wear today is quite remarkable, not only for the wide offering of lens designs and materials available for almost all refractive conditions,

but for the excellent physiologic tolerance achieved. Corneal inflammation is not a common observation in the typical contact lens wearer. When corneal inflammation is observed, however, the clinician must be suspicious of several major potential etiologies: corneal infection, underlying chronic blepharitis or related conditions, lens soiling and deposition, and extended wear.

An important sign of corneal inflammation is the presence of corneal infiltrates. Infiltrates are accumulations of cellular components of leaking serum from nearby limbal vessels. Infiltrates may be observed in a quiet eye without obvious clinical signs of inflammation or in single or multiple locations in a "hot" red eye (Figs. 6-11 and 6-12).[34] Contact lens–induced infiltrates are usually observed

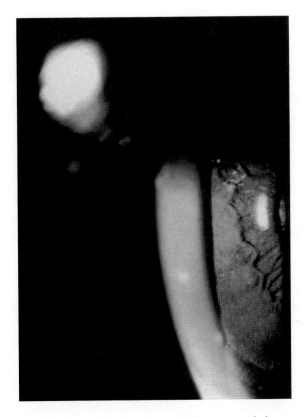

FIG. 6-11. *Infiltrates in a quiet eye with intact epithelium.*

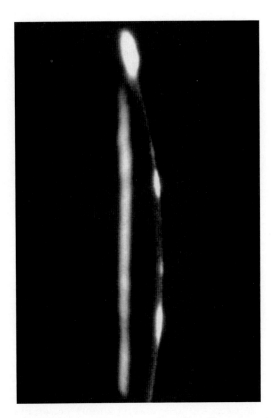

FIG. 6-12. *Multiple infiltrates in a clinically inflamed eye (optic section view).*

within 2 mm of the limbus and may be missed altogether if the upper lid is not raised or if a careful biomicroscopic examination of the limbus, especially superiorly, is not performed. Although speculative, the presence of corneal infiltrates or neovascularization in the superior cornea of hydrogel lens wearers (especially those wearing thick lenses or using lenses on an extended-wear basis) may result from increased hypoxia under the upper lid. The appearance of infiltrates may vary widely, ranging from tiny white or translucent spheric foci in the anterior corneal layers to large, grayish-white *snowball* opacities in the central corneal stroma (Figs. 6-13 and 6-14).[35]

A minimal but ready-to-act level of cellular infiltration may be present in the normal cornea. For example, lymphocytes have been reported in the basal layer of the normal corneal epithelium.[36] Polymorphonuclear leukocytes are known to move easily within the corneal stroma, although their movement is delimited by the presence of Descemet's membrane and an intact corneal epithelium.[37] Stromal keratocytes may also participate in the corneal inflammatory response through their own phagocytic activity.[38]

Cellular infiltration can occur very rapidly as a sign of inflammation, with chemotactic induction of inflammatory cells via the complement pathway, which has been shown to be concentrated in the peripheral cornea.[39] Corneal infiltrates primarily consist of mononuclear cells, such as lymphocytes or polymorphonuclear leukocytes. Viral infection typically induces a lymphocytic response, whereas bacterial infection induces a polymorphonuclear reaction, with neutrophils being the dominant cell type.[40]

One of the more common causes of marginal limbal infiltrates is a response to staphylococcal exotoxins present in chronic blepharitis. These sterile infiltrates are typically associated with generalized conjunctival hyperemia and superficial punctate staining of the inferior cornea, primarily as a consequence of increased concentration and contact time of exotoxins in the inferior cul-de-sac during sleep. The staphylococcal toxins involved are the α, β, γ, and δ toxins, as well as exfoliative toxin and leukocidin, all of which contribute to neutrophilic clouding of the cornea in these marginal areas.[41] Ovoid, grayish-white marginal catarrhal ulcers are actually aggregates of sterile infiltrates. They may be seen inferiorly or circumfer-

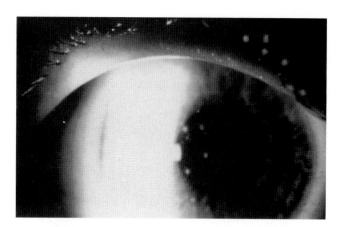

FIG. 6-13. *Infiltrates appearing as small, spheric foci in a white (quiet) eye. (Reprinted with permission from JE Josephson, S Zantos, BE Caffery, et al: Differentiation of corneal complications observed in contact lens wearers. J Am Optom Assoc 59:679, 1988.)*

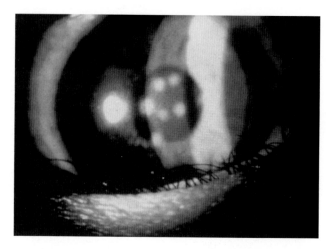

FIG. 6-14. *Infiltrates appearing as large stromal snowball opacities as an inflammatory reaction to long-term exposure to thimerosal. (Reprinted with permission from JA Silbert: Contact lens–related inflammatory reactions. p. 7. In ES Bennett, BA Weissman [eds]: Clinical Contact Lens Practice. Lippincott, Philadelphia, 1991.)*

entially and often exhibit a clear zone separating them from the limbus (Fig. 6-15). Unlike infectious corneal ulcers, these recurrent lesions do not lead to thinning, perforation, or vision loss, and they represent an immune reaction to the presence of staphylococcal toxins.[41]

Phlyctenulosis represents a related but more severe reaction, with pinkish-white limbal nodules and an inflammatory vascular leash or pannus. One or more phlyctenulae may progress into clear cornea, producing thinning, scarring, and vascularization (Fig. 6-16). Healing occurs within 10–15 days. Phlyctenular keratoconjunctivitis is typically bilateral and affects young children and young adults, with a higher incidence in females.[42] Corneal involvement produces pain, photophobia, and sometimes vision loss. Before 1950, the disease was caused primarily by a hypersensitivity reaction to tuberculin protein. Since 1950 and the concomitant decline of tuberculosis in the United States, the primary cause of phlyctenular keratoconjunctivitis has been a local immune reaction to *Staphylococcus aureus* antigens, producing a type IV hypersensitivity reaction.[42–45]

Treatment for blepharitis, marginal ulcers, and phlyctenulae should be directed toward the underlying disease. Blepharitis should be treated aggressively with lid hygiene and topical antibiotics.[46] Marginal infiltrates respond very well to topical steroids, which can be prescribed alone or in combination with a topical antibiotic. Care should be exercised, as with any use of topical steroids, to monitor intraocular pressure. As the therapeutic effect is achieved, treatment should be slowly tapered, and regular lid hygiene is also recommended to

reduce the volume of staphylococcal toxins. With phlyctenulosis, despite favorable response to topical corticosteroid therapy, when treatment is discontinued, the disease often recurs.[47] A study by Culbertson et al. (1993) of 17 young patients with phlyctenular keratoconjunctivitis showed that a prompt and long-lasting remission could be achieved through the use of oral tetracycline or erythromycin.[45] The beneficial effects of these antibiotics were not related to anti-inflammatory effects but rather to the elimination of concurrent microbial infection, primarily *Chlamydia trachomatis* or *Propionibacterium acnes*.

Corneal infiltrates occur more frequently with hydrogel lens wear than with gas-permeable contact lenses.[35] Among wearers of extended-wear hydrogel lenses, corneal infiltrates are commonly observed. They are similar to those seen in association with staphylococcal blepharitis and may indicate a reaction to antigens on the lens surface.[48] Several studies have shown that contact lens wear can increase the level of plasmin in the tear film, a substance which inhibits wound healing and which is also responsible for the chemotaxis of leukocytes.[49–51] Although the open-eye precorneal tear fluid contains lysozyme, lactoferrin, and tear-specific tear albumin, the closed-eye tear proteins are altered such that secretory IgA and albumin become dominant, with activation of complement C3 and plasminogen.[52] Sack et al. (1992) postulated that this subclinical inflammatory environment in the closed eye may serve as a protective function against pathogens trapped under the closed lids and may be exacerbated

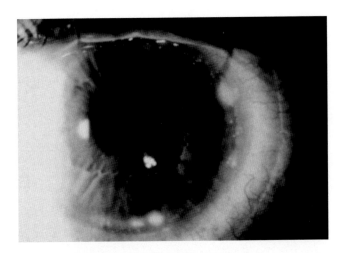

FIG. 6-15. *Marginal catarrhal ulcers ring the cornea as an inflammatory reaction to staphylococcal exotoxins. (Courtesy of Dr. Joshua Josephson.) (Reprinted with permission from JA Silbert: Contact lens–related inflammatory reactions. p. 7. In ES Bennett, BA Weissman [eds]: Clinical Contact Lens Practice. Lippincott, Philadelphia, 1991.)*

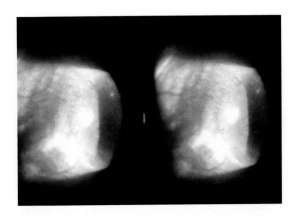

FIG. 6-16. *Phlyctenulosis with scarring and pannus as an inflammatory consequence of staphylococcal exotoxins. (Reprinted with permission from JA Silbert: Ocular inflammation and contact lens wear. p. 221. In A Tomlinson [ed]: Complications of Contact Lens Wear. Mosby–Year Book, St. Louis, 1992.)*

under conditions of overnight wear of hydrogel contact lenses.[53] Indeed, the issues involving alteration of mediators in the precorneal tear fluid and in corneal tissue under conditions of extended wear are very complex and not well understood; they are the subject of intense investigation. The lack of knowledge concerning these issues is illustrated by the paradoxical clinical observation that increased levels of peripheral infiltrates exist among wearers of disposable contact lenses worn on an extended-wear basis compared to those wearing conventional extended-wear lenses. One might predict that if increasing levels of lens deposits and post-lens debris are associated with the development of corneal infiltration, there should be a higher incidence of corneal infiltrates with conventional (nondiscarded) hydrogel lenses. Several investigations, however, have demonstrated trends toward an increased level of infiltration in wearers of disposable extended-wear lenses.[54–60] Many factors may be responsible for these observations, including the use of disposable lenses for longer than the intended period, less stringent criteria exercised by practitioners in prescribing disposable lenses, liberalized lens care regimens advocated by practitioners, lack of lens rubbing during the lens cleaning process, lens edge defects, and a more cavalier attitude demonstrated by patients toward disposable lenses. Until controlled studies can identify the factors responsible for the inflammatory events associated with overnight lens wear of hydrogel lenses or provide the clinician with new lens materials and pharmacologic tools to reduce the inflam-

matory consequences, practitioners must rely on clinical prudence in managing corneal infiltration.

When infiltrates are observed in a patient wearing contact lenses, the patient should temporarily discontinue lens wear until they are resolved. This is unquestionably difficult, particularly when the patient is asymptomatic and the eye appears grossly quiet. Patient education is imperative to obtain good compliance. If the patient is symptomatic, however, the practitioner must rule out infectious keratitis. Corneal infection must be assumed if a corneal epithelial defect exists with an underlying zone of infiltration, and immediate and aggressive therapy should be initiated after cultures are taken (Fig. 6-17).[61] In the absence of infection, lens discontinuance usually leads to resolution of symptoms, often before the infiltrates themselves resolve. Infiltrates in patients who wear hydrogel extended-wear lenses are at higher risk of being infectious or becoming infectious owing to the association of poor tear exchange under these lenses, bacterial adherence to the lenses, and chronic hypoxia.[62,63] Close monitoring of these patients is essential, with lens wear reinstituted only when infiltrates have cleared, and then only on a daily-wear basis with fresh lenses. Disposable lenses are desirable if the patient later resumes extended wear, although their use is not a guarantee that an infiltrative reaction will not recur. Indeed, infiltrative reactions, sterile and infectious, have been observed with disposable extended-wear lenses.[64] Therefore, daily wear is mandatory should a similar reaction recur. In general, after an infiltrative or red-eye episode with disposable hydrogel extended-wear lenses, the best advice to give a patient is that extended wear should be avoided. With the

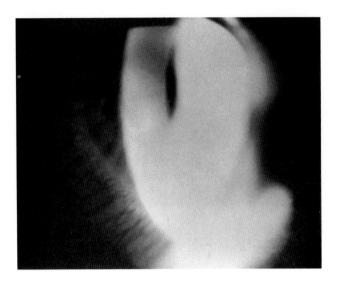

FIG. 6-17. *Infiltrates in ulcerative bacterial keratitis. Note fluorescein staining of epithelial defect overlying the infiltration.*

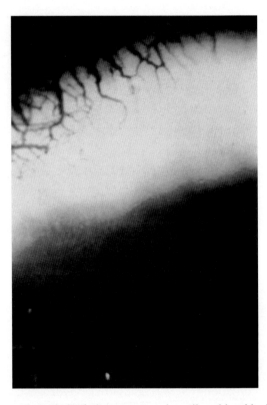

FIG. 6-18. *Early limbal congestion of capillary blood bed.*

introduction of newer high-Dk soft lens polymers for extended wear to reduce the consequences of hypoxia, the rates of inflammatory complications can be compared in controlled studies.

NEOVASCULARIZATION

McMonnies[65] has shown that hypoxia, vascular compression from tight-fitting contact lenses, trauma from damaged lenses, and toxic and inflammatory stimuli are all potential causes of corneal vascularization. Although these problems are much less commonly encountered with more oxygen-transmissive lens materials and generally nonsensitizing lens care systems, vascularization is still observed as a complication of hydrogel lens wear (Figs. 6-18–6-20). In fact, patients who wear hydrogel lenses overnight may develop vascularization from any or all the triggering stimuli.

A chronically dilated limbal vessel plexus is believed to be one of the initial steps in the development of corneal vascularization. This finding is observed commonly among wearers of hydrogel lenses,[66] as is the finding of increased bulbar conjunctival injection.[67,68]

Theories to explain the development of corneal vascularization from contact lens wear have included loss of compactness of limbal tissue from stromal edema[69,70] as well as effects of chemotactic mediators. Studies have shown, however, that edematous stromal softening alone is not an adequate stimulus for vascularization because a

reduced swelling response exists in the peripheral cornea and limbal region compared to the central cornea.[71,72] This further sheds doubt on the theory that peripheral corneal edema is responsible for corneal vascularization.

A vasostimulatory or angiogenic factor is released by existing blood vessels, which triggers the development of fibroblasts, pericytes, smooth muscle cells, and new vascular endothelial cells.[73] Although it is not clear how hypoxia exerts its vasostimulatory effect on the limbal arcades, it is believed that prostaglandins are directly involved in these inflammatory mechanisms.[74] Furthermore, additional evidence exists for plasminogen activator as a factor in the development of corneal vascularization in the use of hydrogel extended-wear lenses.[50,75]

Efron[76] has described a sequence of events in a proposed model of corneal vascularization in which hypoxia and epithelial microtrauma are the triggering factors (Fig. 6-21):

Contact lens hypoxia leads to corneal edema and stromal softening. Microtrauma from contact lens wear releases enzymes that are chemotactic for inflammatory cells. When the cells reach the area of epithelial damage, they, in turn, release angiogenic factors that stimulate new vessel spikes toward the site of injury.

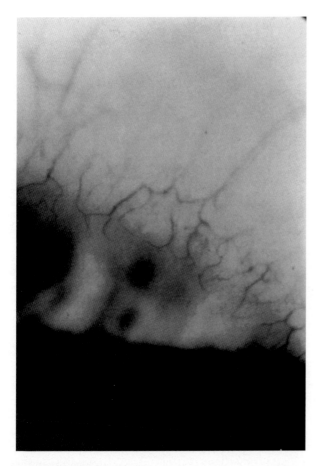

FIG. 6-19. *Vascular spike formation as an angiogenic response in contact lens hypoxia. (Reprinted with permission from JA Silbert: Contact lens–related inflammatory reactions. In ES Bennett, BA Weissman [eds]: Clinical Contact Lens Practice. Lippincott, Philadelphia, 1991.)*

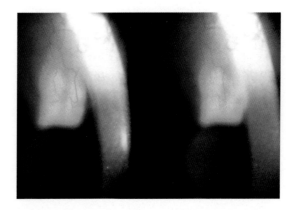

FIG. 6-20. *Advanced neovascularization as a vasostimulatory response to hypoxia in a long-term wearer of hydrogel extended-wear lenses. (Reprinted with permission from JA Silbert: Ocular inflammation and contact lens wear. p. 221. In A Tomlinson [ed]: Complications of Contact Lens Wear. Mosby–Year Book, St. Louis, 1992.)*

Consult Chapter 5 for an in-depth discussion of the effects of vascularization from contact lens wear.

Contact Lens–Induced Acute Red-Eye Syndrome

An acute inflammatory response in some patients wearing extended-wear hydrogel lenses has been termed *contact lens–induced acute red eye*, or CLARE.[77] The patient, wearing a tightly adherent lens, is typically awakened in the early morning hours with severe unilateral ocular pain, photophobia, lacrimation, and injection. Although epithe-

FIG. 6-21. *A dual-etiology model of contact lens–induced corneal vascularization. (Reprinted with permission from N Efron: Vascular response of the cornea to contact lens wear. J Am Optom Assoc 58:836, 1987.)*

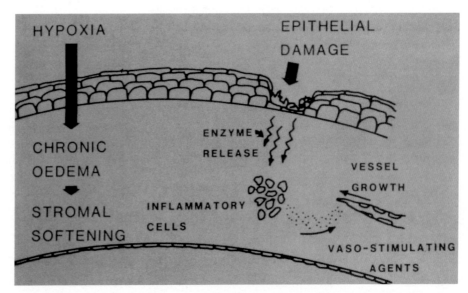

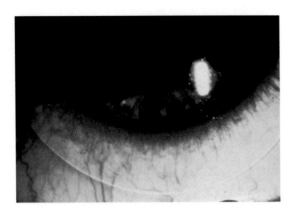

FIG. 6-22. *Tightly adherent hydrogel extended-wear lens in the acute red-eye syndrome. (Reprinted with permission from JA Silbert: Contact lens–related inflammatory reactions. p. 7. In ES Bennett, BA Weissman [eds]: Clinical Contact Lens Practice. Lippincott, Philadelphia, 1991.)*

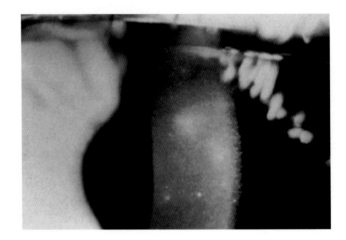

FIG. 6-23. *Infiltrative response in acute red-eye syndrome. (Reprinted with permission from Silbert JA: Microbial infection in contact lens patients. p. 571. In MG Harris [ed]: Problems in Optometry: Contact Lenses and Ocular Disease. Lippincott, Philadelphia, 1990.)*

lial corneal insult is not usually seen, subepithelial or anterior stromal infiltrates are often present in the midperiphery of the cornea or adjacent to the limbus (Figs. 6-22 and 6-23).[78] The majority of cases are unilateral, and may be recurrent if extended wear is not discontinued.[79] In many cases of CLARE reactions, immobile extended-wear lenses or lenses with insufficient movement are observed, suggesting that this is an important contributing factor.[80]

The CLARE syndrome can also be caused by inflammatory toxic effects from post-lens debris and neutrophils under an immobile lens,[81] from mechanical irritation,[82] from dehydration of the tear film during sleep,[83] and from hypersensitivity or toxicity to solution preservatives.[84,85] Although it is almost exclusively a hydrogel lens complication, CLARE syndrome has been reported with persistent lens adherence in extended-wear gas-permeable lens use.[5,86] Vajdic and Holden[87] have documented CLARE syndrome in a patient wearing a bound silicone elastomer lens overnight, indicating that it is unlikely that hypoxia is an etiologic factor.

A number of studies have implicated bacterial contamination or the production of bacterial toxins as etiologic factors in CLARE syndrome.[88,89] Gram-negative bacterial contamination is seen more frequently in patients experiencing a CLARE reaction.[90] This is further supported by a study (Holden et al., 1996)[91] in which inadvertent contamination of hydrogel contact lenses worn overnight led to CLARE syndrome in 33% of subjects, and the production of corneal infiltrates in an additional 42% of subjects.

Because the potential for infectious keratitis is evident in a case of a suddenly painful eye in a patient using extended-wear hydrogel lenses, the clinician must make a careful differential diagnosis when examining such an acutely distressed patient. Because only corneal infiltration without epithelial involvement exists in CLARE syndrome, the syndrome has typically been managed by lens discontinuation and palliative therapy, with infiltrates resolving over a period of several days to a few weeks.[92] Although topical corticosteroids can reduce the inflammatory reaction seen with CLARE syndrome, their use without an antibiotic cover in a patient experiencing acute extended-wear hypoxia is risky.[93] A better approach, in addition to immediate lens discontinuance and palliative measures, is to institute broad-spectrum coverage, either with topical fluoroquinolones (ciprofloxacin or oxyfloxacin) or with topical aminoglycosides (tobramycin or gentamicin) during the initial 24- to 48-hour period after the CLARE reaction.[1]

Lens wear should be resumed only after all signs and symptoms of ocular inflammation have disappeared. Refitting the patient with more loosely fitting hydrogel lenses, preferably on a daily-wear basis, along with a preservative-free peroxide disinfection system is prudent. Disposable extended-wear lenses worn on a weekly replacement schedule can reduce, although not eliminate, the incidence of CLARE syndrome.[94]

Contact Lens–Induced Superior Limbic Keratoconjunctivitis

An inflammatory reaction that has affected some hydrogel lens wearers using thimerosal in their lens care products is known as contact lens–induced superior limbic keratoconjunctivitis (CL-SLK). Although not associated with thyroid disease or with a predilection for middle-aged women, CL-SLK often mimics the clinical appearance of true superior limbic keratoconjunctivitis. The clinical syndrome of CL-SLK includes the following observations[1]:

- Intense hyperemia of the superior bulbar conjunctiva, with radiating vessels
- Epithelial and subepithelial infiltrates
- Superior corneal and limbal punctate staining
- A fine papillary hypertrophy of the superior tarsal conjunctiva

Corneal changes observed in CL-SLK can reduce central acuity because the inflammatory signs often progressively encroach on the visual axis. Of diagnostic assistance is the appearance of a V-shaped wedge of corneal changes, with its apex directed toward the pupil (Fig. 6-24).[1] The condition is typically bilateral and can usually be resolved by temporary lens discontinuation for several weeks to months while corneal signs regress, and total abstinence from thimerosal-containing lens care products. The patient's old lenses should be discarded, whenever possible, rather than attempting to purge the lenses. Empty ghost vessels may remain as the condition subsides, but they should not refill when the patient resumes lens wear with a thimerosal-free disinfection system (preferably a preservative-free hydrogen peroxide system). If the patient had no history of prior thimerosal usage, CL-SLK must be presumed to have a mechanical cause, and refitting with another lens design or polymer is warranted.

Giant Papillary Conjunctivitis

Consult Chapter 7 in this text for an in-depth discussion of the inflammatory and allergic manifestations of contact lens–related papillary conjunctivitis and its more severe form, giant papillary conjunctivitis.

Inflammatory Consequences of Microbial Keratitis

Ocular infection is an ominous finding that suggests pronounced inflammatory signs and symptoms. Nevertheless, microbial infection may not always produce pain or the gross appearance of a red eye. The use of an extended-wear hydrogel lens, for example, may actually mask some signs and symptoms of incipient corneal infection (probably owing to the bandage-like effect of the lens polymer). Clinicians often see the sequelae of prior episodes of corneal

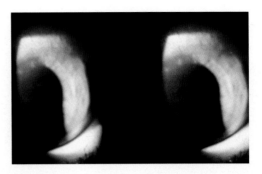

FIG. 6-24. *Contact lens–related superior limbic keratoconjunctivitis (CL-SLK). Note vascularization and infiltrates affecting the superior cornea, with apex of V-shaped zone aimed toward pupil. (Reprinted with permission from JA Silbert: Contact lens–related inflammatory reactions. p. 7. In ES Bennett, BA Weissman [eds]: Clinical Contact Lens Practice. Lippincott, Philadelphia, 1991.)*

ulcers, particularly in the extended-wear patient, in the form of healed round stromal scars, yet the patient denies any history of frank pain or red-eye reactions. It has been seen that the sole presence of corneal infiltrates signifies inflammation rather than infection. For a confirmed diagnosis of infection, the clinician must employ a thorough patient history, careful biomicroscopic examination, laboratory tests, and clinical intuition.

The cornea of a contact lens wearer is exposed to microbial challenge from the lenses themselves, from tears, and from lid margins. In addition, the cornea is also exposed to contaminants in lens cases, in contact lens solutions, and from patients' hands as well as from the effects of lens-related mechanical trauma and hypoxia.

The precorneal tear film contains many antimicrobial substances. These include lysozyme, lactoferrin, ceruloplasmin, lymphocytes, immunoglobulins, and complement, to name just a few. Despite these protective mechanisms, a small epithelial defect is often all that is required to enable opportunistic bacteria in the tear film, in the corneal epithelium, or adherent to the lenses themselves to invade the stroma and set up an infection.[1]

Clinical evidence for infection depends on the presence of an epithelial lesion with an underlying cellular infiltration. The presence of any of the following signs further increases the level of suspicion of microbial keratitis: pain, photophobia, mucopurulent discharge, exudate on the corneal surface, and decreased vision (Figs. 6-25 and 6-26). These signs, however, are nonspecific. Although treatment may be initiated with a potent broad-spectrum topical antibiotic, such as a fluoroquinolone, one is always concerned if such therapy does not stem the infection. As

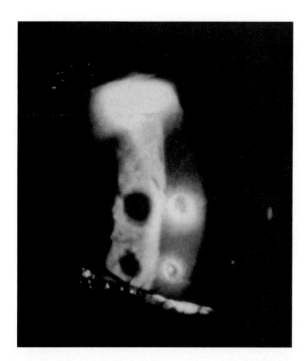

FIG. 6-25. *Paracentral corneal ulcers caused by Staphylococcus aureus in a wearer of hydrogel extended-wear lenses. (Reprinted with permission from JA Silbert: Complications of extended wear. In JG Classé [ed]: Extended Wear Contact Lenses. Optometry Clinics 1:95, 1991.)*

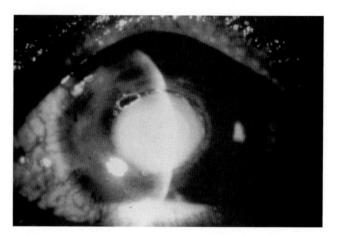

FIG. 6-27. *Immune ring (surrounding central lesion) caused by endotoxins in a patient with a corneal ulcer.*

such, identification of the specific pathogen or pathogens still requires the use of cultures and sensitivities.[95]

Inflammation is heightened in microbial keratitis because associated release of tissue-damaging toxins occurs. Bacteria that are actively replicating elicit exotoxins, whereas endotoxins are released by certain bacteria only after micro-

bial death, producing ring infiltrates and even greater tissue damage.[96] Immune rings or ring-shaped lesions are believed to involve an immune reaction[97] triggered by bacterial endotoxin through the alternate or properdin pathway of complement activation (Fig. 6-27; see also Fig. 6-4).[98,99] Enzymes released by virulent bacteria also contribute to tissue damage. These include collagenases, coagulases, proteases, nucleases, lipases, elastase, fibrinolysins, and hemolysins.[57] A strain of *Pseudomonas aeruginosa*, for example, produces a necrotizing enzyme, proteoglycanase, that breaks down the protective ground substance around collagen.[100] Exotoxin A, which impairs phagocytosis and inhibits cellular protein synthesis, along with the effects of other enzymes, contributes to rapid stromal melting, descemetocele formation, and even corneal perforation in pseudomonal infections.[95]

See Chapter 12 for an in-depth discussion of the diagnosis and management of ulcerative keratitis.

CONCLUSION

This chapter reviews the basic mechanisms of inflammation, with specific reference to the anterior ocular segment and contact lens wear. Inflammation can arise from infectious, allergic, toxic, and mechanical causes. A highly complex sequence of interrelated events is initiated during any inflammatory reaction. Although inflammation is protective in its design, it can be incomplete or excessive in its response, leading paradoxically to actual loss of function of the tissue it was designed to protect. This double-edged sword of inflammation is a complex and still incompletely understood phenomenon.

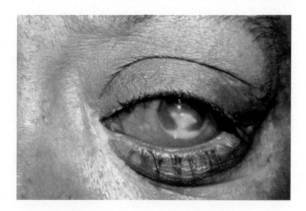

FIG. 6-26. *Ulcerative keratitis caused by Pseudomonas aeruginosa. Note large central infiltration, adherent exudate, hypopeon, and intense bulbar injection.*

The clinical consequences of inflammation are reviewed, with special attention to inflammatory reactions and syndromes affecting the contact lens patient. The judicious use of pharmacologic intervention can be important in reducing the negative sequelae of ocular inflammation and in preserving function and maintaining patient comfort. The eye care practitioner must be vigilant to recognize the signs and symptoms of inflammation, to make an appropriate diagnosis, and to act swiftly in suppressing the adverse reactions associated with the inflammatory response.

REFERENCES

1. Silbert JA: Ocular inflammation and contact lens wear. p. 221. In Tomlinson A (ed): Complications of Contact Lens Wear. Mosby-Year Book, St. Louis, 1992

2. Benjamini E, Sunshine G, Leskowitz S: Immunology: A Short Course, 3rd ed. Wiley-Liss, New York, 1996

3. Allansmith MR: Immunology of the external ocular tissues. J Am Optom Assoc 61:S16, 1990

4. Leopold IH, Gaster RN: Ocular inflammation and anti-inflammatory drugs. p. 67. In Kaufman HE, Barron BA, McDonald MB, Waltman SR (eds): The Cornea. Churchill Livingstone, New York, 1988

5. Rosenbaum JT, Boney RS, Samples JR, et al: Synthesis of platelet activating factor by ocular tissue from inflamed eyes. Arch Ophthalmol 109:410, 1991

6. Majno G, Shea SM, Leventhal M: Endothelial contraction induced by histamine-type mediators: an electron microscopic study. J Cell Biol 42:647, 1969

7. Ryan GB, Majno G: Inflammation. The Upjohn Co, Kalamazoo, MI, 1977

8. Klebanoff SJ: Iodination of bacteria: a bacterial mechanism. J Exp Med 126:1063, 1967

9. Klebanoff SJ: Intraleukocytic microbicidal defects. Annu Rev Med 22:39, 1971

10. Basu PK, Minta JO: Chemotactic migration of leukocytes through corneal layers: an in vitro study. Can J Ophthalmol 11:235, 1976

11. Butrus SI, Abelson MB: Importance of limbal examination in ocular allergic disease. Ann Ophthalmol 20:101, 1988

12. Pfortner T, DeAldama EB, Korbenfeld P, et al: Immunological action of the precorneal tear film with the use of contact lenses. Int Contact Lens Clin 4:65, 1977

13. Meyers RL, Pettit TH: Chemotaxis of polymorphonuclear leukocytes in corneal inflammation: tissue injury in Herpes simplex virus infection. Invest Ophthalmol 13:187, 1974

14. Ward PA, Lepow IH, Neuman LJ: Bacterial factors chemotactic for polymorphonuclear leukocytes. Am J Pathol 52:725, 1968

15. Foster CS: Basic ocular immunology. p. 101. In Kaufman HE, Barron BA, McDonald MB, Waltman SR (eds): The Cornea. Churchill Livingstone, New York, 1988

16. Gell P, Coombs R: Clinical Aspects of Immunology. p.317. Blackwell, Oxford, 1963

17. Jennings B: Mechanisms, diagnosis, and management of common ocular allergies. J Am Optom Assoc 61:S32, 1991

18. Allansmith MR: Giant papillary conjunctivitis. J Am Optom Assoc 61:S42, 1991

19. Allansmith MR, Greiner JV, Baird RS: Number of inflammatory cells in the normal conjunctiva. Am J Ophthalmol 86:250, 1978

20. Allansmith MR: The Eye and Immunology. Mosby, St Louis, 1982

21. Gebhardt B, Hamano H: Ocular surface immune reactions and contact lens wear. p.176. In Hamano H, Kaufman HE (eds): Corneal Physiology and Disposable Contact Lenses. Butterworth–Heinemann, Boston, 1997

22. Brocklehurst WE: The release of histamine and formation of a slow-reacting substance (SRS-A) during anaphylactic shock. J Physiol 151:416, 1960

23. Orange RP, Austen KF: Slow reacting substance of anaphylaxis. Adv Immunol 10:105, 1969

24. Bhattacherjee P, Eakins KE: Inhibition of the PG-synthetase systems in ocular tissues by indomethacin. Br J Pharmacol 15:209, 1973

25. Ambache N, Kavanaugh L, Whiting J: Effect of mechanical stimulation on rabbits' eyes: release of active substance in anterior chamber perfusates. J Physiol 176:378, 1965

26. Silbert JA: Prostaglandins and the ocular inflammatory response. Rev Optom 115:53, 1978

27. Vane JR: Inhibition of prostaglandin synthesis as a mechanism of action for aspirin-like drugs. Nature [New Biol] 231:232, 1971

28. Flower RJ, Blackwell GJ: Anti-inflammatory steroids induce biosynthesis of a phospholipase A_2 inhibitor which prevents prostaglandin generation. Nature 278:456, 1979

29. Frucht-Pery J, Zauberman H: The effect of indomethacin on prostaglandin E_2 in human cornea and conjunctiva. Arch Ophthalmol 110:343, 1992

30. Shlaegel TF: Nonspecific treatment of uveitis. p. 3. In Duane TD (ed): Clinical Ophthalmology. Vol. 4. Harper & Row, Philadelphia, 1986

31. Bartlett JD: Pharmacology of allergic eye disease. J Am Optom Assoc 61:S23, 1990

32. Jaanus SD: Anti-inflammatory drugs. p. 163. In Bartlett JD, Jaanus SD (eds): Clinical Ocular Pharmacology. 2nd ed. Butterworth, Boston, 1989

33. Allansmith MR, Ross RN: Ocular allergy and mast cell stabilizers. Surv Ophthalmol 30:229, 1986

34. Josephson JE, Zantos S, Caffery BE, et al: Differentiation of corneal complications observed in contact lens wearers. J Am Optom Assoc 59:679, 1988

35. Josephson JE, Caffery BE: Infiltrative keratitis in hydrogel lens wearers. Int Contact Lens Clin 6:223, 1979

36. Marshall J, Grindall J: Fine structure of the cornea and its development. Br J Ophthalmol 98:320, 1978

37. Basu PK, Minta JO: Chemotactic migration of leukocytes through corneal layers: an in vitro study. Can J Ophthalmol 11:235, 1976

38. Madigan MC, Penfold PL, Holden BA, Billson FA: Ultra-structural features of contact lens-induced deep corneal neovascularization and associated stromal leucocytes. Cornea 9:144, 1990

39. Mondino BJ, Ratajczak HV, Goldberg DB, et al: Alternate and classical pathway components of complement in the normal cornea. Arch Ophthalmol 98:346, 1980

40. Leibowitz HM. Inflammation of the cornea: basic principles. p. 265. In HM Leibowitz (ed): Corneal Disorders: Clinical Diagnosis and Management. Saunders, Philadelphia, 1984

41. Mannis MJ: Bacterial conjunctivitis. p. 193. In Kaufman HE, Barron BA, McDonald MB, Waltman SR (eds): The Cornea. Churchill Livingstone, New York, 1988

42. Robin JB, Dugel R: Immunologic disorders of the cornea and conjunctiva. p. 545. In Kaufman HE, Barron BA, McDonald MB, Waltman SR (eds): The Cornea. Churchill Livingstone, New York, 1988

43. Mondino BJ, Kowalski HV: Phlyctenulae and catarrhal infiltrates. Arch Ophthalmol 100:1968, 1982

44. Thygeson PL: The etiology and treatment of phlyctenular keratoconjunctivitis. Am J Ophthalmol 9:446, 1975

45. Culbertson WW, Huang JW, Mandelbaum SH, et al: Effective treatment of phlyctenular keratoconjunctivitis with oral tetracycline. Ophthalmology 100:1358, 1993

46. Silbert JA: Contact lens related pathology: Part 1. Rev Optom 121:104, 1984

47. Smith RE, Dippe DW, Miller SD: Phlyctenular kerato-conjunctivitis: results of penetrating keratoplasty in Alaskan natives. Ophthalmic Surg 6:62, 1975

48. Dart JG, Badenoch PR: Bacterial adherence to contact lenses. CLAO J 12:220, 1986

49. Tervo T, van Setten GB, Andersson R, et al: Contact lens wear is associated with the appearance of plasmin in the tear fluid-preliminary results. Graefes Arch Clin Exp Ophthalmol 227:42, 1989

50. van Setten GB, Tervo T, Andersson R, et al: Plasmin and epidermal growth factor in the tear fluid of contact-lens wearers: effect of wearing different types of contact lenses and association with clinical findings. Ophthalmic Res 232:233, 1990

51. Vannas A, Sweeney DF, Holden BA, et al: Tear plasmin activity with contact lens wear. Curr Eye Res 11:243, 1992

52. Vajdic CM, Holden BA: Extended-wear contact lenses. p.127. In: Hamano H, Kaufman HE (eds): Corneal Physiology and Disposable Contact Lenses. Butterworth–Heinemann, Boston, 1997

53. Sack RA, Tan KO, Tan A: Diurnal tear cycle: evidence for a nocturnal inflammatory constitutive tear fluid. Invest Ophthalmol Vis Sci 33:626, 1992

54. Poggio EC, Abelson M: Complications and symptoms in disposable extended wear lenses compared with conventional soft daily wear and soft extended wear lenses. CLAO J 19:31, 1993

55. Boswall GJ, Ehlers WH, Luistro A, et al: A comparison of conventional and disposable extended wear contact lenses. CLAO J 19:158, 1993

56. Baum J, Barza M: *Pseudomonas* keratitis and extended wear soft contact lenses. Arch Ophthalmol 108:663, 1990

57. Port M: A European multicentre extended wear study of the New Vues disposable contact lens. Contact Lens J 19:86, 1991

58. Maguen E, Rosner I, Caroline P, et al: A retrospective study of disposable extended wear lenses in 100 patients: year 2. CLAO J 18:229, 1992

59. Maguen E, Rosner I, Caroline P, et al: A retrospective study of disposable extended wear lenses in 100 patients: year 3. CLAO J 20:179, 1994

60. Efron N, Veys J: Defects in disposable contact lenses can compromise ocular integrity. Int Contact Lens Clin 19:8, 1992

61. Silbert JA: Microbial infection in contact lens patients. p. 571. In Harris MG (ed): Problems in Optometry: Contact Lenses and Ocular Disease. Lippincott, Philadelphia, 1990

62. Stern GA, Zam ZS: The pathogenesis of contact lens-associated *Pseudomonas aeruginosa* corneal ulceration: 1. The effect of contact lens coatings on adherence of *Pseudomonas aeruginosa* to soft contact lenses. Cornea 5:41, 1987

63. Slusher MM, Myrvik QN, Lewis JC, et al: Extended wear lenses, biofilm, and bacterial adhesion. Arch Ophthalmol 105:110, 1987

64. Maguen E, Tsai JC, Martinez M, et al: A retrospective study of disposable extended-wear lenses in 100 patients. Ophthalmology 98:1685, 1991

65. McMonnies CW: Risk factors in the etiology of contact lens-induced vascularization. Int Contact Lens Clin 11:286, 1984

66. Zantos SG: The ocular response to continuous wear of contact lenses. PhD thesis, School of Optometry, University of New South Wales, Sydney, 1981

67. Holden BA: Corneal requirements for extended wear: an update. CLAO J 14:220, 1988

68. Gautier C, Holden B, Terry R: Can contact lens wearers be correctly identified from their "appearance?" Invest Ophthalmol Vis Sci 33(suppl.): 1294, 1992

69. Cogan DG: Vascularization of the cornea. Arch Ophthalmol 41:406, 1949

70. Tomlinson A, Haas DD: Changes in corneal thickness and circumcorneal vascularization with contact lens wear. Int Contact Lens Clin 7:45, 1980

71. Maurice DM, Zauberman H, Michaelson IC: The stimulus to neovascularization in the cornea. Exp Eye Res 5:168, 1966

72. Holden BA, McNally JJ, Mertz GW, Swarbrick HA: Topographical corneal oedema. Acta Ophthalmol (Copenh) 63:684, 1985

73. Larke JR: The Eye in Contact Lens Wear. Butterworth, Boston, 1985

74. Cooper CA, Bergamini MVW, Leopold IH: Use of flurbiprofen to inhibit corneal vascularization. Arch Ophthalmol 98:1102, 1980

75. Berman M, Winthrop S, Ausprunk D, et al: Plasminogen actvator (urokinase) causes vascularization of the cornea. Invest Ophthalmol Vis Sci 22:191, 1982

76. Efron N: Vascular response of the cornea to contact lens wear. J Am Optom Assoc 58:836, 1987

77. Fichman S, Baker VV, Horton HR: Iatrogenic red eyes in soft lens wearers. Int Contact Lens Clin 15:202, 1978

78. Holden BA, Zantos SG: The ocular response to continuous wear of contact lenses. Optician 177:50, 1979

79. Sweeney DF, Grant T, Chong MS, et al: Recurrence of acute inflammatory conditions with hydrogel extended wear. Invest Ophthalmol Vis Sci 34(suppl.):1008, 1993

80. Nilsson SEG, Lindh H: Disposable contact lenses—a prospective study of clinical performance in flexible and extended wear. Contactologia 12:80, 1990.

81. Mertz GW, Holden BA: Clinical implications of extended wear research. Can J Optom 43:203, 1981

82. Weissman BA: An introduction to extended wear contact lenses. J Am Optom Assoc 53:183, 1982

83. Mandell RB: Contact Lens Practice. 4th ed. Thomas, Springfield, IL, 1989

84. Holden BA, Vannas A, Nilsson K, et al: Epithelial and endothelial effects from the extended wear of contact lenses. Curr Eye Res 4:739, 1985

85. Kotow M, Grant T, Holden BA: Avoiding ocular complications during hydrogel extended wear. Int Contact Lens Clin 14:95, 1987

86. Schnider C, Zabkiewicz K, Holden BA: Unusual complications associated with rigid gas permeable extended wear. Int Contact Lens Clin 15:124, 1988

87. Vajdic CM, Holden BA: Extended-wear contact lenses. p. 132. In Hamano H, Kaufman HE (eds): Corneal Physiology and Disposable Contact Lenses. Butterworth–Heinemann, Boston, 1997

88. Phillips AJ, Badenoch PR, Grutzmacher R, Roussel TJ: Microbial contamination of extended-wear contact lenses: an investigation of endotoxin as a cause of the acute ocular inflammation reaction. Int Eye Care 2:469, 1986

89. Dohlman CH, Boruchoff A, Mobilia EF: Complications in the use of soft contact lenses in corneal disease. Arch Ophthalmol 90:367, 1973

90. Baleriola-Lucas C, Grant T, Newton-Howes J, et al: Enumeration and identification of bacteria on hydrogel lenses from asymptomatic patients and those experiencing adverse reactions with extended wear. Invest Ophthalmol Vis Sci 32(suppl.): 739, 1991

91. Holden BA, La Hood D, Grant T, et al: Gram-negative bacteria can induce contact lens-induced acute red eye (CLARE) responses. CLAO J 22:47, 1996

92. Grant T, Terry R, Holden BA: Extended wear of hydrogel lenses. p. 609. In Harris MG (eds): Problems in Optometry: Contact Lenses and Ocular Disease. Lippincott, Philadelphia, 1990

93. Silbert JA: Contact lens-related inflammatory reactions. p. 7. In Bennett ES, Weissman BA (eds): Clinical Contact Lens Practice. Lippincott, Philadelphia, 1991

94. Grant T, Chong MS, Holden BA: Which is best for the eye: daily wear, 2 nights, or 6 nights? Am J Optom Physiol Opt 65:S40, 1988

95. Liesegang TJ: Bacterial and fungal keratitis. p. 217. In Kaufman HE, Barron BA, McDonald MB, Waltman SR (eds): The Cornea. Churchill Livingstone, New York, 1988

96. Mondino BJ, Rabin BS, Kessler E, et al: Corneal rings with gram negative bacteria. Arch Ophthalmol 95:2222, 1977

97. Ellison A, Poirier R: Therapeutic effects of heparin on *Pseudomonas*-induced corneal ulceration. Am J Ophthalmol 82:619, 1976

98. Fine DP: Activation of the classic and alternate complement pathways by endotoxin. J Immunol 112:763, 1974

99. Klein P: Corneal immune ring as a complication of soft extended wear contact lens use. Optom Vis Sci 68:853, 1991

100. Brown SI, Bloomfield SE, Wai-Fong IT: The cornea-destroying enzyme of *Pseudomonas aeruginosa*. Invest Ophthalmol 11:174, 1974

7

Contact Lens–Induced Giant Papillary Conjunctivitis

JANICE M. JURKUS

GRAND ROUNDS CASE REPORT

Subjective:
A 28-year-old woman with chief complaint of soft lens discomfort leading to reduced wearing time. Lenses move excessively, with variable vision, mucus strands, and itching noted after lenses removed. History of 5 years hydrogel use on a "flex-wear" basis (occasional extended-wear use). Current lenses 8 months old. Compliance is poor, with cleaning with surfactant twice weekly, enzyme use every other month, use of whatever is on sale for disinfection. Patient in good health, nonsmoker, takes no medications. Patient refuses to wear glasses.

Objective:
- Best acuity with contact lenses: right eye $^{20}/_{20}$, left eye $^{20}/_{20}$ variable with blink.
- Biomicroscopy: Lenses heavily coated with whitish, translucent protein film. Lenses position superotemporally, with 2-mm lens movement exposing the inferonasal cornea. On lens removal, cornea is clear, with no staining, striae, or vascularization. Bulbar conjunctiva is clear, with no hyperemia. Upper lid eversion reveals hyperemia, macropapillae (>0.3 mm), and giant papillae (>1.0 mm) on zone 1 (area closest to top of tarsal plate).

Assessment:
Stage 3 contact lens–induced giant papillary conjunctivitis (GPC)

Plan:
1. Replace lenses with daily-wear disposable lenses, to be replaced weekly until symptoms cease.
2. Reduce wearing time.
3. Use preservative-free hydrogen peroxide disinfection system, with daily surfactant cleaning.
4. Monitor GPC and lens fitting relationship in 3-week follow-up. Consider pharmacologic intervention.
5. Patient education.

The introduction of frequent replacement and disposable soft contact lenses has allowed patients the opportunity to wear new and cleaner lenses with great regularity. This helps to reduce contact lens–associated problems, but many patients still believe that complaints of mild ocular itching after contact lens removal and the presence of mucus in the nasal canthus is a normal part of contact lens wear. It is now known that these symptoms may herald a condition called *contact lens–induced papillary conjunctivitis*, or GPC. GPC is one of the iatrogenic diseases provoked by the regular use of contact lenses.[1] Although the current use of frequent-replacement and disposable lenses has helped to reduce the clinical incidence of GPC, it is still important to understand this disease. Although the giant papillary response of the superior tarsal conjunctiva has been reported in other circumstances, such as with wearers of an ocular prosthesis,[2] those with corneal elevations consisting of keratin and calcium,[3] those with exposed nylon sutures,[4] and those with contact lenses embedded in the upper fornix,[5] the primary association of GPC is with patients who wear soft or rigid contact lenses.

GPC is easily recognizable by the symptoms of itching, mucoid discharge, and decreased lens tolerance, combined with the characteristic large elevations on the upper tarsal conjunctiva. Other than vernal conjunctivitis, GPC alone is accompanied by superior tarsal lid papillae that are greater than 1 mm in diameter.

Routine lid eversion enables the examiner to see the developing conjunctival changes. Kennedy[6] was one of the first to suggest the investigation of the everted upper lid of the contact lens wearer. Only with routine lid eversion can tarsal conjunctival changes related to contact lens wear be observed and monitored. An Australian report by Spring[7] is largely credited with first describing the large tarsal abnormalities, which he attributed to an allergiclike reaction, in soft contact lens wearers. The seminal work by Allansmith et al.[1] in 1977 produced histologic evidence, described the clinical signs and symptoms, developed a hypothesis concerning the etiology of GPC, and first gave the disease its name.

The reported incidence of GPC varies from a low of 4.23%[8] to a high of 47.5%.[9] The variation can be accounted for by different stages of detection. A 2-year study of 70 patients reported a GPC incidence of 47.5% for soft lens wearers and 21.6% for rigid gas-permeable lens wearers.[9] This study noted that only 15% of the patients had progressed to the stage of GPC at which giant papillae were present (stage 2 or greater). Five percent of patients experienced difficulty wearing contact lenses (stage 3 or 4).[9] All others had mild symptoms and few signs.[9] Because the number of contact lens wearers in the United States is approximately 25 million, some 11 million contact lens wearers could potentially develop GPC. The contact lens fitter can anticipate that as much as 40% of lens wearers may exhibit some stage of GPC, although the stage may be mild because of the advent of frequent replacement lenses.

Knowledge of the disease and of its signs, symptoms, and possible etiology enables the practitioner to prescribe a logical and practical mode of therapy for the patient who has developed GPC.

ETIOLOGY

The etiology of GPC is probably a combination of immune and mechanical mechanisms. By looking at the unique clinical presentation of this condition, the proposed etiology can be developed. The hallmark subjective symptoms of GPC include diminished contact lens wearing time, itching (noted especially after contact lens removal), an increase in mucus secretion, and variable vision while wearing contact lenses. The classic objective signs of GPC consist of the following:

- Tarsal conjunctival papillae of varying size and shape
- Fluorescein staining of the papillary surfaces
- Hyperemia and edema of the upper lid
- Sheets of mucus over and around the papillae
- Protein coatings on contact lens surfaces.

To understand the mechanisms that give rise to the clinical presentation of GPC, the morphology, histology, immunology, and pathophysiology of the conjunctiva must be investigated.

MORPHOLOGIC STUDIES

The shape of the tarsal conjunctiva is investigated with the slit-lamp biomicroscope and electron microscope. A review of the conjunctival morphology of those who do not wear lenses and asymptomatic contact lens wearers aids understanding of the development of GPC.

Slit-Lamp Biomicroscopic Evaluation

Slit-lamp biomicroscopic study reveals that normal superior tarsal conjunctival papillae can be classified into three categories: uniform, satin, and nonuniform. The most common (69%) is the uniform papillary appearance, characterized by mildly elevated papillae of 0.1–0.2-mm diameter, with a uniform distribution (4–8/mm). Satin-smooth appearance devoid of papillae has approximately a 24% incidence, and the nonuniform papillary distribution shows

FIG. 7-1. *Normal palpebral conjunctival papillae:* **(A)** *satin,* **(B)** *uniform, and* **(C)** *nonuniform presentations.*

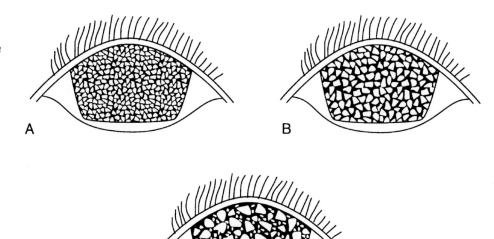

papillae of 0.4–0.8 mm in diameter and has a 7% incidence.[1] Zonular or junctional papillae appear to be unrelated to the conjunctival type, as judged from tarsal conjunctiva, and are not considered in the normal classification of upper conjunctival types (Fig. 7-1).

GPC is identified by the presence of papillae greater than 1 mm in diameter on all or part of the tarsal conjunctival surface. Fluorescein stain allows an outlined view of the papillae (Fig. 7-2).

Electron Microscopic Study of Papillae

Non–Lens Wearers

A morphologic study by Greiner et al.[10] investigating biopsied conjunctival tissue with the scanning electron microscope shows the general surfaces of the three types of normal tarsal conjunctiva to be similar. Surface cell boundaries are outlined by microvillus borders. The surface cell shape is hexagonal, 6–10 μm across. A slight elongation of surface cells exists in the uniform and nonuniform papillary appearance. The microvilli covering the cell surface have a shaglike texture, and mucus particles appear to stick to the microvilli. Light and dark cells, which may represent cells in different stages of development, are normally observed. The lighter cells are smaller, having fewer but longer microvilli, whereas the darker cells have a larger, irregular surface area covered with shorter, denser microvilli.[10] Two types of crypt openings are seen. The majority of the openings are 1–3 μm in diameter, round, surrounded by distinct microvillus borders, and located at the junction of three or four cells. The bases of these crypts contain protoplasmic processes. These small crypts are thought to be the collapsed surfaces of empty goblet cells that open independently onto the conjunctival surface.[11] Larger crypt openings, 10–60 μm in diameter, vary in shape from round to elliptical. These cylindrical infoldings of the conjunctival epithelium, known as the crypts of Henle, contain goblet cells. The walls of the large crypts are lined with microvillus-covered cells, and mucuslike strands protrude from the large crypts (Fig. 7-3).

Asymptomatic Contact Lens Wearers

The conjunctival surface in the normal, asymptomatic contact lens wearer undergoes some dramatic changes, which are thought to be an adaptive response of the surface cells to contact lens wear.[12] Interspersed among normal epithelial cells are cells of smaller diameter with centrally clumped, highly tufted microvilli. These cells are covered with mucus, which may be extruded from the cell onto the cell surface. This is thought to represent the induction of a non–goblet cell secretory function. Small,

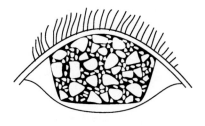

FIG. 7-2. *Contact lens–induced giant papillae.*

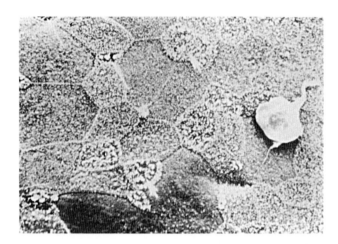

FIG. 7-3. *Normal conjunctiva with light, medium, and dark cell surfaces. Cell boundaries are visible and small crypt openings are present. A large piece of mucinlike material (white structure) is at the right. Shaglike microvilli cover the surface. (Reprinted with permission from JV Greiner, HI Covington, MR Allansmith: Surface morphology of the human upper tarsal conjunctiva. Am J Ophthalmol 83:892, 1977.)*

irregular crypts, as well as the crypts of Henle, are present in the epithelial surface (Fig. 7-4).

CONJUNCTIVAL CHANGES IN GIANT PAPILLARY CONJUNCTIVITIS

The conjunctival surface changes in GPC are striking. At least a twofold increase in epithelial surface area occurs, as well as a dramatic distortion of the epithelial cells.[13,14] The cells are characterized by loss of the hexagonal shape observed in normal and asymptomatic contact lens wearers. Cells are irregular and elongated, and microvilli have balloon-shaped distal ends that adhere to form a white, tufted surface. The tufted structures on top of the papillae are flattened, and it is difficult to distinguish the individual microvilli, whereas the tufts on the sides of the papillae are more elevated and the microvilli are easily seen. As many as 25 tufts per cell exist. The small surface crypts become irregular, and the crypts of Henle are not observed. Mucus-secreting non–goblet cells are increased and the light and dark cells are present, but the dark cell number is increased at the apices of the giant papillae (Fig. 7-5).

Mucus Secretion

Increased mucus secretion is a cardinal sign of GPC and is noted even in the preclinical stage. Mucus in the conjunctival sac is believed to come from three sources:

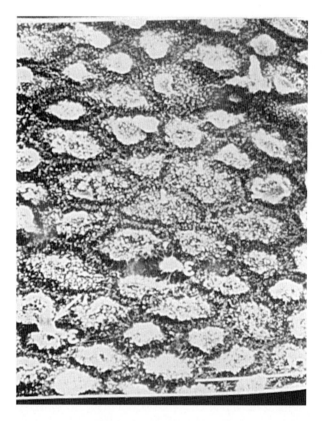

FIG. 7-4. *Conjunctiva of asymptomatic contact lens wearer, showing centralization of microvilli with mucus debris. (Reprinted with permission from JV Greiner, HI Covington, DR Korb, MR Allansmith: Conjunctiva in asymptomatic contact lens wearers. Am J Ophthalmol 86:403, 1978.)*

- The conjunctival goblet cells
- The mucus-secreting acinar cells of the lacrimal gland
- The non–goblet cells of the conjunctiva, which contain mucus secretory vesicles

As shown histologically, the upper tarsal conjunctiva has goblet and non–goblet mucus-secreting cells. Although no significant increase in goblet cell density occurs in GPC, the total number of cells increases because the conjunctival surface thickens and expands several times with the growth of papillae. Greiner et al.[15] have also shown an increase in the number of non–goblet cells containing mucus secretory vesicles. In general, contact lens wearers have an increase in the number of secretory vesicles per cell. These non–goblet epithelial cells contain neutral mucin, sialomucin, and sulfomucin. The specific alterations in the conjunctiva that contribute to the increase in mucus production in GPC are not fully understood but appear to be related to increased mucus production in goblet and non–goblet epithelial cells.[15]

HISTOLOGIC EXAMINATION

Study of conjunctival inflammatory cells and the changes in ultrastructure of the palpebral conjunctiva discloses major differences between normal conjunctiva and that of GPC.

Normal Conjunctiva

The normal palpebral conjunctiva contains a large number of inflammatory cells. Although individual variation is great, the normal upper limit is 56,000 per mm^3 for the epithelium and 410,000 per mm^3 in the substantia propria (stroma).[16] Lymphocytes comprise 69% and neutrophils make up 31% of the inflammatory cells in the upper tarsal conjunctival epithelium. Plasma cells, eosinophils, mast cells, and basophils are not normally found in the epithelial layer of the tarsal conjunctiva.[16]

The substantia propria contains a wider variety of inflammatory cells. Neutrophils are fewer (1%), and lymphocytes make up 66%, mast cells 3%, and plasma cells 30% of the inflammatory cells of the normal substantia propria of the upper tarsal conjunctiva.[17] The normal conjunctiva is also devoid of eosinophils and basophils in the stroma. This is noteworthy because these cells are found in the conjunctiva of patients with GPC.

Asymptomatic Contact Lens Wearers

The contact lens wearer with no evidence of GPC has no significant change in the numbers of inflammatory cells compared to the non–contact lens wearer.[18]

Giant Papillary Conjunctivitis

Histologic studies in cases of GPC reveal thick conjunctiva: approximately 0.2 mm compared with the normal thickness of approximately 0.05 mm. Mast cells, eosinophils, and basophils infiltrate the epithelium. Neutrophils increase to make up approximately 39% of the inflammatory cells in the epithelium. Although no significant change in number of lymphocytes per cubic millimeter occurs, the overall mass increase of the palpebral conjunctival tissue demonstrates that a greater number are present.[13] The stromal tissue shows the presence of eosinophils and basophils, with an increased number of mast cells, plasma cells, and neutrophils.[17]

Contact lens–induced GPC is characterized by three histologic findings regarding inflammatory cells:

- Mast cells in the epithelium
- Eosinophils in the epithelium and substantia propria
- Basophils in the epithelium and substantia propria

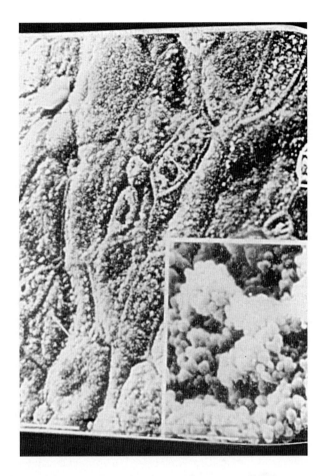

FIG. 7-5. *Conjunctiva of patient with giant papillary conjunctivitis. Note elongated, irregularly shaped cells with clumped microvilli. Inset shows balloon-shaped microvilli, which are clumped at the tips. (Reprinted with permission from JV Greiner, HI Covington, MR Allansmith: Surface morphology of giant papillary conjunctivitis in contact lens wearers. Am J Ophthalmol 85:242, 1978.)*

These inflammatory cells are not found in the described areas of normal palpebral conjunctival tissues (Fig. 7-6).[17]

IMMUNOLOGIC MECHANISMS

Antibodies associated with immunologic mechanisms are found in the tissues of patients with GPC. The antigen-antibody response is characterized by the development of protein globulins manufactured by plasma cells. The presence of Russell bodies, defined as accumulations of immunoglobulins in mature and healthy plasma cells, is considered a regular component of the immune response. Russell bodies have been reported in GPC tissues.[19] The

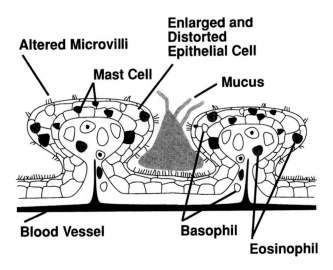

FIG. 7-6. *Distribution of inflammatory cells in giant papillary conjunctivitis. Note mast cells, basophils, and eosinophils in the epithelial layer of papillae.*

five classes of immunoglobulins are IgG, IgA, IgM, IgD, and IgE. Tear IgE, IgG, and IgM levels were found to be higher in patients with GPC than in healthy eyes, and concentrations were higher in eyes that exhibited more severe GPC symptoms.[20] To determine whether the IgE and mast cell migration was related to contact lens wear, soft lenses that had been worn by patients with GPC were placed on healthy monkey corneas. Elevated tear IgE and epithelial mast cells were subsequently induced in these corneas.[21]

Mast cells, specifically tryptase-positive, chymase-positive mast cells, are found in the GPC tissue.[22] These mast cells show various degrees of degranulation, which releases the vasoactive and chemical mediators of inflammation. Type 1 (immediate or anaphylactic reactions) are IgE mediated, releasing histamine, serotonin, heparin, neutral proteases, and acid hydrolases, as well as neutrophil, lymphocyte, and eosinophil chemotactic factors.[23] Mast cell degranulation can cause edema, hyperemia, and itching of palpebral tissue. Because mast cell degranulation is part of the process of GPC, an unusual finding is that the tear histamine level is not elevated in GPC patients. Henriquez et al.[24] suggested that the histamine level in patients with GPC is no greater than in healthy individuals because an insufficient amount of histamine is released or because the released histamine is degraded before it can reach the tear film.

The association of GPC with other atopic or allergic conditions is unclear. GPC has similarities to vernal conjunctivitis, which is an atopic condition, but the presence of histamine in the tear layer and of tryptase-positive, chymase-negative mast cells only in vernal conjunctivitis differentiates the two entities.[22] Allansmith and colleagues did not find a connection between GPC and atopy.[1] Henriquez et al.[24] reported a patient with GPC in whom skin test results for various allergens were negative. Other authors have suggested a higher incidence of GPC associated with seasonal allergies.[8,25] In fact, Molinari[26] considers the presence of allergies a high risk factor for the development of GPC.

PATHOPHYSIOLOGY

The morphologic and histologic evidence relating to GPC suggests that it can result from mechanical trauma, a hypersensitivity reaction to antigens, or a combination of these factors as well as by other factors yet to be identified. The exact etiology and pathogenesis of contact lens–induced GPC are not yet fully understood.

Mechanical Trauma

Reports of GPC development associated with inert stimuli, such as exposed sutures, extruded scleral buckles, cyanoacrylate adhesive, and epithelialized corneal bodies, suggest a mechanical etiology. In these cases, GPC is localized at the area of the tarsal conjunctiva in contact with the offending stimuli. Removal or smoothing of the irregularity relieves the symptoms and signs of this response.[27] The morphologic changes in epithelial cells suggest mechanical trauma. A model of ocular inflammation has been described demonstrating that the trauma of eye rubbing histologically disrupts the epithelium and induces a dramatic increase in the number of neutrophils in the epithelium.[28] This response also occurs in GPC patients.

Hypersensitivity Reaction

The quantitative histologic evaluation of the conjunctiva exhibiting GPC reveals inflammatory cells typically associated with humoral (anaphylactic) and cellular (cutaneous basophil) hypersensitivity.[29] The presence of mast cells, eosinophils, basophils, leukocytes, and lymphocytes in GPC reflects the disturbed nature of the immune apparatus. Signs of immediate type 1 IgE-mediated hypersensitivity reaction and type IV delayed reaction are present. The increased levels of tear IgE suggest a humoral component. As previously noted in the Immunologic Mechansms Section, cell inclusions, such as Russell bodies, are found in immune conditions. Allansmith[30] states that in genetically predisposed individuals, irritation caused by a contact lens combined with an antigen (probably the debris and films on the surface of the lens that grind against the conjunctiva) triggers the hypersensitivity response.

The development and exacerbation of contact lens–induced GPC occur as a result of many different factors. These factors include the following:

- The individual genetic predisposition to protein accumulation
- Increased protein deposition on the contact lens surfaces
- Increased lens wearing time
- Use of the same lenses for months or years
- Individual reaction to a particular lens type

Larger lenses may allow a broader area of adhering antigenic material, which can increase the GPC response.[31]

Contact Lens Surfaces

Contact lens coatings are normal and necessary for proper wetting and comfort, but they can provide a sticky substrate for attraction of bacteria and other environmental particles.[32,33] The amount of protein burden has been related to the material of the lens. Higher protein accumulation was found with lenses having 55% water content than with those having 38% water content.[34,35] Rigid lenses allow less protein accumulation.[36] The single common factor in contact lens–related GPC is the presence of lens surface deposits. The deposits on lenses of patients with GPC are the same as those on lenses of asymptomatic wearers.[37] The similarity of these deposits supports the hypothesis that GPC is more likely to be related to differences among individual contact lens wearers rather than among the type of deposits. Bacteria and protein particles that adhere to the surface of the contact lens expose a constant and significant dose of allergen to the upper tarsal conjunctiva.[38] The predominant protein component on soft lenses is lysozyme, although other normal tear proteins, such as IgA, lactoferrin, and IgG, also adhere to soft lens surfaces.[39] The protein coatings become more complex with increased lens wear. The deposits consist of an underlying layer of cells, a layer of granular, mucus-like material through which the cell outlines are seen, and another layer of cells. The deposition becomes thicker, more convoluted, and irregular with increased wearing time. Anterior and posterior lens surfaces develop coatings, although the posterior surface is markedly smoother than the anterior.[37] The coatings are difficult, if not impossible, to remove completely. Surfactant cleaning removes clumps of deposits, and enzymatic cleaning results in a

so-called eaten appearance and reduction of the protein deposit thickness.[40] A contact lens coated with antigenic deposits can cause mechanical trauma to the superior tarsal conjunctiva, which constitutes the afferent or incoming branch of the immune response. The efferent or outward-bearing branch involves the accumulation of mast cells, basophils, and lymphocytes in the affected area.[41] Hence, it is likely that contact lens deposition actually contributes to mechanical and immunologic factors responsible for the development of contact lens–induced GPC.

CLINICAL PRESENTATION

GPC progresses through various stages. The size of the papillae, the amount of mucus, and the patient's symptoms increase as the disease progresses.[1,42] In the earliest stage, GPC patients may exhibit few, if any, symptoms. As the disease progresses, signs and symptoms may become so pronounced that contact lens wear is not possible.

For diagnosis of GPC, the signs to be evaluated are the presence of lens coatings, size and elevation of papillae, staining characteristics of the papillae, amount of lid hyperemia and edema, presence of excess mucus, and corneal condition. The subjective symptoms associated with GPC include mucus discharge in the morning, itching after lens removal, awareness of the lens during wear, visual fluctuations, decreased wearing time because of discomfort, and excessive lens movement.

Early identification of contact lens–induced GPC allows more effective treatment and rapid resolution of the condition. The stage 1 lid appears to be normal. Symptoms are often recognized only if direct questions about mucus in the nasal corner of the eye on waking and mild itching just after lens removal are answered in the affirmative. Diagnosis of stage 1 contact lens–induced GPC is made on the basis of contact lens wear and symptoms of itching and mucus.

Stage 2 exhibits enlargement of normal papillae and formation of giant papillae. The giant papillae are formed by substructural changes from the deep tarsal conjunctiva. These changes elevate areas containing several overlying papillae rather than representing a simple enlargement of normal papillae.[43] The initial presentation of giant papillae appears to be related to the type of contact lens worn. Rigid lens wear allows the initial development of papillae nearest the lid margin (zone 3) and progressing toward the tarsal plate. Soft lens wear demonstrates a reverse progression, in which the papillae initially develop at the superior tarsal plate area (zone 1) and progress to the lid margin (Figs. 7-7 and 7-8).[14,44]

Patients with stage 2 GPC report increased amounts of mucus and itching as well as mild blurring of vision.

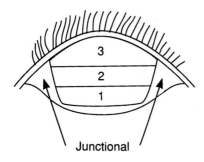

FIG. 7-7. *Trizonal configuration of upper tarsal plate.*

Increased lens awareness and foreign-body sensation may lead to reduction in lens wearing time. The papillae are found on the thickened, edematous, and hyperemic conjunctiva. Fine conjunctival vasculature may be obscured, but the deeper vessels over the tarsal plate are visible. A comparison of the superior and inferior palpebral conjunctiva is useful to determine the degree of edema and hyperemia. In GPC, the lower lid is not affected, thus remaining normal in thickness and color.

Stage 3 GPC generates symptoms of increased mucus production, pronounced itching, and excessive lens movement during the blink. The lens wearer is constantly aware

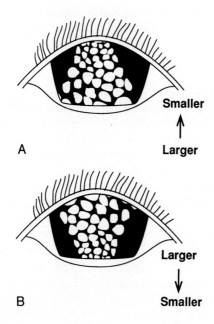

FIG. 7-8. *Presentations of giant papillary conjunctivitis. (A) Changes for soft lens wearers start in zone 1, near superior tarsal area, and progress toward zone 3, near the lash margin. (B) Changes for rigid lens wearers start in zone 3 and progress toward zone 1.*

of the lens on the eye and reports frequent lens removal in an attempt to clean the debris and mucus from the lens surface. The papillae continue to enlarge, and a clover-like morphology develops, with smaller papillae found over the elevated areas. The apices of the giant papillae stain with fluorescein. Mucus often appears in strands that fill the spaces around the papillae.

The patient experiencing stage 4 GPC loses the ability to wear contact lenses because the lenses become coated almost immediately after insertion. Because of lens decentration and excessive movement, foreign-body sensation forces removal of the lenses. Excessive secretion produces strands or sheets of mucus, with a common patient report of eyelids sticking together after sleeping. Stage 4 is an exacerbation of the previous stages, with the papillae enlarging in size and number. Flattening of the apices, which continue to stain with fluorescein, is evident. The giant papillae and hyperemia in severe GPC can lead to development of a lid ptosis.[45,46] In stage 4, the appearance of GPC is nearly identical to that of vernal conjunctivitis. The basis for differential diagnosis includes the report of contact lens use, less severe itching, and rarity of punctate keratitis and Trantas' dots in GPC. Conjunctival scrapings processed with Giemsa stain reveal greater numbers of eosinophils in patients with vernal conjunctivitis than in those with GPC. Symptomatic relief of GPC is obtained by discontinuation of contact lens wear. The symptoms of vernal conjunctivitis do not resolve as rapidly with any single treatment. Vernal conjunctivitis is associated with atopy, occurs most frequently in young men, and follows a seasonal pattern.[47]

Variation exists in the development of symptoms, in contrast to signs, of contact lens–induced GPC.[1] Some patients exhibit giant papillae in all zones of the tarsal plate conjunctiva and have minimal symptoms, thereby allowing continued wearing of contact lenses with little discomfort. Other patients may have itching, increased mucus, conjunctival thickening, and hyperemia leading to lens intolerance, but lid eversion reveals few papillae.[43]

EXAMINATION TECHNIQUES

The examination of the GPC patient involves two major components: case history and slit-lamp biomicroscopic evaluation of the tarsal conjunctiva. Because the initial stage of GPC has few identifiable objective signs, careful elicitation of a complete case history is necessary. The history should include questions about the presence of mucus in the nasal canthus on waking, itching after the lenses are removed, and reduction in contact lens wearing time. Positive responses to these questions suggest stage 1 contact lens–induced con-

TABLE 7-1. *Contact Lens–Induced Giant Papillary Conjunctivitis Case History Questions*

1. Is your vision satisfactory while you are wearing your contact lenses?
2. Are your lenses comfortable while you wear them?
3. Do you notice any mucus or stringy matter in the corner of your eyes when you wake up?
4. Do your eyes itch after you take out your contact lenses? Do you rub your eyes after you remove your lenses?
5. How long do you wear your lenses each day? Has the length of time the lenses are worn decreased lately?
6. How old are the lenses you are wearing? Do you know what kind they are?
7. Describe how you care for your contact lenses. What products do you use?

TABLE 7-2. *Slit-Lamp Biomicroscopic Evaluation of the Lens Wearer with Giant Papillary Conjunctivitis*

Contact lens on the eye: white light, low magnification, direct illumination
  Lens centration
Corneal coverage, lens decentration
  Amount of lens movement with the blink
  Lens surface deposition
Tarsal conjunctiva: white light, low magnification
  Presence of hyperemia, amount of redness
  Presence of conjunctival edema or swelling
  Position of papillae
  Number and size of papillae
  Amount of elevation using a narrow beam width
Tarsal conjunctiva after instillation of fluorescein: cobalt blue filter, high magnification
  Delineation of papillae
  Apical staining or flattering of papillae
  Amount of mucus
Contact lens inspection off the eye: low magnification, white light
  Surface deposits
  Scratches, tears, defects

junctivitis. Because many patients believe that these changes are a normal part of contact lens wear, they may not offer the subjective information unless specifically asked. The age and type of contact lens worn can provide information about the expected condition of the lenses. The patient should be asked about the care products used so that compliance, or lack thereof, can be assessed. Table 7-1 summarizes specific questions to be asked.

The slit-lamp biomicroscope is used to evaluate the contact lenses and to observe the conjunctival integrity of the everted upper lid. If a patient is wearing contact lenses, the lens-cornea fitting relationship and amount of lens movement should be evaluated. Keep in mind that tarsal conjunctival changes can produce increased lens movement with the blink and lens decentration. The condition of the lens surface should be evaluated when the lens is off the eye, although heavy lens coatings can be seen while the lens is worn by using the slit-lamp biomicroscope with white light and indirect illumination.

The tarsal conjunctiva should then be evaluated without a lens on the eye. The everted upper lid should first be examined under low (10–16×) magnification and white light. The presence of hyperemia and edema should be noted, and the general position of the papillae should be documented. The trizonal configuration, dividing the tarsal plate into three zones of equal width, is useful for documentation (see Fig. 7-7). The estimated number and size of papillae should be recorded for future comparison. The papillae diameter can range from 0.3–2.0 mm.[1] Using a narrow slit beam, elevation is determined when the papillae protrude from the surrounding tissue. Surface detail can be examined with higher magnification (25×). If a patient has discontinued lens wear for 3–5 days, the size of the papillae may be decreased. Smaller papillae are more easily observed with the instillation of fluorescein. After white light examination, the lids are returned to the normal posi-

tion and fluorescein is instilled in the usual fashion. The patient is asked to blink at least six times to distribute the fluorescein over the tarsal conjunctival surface. After eversion, the tarsal conjunctiva is inspected with cobalt blue light for the delineation of papillae and apical staining. Fluorescein staining occurs when epithelial cells are mechanically damaged or the apices are flattened and craterlike.[43,44] The upper and lower palpebral conjunctival surfaces should be compared and the amount of mucus should also be noted.

With the lens off the eye, lens surface inspection can be performed with the slit-lamp biomicroscope. The lens should be rinsed with sterile saline to remove surface debris and held with tweezers at the plane of the slit-lamp biomicroscope headrest. White light, coming from a 45–60-degree angle, is used to illuminate the lens, and the lighted lens is viewed against a darker background. By looking through the biomicroscope oculars under low magnification, surface deposits can be seen. The single factor common to all lens wearers with GPC is the presence of deposits on the lens surface. A summary of areas of slit-lamp biomicroscopic inspection is given in Table 7-2.

TREATMENT

No single, totally effective treatment for GPC exists. Treatment modalities for GPC include reducing or eliminating lens wear, replacing contact lenses with new ones of the same material and design, changing lens material and design, altering the care solution, using aqueous lubricants, and prescribing drugs.[48] All treatment methods lead to improvement of the condition. A multimodal plan of therapy may bring the condition under control and allow lens wear for many patients with GPC. Excellent patient cooperation and compliance are needed for effective treatment. The intensity and length of treatment depend on the stage at which GPC is diagnosed. Early detection allows faster, more complete resolution of the condition.

The four general steps in the treatment of GPC are to replace the lenses with a more suitable lens design and material, modify lens use, improve lens and ocular hygiene, and, if necessary, treat the conjunctival inflammation with pharmacologic agents.

Lens Replacement

Opinions vary about the type of lens most suitable for the patient with GPC.[26,49–53] The soft lens type (ionic versus nonionic), water content (low versus high), material (HEMA versus non-HEMA), edge (design and thickness), and manufacturing technique (lathe-cut versus molded) have been investigated with conflicting reports.[46,52,54–57] The single constant in all reports is that the lens that remains clean with minimal deposition is the most appropriate type. The disposable or frequent-replacement soft lens modality addresses many causes of GPC.[58] As previously stated in the Etiology Section, the GPC reaction is linked to lens deposition, particularly to protein coating on lenses. Protein deposits increase in magnitude with increased wear and are not completely removed with surfactant and enzymatic cleaning. Therefore, daily or weekly replacement with new, clean contact lenses minimizes the surface buildup that becomes intolerable for soft lens wearers with GPC. Watanabe and Hamano concluded that the reduced buildup of deposits with disposable lenses made them safer for patients with GPC.[59] Disposable soft lenses have been reported to be an effective management tool for GPC patients when they are used on either an extended-wear or a daily-wear basis.[54–56] Bucci et al.[60] compared the performance of three types of disposable lenses worn on a daily-wear basis by patients with GPC. They did not find a specific brand of disposable lenses superior with regard to difference in papillary changes or overall lens performance.

Selection guidelines for the type of disposable lens are similar to those for conventional lenses. Disposable or frequent-replacement lenses are now manufactured in all U.S. Food and Drug Administration material groups. The majority of the polymer materials used are in group 1 (low-water, nonionic), group 4 (high-water, ionic polymers), or lenses in group 2 (high-water, nonionic). Daily-wear use of disposable lenses requires the daily use of a surfactant cleaner as well as daily disinfection, unless the patient is wearing a 1-day single-use lens. Hydrogen peroxide is a preservative-free disinfection solution that may eliminate the possibility of added preservative intolerance. Patients using disposable lenses who wish to keep using the same lenses for more than the prescribed number of days should be cautioned that GPC symptoms may reappear if lenses are allowed to develop protein coatings, which would defeat the purpose of using disposable lenses.

In the early stages of GPC, lens replacement with the same polymer and design previously worn plus improved lens hygiene and regular replacement of lenses may be all that is required. Replacement of conventional lenses at least every 6–12 months often controls GPC.[29] If this treatment is not successful, prescribing a soft lens of a dramatically different design and polymer is suggested. The prescription of different lenses for each eye, such as a low–water content lens fit on one eye and a high–water content lens fit on the other eye, maximizes efficiency in the process of new lens selection. The lens type that decreases more of the symptoms and signs of GPC, therefore, is the most appropriate for that individual. The key is to prescribe a lens that is dramatically different from the type that triggered the GPC.[29]

The treatment of GPC for patients who wear rigid lenses is similar to that for soft lens wearers. The difference is that polishing rigid contact lenses can obviate the need for lens replacement. Professional polishing yields a smooth surface that minimizes the attraction of deposits. Smooth, thinner edge designs are less likely to provoke mechanical lid irritation and deposition of debris. An inverse relationship is reported between the lens material permeability value, Dk value, and onset time of rigid gas-permeable lens–induced GPC.[61] Rigid gas-permeable lenses that attract protein deposition are more likely to cause development of GPC. A change of lens design (i.e., soft to rigid or vice versa) may be required in more resistant cases of GPC.

It is important to explain to the patient that the GPC may never completely disappear. The symptoms can be eliminated and the signs minimized, but the papillae, which decrease in size, enlarge again when they are exposed to the allergic stimulus, specifically, protein deposition on the surface of a contact lens.[51,62]

Modification of Lens Use

Relief of symptoms can be achieved when lens wear is discontinued. Most patients with GPC become asymptomatic within 5 days of lens removal.[63] Discontinuation of lens wear is often impractical, however, because patients desire or need (as in the case of the patient with keratoconus) to continue wearing contact lenses. In more advanced stages of GPC, patients should stop wearing contact lenses until the hyperemia, excessive mucus production, and itching resolve before obtaining new lenses. This may require the discontinuation of lens wear for more than 3–5 days. The enlarged papillae may still be present. If after approximately 1 week of not wearing lenses the mucus production, hyperemia, and itching decrease, resumption of contact lens wear with new lenses may be possible. Total regression of giant papillae may take several months or even years (Fig. 7-9).[30] Once lens wear is resumed, daily wear and frequent replacement are recommended.

Lens and Ocular Hygiene

Proper contact lens care involves surfactant cleaning, disinfection, conditioning, and enzymatic cleaning procedures. Each procedure addresses a different part of lens hygiene. Lens wearers in the preclinical or early stages of GPC may achieve resolution by methodical application of each care procedure. Routine cleaning with proteolytic enzymes has been reported to be beneficial for wearers of rigid and soft lenses.[40,64] It is important to instruct the patient to clean the lenses with surfactants before and after the enzymatic treatment. Each individual produces lens deposits at different rates. Therefore, the practitioner must decide on the frequency of enzyme treatment.[49,50] The minimal suggested frequency of enzyme tablet use is once a week. To reduce the possibility of a compounding sensitivity reaction to the preservatives in soft lens solutions, preservative-free hydrogen peroxide disinfection has been recommended for soft lens wearers.[51] The introduction of daily liquid enzyme removers and disinfectants that retard protein formation help fight the protein development.

Ocular hygiene can be aided by conjunctival irrigation with an irrigating solution or sterile saline. The frequency of required irrigation varies with the severity of the GPC. Two or more times, specifically 15 minutes before lens insertion and immediately after lens removal, is suggested. Dilution of GPC protein antigens is achieved by the flushing action of the irrigation.[52]

Drug Therapy for Conjunctival Inflammation

Pharmacologic treatment of GPC can take several forms. Antiallergy agents, specifically mast cell stabilizer, topical corticosteroids, and nonsteroidal anti-inflammatory agents have been used to reduce the conjunctival inflammation.[57,65–67] A clear consensus about which is most effective does not exist.

Antiallergy Agents

Mast cell stabilizers, such as cromolyn sodium (Crolom 4%, Bausch & Lomb, Rochester, NY) and lodoxamide tromethamine (Alomide 0.1%, Alcon Laboratories, Inc., Fort Worth, TX) stabilize mast cell membranes, thus pre-

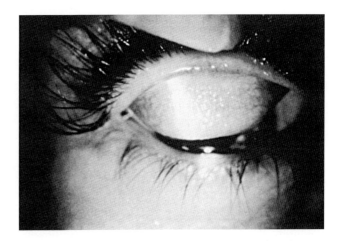

FIG. 7-9. *Papillae of a patient who had discontinued contact lens wear for 3 months. Before stopping lens wear, patient was diagnosed as having stage 3 giant papillary conjunctivitis.*

venting the release of histamine and other biochemical mediators. When topically applied in stage 1 or stage 2 GPC, these agents can prevent the signs and symptoms associated with type 1 allergic reactions, including the GPC reaction.[68–70] The common dosage is 1–2 drops four times per day for a month, then twice per day for a month.[65,71] Donshik et al.[62] concluded that topical cromolyn appears to help in the treatment of difficult-to-manage GPC. These authors used 2% cromolyn sodium drops four times a day, along with new contact lenses, in refractory patients who remained symptomatic after lens replacement, and found that these patients were able to maintain contact lens wear. Another retrospective study had a 70% overall success rate when 4% cromolyn sodium was prescribed for patients who remained symptomatic after the application of new lenses.[69] Case reports by Meisler et al.[72] indicated that five patients with GPC who used 2% or 4% cromolyn sodium four times a day had relief of symptoms and less prominent giant papillae. The dosage was tapered to once a day for two of the patients.

The question of instilling mast cell stabilizers during contact lens wear has been debated. More advanced stages of GPC must first be brought under control by better lens hygiene; the use of new, clean lenses; and temporary discontinuation of lens wear for approximately 3–5 days. When lens wear is reinstated, mast cell stabilizers can be used as part of the maintenance therapy.[25] The side effects of sodium cromolyn and lodoxamide are minimal. They include transient stinging or burning on insertion.[73,74] Benzalkonium chloride (BAK) is the preservative in both formulations. BAK has been shown to be a causative factor in the development of GPC and is known to bind to soft lens polymers.[75] Roth[76] reported that preserved sodium cromolyn did not produce remission of GPC after 6 weeks of use, whereas a preservative-free formulation of 3% sodium cromoglycate applied two to five times daily relieved symptoms within 14 days. Conversely, a study by Iwasaki et al.[77] indicated that a specific 2% disodium cromoglycate (Intal), which is preserved with BAK, did not accumulate in soft lenses and was safe for application while lenses were worn.

Clinical use of olopatadine hydrochloride (Patanol 0.1%, Alcon Laboratories, Inc., Fort Worth, TX) has been reported to be effective. The recommended dosage is twice per day. One drop usually gives approximately 8 hours of symptomatic relief. The combined effect of an antihistamine and a mast-cell stabilizer in this product are favorable for the control of the chronic allergic response and for symptomatic relief in acute cases of GPC.[78,79] The acute itching and mucus associated with GPC have also been treated with topical antihistamines, such as levocabastine hydrochloride (Livostin 0.05%, CIBA Vision, Duluth, GA) and decongestants, such as naphazoline.[78]

Steroids

Traditionally, topical steroids have been reserved for use in cases of severe inflammation. Because GPC is a self-induced iatrogenic disease, the potential risks associated with routine use of steroidal agents outweigh the benefits. The documented risks of steroid use include increased intraocular pressure, cataract formation, and propensity for suprainfection. Limited use of topical steroids has been suggested in severe cases of GPC to minimize the vast amounts of mucus, extreme hyperemia, cellular infiltrates, and mediator substances in the tear film present in stage 4 GPC so that conventional intervention can be used.[65] A report of short-term use of a topical steroid (0.10% fluorometholone) showed 90% improvement in objective findings and a 70% general improvement in 10 GPC patients who underwent seasonal exacerbation. The dosage was 1 drop four times a day for 1 week, 1 drop three times a day for the next week, tapering to 2 drops per day for 1 week, and then 1 drop per day for the final week of therapy.[66] It should be remembered that steroidal agents do not treat the cause of GPC; they merely control the symptoms. The risk-benefit ratio must be carefully weighed before topical steroids are prescribed. Abuse and noncompliance may cause irreversible, damaging side effects. A new soft drug, loteprednol etabonate (Lotemax 0.5%, Bausch & Lomb, Rochester, NY), which is an analogue of the steroid prednisolone, has been reported to reduce significantly more primary signs of GPC than a placebo in a study of 37 patients.[80] This new drug is promising. Its site-active components should not have the potential steroidal side effect of increasing intraocular

pressure because it is rapidly and predictably transformed into an inactive metabolite in the anterior chamber. Another study included 220 adults with contact lens–associated GPC treated with loteprednol etabonate or a placebo, four times per day for 6 weeks. Symptoms of GPC, such as papillae, itching, and lens intolerance plus intraocular pressure were measured. Loteprednol etabonate subjects showed at least one grade improvement in papillae and a reduction in itching and lens intolerance. This was not so with the placebo subjects. Only three subjects using loteprednol etabonate had an intraocular pressure elevation 10 mm or higher from baseline. The authors concluded that loteprednol etabonate is an appropriate treatment for GPC owing to rapid therapeutic response combined with the low incidence and transient nature of intraocular pressure changes.[81,82]

Nonsteroidal Anti-Inflammatory Agents

Nonsteroidal anti-inflammatory agents have been used to treat vernal conjunctivitis, which is similar to GPC.[83] A multicenter study reported a greater reduction in signs and symptoms of GPC for patients using suprofen (Profenal 1%, Alcon Laboratories, Inc., Fort Worth, TX) rather than a placebo. Suprofen inhibits prostaglandin synthesis by inhibiting the cyclooxygenase system. Forty-eight percent of the subjects tested reported ocular side effects of stinging and burning.[67]

No pharmacologic treatment alone has been consistently effective in the treatment of contact lens–induced GPC.

Other Agents and Tests

The use of an aqueous preparation of antioxidant polysorbate 80 and vitamin A, retinol 0.012% (Viva-Drops, Vision Pharmaceuticals, Inc., Mitchell, SD) has been proposed as a treatment for GPC.[84] A subjective improvement in GPC was reported with the use of topical application three to four times a day. All patients wore new lenses during the study. Treatment continued for 60 days and produced an 87.5% success rate.

One of the keys to successful treatment of contact lens–induced GPC is early diagnosis of the disease. A careful case history, asking specifically about itching and mucus discharge after contact lens wear, can allow preventive measures, such as improved lens cleaning or frequent lens replacement, to minimize the progression of GPC. An in-office tear testing technique (Touch Tear MicroAssay System, Touch Scientific Inc., Raleigh, NC) measures IgE levels in the tear layer. An increase of tear IgE from baseline indicates the need for lens care intervention or lens polymer changes.

Careful examination and early intervention can facilitate the treatment of GPC. Figures 7-10–7-13 in Table 7-3 summarize the signs, symptoms, and treatments recom-

TABLE 7-3. *Giant Papillary Conjunctivitis Signs, Symptoms, and Treatment*

	Figure	Signs	Symptoms	Treatment
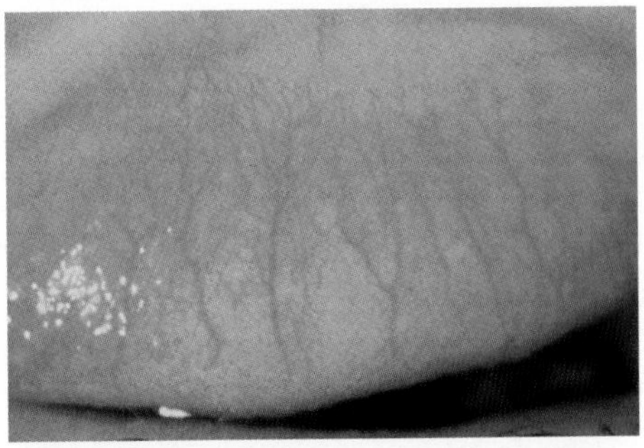	Fig. 7-10	None	Mild itching, lenses off Some morning mucus	Improve lens care Enzyme often
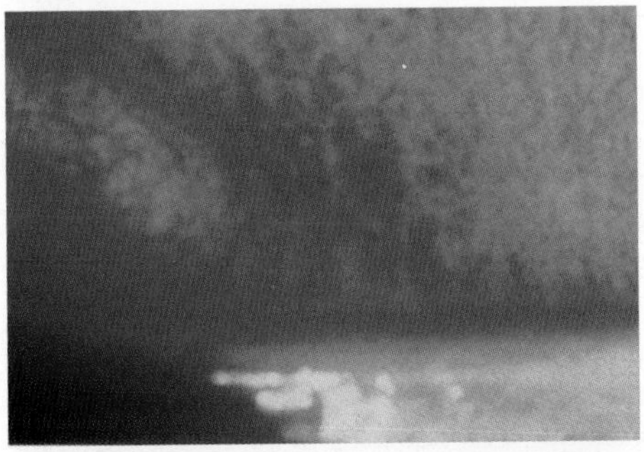	Fig. 7-11	Papillae enlargement Mucoid strands Lid hyperemia Lens deposits	Itching, lenses off More mucus Lens awareness late in day Blurry vision late in day	Replace lenses Irrigate eyes Improve lens care Change lens design Drugs (mast cell stabilizer)
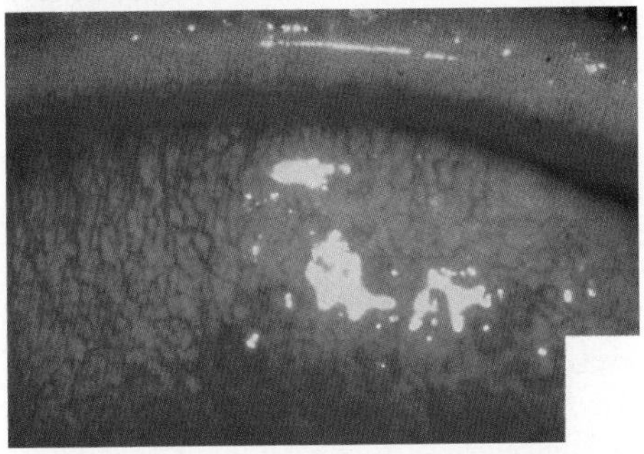	Fig. 7-12	Papillae >1 mm Mucoid strands or sheets Lid edema, hyperemia Heavy lens deposits Lens decentration, superior Superior corneal staining (rare)	Moderate to severe itching, lenses off or on More mucus Lens discomfort Reduced wearing time Excessive lens movement Variable vision with lenses on	Reduce or stop lens wear Disposable lenses; change design Improve hygiene Drugs (mast cell stabilizer) Irrigate eyes
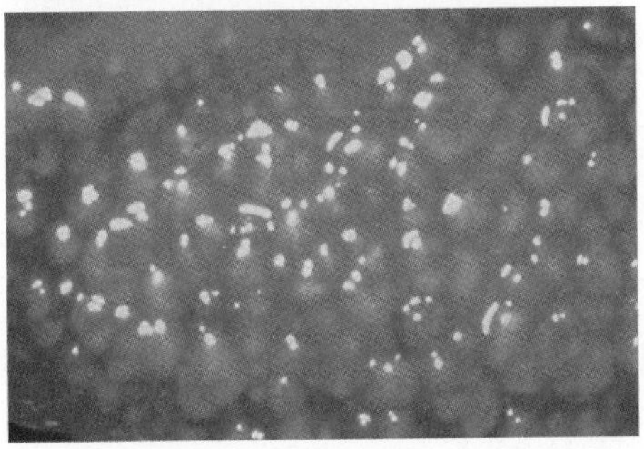	Fig. 7-13	>1-mm, mushroom-shaped papillae Lid edema, hyperemia Heavy mucoid strands Severe lens coating Superior punctate staining, infiltrates	Severe itching Lens intolerance Severe mucus Blurred vision, lenses on Lens decentration	Lens removal New lenses Irrigate eyes Disposable lenses, rigid gas-permeable lenses Improve lens care Drugs (steroids)

mended for each stage of GPC. The sooner the condition is diagnosed, the more effective the therapy.

The length of time soft lenses can be worn before GPC develops can be as short as 3 weeks to as long as 4 years, whereas presentation time of GPC in rigid lens wearers is after approximately 14 months.[85] Special care should be taken with patients who have had contact lens–induced GPC in the past. Recurrent GPC is not rare, and the time interval between episodes can vary. As with other allergic reactions, patients with GPC are prone to recurrence, although they may recognize the symptoms earlier and seek treatment sooner.

The time required for complete recovery from GPC varies. More severe GPC takes significantly longer to resolve than does early GPC. In the early-to-moderate stages, the symptoms usually abate after approximately 1 week of treatment. Resolution of the signs, particularly the reduction of papillae size, may take up to 6 months or longer. Treatment and monitoring of the more severe stages may require up to a year before resolution is achieved.[86]

SUMMARY

Contact lens–induced GPC is a common complication of contact lens wear. The early stages are often ignored and undiagnosed because the development of large papillae occurs only in later stages of the disease. Although the exact etiology is not known, prevention or minimization of the condition can be achieved by removing the antigen (lens-attached protein) from the eye. Scrupulous compliance with lens care and frequent replacement of lenses can help to minimize the potential for GPC. The best treatment is education for prevention. When stage 2 or greater GPC is evident, lens changes, improved ocular hygiene, and possible pharmacologic intervention can bring this disease under control.

REFERENCES

1. Allansmith MR, Korb DR, Greiner JV: Giant papillary conjunctivitis in contact lens wearers. Am J Ophthalmol 83:697, 1977
2. Srinivasan BD, Jakobiec FA, Iamoto T, et al: Giant papillary conjunctivitis with ocular prostheses. Arch Ophthalmol 83:892, 1979
3. Dunn JP, Weissman BA, Mondino BJ, Arnold AC: Giant papillary conjunctivitis associated with elevated corneal deposits. Cornea 9:357, 1990
4. Reynolds RM: Giant papillary conjunctivitis. Trans Ophthalmol Soc NZ 32:92, 1980
5. Stenson S: Focal giant papillary conjunctivitis from retained contact lenses. Ann Ophthalmol 14:881, 1982
6. Kennedy JR: A mechanism of corneal abrasion. Am J Optom 47:564, 1970
7. Spring TF: Reaction to hydrophilic lenses. Med J Aust 1:449, 1974
8. Soni PS, Hathcoat G: Complications reported with hydrogel extended wear contact lenses. Am J Physiol Opt 65:545, 1988
9. Alemany AL, Redal AP: Giant papillary conjunctivitis in soft and rigid lens wear. Contactologia 13E:14, 1991
10. Greiner JV, Covington HI, Allansmith MR: Surface morphology of the human upper tarsal conjunctiva. Am J Ophthalmol 83:892, 1977
11. Kessing SV: Mucus gland system of the conjunctiva: a quantitative normal anatomical study. Am J Ophthalmol 95(suppl):61, 1968
12. Greiner JV, Covington HI, Korb DR, Allansmith MR: Conjunctiva in asymptomatic contact lens wearers. Am J Ophthalmol 86:403, 1978
13. Richmond PP, Allansmith MR: Giant papillary conjunctivitis. Int Ophthalmol Clin 21:65, 1981
14. Greiner JV, Covington HI, Allansmith MR: Surface morphology of giant papillary conjunctivitis in contact lens wearers. Am J Ophthalmol 85:242, 1978
15. Greiner JV, Weidman TA, Korb DR, Allansmith MR: Histochemical analysis of secretory vesicles in nongoblet conjunctival epithelial cells. Acta Ophthalmol 63:89, 1985
16. Allansmith MR, Greiner JV, Baird RS: Number of inflammatory cells in the normal conjunctiva. Am J Ophthalmol 86:250, 1978
17. Allansmith MR, Korb DR, Greiner JV: Giant papillary conjunctivitis induced by hard or soft contact lens wear: quantitative histology. Ophthalmology 85:766, 1978
18. Allansmith MR, Baird RS, Greiner JV: Number and type of inflammatory cells in conjunctiva of asymptomatic contact lens wearers. Am J Ophthalmol 87:171, 1979
19. Henriquez AS, Allansmith MR: Russell bodies in contact lens associated giant papillary conjunctivitis. Arch Ophthalmol 97:473, 1979
20. Donshik PC, Ballow M: Tear immunoglobulins in giant papillary conjunctivitis induced by contact lenses. Am J Ophthalmol 96:460, 1993
21. Ballow M, Donshik PC, Rapacz P, et al: Immune responses in monkeys to lenses from patients with contact lens induced giant papillary conjunctivitis. CLAO J 15:64, 1989
22. Irani AA, Butrus SI, Tabbara KF, Schwartz LB: Human conjunctival mast cells: distribution of MC_T and MC_{TC} in vernal conjunctivitis and giant papillary conjunctivitis. J Allerg Clin Immunol 86:34, 1990
23. Allansmith MR: Immunology of the external ocular tissues. J Am Optom Assoc 61(suppl):S16, 1990
24. Henriquez AS, Kenyon KR, Allansmith MR: Mast cell ultrastructure. Arch Ophthalmol 99:1266, 1981
25. Begley CG, Riggle A, Tuel JA: Association of giant papillary conjunctivitis with seasonal allergies. Optom Vis Sci 67:192, 1990

26. Molinari JF: The clinical management of giant papillary conjunctivitis. Am J Optom Physiol Opt 58:886, 1981

27. Freidlander MH: Some unusual nonallergic causes of giant papillary conjunctivitis. Trans Am Ophthalmol Soc 88:343, 1990

28. Greiner JV, Peace DG, Baird RS, Allansmith MR: Effects of eye rubbing on the conjunctiva as a model of ocular inflammation. Am J Ophthalmol 100:45, 1985

29. Richmond PP: Giant papillary conjunctivitis—a closer look. J Am Optom Assoc 51:252, 1980

30. Allansmith MR: Giant papillary conjunctivitis. J Am Optom Assoc 61(suppl):S42, 1990

31. Allansmith MR, Ross RN: Ocular allergy. Clin Allerg 18:1, 1988

32. Fowler SA, Allansmith MR: Evolution of soft contact lens coatings. Arch Ophthalmol 98:95, 1980

33. Fowler SA, Allansmith MR: The surface of the continuously worn contact lens. Arch Ophthalmol 98:1233, 1980

34. Barr JT, Dugan PR, Reindel WR, Tuovinen OH: Protein and elemental analysis of contact lenses of patients with superior limbic keratoconjunctivitis or giant papillary conjunctivitis. Opt Vis Sci 66:133, 1989

35. Fowler SA, Korb DR, Allansmith MR: Deposits on soft contact lenses of various water contents. CLAO J 11:124, 1985

36. Fowler SA, Korb DR, Finnemore VM, Allansmith MR: Surface deposits on worn hard contact lenses. Arch Ophthalmol 102:757, 1984

37. Fowler SA, Greiner JV, Allansmith MR: Soft contact lenses from patients with giant papillary conjunctivitis. Am J Ophthalmol 88:1056, 1979

38. Fowler SA, Greiner JV, Allansmith MR: Attachment of bacteria to soft contact lenses. Arch Ophthalmol 97:659, 1979

39. Gudmundsson OG, Woodward DF, Fowler SA, Allansmith MR: Identification of proteins in contact lens surface deposits by immunofluorescence microscopy. Arch Ophthalmol 103:196, 1985

40. Fowler SA, Allansmith MR: The effect of cleaning soft contact lenses: a scanning electron microscopic study. Arch Ophthalmol 99:1382, 1981

41. Lustine T, Bouchard CS, Cavanagh HD: Continued contact lens wear in patients with giant papillary conjunctivitis. CLAO J 17:104, 1991

42. Korb DR, Allansmith MR, Greiner JV, et al: Prevalence of conjunctival changes in wearers of hard contact lenses. Am J Ophthalmol 90:336, 1980

43. Greiner JV, Fowler SA, Allansmith MR: Giant papillary conjunctivitis. p. 431. In Dabezies O (ed): Contact Lenses: The CLAO Guide to Basic Science and Clinical practice. Grune & Stratton, Orlando, FL, 1984

44. Korb DR, Allansmith MR, Greiner JV, et al: Biomicroscopy of papillae associated with hard contact lens wearing. Ophthalmology 88:1132, 1981

45. Sheldon L, Biedner B, Geltman C, Sachs U: Giant papillary conjunctivitis and ptosis in a contact lens wearer. J Pediatr Ophthalmol Strabismus 16:136, 1979

46. Luxenberg MN: Blepharoptosis associated with giant papillary conjunctivitis. Arch Ophthalmol 104:1706, 1986

47. Mondino BJ, Salamon SM, Zaidman GW: Allergic and toxic reactions in soft contact lens wearers. Surv Ophthalmol 26:337, 1982

48. Molinari J: Giant papillary conjunctivitis management: a review of management and a retrospective clinical study. Clin Eye Vis Care 3:68, 1991

49. Herman JP: Clinical management of GPC. Contact Lens Spectrum 2:24, 1987

50. Fowler SA, Allansmith MR: Removal of soft contact lens deposits with surfactant-polymeric bead cleaner. CLAO J 10:229, 1984

51. Allansmith MR: Pathology and treatment of giant papillary conjunctivitis. I: The U.S. perspective. Clin Ther 9:443, 1987

52. Farkas P, Kasalow TW, Farkas B: Clinical management and control of giant papillary conjunctivitis secondary to contact lens wear. J Am Optom Assoc 57:197, 1986

53. Weintraub MS: Resolution of grade 4 giant papillary conjunctivitis while wearing Allergan Advent™ (Flurofocon A) contact lenses. Int Contact Lens Clin 17:40, 1990

54. Strulowitz L, Brudno J: The management and treatment of giant papillary conjunctivitis with disposables. Contact Lens Spectrum 4:45, 1989

55. Hart DE, Schkolnick JA, Bernstein S, et al: Contact lens induced giant papillary conjunctivitis: a retrospective study. J Am Optom Assoc 60:195, 1989

56. Cho MH, Norden LC, Chang FW: Disposable extended-wear soft contact lenses for the treatment of giant papillary conjunctivitis. South J Optom 6:9, 1988

57. Schultz JE: Treating giant papillary conjunctivitis while wearing contact lenses. Int Contact Lens Clin 17:139, 1990

58. Meisler DM, Keller WB: Contact lens type, material, and deposits and giant papillary conjunctivitis. CLAO J 21:1. 1995

59. Watanabe K, Hamano H: Disposable contact lenses. p. 149. In: Hamano H, Kaufman H (eds): Corneal Physiology and Disposable Contact Lenses. Butterworth–Heinemann, Boston, 1997.

60. Bucci FA, Lopatynsky MO, Zloty P: The clinical performance of the ACUVUE, NewVues, and SeeQuence disposable contact lenses in patients with giant papillary conjunctivitis. ICLC 22:80, 1995

61. Douglas JP, Lowder CY, Lazorik R, Meisler DM: Giant papillary conjunctivitis associated with rigid gas permeable contact lenses. CLAO J 14:143, 1988

62. Donshik PC, Ballow M, Luistro A, Samartino L: Treatment of contact lens induced giant papillary conjunctivitis. CLAO J 10:346, 1984

63. Hill DS, Molinari JF: A review of giant papillary conjunctivitis associated with soft contact lens wear. Int Contact Lens Clin 8:45, 1981

64. Korb DR, Greiner JV, Finnemore VM, Allansmith MR: Treatment of contact lenses with papain. Arch Ophthalmol 101:48, 1983

65. Allansmith MR, Ross RN: Giant papillary conjunctivitis. Int Ophthalmol Clin 28:309, 1988

66. DePaolis MD, Aquavella JV: Giant papillary conjunctivitis—treatment without cromolyn sodium. Contact Lens Spectrum 6:11, 1991

67. Wood TS, Stewart RH, Bowman RW, et al: Suprofen treatment of contact lens associated giant papillary conjunctivitis. Ophthalmology 95:822, 1988

68. Sorkin EM, Ward A: Ocular sodium cromoglycate: an overview of its therapeutic efficacy in allergic eye disease. Drugs 31:131, 1986

69. Kruger CJ, Ehlers WH, Luistro AE, Donshik PC: Treatment of giant papillary conjunctivitis with cromolyn sodium. CLAO J 18:46, 1992

70. Pascucci S, Shovlin J: How to beat giant papillary conjunctivitis. Rev of Ophth June, 87, 1994

71. Supplement: Drugs to treat ocular allergic disease. Rev of Optom June, 34A, 1998

72. Meisler DM, Berzins UJ, Krachmer JH, Stock EL: Cromolyn treatment of giant papillary conjunctivitis. Arch Ophthalmol 100:1608, 1982

73. Goen TM, Sieboldt K, Terry JE: Cromolyn sodium in ocular allergic diseases. J Am Optom Assoc 57:526, 1986

74. Antiallergy and decongestant agents. p.73. In Bartlett JD (ed): Drug Facts. Facts and Comparisons. A Wolters Keuwer Company, St. Louis, 1998

75. Chapman JM, Cheeks L, Green K: Interaction of benzalkonium chloride with soft and hard contact lenses. Arch Ophthalmol 108:244, 1990

76. Roth HW: Studies on the etiology and treatment of giant papillary conjunctivitis in contact lens wearers. Contactologia 13E:55, 1991

77. Iwasaki W, Kosaka Y, Momose T, Yasuda T: Absorption of topical disodium cromoglycate and its preservative by soft contact lenses: CLAO J 14:155, 1988

78. Marren SE: Clinicians favor Livostin, Patanol among newer anti-allergy agents. Prim Care Optom News April:18, 1998

79. Trocme SD: GPC doesn't have to end contact lens use. Ophth Times Oct:8, 1996

80. Laibovitz RA, Ghormley NR, Insler MS: Treatment of giant papillary conjunctivitis with loteprednol etabonate: a novel corticosteroid. Invest Ophthalmol Vis Sci 32(suppl):734,1991

81. Asbell P, Howes J: A double-masked, placebo-controlled evaluation of the efficacy and safety of loteprednol etabonate in the treatment of giant papillary conjunctivitis. CLAO J 23:31, 1997

82. Friedlaender MH, Howes J: A double-masked, placebo-controlled evaluation of the efficacy and safety of loteprednol etabonate in the treatment of giant papillary conjunctivitis. Am J Opthalmol 123:455, 1997

83. Syrbopoulos S, Gilbert D, Easty DL: Double-blind comparison of a steroid (prednisolone) and a nonsteroid (tolmetin) in vernal kerato-conjunctivitis. Cornea 5:35,1986

84. Butts BL, Rengstorff RH: Antioxidant and vitamin A eyedrops for giant papillary conjunctivitis. Contact Lens J 18:40, 1990

85. Mondino BJ, Brawman-Mintzer O, Boothe WA: Immunological complications of soft contact lenses. J Am Optom Assoc 58:832, 1987

86. Shadbolt H: Contact lens associated papillary conjunctivitis. Disp Opt 6:8; 1991

8

Complications of Lens Care Solutions

BARBARA E. CAFFERY AND JOSHUA E. JOSEPHSON

GRAND ROUNDS CASE REPORT

Subjective:
A 22-year-old woman, in good health, taking birth control pills and occasional antihistamines during allergy season. Complaints of reduced acuity both eyes (OU) with and without contact lenses, chronic redness, reduced wearing time. Has worn soft lenses for 1 year, using Hydrocare (Allergan, Irvine, CA) chemical disinfection system.

Objective:
- Acuity with contact lenses: right eye (OD) $^{20}/_{25}$, left eye (OS) $^{20}/_{30}$ (distance and near)
- Lids, lashes, and meibomian glands clear OU
- OD: Dilatated limbal vasculature with Trantas' dots
  Superior cornea is lusterless and uneven.
  Cornea stains with fluorescein and rose bengal.
  Bulbar conjunctiva is markedly hyperemic superiorly OU.
  Tarsal conjunctiva is hyperemic with follicles.
- OS: Superior cornea has moderate pannus and fibrosis extending into pupillary zone in a triangular fashion (V-shaped, with apex toward pupil)
  Stains with fluorescein and rose bengal.
  Bulbar conjunctiva very hyperemic and chemotic, especially superiorly.
  Epithelial and anterior stromal infiltrates in superior corneal zone.
- Other findings
  Manifest spectacle refraction gives best acuity of OD $^{20}/_{25}$, OS $^{20}/_{30}$, with no improvement with pinhole.
  Keratometric readings distorted OU.
  All other ocular health findings normal OU.

Assessment:
Contact lens–induced superior limbic keratoconjunctivitis (SLK)

Plan:
1. Immediate cessation of lens wear.
2. Preservative-free ocular lubricants for symptomatic relief.
3. Patch test for thimerosal (was found to be positive).
4. Reassess 2 weeks (signs and symptoms much improved; continued abstinence from lenses and solutions containing thimerosal).
5. At 6 weeks, fully resolved, although residual V-shaped corneal fibrosis remains OS.
6. Refit with gas-permeable contact lenses.

Contact lens solutions must serve multiple purposes: to clean debris from the surface of lenses, to kill organisms, to keep lenses hydrated, to condition lens surfaces, and to maintain lens compatibility with the tear film and ocular surface. This is a tall order, considering that they must do all these things without changing the physiology of the anterior ocular segment. Finally, they must remain stable and free of organisms between uses.

It is no wonder, then, that solution-related problems are encountered in contact lens practice. Examples of patient-related solution problems include not following the necessary steps in each system, changing and mixing incompatible solutions, and contamination of bottles or use of open bottles for too long.

The lens care solutions themselves can cause problems in the anterior segment. A chemical that can kill a cellular organism, such as a bacterium, has the potential to interact adversely with the cells of body tissues. Regular, continuous exposure to any chemical can lead to an untoward physiologic or pathologic response. In addition, a chemical that the immune system recognizes from a previous exposure can cause an allergic response. Furthermore, solutions are facing new challenges. Some so-called smart bacteria learn to survive the normal effects of disinfection by secreting a protective biofilm that enables them to live in a contact lens case for prolonged periods. As a result, clinicians may have reason to fear more frequent eye infections in compliant contact lens wearers.

Understanding the effects of solutions on the ocular surface can be difficult. Each solution has many components, and any single component can affect patient response. For example, although residual hydrogen peroxide may be blamed for the symptom of stinging after insertion and placement of a contact lens, the stinging may actually be the result of solution pH. The vehicle's composition can also affect the patient's response. The osmolarity and electrolyte composition of solutions that are constantly in contact with the ocular surface can also cause physiologic changes.[1]

Understanding of the effects of solutions may also be confounded by various investigational methods. For example, the definition of an adverse ocular response to a solution, as well as the severity ratings, may vary with different study criteria. Therefore, the prevalence of adverse responses to chemical solutions can vary greatly, depending on these criteria. In addition, so many variables are present at a given time in the individual and in the contact lens system that it is difficult to identify the solution alone as causative. The physical condition of the contact lens, for example, can surely confound the diagnosis. In this situation, one must consider whether the presenting adverse response is related to a lens problem or to a care product problem.

Finally, the effects of solutions on the eyes of experimental animals, such as the rabbit, are difficult to extrapolate directly to human eyes. The ocular differences between the two species are well known. One of the most obvious differences is the significantly reduced blink rate of the rabbit. In rabbits, the chemical has prolonged contact time because it is not washed or wiped away as efficiently as in humans. Experimental methods also yield conflicting results. If simple drop formulations are used, the dosage and repeat exposure times may vary from study to study. Studies that are more true to life use experimental methods in which hydrogel lenses are soaked in solutions, and these types of studies often produce different results.

Baker et al.[2] found that preserved solutions cause significant physiologic changes in the rabbit cornea and conjunctiva. These authors also produced mild physiologic changes by using simple saline solutions without preservatives. Perhaps the very presence of any solution on the surface of the eye, other than tears, can disturb the natural balance.

Individual ocular characteristics can also influence the effect of these solutions. For example, compromised epithelial surfaces may have an exaggerated response to active ingredients or preservatives.[3] For this reason, it is good practice to take a thorough dry eye and allergy history from all potential contact lens wearers and to avoid the use of care systems that leave residual chemicals in the lenses of potentially sensitive patients.

Therefore, because of the many variables involved, the subject of adverse response to solutions must be approached with a suitable amount of credence as well as skepticism. As clinicians, a differential diagnostic mindset must be in place so that all possible etiologies can be entertained, including solution reactions, when solving patient problems.

TYPES OF ADVERSE RESPONSES

Allergy

An allergic reaction to the chemicals used in contact lens solutions can occur in certain individuals. Clinically, patients present with palpebral conjunctival papillary hypertrophy, eosinophilia, occasional follicular reaction, mucous discharge, eczema of lids and surrounding tissue, and symptoms of itching.[4]

The type of allergic response most often seen in contact lens–related cases is delayed hypersensitivity,[5] which is a cell-mediated, T cell–dependent reaction that is confirmed by the use of an intradermal or occlusive patch test.[6] This type of response can develop after repeated and prolonged exposure to a specific chemical or through previous parenteral exposure from other drugs or inocula containing the same chemical. In contact lens wear, patients are easily re-exposed to the same chemicals through repeated insertion of lenses soaked in solution. Many patients may also have been pre-exposed to chemicals, such as thimerosal, which is found in many inocula (e.g., booster shots).

Toxicity

Any chemical in sufficiently high concentration can be toxic to living tissue.[7] Chemical toxicity causes irritation and tissue damage because of its biological activity.[8] Thus, morphology and function of tissues are affected in a toxic response. A toxic response is typically immediate. The contact lens provides the ocular surface with a prolonged exposure time to solution components, thus increasing the risk for toxic embarrassment.[9] Prolonged use of these topically applied agents can also cause a cumulative cytotoxic effect, resulting in iatrogenic corneal disease or medicamentosa.

Adverse Ocular Response

Many of the preservatives and disinfectants that were used in the past and are being used in the present can cause either allergic or toxic effects on the corneal and conjunctival epithelium. The solution pH may also play a role. Clinicians rarely pursue these adverse responses to the point of patch testing or retesting to prove an allergic or toxic response. Therefore, practitioners commonly refer to these clinical scenarios as adverse ocular responses.

CLINICAL PRESENTATION OF ADVERSE OCULAR RESPONSE TO SOLUTIONS

Symptoms

The patient most often presents with symptoms of redness, stinging, photophobia, tearing, discomfort on insertion, decreased lens wearing time, and, in cases of allergic response, itching. Many of these symptoms can be attributed to other contact lens or systemic etiologies, such as soiled lenses or influenza, and clinicians must rule out these issues before attributing them to contact lens solutions.

Signs

The conjunctiva and the cornea may react to the presence of chemicals in specific ways. The clinical presentation may include conjunctival and limbal hyperemia, conjunctival chemosis, follicles or papules, SPK, corneal edema, microcysts, perilimbal infiltrates, epithelial or stromal corneal infiltrates, and epiphora.

Conjunctival Response

The conjunctiva reacts to stimuli much like other mucous membranes do.[10] The conjunctiva is a lymphoid mucous membrane that possesses its own first line of defense. Within the conjunctival epithelium are many goblet cells, which secrete mucin and serve as a lubricant for ocular wetting. Goblet cells tend to increase in number and degree of secretion during conjunctival inflammation. Relatively mild inflammation results in the accumulation of gray-white mucoid discharge floating in the tears. Beneath the conjunctival epithelial layer lies the submucosal lymphoid layer. During inflammation, this tissue may proliferate, causing irregularities in the mucous membrane surface. The conjunctiva has a rich vascular supply that serves as a route for inflammatory cells during inflammation. The pericorneal plexus of vessels contains two layers of diagnostic significance: the superficial conjunctival layer and the deep episcleral layer. The superficial layer becomes injected in corneal epithelial inflammation, such as in adverse response to solutions, whereas the episcleral layer does so in deep corneal, iris, and ciliary body inflammation, which are much less commonly seen in adverse responses to solution.

The conjunctiva has a lymphatic system that drains toward the lymphatic vessels emerging from the lids. Drainage occurs from the lateral side to the preauricular lymph nodes and from the medial side to the submaxillary lymph nodes.

The signs and symptoms of conjunctival inflammation include follicles, papillae, hyperemia, irritation, tearing, and discharge. The degree of irritation experienced is highly variable between patients. Mild stimulation causes an itching sensation, whereas stronger stimulation may yield pain. The variability in clinical presentation occurs because of individual variations in inflammatory response and interpretation of sensation.

Because of the loose structure of the conjunctival mucous membrane, this anterior segment structure is strongly predisposed to visible swelling during inflammation. In allergic responses, the associated serum leakage causes the predominant sign of conjunctival chemosis.

The submucosal lymphoid tissue often proliferates during inflammation to form miniature lymph nodes. The newly formed germinal centers in this tissue yield primarily mononuclear inflammatory cells (lymphocytes) to combat the invading agents. As these germinal centers grow, they create elevations or bumps on the mucous membrane surface and are called *follicles*. Follicles usually are approximately one-half millimeter to several millimeters and show slight gray-white discoloration. Because of the loose attachment of the conjunctiva to the tarsal plate, follicles usually appear only in the inverted lower lids. In more severe inflammation, the follicles enlarge, and some may become visible in the upper lids. The superior lid is the main conjunctival site for mast cell production. This occurs within elevated areas that are often larger than follicles, known as *papillae*. Papillae usually signify delayed allergic response.

Limbal Response

The limbal area is very responsive to toxic and allergic stimuli. Chemicals in contact lens solutions are typical stimulants associated with contact lens wear.[11,12] A massive lymph network exists in this area. The presence of Trantas' dots, or tiny limbal follicles, should alert the practitioner to suspect an allergic reaction. The limbal blood vessels dilate and release inflammatory serum and cells that may gather in the form of limbal infiltrates or exudates and then move inward, toward the central cornea.

The superior limbus seems particularly prone to react in this manner. This may relate to the availability of extravascular inflammatory mediators in the overlying tarsal conjunctiva. An extreme reaction to a solution preservative in the superior limbal area is known as contact lens–induced SLK (CL-SLK), which is described in the section Superior Limbic Keratoconjunctivitis.

The perilimbal area may also have an irregular bumpy appearance on specular reflection. The limbal area may stain with fluorescein as well, indicating a separation and disturbance of the underlying epithelial cells.

Corneal Response

The response of the normally avascular cornea is usually limited to a much subtler inflammation.[13] The earliest response of the cornea to chemical adversity is disruption of epithelial cell interdigitation, presenting in the form of SPK. Further and prolonged exposure to these chemicals leads to depressed corneal metabolism, causing edema, vacuole formation, and cellular death. In addition, inflammatory cells from the limbus and tear film may congregate in the epithelium or anterior stroma to form infiltrates.

Vital Staining

Fluorescein is the most widely used stain in contact lens practice. It is a high-molecular-weight molecule that does not enter individual cells but rather penetrates between epithelial cells that have become sufficiently disturbed to separate slightly from their neighbors.[14] SPK is most often the first sign of solution-related adverse response. SPK has a mild, diffuse staining pattern that often occurs early in the adverse response. This situation, left unattended, may result in coalesced dense staining.

Rose bengal is another high-molecular-weight vital stain that stains cells that have lost their mucous coating.[14] This typically occurs in dry eye states and in long-standing solution-related adverse responses. One of the more common presentations is the superior triangular shape stain seen in CL-SLK.

Epithelial Microcysts

Epithelial microcysts are associated with depressed corneal metabolism sustained over some period.[3,15] Clinicians see epithelial microcysts in chronic hypoxia and in long-standing chronic solution-related adverse response for which the patient has not sought a resolution. Microcysts appear as minute translucent dots, usually toward the center or midperiphery of the cornea.[16] They are typically irregular in shape and vary in diameter from 15 to 50 μm. Microcysts may be present anywhere in the epithelium, from the deep layers to the most anterior layers. They do not stain with fluorescein as long as the anterior corneal surface is intact. These microcysts probably represent pockets of cell debris and disorganized cell growth. Over time, the pockets of debris move anteriorly to the corneal surface, where they eventually break through and present as punctate staining when fluorescein is instilled.

Corneal Infiltrates

The appearance of corneal infiltrates (aggregates of inflammatory cells) is typically associated with allergic or toxic reactions to contact lens solution preservatives. They can also be seen in adenovirus infections, chlamydial infections, and staphylococcal exotoxin hypersensitivity.[17,18] Corneal infiltrates can occur in the epithelium, in the stroma, or in both layers simultaneously.[16] In the center of the infiltrates, the inflammatory cells are densely packed and become less dense toward the periphery of the infiltrate. Localized mild edema and aggregation of the inflammatory cells give infiltrates in the cornea a translucent appearance.

Corneal infiltrates can be viewed with direct or indirect retroillumination. With direct illumination, infiltrates are seen as nummular, cloudy, and somewhat amorphous bodies with slightly denser centers. Stromal infiltrates appear snowball-like and are densely white or buff colored centrally with a diaphanous border.[19] Epithelial infiltrates often take the form of single or multiple discrete small gray or whitish patches. When epithelial corneal infiltrates are viewed under high magnification with high-intensity marginal retroillumination, it is possible to observe minute refractile or gray bodies in the infiltrate patch. When stromal infiltrates are observed in this way, no similar defined bodies can be observed in the infiltrate.

The limbus is a key area for observing corneal infiltrates. They are often very small and subtle in presentation and usually overlie limbal vessels. Another limbal presentation is that of band infiltrates, seen as patches of infiltrates along the limbus. Serum leakage along terminal limbal vessels that project into the normally transparent cornea causes the immediate areas surrounding these vessels to appear somewhat cloudy. Very small epithelial infiltrates are sometimes observed with this presentation, located near the terminal ends of these vessels.

SUPERIOR LIMBIC KERATOCONJUNCTIVITIS

Theodore first described SLK in patients who did not wear contact lenses.[20] It is a disease of unknown etiology, characterized by hyperemia and papillary hypertrophy of the superior tarsal conjunctiva and the superior limbus, with gray thickening of the superior corneal epithelium. Fine punctate epithelial staining is observed on the perilimbal conjunctiva and cornea, and blood vessel infiltration of the superior cornea is seen. Giemsa staining of scraped cells from the area shows keratinized epithelial cells and polymorphonuclear cells without eosinophils. This condition is most common in women older than age 40 years, who often have thyroid disease.

Hydrogel lens wearers with CL-SLK show many similar signs.[21] The clinical presentation includes superior bulbar conjunctival hyperemia, punctate staining of the superior cornea and limbus, mild superior tarsal papillary hypertrophy, grayish-white subepithelial and intraepithelial opacities, and superior vascularization of the cornea. The symptomatic presentation includes photophobia, foreign-body sensation, redness, and an inability to wear contact lenses comfortably. Clinical differences exist between the two SLK entities in that CL-SLK has no particular patient population and is not associated with any systemic disease. Patients with Theodore's SLK tend to have more tarsal papillae and corneal filaments than patients with contact lens–induced SLK. CL-SLK has been associated in some patients with the use of thimerosal-preserved solutions.[21,22]

Treatment of contact lens–related SLK includes abstinence from thimerosal-containing solutions and cessation of lens wear until the active signs of the pathology have disappeared. Preservative-free ocular lubricants are often helpful in reducing symptoms. In severe cases, corneas have been treated with silver nitrate to remove the affected cells and to promote the regrowth of new, healthy epithelium. Once the condition is resolved, patients may be refitted with gas-permeable lenses and, in some cases, well-fitted hydrogel lenses. Patients should be placed on a preservative-free care system and monitored carefully after lens wear is resumed.[23]

COMPONENTS OF DISINFECTANT AND SALINE SOLUTIONS

Solutions used in rigid and hydrogel lens care systems are complex. The characteristics of solutions that may be important in producing adverse responses include the buffering system, preservatives, and disinfectants.[24] The osmolarity, pH, and viscosity of a solution are characteristics that can make it physiologically acceptable or unacceptable to an individual patient.[25] The appendixes to this chapter contain a list of all the solutions available on the North American market as of 1998. The preservatives and disinfectants found in each are also provided.

Buffers and pH

The common buffers used in ophthalmic solutions are boric acid, boric acid plus sodium borate, boric acid plus sodium carbonate, boric acid plus sodium phosphate, barbital plus sodium barbital, disodium phosphate plus disodium acid phosphate, potassium borate plus potassium bicarbonate, sodium citrate, and sodium phosphate plus sodium biphosphate.

Demas[26] examined the pH of several saline solutions and found them to differ greatly. Those without any buffer at all were more acidic than those with a buffer. When the pH differs dramatically from that of the tear film, stinging can ensue. Solutions whose tonicity falls dramatically out of the range of the tear film also cause obvious damage, as can be seen from either alkali or acid burns of the cornea and conjunctiva. It is possible that patients who present with stinging on insertion may be using a saline that is not buffered to their tear pH, and a change in saline solution may increase their comfort.[25] Solutions can demonstrate changes in pH as they age.[27] In these circumstances, a fresh bottle of the same saline can eliminate symptoms of stinging.

Disinfectants and Preservatives

Thimerosal

Thimerosal is a mercurial antibacterial agent that works by binding mercury ions to the sulfhydryl groups of enzymes and other proteins that microbes use to survive. Thimerosal by itself is not the most efficient antibacterial chemical, but it does have marked antifungal activity.[28] It is, therefore, often combined with other preservatives and disinfectants in contact lens solution formulations.

The presentation of thimerosal hypersensitivity is becoming a historic footnote in North America because almost all solutions have been changed to include other forms of preservatives. In an attempt to obviate such adverse responses, the pharmaceutical industry has worked hard to find preservatives that are less toxic and has certainly managed to reduce the number of obvious clinical presentations. However, this does not mean that we are not presented with more subtle and less easily explained adverse responses to the solutions presently in use.

Clinicians whose patients still use solutions preserved with thimerosal see allergic reactions. In fact, it was often much easier to identify adverse responses in patients when contact lens solution preservatives such as thimerosal were in common use. Wilson[29] described 18 patients wearing hydrogel lenses with confirmed adverse responses to thimerosal. These patients presented with red, irritated eyes, light sensitivity, reduced vision, and foreign-body sensation. Objectively, he noted conjunctival inflammation, ciliary injection, limbal follicles, and corneal changes, including gray, infiltrated epithelium, SPK, and, if left untreated, neovascularization. Wilson patch tested these patients and found them all to test positive. He presumed this to be a true example of thimerosal hypersensitivity, noting that the incidence of hypersensitivity was well documented in the dermatologic literature. In the United States, 6.5–8.0% were found to be sensitive, whereas in Scandinavia, numbers as high as 10–26% had been reported. These contact lens patients clearly had prior exposure to thimerosal. Their exposure came through inoculations in childhood in which the antisera were preserved with chemically related mercurial agents and through topical applications of drugs, such as merbromin (Mercurochrome).

Later, Cai et al.[30] demonstrated in rabbits the pathophysiology of immediate and delayed hypersensitivity with thimerosal. These authors suggested that toxic and hypersensitivity reactions were involved in these adverse responses. Tosti and Tosti[31] also reported on 36 patients with confirmed positive patch-test reactions to thimerosal who presented in their clinic with a follicular red eye. Five of them also had contact dermatitis of the lids. Other clinicians and researchers have reported eyelid dermatitis associated with thimerosal-preserved solutions.[32,33]

Chlorhexidine

Chlorhexidine is a cationic biguanide germicide with bactericidal properties against a wide range of micro-organisms.[34] It acts at the level of the cytoplasmic membrane

by interacting with acid lipid components to cause a change in membrane permeability. This change leads to a loss of intracellular potassium and phosphates and ultimately to the death of the organism.[34] It is most commonly used as a 0.004% formulation in contact lens solutions, but it has also been used in formulations of 0.0025% in Europe, especially in the United Kingdom.

Chlorhexidine digluconate was at one time the most common agent used in hydrogel lens solutions. It can bind strongly to the backbone of many hydrogel polymers.[35] There may be some competition between chlorhexidine and the smaller components of the tear fluid for the available binding sites on the hydrogel polymer hydroxyethylmethacrylate (polyHEMA). When desorbed from the lens, chlorhexidine can complex with tear proteins to prolong its exposure to the ocular epithelium.

Patients can and do present with adverse ocular responses to chlorhexidine-preserved solutions. In the dermatologic world, reported cases exist of delayed and immediate hypersensitivity to chlorhexidine.[36–39] Delayed eczematous contact dermatitis, contact urticaria, and combined dermatitis, urticaria, and anaphylaxis have been reported because this preservative is widely used in obstetric creams, in chlorhexidine digluconate (Hibitane), and in throat lozenges.

Ocular chlorhexidine hypersensitivity presents similarly to thimerosal hypersensitivity. Because these agents are often used in combination, however, it is difficult to determine which chemical is the true culprit. Studies in humans on the incidence of hypersensitivity to chlorhexidine range from as high as 33% to as low as 0.1%.[6]

Toxicity studies in rabbits have also yielded mixed results. Bonatz and Brewitt[40] found no cell desquamation at 0.15% concentration but did find evidence of cell loss at 0.25%. Dormans and van Logten,[41] on the other hand, found complete loss of cells at 0.1%. Using drops two times per day, Gasset and Ishi[42] found that up to 2% chlorhexidine produced no damage to rabbit corneas. These studies highlight the fact that it is difficult to simulate human cell toxicity in normal contact lens–wearing conditions using a rabbit eye model in the laboratories.

Soft lenses hold approximately 150 mg of chlorhexidine on initial insertion, and 20% of this may desorb into the tears within 8 hours (i.e., a rate of 4 mg per hour).[43] Thus, the maximum concentration at any one time is 70 mg/ml. Green et al.[43] believe that this is a nontoxic dose. However, it is clear that the contact time of this chemical is prolonged. This prolonged contact time, exacerbated by chlorhexidine binding to ocular surface proteins with detection up to 7 days after the use of a single drop, increases its ability to cause ocular irritation. Chlorhexidine is very toxic to the endothelium at very low concentrations, but this level cannot be reached through topical use.[43]

Chlorhexidine bound to tear proteins inactivates them and reduces their antimicrobial activity. This agent may also bind with mucin (glycoproteins) to form lens surface deposits that produce their own ocular complications.

Benzalkonium Chloride

Benzalkonium chloride (BAK) is a quaternary ammonium compound effective against gram-positive and gram-negative organisms. In contact lens solutions, it is used in 0.002–0.004% solution.

It is generally believed that BAK adsorbs to rigid gas-permeable and polymethylmethacrylate lenses in small percentages but is absorbed by hydrogels in an extreme fashion.[44,45] For this reason, it is not used in soft lens storage solutions. However, Rosenthal et al.[46] suggest that BAK can bind to silicone-acrylate lenses and that this binding can reach a toxic level. BAK is absorbed by self-aggregation, whereby molecules of BAK bind to each other in layers. BAK is a positively charged molecule. Initial adsorption may be charge related, but its longer hydrophobic chain may orient itself on the lens surface to create a template to which the hydrocarbon tails of adjacent BAK can adhere by hydrophobic interaction. BAK is unusual in that friction on the surface of the lens does not always remove it. Therefore, it can reach toxic concentrations even though lenses are being cared for properly.

BAK is a component of cosmetics, deodorants, mouthwashes, and topical skin medications; therefore, many patients have been sensitized to it. Allergic responses, however, are rarely reported. Hatiner et al.[47] described the allergic response of some glaucoma patients to BAK-preserved medications. Andersen and Rycroft[6] reported on several BAK-sensitivity studies in the literature. When it does occur, the mechanism is a hapten-binding, T cell–dependent reaction. Fisher[48] tested eight patients over 1 year for sensitivities and found BAK to show a rare incidence of allergy. Sterling and Hecht[49] reported on two cases with SPK, reduced acuity, epithelial edema, bulbar conjunctival hyperemia, and grade I papillary hypertrophy.

The most common clinical presentation of adverse response to BAK is toxicity. BAK is lipophilic and, therefore, binds to ocular tissue immediately after application. At high concentrations, it can cause morphologic disruption of the epithelium. At normal clinical concentrations, BAK may change the ionic resistance of the cornea by intercalating into cell membranes, thus increasing epithelial permeability.

Chapman et al.[44] suggested that contact lens wear accentuates the toxic effect of BAK because of the increased contact time provided to the ocular surface. Norn and Opauszki[50] also noted its effect on the tear film in that it caused a 50% decrease in tear breakup time.

The prevalence of toxicity varies depending on the method used and the population studied. Hatiner et al.[47] reported that 0.01% BAK caused marked damage to human corneal epithelial cells 4 hours after exposure. Dreifus and Wobman[51] reported 15–20% toxicity (defined as irritation) in 15–20% of human subjects. Gasset[52] reported on a case in which hydrogels were mistakenly soaked in rigid lens solution preserved with BAK. There was significant red and injected bulbar conjunctiva, SPK, inflammatory keratitis, and flare.

Studies on rabbit corneas using a variety of techniques have described a wide variety of adverse effects from BAK, including conjunctival hyperemia, blepharoedema, vascularization of corneal epithelium and dilated intercellular spaces,[51] loss of cell layers,[53] damage to all cell components,[54,55] increased ion transport and decreased epithelial resistance,[56] lysis of plasma membranes,[56] retardation of corneal healing and migration rates,[57] prolonged tissue retention,[58] and subjective irritation.[59] BAK can also affect the corneal endothelium negatively,[60] but it is unlikely that normal contact lens solution ever reaches sufficient concentrations to affect the endothelium.

Chlorobutanol

Chlorobutanol is rarely used in contact lens solutions. It is limited to the preservative in one lubricating drop for rigid lenses and is incompatible with hydrogel lens solutions. Burstein[9] found little toxic effect in rabbit corneas, but Collin and Grabsch[56] and later Burstein and Klyce[61] demonstrated surface cell disruption and decreased electron potential in rabbit epithelia. Kerr[62] found a 47% increase in adverse responses in patients using chlorobutanol-preserved solutions.

Benzyl Alcohol

Benzyl alcohol is a preservative used in one gas-permeable rigid lens disinfectant solution. It has been suggested as an alternative for patients who react to the preservatives in other rigid lens solutions, such as chlorhexidine. It is used in a 0.5% concentration and has caused very few adverse responses in patients.[6]

Sorbates

Sorbic acid has antibacterial and antifungal properties. It is active against molds and yeast but less active against bacteria. It is used mainly as a preservative in contact lens saline solutions. As a preservative in skin creams, it has been found to cause dermatitis in some patients.[63] Its effect on contact lenses is to discolor them yellow once protein has become adsorbed to the lens surface. Heating the lens in the saline exacerbates this process. The corneal epithelium can be affected occasionally by solutions containing sorbic acid.[64]

Fisher has reported actual allergic sensitivities to sorbates.[65] Andersen and Rycroft[6] reported three studies of dermal testing showing 1/260, 1/627, and 1/465 as the incidence of sorbic acid sensitivity.

The most common presentation associated with sorbic acid in contact lens practice is that of stinging on insertion, which may represent a toxic reaction or may relate to the pH of the solution. Caffery and Josephson[66] reported a reaction in 15% of patients using 0.1% solution. Adverse response was defined as discomfort or stinging on insertion with sorbic acid–preserved saline, which resolved when the patient switched to nonpreserved saline solution.

Disodium Ethylenediaminetetraacetic Acid

Disodium ethylenediaminetetraacetic acid (Na_2EDTA) is a preservative used in conjunction with thimerosal, sorbates, and BAK in contact lens products, usually in a 0.1% concentration. No human clinical studies exist that implicate this product as the cause of adverse ocular response. However, guinea pig studies by Collin et al.[67] showed endothelial and stromal cell changes with 0.2% Na_2EDTA.

Hydrogen Peroxide

The introduction of hydrogen peroxide for disinfection changed the face of contact lens care systems dramatically. Thermal disinfection systems had lost favor because of the contamination factor in salt tablet saline preparations, the high incidence of giant papillary conjunctivitis, discoloration of lenses, more frequent use of high–water content (unheatable) lenses, and inconvenience. The only available cold disinfection systems were fraught with problems related to the toxic and allergic responses produced by prolonged use of thimerosal or chlorhexidine preparations. The stage was set for safer cold disinfection systems.

The efficacy of hydrogen peroxide as a disinfectant has been well studied.[68] This chemical was first prepared in 1918, and when it was found unstable, phosphoric acid was added to stabilize it. O'Driscoll and Isen[69] first discussed it in conjunction with soft lens disinfection.

Fears about hydrogen peroxide concern the adverse effects of free radical reactions.[70,71] Many evolutionary changes occurred as a result of the effects of free radicals on molecules, causing cell mutation and death. The aging process of cells involves the deleterious effects of free radicals throughout the body.[72] Imlay et al.[70] describe the reaction of hydrogen peroxide with ferrous ions to produce reactive radicals, which must be removed from the cell to prevent DNA damage.

One expressed fear is that corneal epithelial cells exposed to hydrogen peroxide lose their interleukin-1 and, thus, are unable to respond in an immune fashion to protect the ocular surface.[73] Further concerns are that excess hydrogen peroxide reaches the crystalline lens and induces cataract.[70] In addition, corneal endothelial cells are vulnerable to physiologic damage from hydrogen peroxide exposure.[68]

The human body has a very efficient mechanism to protect its cells from the effects of hydrogen peroxide.[74] Three enzymes—catalase, superoxide dismutase, and glutathione peroxidase—are present in all cells.[68] The corneal and conjunctival epithelium and the tear film have these enzymes available to neutralize any excess hydrogen peroxide on the ocular surface. Catalase appears to be present because 90% of hydrogen peroxide is removed from the surface of the eye in 30 seconds.[75]

Peroxide-based care systems are formulated to leave the contact lens and solutions as free as possible of hydrogen peroxide before insertion.[76] Catalase and sodium pyruvate are two enzymes used to eliminate hydrogen peroxide, and platinum disks act as catalysts in two systems and dilution in another. Gyulai et al.[77] measured the amount of hydrogen peroxide remaining in the solution in the contact lens case after neutralization. Catalase left 0–1.0 part per million (ppm), sodium pyruvate left 1.0 ppm, AOSept (CIBA Vision, Duluth, GA) 15.0 ppm, Lensept (CIBA Vision, Duluth, GA) 1.8 ppm, and Quicksept (CIBA Vision, Duluth, GA) 200 ppm. Kelly et al.[78] tested Permaflex (CooperVision, Inc., Fairport, NY) nonionic 74%-water content lenses to determine the percentage of hydrogen peroxide left after neutralization in solution and in lenses. The results are noted in Table 8-1.

Several studies have been conducted to determine the levels of hydrogen peroxide that produce symptoms and toxicity.[79] Riley suggests that no toxicity can occur in normal usage.[80] McNally[71] used drops of various dilutions to determine the threshold sting sensitivity in 10 subjects. The mean threshold was 267 ppm for lenses with 55% water content and 282 ppm for those with 38% water content. He also tested the effect of hydrogen peroxide on corneal permeability. In topical form, 50–500 ppm did not change corneal permeability from that of controls.

Chalmers and McNally[81] rated the human drop threshold at 490–1,470 ppm and the lens-soaked threshold as 210–408 ppm. Their belief is that most patients are more sensitive to pH than to hydrogen peroxide. Work by Harris and others adds support to this hypothesis.[82–84]

Paugh et al.[85] tested eight subjects with presoaked contact lenses, keeping the pH equal. Toxicity was defined as subjective discomfort, conjunctival hyperemia, corneal and conjunctival staining, and corneal oxygen uptake. The limit was 100 ppm with respect to symptoms. Even at 800 ppm, no staining occurred. Boets et al.[86] found no change in epithelial barrier function tested by flourophotometry in 30 healthy contact lens wearers.

Researchers have studied the direct effect of hydrogen peroxide concentrations on the rabbit epithelium.[45,64,87] Williams et al.[87] showed in rabbits, however, that hydrogen peroxide caused metabolic changes at lower concentrations than those that typically produce clinical symptoms in humans. Wilson and Chalmers[88,89] demonstrated that stromal swelling and light scatter occurred in the stroma of rabbits exposed to 72–153 ppm of hydrogen peroxide. Tripathi and Tripathi[90] cultured human epithelial cells and used single doses of 30–100 ppm of hydrogen peroxide. They found that even 30 ppm caused cell retraction and changes in function and morphology that were dose and time dependent. It is their belief that contact lens wearers may be subject to deleterious effects of peroxide without being aware of their presence.

Acute clinical toxicities have been reported[91] and have probably been seen by most practitioners whose patients have inadvertently inserted lenses that were soaked in 3% hydrogen peroxide and were not neutralized. Lavery et al.[92] reported an aphakic patient who presented with a clear white anterior stromal lesion consisting of bubbles that split the stromal lamella. The lesion was gone within 3 hours.

Epstein and colleagues[93,94] reported on four patients who presented with punctate, coalesced staining after normal use of hydrogen peroxide solutions. These lesions were absent when patients were switched to solutions that did not contain hydrogen peroxide.

Although there have been concerns about effects on the endothelium,[95] Riley and Kast[96] found it impossible to transfer even 680 ppm across an intact rabbit epithelium. They concluded that in the normal clinical situation with an intact epithelium and normal contact lens use, neither corneal endothelium nor intraocular tissue is damaged by residual concentrations of hydrogen peroxide up to 680 ppm, whether by single incidence or daily events.

Poly Biguanides

Polyaminopropyl biguanide (PAPB) (also known as Dymed, Bausch & Lomb, Inc., Rochester, NY) and polyhexamethylene biguanide HCl (PHMB) are two common multipurpose solution disinfectant chemicals used in rigid and hydrogel lens solutions. They are used in concentrations of 0.00003% in saline solutions and 0.00005% in storage solutions. PAPB is used at 0.00015% in one solution for rigid gas-permeable lenses.

These disinfectants are considered an improvement over previous disinfectants such as thimerosal because of their

TABLE 8-1. *Comparison of Residual Peroxide in Solution and on Lenses*

Product (Neutralization)	Solution (ppm)	Lenses (ppm)
Oxysept[a] (catalase)	<1	<1
Omnicare[a] (catalase)	<1	<1
Mirasept[b] (Na pyruvate)	1	3
AOSept[b] (platinum disk)	12	10
Puresept[c] (dilution)	196	55
Quicksept[c] (dilution)	203	216

ppm = parts per million.
[a]Manufactured by Allergan, Irvine, CA.
[b]Manufactured by CIBA Vision, Duluth, GA.
[c]Discontinued.
Source: Adapted from W Kelly, G Ward, W Williams, A Dziabo. Eliminating hydrogen peroxide residuals in solutions and contact lenses. Contact Lens Spectrum 5:41, 1990.

larger molecular size. This prevents penetration into the hydrogel lens matrix, reducing the dosage received by the ocular anterior segment. However, Rosenthal[97] has suggested that some accumulation occurs in the lens.

Begley et al.[98] studied the toxic effects of PAPB on rabbit corneas and demonstrated significant toxicity to the epithelium at only 10–100 times the concentration found in normal soft contact lens solutions. Thus, the rigid lens solution that was tested, in its higher-concentration format, did demonstrate higher toxicity in the rabbit eye than did the soft lens variety.[64] Bergmanson and Ross[99] found no significant toxic effects on rabbit corneas. Boets et al.[86] found no effect on corneal barrier function.

Clompus[100] described a clinical situation in which dermatitis presented as a red stripe down a patient's face, which exactly followed the route of the excess PAPB-preserved solution. It appears that the skin can react even more quickly than the conjunctiva to this chemical, but the incidence of adverse responses clinically is very small.[101] Soni et al.[102] found increased corneal staining and inflammatory response in an adolescent population followed for 3 years with ReNu Multi-Purpose Solution (Bausch & Lomb , Inc., Rochester, NY) compared to a hydrogen peroxide solution.

Polyquaternium-1

Another of the modern hydrogel lens disinfectants is polyquaternium-1 (Polyquad, Alcon Laboratories, Ft. Worth, TX), a molecule of large diameter (225 Å).[103] The larger diameter prevents it from entering the lens matrix, thus reducing the dosage and time of contact with the ocular surface.[97] Polyquaternium-1 is used in various Optifree (Alcon Laboratories, Inc., Fort Worth, TX) systems at a concentration of 0.001%,[103] which is a relatively low concentration. In a challenge study, even higher concentrations provoked few adverse responses in healthy contact lens wearers who used the solution over a 3-month period.[104] Its formulation has been changed by using a citrate buffer, from the original OptiSoft (Alcon Laboratories, Inc., Fort Worth, TX) version, which was not suitable for some hydrogel materials.[105] Gordon[103] reported clinical success with 99.5% of patients, and Schachet et al.[106] reported 98.7% success in 303 patients.

When adverse responses do present, patients report irritation and redness, and practitioners observe hyperemia and occasional punctate keratitis. Gibbs et al.[107] reported one patient in 51 to be intolerant. Davis et al.[108] reported one in 65 previously preservative-sensitive patients to be symptomatic with polyquaternium-1. Soni et al.[102] did find more adverse corneal and conjunctival effects in an adolescent population who used solutions preserved with polyquaternium-1 compared to hydrogen peroxide solutions.

The immunogenicity of the high-molecular-weight polyquaternium-1 molecule is considered very low, and its cytotoxic effects are also considered very low. However, Adams et al.[109] studied the effects of several preservatives on the corneal epithelium and found that polyquaternium-1 and EDTA produced changes in cell shape that may represent a compromise in barrier function of the epithelium. Begley et al.[98] also found some epithelial effects on the rabbit cornea from components of cleaning solutions.

COMPONENTS OF CLEANING SOLUTIONS

Enzymes

Three enzymes used in hydrogel lens cleaning are papain, pancreatin, and subtilisin. Enzymes are typically used with conventional (repeated-usage) contact lenses to maintain the lens surfaces free of protein filming and to prevent the adverse effects of protein buildup leading to conjunctival alterations, such as giant papillary conjunctivitis. With widespread use of disposable and frequent-replacement hydrogel contact lenses, the use of enzyme products has greatly diminished. Rigid gas-permeable lenses also benefit from protein removal afforded by enzymes. Although enzyme tablets originally formulated for soft lenses have been adapted and formulated for rigid gas-permeable lenses, the introduction of a liquid enzyme (Boston Liquid Enzyme, Polymer Technology, Inc., Rochester, NY) holds promise of improving patient compliance and in making the use of enzymes with these lenses much easier.

Papain

The first enzyme introduced for hydrogel lenses was papain. This is a microcrystalline powder enzyme extracted from the green fruits of Carica papaya. It denatures proteins and renders them easily cleaned from a lens surface. Papain should be fully removed from a contact lens surface before insertion. This is accomplished by surfactant cleaning, followed by thorough rinsing with saline solution. Residual papain on a lens can cause reactions when the lens is inserted. Papain sensitivities have been demonstrated on the hands of personnel who manufacture the tablets.[110]

In contact lens use, Davis[111] reported on 30 patients with mild-to-severe discomfort after papain use. Santucci et al.[110] documented a case of hand and ocular reactions to the enzyme, which was an allergic response confirmed with patch testing. Bernstein et al.[112] reported on a documented immunoglobulin E–mediated sensitization to papain, producing conjunctivitis and ocular angioedema, which took 1 year to develop.

Patients using papain who have discomfort with lenses after insertion should be advised to clean and rinse their lenses well before insertion. If the irritation continues, change to another enzyme or discontinuation of enzyme use is suggested.

Pancreatin

Pancreatin, a naturally occurring enzyme derived from porcine tissue, serves to break down proteins adherent to the soft lens surface. A low level of toxicity and sensitivity to pancreatin has been reported.[113] Davis, however, found that 30 papain-sensitive patients could use pancreatin without complication.[111]

Subtilisin

Subtilisin is a larger molecule used to break down protein. Three incidences of allergy to this chemical have been reported by Zetterstrom and Wide.[114] A 19% sensitivity rate was found in Scandinavia. Those with a history of atopy were even more sensitive.

The reaction to these chemicals depends on dosage and exposure time, which are closely related to patient handling, compliance, and soiling level of the lenses. Patients with consistent symptoms of adverse response on the morning after an enzyme treatment should change enzymes or discontinue use of the product and replace their lenses more often.

Surfactant Cleaners

In general, it is believed that if patients thoroughly rinse surfactant cleaners off lens surfaces, no effect of the solution occurs on the ocular surface and, therefore, no effect on patient comfort. No guarantees exist that patients are complying with this directive, and clinicians, therefore, have observed adverse responses to lens wear that seem to be directly related to the cleaner. The most common examples are Miraflow and AOFlow (CIBA Vision, Duluth, GA), which are excellent cleaners containing isopropyl alcohol. Patients who do not rinse this surfactant thoroughly are especially likely to report stinging on insertion. The original version of Opticlean (Alcon Laboratories, Inc., Fort Worth, TX), with its cleaning granules, also provided above-average cleaning effects but was responsible for some reports of stinging on insertion. This product has since been reformulated, and this change has been clinically observed to resolve the problem.

Surfactants are necessary for proper lens care, for their cleaning properties and for the effect on the microbial count on the lenses, but if patients do not rinse their lenses thoroughly before insertion, they may experience problems.

LUBRICATING AND REWETTING DROPS

The formulations of lubricating drops can also be suspect in the etiology of red and irritated eyes. Most of these drops are multipurpose and, therefore, are preserved with chemicals similar to those in other contact lens solutions. Because lenses are not stored in these solutions, their chemical agents may not have as prolonged a contact time in the tear film. However, excessive use of these drops can increase the frequency of exposure.

Because many patients are not accurate when instilling drops, the irritation in susceptible patients appears on the lids and even on the cheeks more often and earlier than on the conjunctiva. Symptoms may include stinging on application, red and crusty lid margins, and red patchy facial skin lesions.

Patients who use glaucoma medications often describe reactions from drop applications. The culprit in most circumstances seems to be the preservatives. This also appears to be true of artificial tear formulations.[115,116] Contact lens–wearing patients with symptoms of dryness had greater relief with nonpreserved eye drops than with preserved drops.[6] Sorbic acid, polyquaternium-1, PAPB, thimerosal, EDTA, and potassium sorbate have all been used in soft lens lubricating drops.

COMPLICATIONS OF MIXING SOLUTIONS

The confusion that surrounds the use of contact lens care products leads to their misuse. Some of the chemical combinations thus created can lead to toxic adverse responses.

Sibley and Shovlin[117] warn against mixing polyvinyl alcohol and boric acid or hydrogen peroxide and potassium sorbate when lenses are soiled with protein.

Rakow[118] warns that cationic molecules, such as chlorhexidine, polyquaternium-1, and PAPB should never be mixed with anionic molecules, such as sorbic acid. Thimerosal and chlorhexidine should never be mixed with either alkyl tri-ethanol ammonium chloride or BAK. Chlorhexidine mixed with hydrogen peroxide can cause chlorhexidine to precipitate.

Various peroxide neutralizers mixed together cause precipitates and adverse responses (i.e., sorbic acid and thiosulfate, pyruvate and thiosulfate). Polaxymer 407 (found in Pliagel, and Miraflow and AOFlow, CIBA Vision, Duluth, GA) should not be used with Barnes-Hind Softmate (Wesley-Jessen, Des Plaines, IL) leaner because this forms a cloudy precipitate.

Because Collins and Carney[119] found only 26% of patients surveyed to be compliant with lens care, some adverse responses in lens wear result from improper mixing of chemicals.

ISSUE OF BIOFILMS

The most important goal of contact lens care is to ensure that the patient remains free from sight-threatening infection. This entails keeping lenses clean and keeping the ocular surface free of infectious micro-organisms. The U.S. Food and Drug Administration has developed a rigorous set of criteria for disinfection, and all solution systems on the market have met these criteria. Many, however, fear that the criteria no longer apply to the reality of the state of micro-organisms in contact lens care systems. Wilson et al.[120] and others have described the state of some so-called smart bacteria in lens cases. These bacteria secrete a sticky substance, called a glycocalyx, that protects them from the effects of disinfectant chemicals for up to 2 years. It is a serious flaw in the present systems if these bacteria are viable and can be transferred from the wall of the case to the ocular surface, potentially causing infection. Whether these protected bacteria can actually cause serious infection is not known, but the possibility is an issue with which the pharmaceutical industry is dealing and of which practitioners must be aware.

Until this issue is resolved, practitioners must reinforce the importance of proper lens case care at each visit. Patients should be advised to change their lens cases frequently and to allow them to air-dry while their lenses are being worn. Scrubbing the case on a weekly basis with a brush, using hot water and dish soap, is also a good idea. Solution manufacturers are responding by packaging cases with their disinfection solutions, and practitioners should encourage frequent case replacement. It is hoped that cases resistant to biofilms and solution systems or devices such as ultraviolet or microwave sterilizers can be made available to lens wearers to keep their cases free of these biofilms.

SUMMARY

The formulations of contact lens materials and the associated care systems are constantly evolving and changing. The past numerous, occasionally severe adverse responses to solutions is at an end, thanks to the response of the pharmaceutical industry and the trend toward more frequent replacement of lenses. However, the contact lens practitioner must remain alert to the realities of the more subtle adverse responses that present clinically. Patients with symptoms of reduced wearing time, stinging, redness, and itching may indeed be experiencing an adverse response to their solutions. After ruling out lens-related or systemic etiologies, changing the patient to a preservative-free care system with buffered saline is appropriate.

Perhaps the more common clinical problems associated with contact lens solutions are those associated with noncompliance. Practitioners must review care systems and procedures with each patient at every visit to reinforce the importance of hygiene and disinfection as well as the purpose of each solution. This should reduce the prevalence of adverse responses related to solution misuse and the mixing of incompatible solutions.

The present standards set for contact lens solutions may not be realistic in the world of so-called smart bacteria. Practitioners must insist that the pharmaceutical industry respond to these changes. As has always been the case, the contact lens practitioner must deal with each patient as a unique challenge. The choice of care systems must consider each patient's particular ocular characteristics. The practitioner must stress and continually monitor each patient's compliance level and upgrade the lens solutions as the pharmaceutical industry develops even safer and more effective care systems.

REFERENCES

1. Gilbard JD, Rossi SR, Heydfa KG: Ophthalmic solutions, the ocular surface, and a unique therapeutic artificial tear formulation. Am J Ophthalmol 107:348, 1989
2. Baker JC, Balodis L, Currie JP, et al: A comparative study of human tears and various ophthalmic products: ionic composition and physiological effects. p. 551. AVRO (Association for Research in Vision and Ophthalmology) Annual Meeting Abstracts, Bethesda, MD, 1990
3. Holden BA, Sweeney DF, Vannas A, et al: Effects of long-term extended contact lens wear on the human cornea. Invest Ophthalmol Vis Sci 26:1489, 1985
4. Goldstein JH: Effects of drugs on cornea, conjunctiva and lids. Int Ophthalmol Clin 11:13, 1971
5. Abelson MB, Allansmith MR: Ocular allergies. p. 307. In Smolin G, Thoft RA (eds): The Cornea. 2nd ed. Little, Brown, Boston, 1987
6. Andersen KE, Rycroft RJ: Recommended patch test concentrations for preservatives, biocides and antimicrobials. Contact Dermatitis 25:1, 1991
7. Sendele DD: Chemical hypersensitivity reactions. Int Ophthalmol Clin 26:25, 1986
8. Pfister RR: The effects of chemical injury on the ocular surface. Ophthalmology 90:601, 1983
9. Burstein NL: Preservative cytotoxic threshold for benzalkonium chloride and chlorhexidine digluconate in cat and rabbit corneas. Invest Ophthalmol 19:308, 1980
10. Duke-Elder S: Inflammation of the conjunctiva and associated inflammations of the cornea. p. 47. In System of Ophthalmology. Vol. VIII. Diseases of the Outer Eye. Part 1. Diseases of the Conjunctiva and Associated Diseases of the Corneal Epithelium. Henry Klimpton, London, 1965
11. Friend J, Kenyon K: Physiology of the conjunctiva: metabolism and chemistry. p. 52. In Smolin G, Thoft RA (eds): The Cornea. 2nd ed. Little, Brown and Company, Boston, 1987
12. Meisler DM, Zaret CR, Stock EL: Trantas' dots and limbal inflammation associated with soft contact lens wear. Am J Ophthalmol 89:66, 1980
13. Kenyon KR: Morphology and pathological responses of the cornea to disease. p. 63. In Smolin G, Thoft RA (eds): The Cornea. 2nd ed. Little, Brown, Boston, 1987
14. Feenstra RC, Tseng SG: What is actually stained by rose bengal? Arch Ophthalmol 110:984, 1992
15. Hamano H, Hori M: Effects of contact lens wear on the mitosis of corneal epithelial cells. Preliminary report. CLAO J 9:133, 1983
16. Josephson JE, Zantos S, Caffery BE, Herman JP: Differentiation of corneal complications observed in contact lens wearers. J Am Optom Assoc 59:679, 1989
17. Josephson JE, Caffery BE: Infiltrative keratitis in hydrogel lens wearers. Int Contact Lens Clin 6:223, 1979
18. Jones BR: Adenovirus infections of the eye. Trans Ophthalmol Soc UK 82:621, 1962
19. Litvin M: Subepithelial infiltrates in soft lens wearers. J Br Contact Lens Assoc 1:31, 1978
20. Theodore F: Superior limbic keratoconjunctivitis. Ear Nose Throat J 42:25, 1963
21. Fuerst DJ, Sugar J, Wrobec S: Superior limbic keratoconjunctivitis associated with cosmetic soft contact lens wear. Arch Ophthalmol 101:1214, 1983
22. Sendale DD, Kenyon KR, Mobilia F, et al: Superior limbic keratoconjunctivitis in contact lens wearers. Ophthalmology 90:616, 1983
23. Silbert JA: Contact lens related pathology: part II. Rev Optom 121:51, 1984

24. Hopkins GA: Pharmaceutical aspects of soft contact lens wear. Optician 192:20, 1986

25. Carney LG, Brezinski SD, Hill RM: Finding solutions' buffering capacity. Contact Lens Spectrum 1:50, 1986

26. Demas GN: pH consistency and stability of contact lens solutions. J Am Optom Assoc 60:732, 1989

27. Carney LG, Hill RM, Habenicht BL: Ageing lubricant solutions: a clinical comment. Contact Lens J 18:157, 1990

28. Bathy I, Harris E, Gasson A: Preservatives and biological reagents. International Symposium on Bifocal Products 1973. Dev Biol Stand, 1974

29. Wilson LA: Thimerosal hypersensitivity in soft contact lens wearers. Contact Lens J 9:21, 1980

30. Cai F, Backman HA, Baines MG: Thimerosal: an ophthalmic preservative which acts as a hapten to elicit specific antibodies and cell mediated immunity. Curr Eye Res 7:341, 1983

31. Tosti A, Tosti G: Thimerosal: a hidden allergen in ophthalmology. Contact Dermatitis 18:268, 1988

32. DeGroot AC, van Wignen WG, van Wignen-Vos M: Occupational contact dermatitis of eyelids without ocular involvement from thimerosal in contact lens fluid. Contact Dermatitis 23:195, 1990

33. Sertoli T, DiFonzo E, Spallanzani P, Panconesi E: Allergic contact dermatitis from thimerosal in a soft contact lens wearer. Contact Dermatitis 6:292, 1980

34. Chawmer JA, Gilbert P: A comparative study of the bacterial and growth inhibitory activities of the biguanides alexidine and chlorhexidine. J Appl Bacteriol 66:243, 1989

35. Refojo MF: Reversible binding of chlorhexidine gluconate to hydrogel contact lenses. Contact Intraocul Lens Med J 2:47, 1976

36. Fisher AA: Contact urticaria from chlorhexidine. Cutis 43:17, 1989

37. Knudsen BB, Avnstorp C: Chlorhexidine gluconate and acetate in patch testing. Contact Dermatitis 24:45, 1991

38. Reynolds NJ, Harman RR: Allergic contact dermatitis from chlorhexidine diacetate in a skin soap. Contact Dermatitis 22:103, 1990

39. Wong WR, Goh GL, Chan KW: Contact urticaria from chlorhexidine. Contact Dermatitis 22:52, 1990

40. Bonatz E, Brewitt H: Morphological studies of corneal epithelium before and after the application of topical ophthalmic drugs. p. 280. In Holly FJ (ed): The Preocular Tear Film in Health, Disease, and Contact Lens Wear. Dry Eye Institute, Lubbock, TX, 1986

41. Dormans JAMA, van Logten MJ: The effects of ophthalmic preservatives on corneal epithelium of the rabbit: a scanning electron microscopical study. Toxicol Appl Pharmacol 62:251, 1982

42. Gasset AR, Ishi Y: Cytotoxicity of chlorhexidine. Can J Ophthalmol 10:98, 1975

43. Green K, Livingston V, Bowman K, Hall DS: Chlorhexidine effects on corneal epithelium and endothelium. Arch Ophthalmol 98:1273, 1980

44. Chapman JM, Cheeks L, Green K: Interactions of benzalkonium chloride with soft and hard contact lenses. Arch Ophthalmol 108:244, 1990

45. Wong MR, Dzaibo AJ, Kiral RM: Adsorption of benzalkonium chloride by RGP lenses. Contact Lens Forum 11:25, 1986

46. Rosenthal P, Chou MH, Salamone JC, Israel SC: Quantitive analyses of chlorhexidine gluconate and benzalkonium chloride absorption on silicone acrylate polymers. CLAO J 12:43, 1986

47. Hatiner A, Terasvirta M, Fraki JE: Contact allergy to components in topical ophthalmologic preparations. Acta Ophthalmol 63:424, 1985

48. Fisher AA: Cutaneous reactions to sorbic acid and potassium sorbate. Cutis 25:350, 1980

49. Sterling JL, Hecht AS: BAK induced chemical keratitis? Contact Lens Spectrum 3:62, 1988

50. Norn MS, Opauszki A: Effects of ophthalmic vehicles on the stability of the precorneal tear film. Acta Ophthalmol 55:23, 1977

51. Dreifus M, Wobman P: Influence of soft contact lens solutions on rabbit cornea. Ophthalmol Res 7:140, 1975

52. Gasset AR: Benzalkonium chloride toxicity to the human cornea. Am J Ophthalmol 84:169, 1977

53. Pfister RR, Burstein W: The effects of ophthalmic drugs, vehicles and preservatives on corneal epithelium. A scanning electron microscope study. Invest Ophthalmol Vis Sci 15:246, 1976

54. Neville R, Dennis P, Sens D, Crouch R: Preservative cytotoxicity to cultured corneal epithelial cells. Curr Eye Res 5:367, 1986

55. Gasset A, Ishi Y, Kaufman H, Miller T: Cytotoxicity of ophthalmic preservatives. Am J Ophthalmol 78:98, 1974

56. Tonjum AM: Effects of benzalkonium chloride upon the corneal epithelium studied with scanning electron microscopy. Acta Ophthalmol 53:358, 1975

57. Collin HB, Grabsch BE: The effect of ophthalmic preservatives on the healing rate of the rabbit corneal epithelium following keratectomy. Am J Optom Physiol Opt 59:215, 1982

58. Champeau EJ, Edelhauser HF: Effect of ophthalmic preservatives on ocular surface; conjunctival and corneal uptake and distribution of benzalkonium chloride and chlorhexidine digluconate. p. 292. In Holly FJ (ed): The Preocular Tear Film in Health, Disease and Contact Lens Wear. Dry Eye Institute, Lubbock, TX, 1986

59. Barkman R, Germanis M, Karpe G, Malmborg AS: Preservatives in eye drops. Acta Ophthamol 47:461, 1969

60. Lemp MA, Zimmerman LE: Toxic endothelial degeneration in ocular surface disease treated with topical medications containing benzalkonium chloride. Am J Ophthalmol 105:670, 1988

61. Burstein NL, Klyce SD: Electrophysiologic and morphologic effects of ophthalmic preparations on the rabbit corneal epithelium. Invest Ophthalmol Vis Sci 16:899, 1977

62. Kerr C: 3 and 9 o'clock staining: a simple solution. Optician 195:25, 1988

63. Hjorth N, Trolle-Lassen C, Shen S: Reactions to preservatives in creams. Am Perfumer Cosmet Oct:146, 1962

64. Begley CJ, Waggoner PJ, Hafner GS, et al: Effect of rigid gas permeable contact lens wetting solutions on the rabbit corneal epithelium. Optom Vis Sci 68:189, 1991

65. Fisher AA: Allergic reactions to contact lens solutions. Cutis 209, 1985

66. Caffery BE, Josephson JE: Is there a better comfort drop? J Am Optom Assoc 61:178, 1990

67. Collin HB, Grabsch BE, Carroll N, Hammond VE: Morphological changes to keratocytes and endothelial cells of the isolated guinea pig cornea due to thimerosal. Int Contact Lens Clin 9:275, 1982

68. Chalmers RL: Hydrogen peroxide in anterior segment physiology: a literature review. Optom Vis Sci 66:796, 1989

69. O'Driscoll FK, Isen AA: United States Patents 3,841,9851 (1974) and 3,700,761 (1974)

70. Imlay JA, Chin SM, Linn S: Toxic DNA damage by hydrogen peroxide through the Fenton reaction in vivo and in vitro. Science 240:640, 1988

71. McNally JJ: Clinical aspects of topical applications of dilute hydrogen peroxide solution. CLAO J 16:546, 1990

72. Hinshaw DB, Sklar LA, Bohl B, et al: Cytoskeletal and morphologic impact of cellular oxidant injury. Am J Pathol 123:454, 1986

73. Grabner G, Luger TA, Smolin G, et al: Corneal epithelial cell–derived thymocyte-activating factor (CETAF). Invest Ophthalmol Vis Sci 23:757, 1982

74. McCord JM, Fridovich I: Superoxide dismutase: an enzymatic function for erythrocuprein and hemocuprein. J Biol Chem 244:6049, 1969

75. Chalmers RL, Tsao M, Scott G: The rate of in vivo residual H_2O_2 from hydrogel lenses. Contact Lens Spectrum 4:21, 1989

76. Muton JW, Phillips JH: Patient comfort comparisons of hydrogen peroxide systems. Contact Lens Spectrum 3:48, 1988

77. Gyulai P, Dziabo A, Kelly W, et al: Relative neutralization ability of six hydrogen peroxide disinfection systems. Contact Lens Spectrum 2:61, 1987

78. Kelly W, Ward G, Williams W, Dziabo A: Eliminating hydrogen peroxide residuals in solutions and contact lenses. Contact Lens Spectrum 5:41, 1990

79. McKenney CH, Chalmers RL, Burstein N: Human corneal epithelial permeability after instillation of hydrogen peroxide (abstract). Ophthalmol Vis Sci 66(suppl):239, 1989

80. Riley MV, Wilson G: Topical hydrogen peroxide and the safety of ocular tissues. CLAO J 19:186, 1993

81. Chalmers RL, McNally JJ: Ocular detection threshold for hydrogen peroxide; drops vs lenses. Int Contact Lens Clin 15:351, 1988

82. Harris MG, Meican C, Lony DA, Cushing LA: The pH of over the counter hydrogen peroxide in soft lens disinfection systems. Optom Vis Sci 66:839, 1989

83. Harris MG, Torres J, Tracewell L: pH and H_2O_2 concentration of hydrogen peroxide disinfection systems. Am J Optom Physiol Opt 65:527, 1988

84. Harris MG, Hernandez GN, Nuno DM: The pH of hydrogen peroxide disinfection systems over time. J Am Optom Assoc 61:171, 1990

85. Paugh JR, Brennan NA, Efron N: Ocular response to hydrogen peroxide. Am J Optom Physiol Opt 65:91, 1988

86. Boets EP, Kerkmeer MJ, vanBest JA: Contact lens care solutions and corneal epithelial barrier function: a flourophotometric study. Ophthalmic Res 26:129, 1994

87. Williams W, Baker J, Currie J, Weiss G: Investigation of the effects of hydrogen peroxide on corneal metabolism using nuclear magnetic resonance (NMR) spectroscopy. Invest Ophthalmol Vis Sci 29:60, 1988

88. Wilson GS, Chalmers RL: Effect of H_2O_2 concentration and exposure time on stromal swelling: an epithelial perfusion model. Optom Vis Sci 67:252, 1990

89. Wilson G: Effects of hydrogen peroxide on epithelial light scattering and stromal detergesecence. CLAO J 16(suppl): S11, 1990

90. Tripathi BJ, Tripathi RC: Hydrogen peroxide damage to human corneal epithelial cells in vitro. Implications for contact lens disinfection systems. Arch Ophthalmol 107:1516, 1989

91. Knopf HLS: Reaction to hydrogen peroxide in a contact lens wearer. Am J Ophthalmol 97:796, 1984

92. Lavery KT, Cowden JW, McDermott ML: Corneal toxicity secondary to hydrogen peroxidesaturated contact lens. Arch Ophthalmol 109:1352, 1991

93. Epstein AB, Donnenfeld ED, Van Valkenburg K: Interaction between lens material and solution causes punctate keratitis. Contact Lens Forum 15:54, 1990

94. Epstein AB, Freedman JM: Keratitis associated with hydrogen peroxide disinfection in soft contact lens wearers. Int Contact Lens Clin 17:74, 1990

95. Polansky JR, Fauss DJ, Hydorn I, Bloom E: Cellular injury from sustained vs. acute hydrogen peroxide exposure in cultured human corneal endothelium and human lens epithelium. CLAO J 16:523, 1990

96. Riley MV, Kast M: Penetration of hydrogen peroxide from contact lenses or tear-side solution to the aqueous humor. Optom Vis Sci 68:546, 1991

97. Rosenthal RA, McDonald MM, Schlitzer RL, et al: Loss of bacterial activity from contact lens storage solutions. CLAO J 23:57, 1997

98. Begley CG, Naggoner PJ, Jani NB, Meetz RE: The effects of soft contact lens disinfection solutions on rabbit corneal epithelium. CLAO J 20:52, 1994

99. Bergmanson JP, Ross RN: A masked quantitative cytologic study of the safety of a multipurpose contact lens solution applied to the in vivo rabbit eye. J Am Optom Assoc 64:308, 1993

100. Clompus R: New care products for soft contact lenses. In Making Contact. American Optometric Association (ADA) Cont Lens Section 6:15, 1988

101. Bergmanson JP, Barbeito R: Clinical assesment of ocular response to a multipurpose contact lens solution. Ophthalmic Physiol Opt 15:535, 1995

102. Soni PS, Horner DG, Ross J: Ocular response to lens care systems in adolescent soft contact lens wearers. Optom Vis Sci 73:70, 1996

103. Gordon KD: Optifree—Alcon's new soft contact lens disinfecting solution. Optical Prism 15:35, 1989

104. Morgan JF, Perry DL, Stein JM, Randeri KJ: The margin of safety of polyquaternium-1–preserved lens care solutions: a phase I clinical study. CLAO J 14:76, 1988

105. Annunziato T, Aquavella J, Blackhurst R, et al: Opti-Soft: shown effective for maintenance of low water contact lenses in a one year study. Int Contact Lens Clin 14:470, 1987

106. Schachet J, Lowther GE, Lavaux JE, et al: Clinical evaluation of the Opti-free disinfection system. Contact Lens Spectrum 5:37, 1990

107. Gibbs DE, Stein JM, Rockett J, et al: Opti-free chemical disinfectant: a safety study with various soft contact lenses. CLAO J 15:57, 1989

108. Davis R, Hansen D, Lowther G, et al: Clinical evaluations of Opti-free among preservative sensitive patients. Contact Lens Spectrum 4:73, 1989

109. Adams JL, Wilcox MJ, Trousdale MD, et al: Morphological and physiological effects of artificial tear formulations on corneal epithelial derived cells. Invest Ophthalmol Vis Sci (suppl.)30:523, 1989

110. Santucci B, Cristaudo A, Picardo L: Contact urticaria for papain in a soft lens solution. Contact Dermatitis 12:233, 1981

111. Davis RL: Animal versus plant enzyme. Int Contact Lens Clin 10:277, 1983

112. Bernstein DI, Gallagher JS, Groam M, Bernstein I: Local ocular anaphylaxis to papain enzyme contained in a contact lens cleaning solution. J Allerg Clin Immunol 74:258, 1984

113. Breen W, Fontana F, Hansen D, Thomas E: Clinical comparison of pancreatin-based and subtilisin-based enzymatic cleaners. Contact Lens Forum 15:32, 1990

114. Zetterstrom O, Wide L: IgE antibodies and skin test reaction to a detergent enzyme in Swedish consumers. Clin Allerg 4:23, 1974

115. Berdy GT, Abelson MB, Smith LM, George MA: Preservative free artificial tear preparations. Arch Ophthalmol 110:528, 1992

116. Fassihi AR, Naidon NT: Irritation associated with tear replacement ophthalmic drops. S Afr Med J 75:233, 1989

117. Sibley MJ, Shovlin JP: Are you having mixed reactions? Rev Optom 127:52, 1990

118. Rakow PL: Solution incompatibilities. Contact Lens Forum 13:41, 1988

119. Collins MJ, CarneyLG: Patient compliance and its influence on contact lens wearing problems. Am J Optom Physiol Opt 63:952, 1986

120. Wilson LA, Sarvant AD, Simmons RB, Ahearn DG: Microbial contamination of contact lens storage cases and solutions. Am J Ophthalmol 110:193, 1990

Appendix 8-1

Soft Contact Lens Care Systems and Their Preservatives—1999

Laboratory	Lens care system	Available products in lens care system	Preservative
Alcon	Opti-Free	*Opti-Free Multi-Action Solution	EDTA, PQ
		*Opti-Free Daily Cleaner	
		*Opti-Free Rewetting Drops	PQ
		*Opti-Free Enzymatic Cleaner	
Alcon	Opti-Free Express	*Opti-Free Express	PQ, AD
		*Opti-Free SupraClens	
		*Opti-Free Rewetting Drops	PQ
Alcon	Opti-One Multi-Purpose Solution	*Opti-One Multi-Purpose Solution	PQ
		*Opti-Free Enzymatic Cleaner	
		*Opti-One Rewetting Drops	PQ
Allergan	Complete or Complete Comfort Plus Multi-Purpose Solution	*Complete Multi-Purpose Solution	Trischem
		*Complete Comfort PLUS Solution	
		*Complete Weekly Enzymatic Tablets	
		*Complete Lubricating & Rewetting Drops	
Allergan	Hydrocare	*Hydrocare Cleaning & Disinfecting Solution	T, A1
		*Lens Plus Aerosol Saline	
		*Allergan Enzymatic Tablets	
		*LC-65 Surfactant Cleaner	
		*Allergan Lens Plus Rewetting Drops	
Allergan	Omnicare	Omnicare Daily Cleaner	
		Omnicare Disinfectant Solution	HP
		Omnicare Neutralizing Tablets	
		*Lens Plus Aerosol Saline	
		*Ultrazyme Enzymatic Cleaner	
Allergan	Oxysept	*Lens Plus Daily Cleaner; Lens Plus Rewetting Drops	
		*Oxysept #1	HP
		*Oxysept #2	SA, EDTA
		*Lens Plus Aerosol Saline	
		*Ultrazyme Enzymatic Cleaner	
Allergan	Ultracare	*Lens Plus Daily Cleaner; Lens Plus Rewetting Drops	
		*Ultracare Disinfectant	HP
		*Ultracare Neutralizing Tablets	
		*Lens Plus Aerosol Saline	
		*Ultrazyme Enzymatic Cleaner	
Allergan	Consept	*Consept Cleaner and Disinfectant	HP
		*Consept Rinse and Neutralize	CHX
		Advantage Enzyme Plus Surfactant Tablet	
Allergan	Soft Lens	Soft Lens Cleaner	CHX, EDTA
		Storage	CHX, EDTA
		Premixed Protein Remover	
Bausch & Lomb	ReNu Multi-Purpose Solution	*ReNu Multi-Purpose Solution	Dymed
		*ReNu Rewetting Drops	
Bausch & Lomb	ReNu Multi-Plus Solution	*ReNu Multi-Plus Solution with Hydranate Protein Remover	Dymed
		*ReNu Rewetting Drops	
CIBA Vision	AOSept	*Miraflow (U.S.) or AOFlow	
		*SoftWear Saline	HP
		*AOSept	HP
		*CIBA Vision Lens Drops	SA, EDTA

Laboratory	Lens care system	Available products in lens care system	Preservative
CIBA Vision	Pure Eyes	*Pure Eyes Disinfectant/Soaking	HP
		*Pure Eyes Cleaner/Rinse	
		*CIBA Vision Lens Drops	
		Any non-thermal enzymatic cleaner	
CIBA Vision	Quick-Care	*Quick-Care Starting Solution	
		*Quick-Care Finishing Solution	B
		*CIBA Vision Lens Drops	
		*Any nonthermal enzymatic cleaner	
CIBA Vision	Solo-Care Multi-Purpose Solution	*SOLO-Care Soft	PHMB
		Any nonthermal enzymatic cleaner	
CIBA Vision	Insta-Care	INSTA-Care Starting Solution	
		INSTA-Care Finishing Solution	B
CIBA Vision	In A Wink	In-A-Wink Daily Cleaner	SA, EDTA
		In-A-Wink Disinfectant	HP
		In-A-Wink Neutralizer	SA, EDTA
		In-A-Wink Refreshing Drops	SA, EDTA
CIBA Vision	Mirasept	Miraflow	HP
		Mirasept 1	SA, EDTA
		Mirasept 2	
		Clerz	SA, EDTA

AD = ALDOX (Alcon Laboratories, Ft. Worth, TX); Al = alkyl triethanol ammonium chloride; B = sodium borate, boric acid, and soium perborate generating up to 0.006% hydrogen peroxide; BA = benzyl alcohol; BC = benzalkonium chloride; CHX = chlorhexidine digluconate; Dymed (Bausch & Lomb, Rochester, NY) = polyaminopropylbiguanide; EDTA = disodium edetate; HP = hydrogen peroxide; PAPB = polyaminopropylbiguanide; PHMB = polyhexamethylene biguanide; PQ = polyquaternium-1 (Polyquad); SA = sorbic acid; T = thimerosal; Trischem = polyhexamethylne biguanide.
Note: North American market; products listed with asterisk are available in the United States.

Appendix 8-2

Rigid Contact Lens Solution Systems—1999

Laboratory	Lens solution system	Available products in lens solution system	Preservative
Alcon	Opti-Soak	*Opti-Soak Conditioning Solution	PQ
		*Opti-Clean II Daily Cleaner (for silicone and fluorosilicone acrylates) or Opti-Soak Daily Cleaner (for silicone/acryl and fluorosilicone/acryl copolymers) (both can use *Opti-Zyme and Opti-Tears)	EDTA, PQ
Alcon	Soaclens (for polymethyl-methacrylate lenses)	*Soaclens	T, EDTA
Allergan	Comfort Care	*Barnes-Hind Comfort Care GP Wetting and Soaking Solution	BC, EDTA
		*Barnes-Hind Comfort Care Dual Action Daily Cleaner tablets	
		*Barnes-Hind GP Daily Cleaner	
		*Barnes-Hind Comfort Care Comfort Drops	
Allergan	Wet N Soak	*Wet N Soak PLUS	CHX, EDTA
		*LC-65 Surfactant Cleaner	
		*Wet N Soak Rewetting Drops	
Allergan	Duracare	Duraclean	
		Duracare	BC, EDTA
		Hydrocare Protein Tablets	
Allergan	Total	LC-65	T, EDTA
		Total	BC, EDTA
Bausch & Lomb		*B&L Wetting & Soaking Solution	CHX, EDTA
		*B&L Concentrated Cleaner	
CIBA	Solo-Care Hard	*Solo-care Hard	Polyhexanide
		*CIBA Vision Lens Drops	
Excel	Luxicon Care System	Fluoro-Stat	BA
		Fluo-o-Wet	BA, SA
Lobob	Optimum	*Optimum Extra Strength Cleaner	
		*Optimum Cleaning, Disinfecting and Storage	BA
		*Optimum Wetting & Rewetting Drops	
Menicon/Allergan	Claris	*Claris Cleaning & Soaking Solution	BA
		*Claris Rewetting Drops	
Polymer technology	Original Formula Boston Care System	*Boston Cleaner	
		*Original Boston Conditioning Solution	CHX, EDTA
		*Boston Rewetting Drops	CHX, EDTA
Polymer technology	Boston Advance Care System	*Boston Advance Cleaner	CHX, PAPB
		*Boston Advance Conditioning Solution	EDTA
		*Boston Rewetting Drops	
*Polymer technology	Boston Simplicity	*Boston Simplicity Multi-action Solution	CHX, PAPB
		*Boston Rewetting Drops	

Al = alkyl triethanol ammonium chloride; BA = benzyl alcohol; BC = benzalkonium chloride; CHX = chlorhexidine digluconate; Dymed = polyaminopropylbiguanide; EDTA = disodium edetate; HP = hydrogen peroxide; PAPB = polyaminopropylbiguanide; PHMB = polyhexamethylene biguanide; PQ = polyquaternium-1 (Polyquad); SA = sorbic acid: T = thimerosal.
Note: North American market; products listed with asterisk are available in the United States.

Appendix 8-3

Weekly Enzyme Cleaners—1999

Laboratory	Enzyme cleaner	Active Ingredient
Alcon	*Opti-Free Enzymatic Cleaner	Pancreatin
	*Optizyme	Pancreatin
Allergan	*Complete	Subtilisin
	*Allergan Enzymatic	Papain
	*Profree/GP (for rigid gas-permeable lenses)	Papain
	*Ultrazyme	Subtilisin
	Advantage	Subtilisin
	Premixed Protein Remover	Subtilisin
Bausch & Lomb	Efferzyme	Subtilisin
	*ReNu Effervescent Enzyme	Subtilisin
	*ReNu One-Step Enzymatic	Subtilisin
CIBA	*Unizyme	Subtilisin
Polymer Technology	*Boston One-Step Liquid Enzyme Cleaner (for rigid gas-permeable lenses)	Subtilisin

Note: North American market; products listed with an asterisk are available in the United States.

III

Complications Affecting Lids and Adnexa

9

Dermatologic Complications of the Lids and Adnexa

PATRICK J. CAROLINE, MARK P. ANDRE, AND RODGER T. KAME

GRAND ROUNDS CASE REPORT

Subjective:
A 31-year-old woman presents with a 6-month history of decreasing lens tolerance, dryness, and foreign-body sensation. Patient has a 3-year history of uneventful soft contact lens wear with habitual wearing time of 12–14 hours per day. Maximum wearing time is reduced to 6–8 hours per day. The patient reports slight mattering along lid margins in the morning.

Objective:
- Best acuity with contact lenses: $^{20}/_{20}$ right eye (OD), left eye (OS), both eyes (OU)
- Biomicroscopy:
  Corneas: Mild inferior epithelial punctate staining OU
  Conjunctiva: Grade 1 tarsal papillary hypertrophy OU
  Tear film: Foamy tears at outer canthus; tear breakup time (TBUT) 8 seconds OU
  Lid margins: Mild seborrheic blepharitis OU
  Meibomian glands: Gland orifices show slight dilatation and pouting OU; glandular expression difficult, preceded by extrusion of an inspissated plug

Assessment:
Grade 2 meibomian gland dysfunction (MGD) OU with mild anterior seborrheic blepharitis. Superficial punctate keratitis (SPK) secondary to dry eyes induced by anterior and posterior lid margin disease.

Plan:
1. Hot compresses twice a day OU for 5–10 minutes.
2. Lid scrubs twice a day.
3. In-office expression of meibomian glands.
4. Antibiotic ointment to treat anterior blepharitis.
5. Continue periodic lens wear, with wear schedule determined by symptoms and individual response to treatment.
6. Return for follow-up in 2 weeks to assess MGD status and possible use of oral doxycycline therapy if unresponsive to therapy.

Within the broad spectrum of ocular disorders, chronic lid margin disease is one of the most frequently encountered ocular anomalies. Despite its frequency, it remains one of the most overlooked and underdiagnosed conditions by eye care specialists. Chronic lid margin disease is also among the most frustrating of diseases to treat because, like most dermatologic anomalies, it has no cure. At best, the treatment goal is to manage the involved areas with a minimal amount of medication once acute therapy has established initial control.

CLASSIFICATION

For purposes of clarity, lid margin disease can be divided into the following clinical entities:

1. Seborrheic dermatitis or blepharitis
2. Staphylococcal blepharitis
3. Angular blepharitis
4. MGD
5. Rosacea blepharitis
6. Parasitic blepharitis

These conditions can occur individually or in tandem with one another. A review of the dermatologic anomalies of the lids and adnexa is helpful to the contact lens specialist in that much of the intolerance and complications associated with lens wear are often found to be dermatologic in origin.

SEBORRHEIC DERMATITIS

Classic seborrheic dermatitis is a condition that affects a large percentage of the population at some time in life.[1] Infantile seborrheic dermatitis most frequently involves the scalp with yellowish, greasy scaling known as *cradle cap*. Yellow-red scaly patches on the face and diaper area may also be seen. The condition usually presents between the ages of 2 and 12 weeks and virtually always resolves by age 8–12 months.[2] Adult-onset seborrheic dermatitis almost exclusively affects males. It most frequently manifests as erythema and scaling, primarily involving the scalp and face. Often the patients' primary concerns are cosmetic because of their oily complexion.[3] The scales in seborrheic dermatitis are greasy, yellow, and fairly nonadherent. In certain groups of individuals, seborrheic dermatitis tends to be exceedingly common and more severe (i.e., in patients with human immunodeficiency virus; individuals with neurologic disorders, especially Parkinson's disease; and

in alcoholics). As many as 80% of individuals with acquired immunodeficiency disease have seborrheic dermatitis.[4,5] This suggests a possible immunologic mechanism involved in the dermatitis.

Seborrheic dermatitis is a chronic disease, in which exacerbations and remissions are common. Individuals afflicted with seborrheic dermatitis have more severe involvement in the winter months. Emotional stress and illness can also aggravate the condition.[1]

SEBORRHEIC BLEPHARITIS

Seborrheic blepharitis is the ocular manifestation of classic seborrheic dermatitis. The condition is frequently classified into three categories: primary seborrheic blepharitis, mixed staphylococcal and seborrheic blepharitis, and seborrheic blepharitis with secondary MGD.

Primary seborrheic blepharitis commonly presents in an older age group (mean age of 50). Its hallmark is increased meibomian gland secretion and mild-to-moderate inflammation of the eyelid margins.[6] Oily debris and scales are seen clinging to the lashes and form collarettes that encircle the cilia (Fig. 9-1). As the lashes grow, the collarettes move away from the base of the lash. Injection of vessels at the lid margin and in the adjacent conjunctiva is frequently seen (Fig. 9-2). Subjective symptoms include mattering of the lashes, burning, and a foreign-body sensation. Mild cases frequently go undiagnosed because of the lack of associated symptoms.

Some patients experience an associated keratitis or conjunctivitis. The keratitis is characterized by punctate epithelial erosions, either in the interpalpebral fissure or across the lower third of the cornea (Fig. 9-3). The keratitis results in patient symptoms of mild photophobia, chronic foreign-body sensation, and tearing. The conjunctivitis is characterized by bulbar injection and either follicular or papillary hypertrophy of the inferior tarsal conjunctiva.

The diagnosis of seborrheic blepharitis is best made by clinical examination of the eyelids using the slit lamp. The clinical signs include atopic changes associated with seborrheic dermatitis; flaky, oily debris on the lid margins and lashes, called *scurf*; and lid inflammation. A critical part of the examination for blepharitis involves meibomian gland expression using digital pressure to the tarsal plate. These secretions are examined for their volume, viscosity, and color. In seborrheic blepharitis and MGD, the glands are engorged and filled with a retained, semiopaque or yellowish liquid called *meibum*, which can be easily expressed on eyelid massage.[2] These patients frequently have symptoms of dry eyes and burning, especially in the morning hours. The dry eye symptoms are

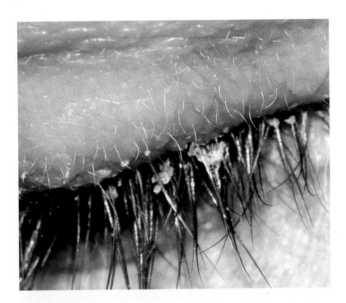

FIG. 9-1. *Seborrheic blepharitis with oily debris and scales clinging to the lashes.*

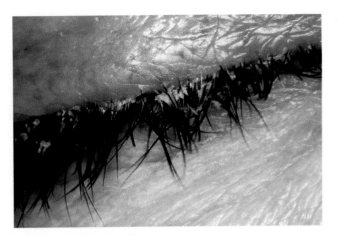

FIG. 9-2. *Lid inflammation associated with seborrheic blepharitis.*

most likely related to tear film instability secondary to the retention of meibum in the meibomian glands.[7,8] The tear film may have a foamy appearance that is most noticeable in the lateral canthal region.

In patients with seborrheic blepharitis, it is important to look carefully for concurrent seborrheic dermatitis. The degree and distribution of involvement vary greatly from patient to patient. Involvement of the scalp, retroauricular, nasolabial, brow, and sternal regions has been reported in patients with primary seborrheic blepharitis. In patients with significant dermatitis, consultation with a dermatologist is suggested.[9]

Pathogenesis of Seborrheic Blepharitis

Although the definitive cause of seborrheic blepharitis is unknown, the yeast *Pityrosporum ovale* is thought by some investigators to play a role in its development.[10,11] Other pathophysiologic factors may include bacterial lipases and variations in the biochemical components of meibum.[12-14] Other epidemiologic factors that may contribute to seborrheic blepharitis include a variety of neurologic disorders, psychological stress, depression, and climate influences in that the condition is frequently worse in the winter and improves in the summer.

Contact Lens Wear

Patients with significant seborrheic blepharitis should be cautioned about contact lens wear. This condition is usu-

ally chronic and may result in significant lens deposition as well as secondary ocular infections. Patients with mild, well-controlled seborrheic blepharitis may be considered for contact lenses if they are well supervised and compliant with the ongoing management of their condition. However, caution should be exercised in these patients.[15]

Management

The most significant aspect in treating chronic lid margin disease is educating the patient that the condition has no

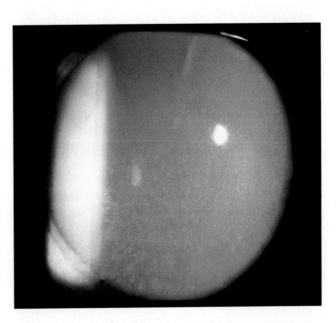

FIG. 9-3. *Punctate epithelial erosions across the lower one-third of the cornea.*

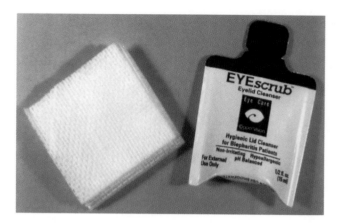

FIG. 9-4. *Commercially available eyelid scrub consisting of a sterile, premoistened cleaning pad.*

cure and requires constant self-maintenance. Frequent exacerbations of the signs and symptoms are common because this form of blepharitis is influenced by numerous extraneous factors. The goals of all blepharitis treatment are to control the disease, maintain vision, and avoid secondary complications. This frequently requires two phases of therapy. The first phase is an aggressive treatment tailored to bringing the disease under control. This is eventually tapered and followed by the minimum treatment necessary to provide long-term control of the chronic disease process.[9]

The treatment for seborrheic blepharitis centers on eyelid hygiene. These techniques must be carefully explained and demonstrated to the patient to guarantee proper compliance and performance. The major objectives of these maneuvers are to reduce the amount of scurf formation at the lid margins, lyse the bacterial membranes, and help to restore normal meibomian secretion.[9] The techniques for lid margin hygiene have been outlined by Halsted and McCulley[9] and include the following steps:

1. A hot compress is used to loosen lid margin debris and liquefy the meibum in congested meibomian glands. This is accomplished by placing a facecloth under a flow of water as warm as can be tolerated by the patient. The cloth is applied to the closed eyelids for 5–10 minutes. As the compress cools, it should be rewarmed with fresh water to maintain the warm temperature.

2. Patients with a meibomian gland component to their blepharitis should follow the warm compresses with expression of the meibomian glands. This is best accomplished by rotating the tip of the finger placed just out-side the lashes and applying enough pressure to the tarsus against the globe to express the contents of the glands onto the lid margin. This should be performed along the entire course of the meibomian glands, massaging the upper and lower lids. In patients with meibomian gland involvement, it is hoped that the warm compresses raise the temperature of the lid sufficiently to surpass the melting point of the abnormal, retained meibum.

3. Loose debris can then be scrubbed from the lid margins with a commercially available eyelid scrub or a clean face cloth saturated with a few drops of a nonirritating baby shampoo (Fig. 9-4). The soap is applied to the upper and lower lids and to the eyebrows in a scrubbing, left-to-right motion. Some advise using diluted baby shampoo, but full-strength shampoo is recommended. The lids are then rinsed until free of soap.

Initially, lid hygiene may be required as often as four times a day. This can be tapered to once or twice a day, usually on awakening and at bedtime. The most important time to perform lid hygiene is in the morning because debris collects and builds up on the closed lids during sleep.

In patients with suspected seborrheic blepharitis, lid margin cultures can be performed to rule out a simultaneous bacterial infection. Topical antibiotics may be of some benefit in certain cases of mixed seborrheic and staphylococcal blepharitis or seborrheic blepharitis with secondary MGD. The role of antibiotics in the treatment of primary seborrheic blepharitis is less clear because the condition is not associated with a bacterial process.

Systemic antibiotics, such as tetracycline, erythromycin, or doxycycline, may be indicated in patients with a secondary MGD, especially if the patient is unresponsive to local lid therapy. Mild topical corticosteroids may be used initially on individuals who have a significant degree of lid inflammation; chronic use of steroids, however, is generally not recommended.

STAPHYLOCOCCAL BLEPHARITIS

Staphylococcal blepharitis is a primary bacterial infection of the eyelids and a common cause of chronic conjunctivitis and recurrent epithelial keratitis.[6,16] The condition is characterized by a relative lack of dermatologic abnormalities. The signs and symptoms of chronic staphylococcal blepharitis are almost always bilateral and often wax and wane throughout its course. Patients are frequently younger (mean age of 42 years), and the con-

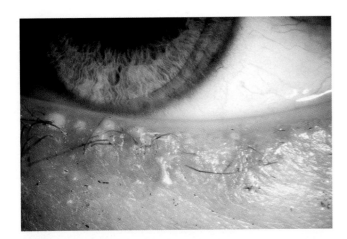

FIG. 9-5. *Staphylococcal blepharitis with ulcerations at the base of the eyelashes. Note the whitish fibrin surrounding the individual cilium. The fibrin exudes from the base of the ulcer, masking its presence.*

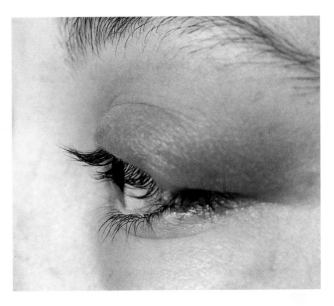

FIG. 9-6. *A hordeolum secondary to staphylococcal infection in a meibomian gland.*

dition is significantly more common in females.[17] The subjective symptoms include itching, burning, photophobia, tearing, redness, blurred vision, and mild discharge.

Pathogenesis

Aerobic and anaerobic cultures from the lids and conjunctiva have shown the presence of *Staphylococcus aureus* and *Staphylococcus epidermidis*. The staphylococcus organism is present throughout life in the nasopharyngeal tissue and can cause a number of infections.[18] It can remain viable for some interval and can produce chronic and smoldering infections of long duration, as seen in chronic staphylococcal blepharitis.[19] Other organisms that have been cultured include *Corynebacterium* species, *Propionibacterium acnes*, and other *Propionibacterium* species.

Staphylococcal blepharitis is generally characterized by one or more of the following clinical features:[20,21]

- *Ulcerations at the base of the eyelash* (Fig. 9-5). In most cases, a characteristic hyperemia and irregularity (tylosis) of the lid margins exist, with matted hard crusts, consisting of fibrin, surrounding the individual cilium. The fibrin, which exudes from the base of the ulcer, usually masks the presence of the ulcer. When the fibrin crusts are removed, the small ulcers can be seen and may even bleed.
- *Collarettes.* Collarettes are small, thin, fibrinous scales that surround the eyelash, like a small piece of paper

impaled on a stick. Collarettes are formed by the fibrin that covers the base of the ulcer. It usually surrounds the eyelash and may be carried away from the surface of the skin as the lash grows. The scales are hard, brittle, and less greasy than those seen in seborrheic blepharitis.
- *Poliosis.* Poliosis is a localized area of white-pigmented lashes caused by damage to the pilosebaceous unit by the staphylococcal organism.
- *Short, misdirected, broken, sparse, or missing eyelashes.* This anomaly is caused by direct damage to the follicles by the staphylococcal infection. Large areas where eyelashes are absent (madarosis) are commonly found.
- *External hordeolum (stye).* An external hordeolum represents an abscess of a gland of Zeis. The signs and symptoms include localized redness and swelling with pain, which is usually proportional to the degree of swelling.
- *Internal hordeolum.* An internal hordeolum may result from the staphylococcal infection. The infection occurs within the meibomian gland and often produces intense pain and swelling. The lesion may eventually drain through the skin or conjunctiva (Fig. 9-6).
- *Multiple, recurrent chalazia.* Multiple or recurrent chalazia are often caused by staphylococcal infections of the meibomian glands. The infection causes inflammation and edema of the gland, resulting in inspissation of the meibum and eventual chalazion formation.

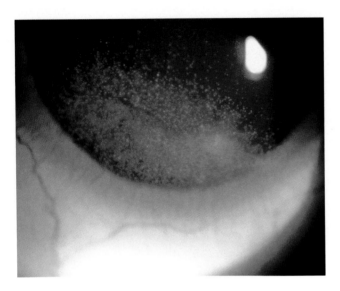

FIG. 9-7. *Toxic, epithelial keratitis in the lower one-third of the cornea secondary to staphylococcal blepharitis.*

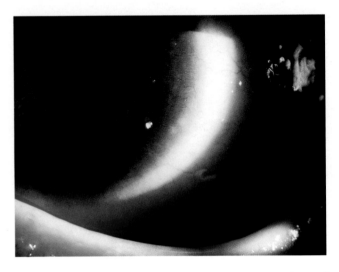

FIG. 9-8. *Marginal stromal infiltrates caused by the release of potent staphylococcal exotoxins in staphylococcal blepharitis.*

- *Toxic, epithelial keratitis* (Fig. 9-7). The chronically infected lids are in close apposition to the globe, and often the conjunctiva and cornea become secondarily infected. A fine epithelial keratitis across the lower one-half of the cornea is commonly associated with staphylococcal blepharitis. The keratitis is secondary to the concentration of staphylococcal antigens, which accumulate in the tears and on the lid margins during sleep. This explains why the keratitis is more severe in the morning and often clears during the daytime.
- *Recurrent conjunctivitis.* Staphylococcal infection can result in chronic papillary conjunctivitis with a mild mucopurulent discharge containing polymorphonuclear leukocytes. The conjunctivitis and its symptoms are often worse on awakening.
- *Marginal corneal infiltrates or ulcers* (Fig. 9-8). Marginal stromal infiltration begins with a hypersensitivity reaction caused by the release of potent exotoxins from the staphylococcus bacterium. Marginal corneal infiltrates usually occur at the 2- to 4-o'clock or 8- to 10-o'clock areas of the peripheral cornea. They are usually separated from the limbus by a lucid interval and progress to ulceration of the overlying epithelium. These lesions are sterile and represent an immunologic response to bacterial antigens. On instillation of fluorescein, the epithelial defect shows pooling, followed by a subsequent diffuse seepage into the anterior stroma. The surrounding area takes on a whitish-gray haze as stromal edema occurs. After healing, there may be a peripheral wedge of pannus at the ulcer site.

MIXED SEBORRHEIC AND STAPHYLOCOCCAL BLEPHARITIS

Description

Mixed blepharitis is caused by a staphylococcal infection in the presence of underlying seborrheic condition. It probably represents the most frequently encountered form of blepharitis. Mixed blepharitis has an equal male and female distribution. The condition is characterized by the signs and symptoms of seborrhea and staphylococcal infection, which include underlying seborrheic dermatitis, oily and flaky lid margin debris, dry eyes, bulbar injection, and punctate epithelial keratitis across the inferior one-third of the cornea.[17]

Treatment

The treatment of staphylococcal or mixed seborrheic and staphylococcal blepharitis usually requires 2–8 weeks of intense therapy, which can be tapered after the initial, more severe signs and symptoms have resolved. Treatment begins with lid margin hygiene, which includes warm compresses and lid scrubs to loosen the crusty, scaly debris that clings to the base of the lashes.

On the initial presentation, it can be difficult to determine the exact form of blepharitis that is present. Therefore, when this question exists, a topical antibiotic can be prescribed. The antibiotics of first choice are frequently bacitracin or erythromycin, which are both highly effective against the gram-positive staphylococci and have a low incidence of associated allergic reactions.

After lid hygiene, the patient should be instructed to place a small amount of the antibiotic on a clean fingertip and rub the ointment into the lid and lashes. This is done two to four times a day, depending on the severity of the condition. Additionally, one-fourth inch of ointment can be instilled into the inferior cul-de-sac at bedtime.

If significant infection exists with some concern about corneal involvement, an aminoglycoside, such as tobramycin or gentamicin, can be used. In addition to being more potent, aminoglycosides can be applied topically in drop form to the globe as well as topically to the lids in the form of an ointment. Patients who are also diagnosed with keratoconjunctivitis sicca should be treated with topical preservative-free artificial tear therapy. After the initial inflammatory signs resolve, the therapy can be tapered to a frequency that keeps the condition stable.

ANGULAR BLEPHARITIS

Angular blepharitis is an ulcerative infection of the conjunctiva and eyelid margins usually confined to the medial and lateral canthal regions of one or both eyes. Angular blepharitis has been reported in all age groups, although it occurs more frequently in adults. There does not appear to be any gender or race predilection.[22]

The condition typically begins in one eye and inevitably spreads to the other eye within a week.[23] On external examination, the skin surrounding the canthi is characteristically red, scaly, thickened, and often macerated.[24] In more severe cases, the skin in the canthal regions takes on a characteristic fanlike appearance (Fig. 9-9).[25] The inflamed conjunctiva produces a mild grayish-yellow mucoid discharge that adheres to the eyelashes and accumulates at the canthal angles. The condition may be accompanied by punctate keratitis, marginal corneal infiltrates, and rarely, ulcerative keratitis.[26,27]

The ocular symptoms are often mild and nonspecific and may include mild irritation, burning, itching, photophobia, and tearing. Angular blepharitis usually runs a benign but chronic course, lasting 6 weeks to 6 months unless treated. Appropriate treatment typically results in rapid resolution of the symptoms, and the eyelid changes are fully reversible.[23,25]

Etiology

Moraxella and *Staphylococcus aureus* have been identified as the causative factor in angular blepharitis.

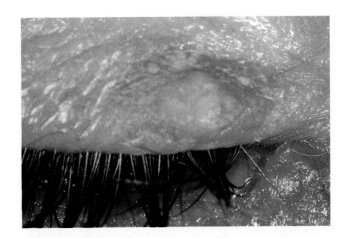

FIG. 9-9. *Angular blepharitis with the characteristic red, scaly macerated skin in the medial canthal region.*

Treatment

The treatment for angular blepharitis should be based on smears and bacterial cultures performed at the time of the initial examination. *Moraxella* species are usually sensitive to all commercially available topical ophthalmic antibiotic preparations and can be used four times a day for 7–10 days.[28,29] Topical antibiotic ointment should be applied to the eyelid margins two to three times a day. Local lid margin hygiene (the same as for seborrheic and staphylococcal blepharitis) is an important adjunctive therapy to prevent future recurrences.

MEIBOMIAN GLAND DYSFUNCTION

MGD is a perplexing condition with an obscure etiology. It is believed to be a congestion of the meibomian glands with chronic stagnation of meibum (meibomian gland oils).[30] The condition appears to have a combined staphylococcal, immunologic, and mechanical etiology.[31] The spectrum of MGD can range from minimal clinical significance to sight-threatening ocular rosacea. In addition, MGD has been suggested as an important factor in the pathogenesis of several ocular conditions, including chronic blepharitis, hordeola, chalazia, and even contact lens intolerance.[32,33]

MEIBOMIAN GLANDS

Tarsal glands were first adequately described by Meibomius in 1666.[34] They are enormously developed sebaceous glands that belong to a category of holocrine

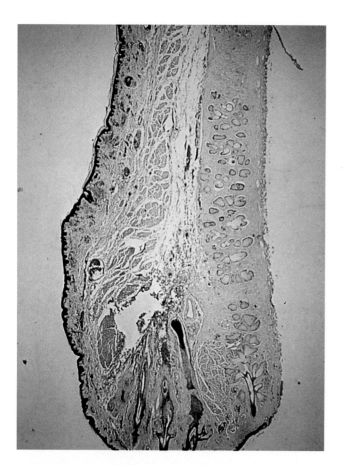

FIG. 9-10. *Light micrograph cross section of an upper lid.*

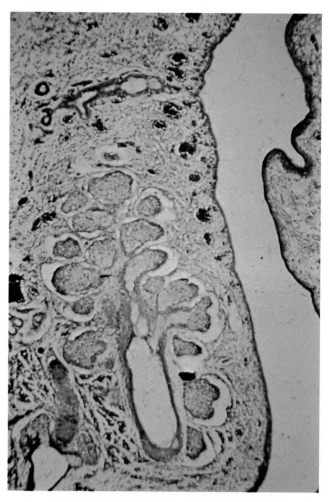

FIG. 9-11. *Light micrograph transverse section of an upper lid and meibomian gland. Note the numerous acini connected to the central duct by short ductules. The gland's meibum is produced within the acini.*

glands whose secretions are composed of entire cells that are released on maturation.[32] The meibomian glands are arranged vertically, parallel with each other, numbering approximately 25 in the upper lid and 20 in the lower lid. The glands of the upper lid are larger than those in the lower lid owing to the larger size of the upper tarsal plate.

Each gland consists of a central canal, into the sides of which open many acini (rounded lateral ducts) numbering 30–40 in the larger glands (Fig. 9-10). The gland is closed at the inner end, and at the outer end lies an excretory duct. Each excretory duct is lined by four layers of squamous epithelial cells situated on a basement membrane. This epithelial layer increases to six cells as the duct approaches the lid margin. The keratinization of these squamous ductal cells is responsible for much of the obstruction of the glands in MGD. The duct mouth opens to form small orifices at the margin of the lid on the inner side of its posterior border. The glands are surrounded by lymph spaces and are supplied by nerves and blood vessels that traverse the tarsus to reach them.[35]

The oily meibum originates in the most remote part of the gland, in the acini, where the cell's cytoplasm accumulates minute droplets of sebaceous material. The sebaceous secretion is expelled into the excretory duct, where it mixes with the desquamated epithelial cells from the duct lining (Fig. 9-11).[32,36] The viscous meibum collected in the excretory duct is then delivered to the tear film through the orifices at the lid margin. Owing to the location of the glands, between the tarsal plates in each lid, the simple act of blinking is sufficient for expression of meibomian secretion into the tear film. Andrews[37] has observed that the thick meibum may be spread on the aqueous surface of tears by a surfactant or solvent component in either the meibum or the tear film.

The major functions of meibum in the tear film are as follows:

- To provide lubrication between the lid margin and the cornea
- To ensure an airtight closure of the lids
- To prevent tears from macerating the skin
- To supply a limiting hydrophobic oily film for the tear film to retard evaporation

BIOCHEMISTRY OF MEIBUM

Many researchers have performed analytical testing of human meibomian secretions. Early investigations by Pez (1897) and by Linton, Curnow, and Riley (1961) were largely qualitative, with only rough indications of the relative magnitudes of lipid components.[38] In the 1960s, further biochemical analyses by thin-layer and gas-liquid chromatography revealed a more complete picture of the makeup of human meibum.[39,40] Today, meibum is generally considered a combination of waxy esters, cholesterol esters, triglycerides, fatty acids, hydrocarbons, fatty alcohols, cholesterol, and phospholipids. There appear to be great variations in the relative makeup of individual meibum components. For this reason, Tiffany[38] concluded that no typical composition for human meibomian oil exists and that mean values are meaningless. Therefore, the synthetic mixing of an artificial tear based on the average meibum composition is not desirable.

MEIBOMIAN GLAND DYSFUNCTION

MGD can be simply defined as physical obstruction of the glands by plugging of the excretory ducts. The blockage causes stagnation of the gland secretions, initiating a wide variety of clinical complications (Fig. 9-12). The mechanism for this blockage appears to be located at the level of the epithelium lining the excretory duct. The excretory duct of the meibomian glands is lined by the same type of epithelium as the surface of the skin. Therefore, excretory duct obstruction could occur under circumstances of increased epithelial turnover, in which cells are detached in the form of small scales, similar to dandruff, or abnormal keratinization or hyperkeratinization of the duct epithelium (including sloughing of keratin and narrowing of the duct), or both.

Increased Epithelial Turnover

Certain dermatologic conditions, such as seborrheic dermatitis and acne rosacea, are characterized by increased

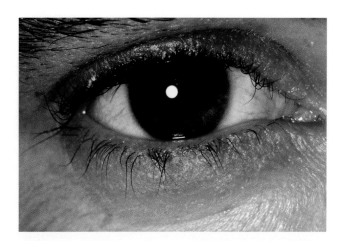

FIG. 9-12. *A 32-year-old man with meibomian-seborrheic blepharitis. Note the scurf at the base of the lashes and the red-rimmed appearance secondary to inflammation of the meibomian glands.*

epidermal turnover. Large amounts of cells are produced that detach from the epidermal surface in the form of small scales. The mechanism is similar to that of dandruff production. Therefore, it is reasonable to assume that duct obstruction is more likely to occur under circumstances of increased epithelial turnover, owing to accumulation of desquamated epithelial cells.

Keratinization of the Meibomian Gland Duct

Studies have indicated that glandular dysfunction may result from hyperkeratinization of the duct epithelium.[30] This keratinization does not end at the orifice but extends more posteriorly throughout the gland duct.[41] In a histopathologic study of seven patients with MGD, Gutgesell et al.[31] found signs of obstruction and dilatation of the meibomian gland ducts, along with acinar enlargement and hyperkeratinization of the duct epithelium.

These changes are not always accompanied by pouting of the orifices or inflammatory signs along the lid margin, and the condition is often overlooked. Under these circumstances, however, expression of the gland often releases an inspissated material. This phenomenon, combined with the patient symptoms, is critical in making the diagnosis of MGD. Observations concerning MGD and keratinization of the meibomian gland may be the counterpart to the well-recognized relationship between skin disease and sebaceous gland dysfunction. Knutson[42] has shown that keratinization of the sebaceous gland duct leading into the pilosebaceous canal is the critical step in the development of clinical acne vulgaris.

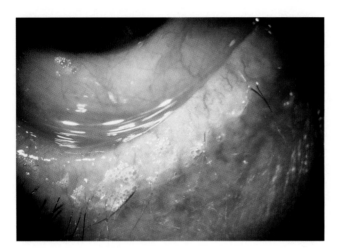

FIG. 9-13. *Centrally located foamy tears in a patient with meibomian gland dysfunction.*

Gland Stagnation

Physical obstruction of the meibomian gland ducts (either partial or total) results in two complications: stagnation and possible infection. Studies of meibomian gland composition have shown that the meibomian lipids in patients with MGD do not differ significantly from those of healthy subjects.[43] It appears that gland health and structure are unaffected by the meibum makeup in MGD. Gutgesell et al.[31] concluded that stagnation of meibum causes an increase in pressure in the gland and that this factor may be responsible for the wide variety of histologic changes seen in MGD. Therefore, the health of the meibomian glands may be best determined by evaluating glandular morphology rather than meibum composition.

In vivo gland structure is best viewed through a modified slit-lamp technique, using a standard transillumination light source. The patient's lower lid is gently everted over the transillumination light probe, which allows direct visualization of the meibomian glands through the palpebral conjunctiva.[30,44] The gland morphology can be photographically documented with high-speed infrared film. This technique appears to be less subjective and provides a greater degree of glandular detail than standard slit-lamp examination.

SIGNS AND SYMPTOMS OF MEIBOMIAN GLAND DYSFUNCTION

The possibility of MGD is usually not investigated unless the patient presents with significant symptoms or gross signs.[36] The signs and symptoms of MGD are usually bilat-

eral and demonstrate little asymmetry.[45] The lid margins may be normal in the early stages of MGD. In the later stages, they become thickened and rounded, with telangiectatic blood vessels crossing the lid margins.

MGD may or may not present with ocular surface involvement in the form of SPK, which is greatest in the interpalpebral space. The SPK has the appearance of that seen in other conditions secondary to an unstable tear film. It is not similar to the keratitis that has been described secondary to *Staphylococcus* toxin, which is more typically seen in association with anterior bacterial blepharitis. The finding of an unstable tear film in patients with posterior blepharitis most likely accounts for this keratopathy without having to postulate the presence of a bacterial exotoxin.[45] Studies by Korb and Henriquez[32] found an incidence of corneal staining in 41 (57.7 percent of symptomatic (probable MGD) eyes and in only eight (10 percent) of control (normal) eyes. The corneal and conjunctival superficial punctate staining may not be seen with the initial instillation of a single drop of 2 percent sodium fluorescein. However, sequential instillation of fluorescein at 5-minute intervals for 20 minutes may reveal an underlying epitheliopathy.[46]

Patient symptoms may not be present unless the integrity of the tear film is stressed by changes in humidity and temperature or by the presence of a contact lens. The stagnation of the meibomian glands may account for the tear film instability. This is suggested by the fact that stabilization of the tear film occurs when fresh secretions from deep within the glands are added by expressing them directly into the tear film. The observed instability cannot be ascribed to a quantitative decrease in the tear lipid layer because these patients have normal or increased interference patterns in the tear film, indicating that no shortage of lipid exists.[47]

Another common tear film finding in MGD is the presence of foamy tears (Fig. 9-13). Andrews[37] has suggested that the frothy secretion may be related to an overproduction of irritative fatty acids secondary to the lid infection or inflammation. Korb and Henriquez[32] reported the finding of foamy tear film at the lower lid margin or the lateral canthus in 47 eyes with MGD (66.2%) and in only three control eyes (3.7%).

In the more advanced stages of MGD, small (2- to 3-mm) microchalazia can be noted in the meibomian glands. The exact histopathologic composition of these spots is unknown, but the presence of a microchalazion may be the earliest change leading to a frank chalazion. They often present 1–2 mm posterior to the lid margin on the conjunctival side. They must be distinguished from concretions, which are inclusions in cystic structures in the conjunctiva, whereas microchalazia are deeper and have a mounded configuration.

GRADE 0 MGD

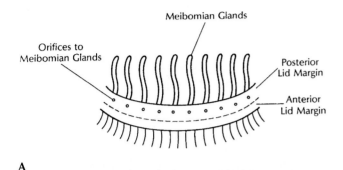

A

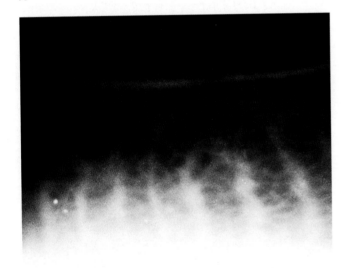

B

FIG. 9-14. *(A) Grade 0 meibomian gland dysfunction. (B) Transilluminated slit-lamp infrared photography of a lower lid with grade 0 meibomian gland dysfunction. The gland complexes are thin and relatively straight. The clusters of small dark spots probably represent acini.*

Classification of Meibomian Gland Dysfunction

Clinical classification of MGD is difficult because of the diversity of morphologic features and varying subjective symptoms. In addition, a frequent association exists of MGD with other underlying dermatologic conditions (e.g., acne rosacea and staphylococcal blepharitis). These must be considered when patients are being evaluated for MGD.

The following classification system is based on objective changes in the meibomian gland structure as viewed through lower lid transillumination. The appearance of

GRADE 1 MGD

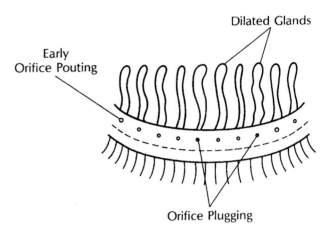

FIG. 9-15. *Grade 1 meibomian gland dysfunction.*

the orifices, tear meniscus, and conjunctiva are examined by standard biomicroscopy techniques.

Grade 0 Meibomian Gland Dysfunction: Normal

Signs *Meibomian glands*: The glands are uniform with a piano key appearance. No engorgement or stagnation of gland structure is present (Figs. 9-14A,B).

Meibomian gland orifices: Orifices appear as tiny holes or only potential openings. No pouting or plugging is present; clear meibum can be seen on gentle expression.

Tear film: No foaming is observed, and the tear meniscus is normal.

Conjunctiva: No congestion or injection is observed.

Symptoms Patients are usually asymptomatic.

Grade 1 Meibomian Gland Dysfunction: Minimal

Signs *Meibomian glands*: Some glands appear normal, whereas others appear slightly engorged by the early stagnation of meibum (Fig. 9-15).

Meibomian gland orifices: The orifices are more obvious, with some mild pouting and plugging. An abundance of clear oily excretion on gentle expression may exist.

Tear film: The tear film is clear but may have some foaming in central areas of the meniscus.

Conjunctiva: Trace congestion and injection may be present with some mild papillary hypertrophy.

Symptoms Patients are often asymptomatic or may experience a nonspecific foreign-body sensation (greater in the morning). Transient symptoms of a burning sensation as well as ocular dryness may exist.

GRADE 2 MGD

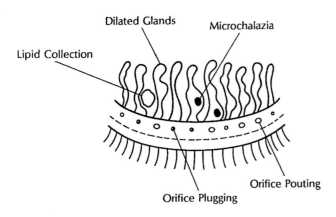

FIG. 9-16. *Grade 2 meibomian gland dysfunction.*

GRADE 3 MGD

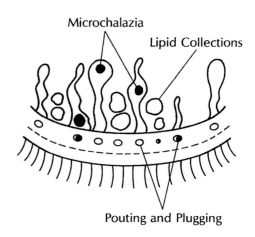

FIG. 9-17. *Grade 3 meibomian gland dysfunction.*

Grade 2 Meibomian Gland Dysfunction: Mild

Signs   *Meibomian glands*: Many glands are dilated and engorged, with obvious stagnation of meibum. Increased irregularity of gland shape occurs, especially near the lid margin. Subconjunctivally, discrete collections of lipid (not solid microchalazia) exist. The patient may have one to three true microchalazia per lid (Fig. 9-16).
Meibomian gland orifices: Most orifices are obvious and slightly dilated, with pouting and plugs. Mild inflammation around the orifices may exist. The glands contain an abundance of oily material, which may appear whitish-yellow on expression.
Tear film: The tear film may be clear with some foam present at the inner or outer canthus, or both.
Conjunctiva: The conjunctiva may exhibit mild congestion and injection with increased papillary changes and mild conjunctival staining.

Symptoms   Patient symptoms may include a slight foreign-body sensation, burning, itching, and dry eyes. Patients may also report red eyes with mattering or crusting along the lid margins.

Grade 3 Meibomian Gland Dysfunction: Moderate

Signs   *Meibomian glands*: Gross enlargement of many glands secondary to meibum stagnation may occur. Multiple collections of lipid may be present subconjunctivally with three or more microchalazia in the lower lid (Fig. 9-17).
Meibomian gland orifices: The orifices exhibit increased pouting and plugging, with inspissation in most. Glandular expression is difficult and is often preceded by the extrusion of an inspissated plug, followed by whitish-yellow or abundant clear oily material. The lid margins may be irregular, edematous, and inflamed.

Tear film: Tear film debris may be present along the lower lid margin with foam present centrally and at the inner or outer canthus.
Conjunctiva: Moderate conjunctival congestion and injection are present overlying the affected glands. Moderate papillary hypertrophic changes occur, with increased conjunctival staining.

Symptoms   Symptoms include moderate irritation, foreign-body sensation, tearing, mattering, redness, burning, and itching with increasing symptoms of ocular dryness. The patient may have cosmetic concerns because of the red rim around the eyes and may have a history of chalazia.

Grade 4 Meibomian Gland Dysfunction: Severe

Signs   *Meibomian glands*: Numerous collections of lipid are noted, with increased numbers of microchalazia as well as frank chalazia (Figs. 9-18A,B).
Meibomian gland orifices: The lid margins are irregular, edematous, and inflamed with increased pouting, plugging, and inspissation. Glandular expression is difficult, owing to near complete blockage at the gland orifices.
Tear film: Obvious foamy discharge in the tear film is present, with excessive debris and rapid TBUT.
Conjunctiva: Moderate to severe congestion and injection exist, with increased papillary hypertrophy.

Symptoms   The patient has chronic symptoms, which include irritation, redness, discharge, foreign-body sensation, tearing, burning, itching, dry eyes, and often a history of recurrent chalazia.

GRADE 4 MGD

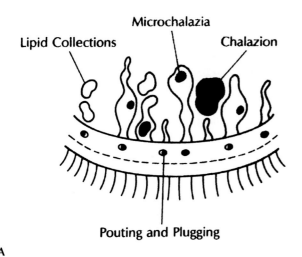

A

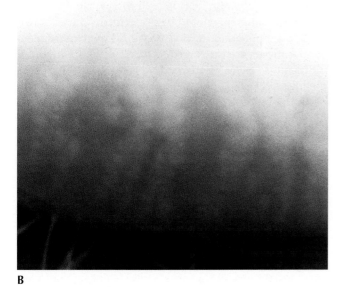

B

FIG. 9-18. *(A) Grade 4 meibomian gland dysfunction. (B) Slit-lamp infrared photograph of lower lid meibomian glands in a patient with grade 4 meibomian gland dysfunction. The gland complexes are dilatated and distorted; however, no significant area of lid is devoid of visible glands. Two microcysts (whitish spots) are noted.*

Glandular Expression

Under normal circumstances, the meibomian glands secrete clear viscous oil with gentle digital pressure on the lower lid. In MGD, the sebaceous material and cell debris from within the meibomian gland and the duct epithelium become cloudy or absent on expression. Inspissated secretions may appear as follows:

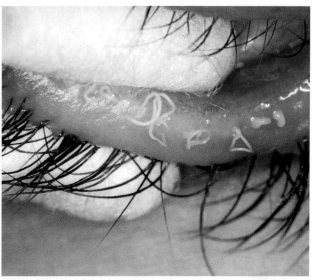

FIG. 9-19. *Meibomian gland expression performed by massaging the lower lid between two sterile swabs. Note the column form (toothpaste appearance) of inspissated meibum in a patient with grade 2 meibomian gland dysfunction.*

- Very fine, translucent filamentary secretion
- Secretion in column form (toothpastelike)
- Creamy secretion (puslike)

Inspissated secretions can be revealed only by more aggressive pressure directed on the lower lid. Aggressive glandular expression can be performed by pressing a rounded glass or plastic rod upward against the lid toward the globe.[48] In addition, the glands can be expressed by squeezing (pinching) the lower lid between the thumb and forefinger.

Korb and Henriquez[32] describe an additional technique for forceful glandular expression, which begins with the instillation of 2% proparacaine into the inferior cul-de-sac. Expression is performed by compressing the lower lid with moderate force between a sterile cotton swab on the palpebral conjunctival surface and the thumb on the surface of the skin. A similar technique of glandular expression is performed by massaging the lid between two sterile swabs[6] (Fig. 9-19).

Studies by Norn[49] found that in apparently healthy subjects, only 44% of the meibomian glands were discharging secretions into the tear film at any given time. On the basis of these data, it appears that very little glandular secretion is necessary to allow normal lipid tear film synergy.

Korb and Henriquez found a high incidence of absent secretion on gentle expression in 26 (36.6%) symptomatic eyes suspected of having MGD. Secretion was absent in only two (2.5%) control eyes that were thought to be healthy.[32]

Bacteriology

The dead and desquamated epithelial cells in the stagnated secretions of the meibomian glands may provide an excellent culture medium for bacteria and represent a continuous source of irritation to the ocular surface.

Bacteriologic studies by Korb and Henriquez[32] indicate that the most frequent organisms identified in MGD are *Staphylococcus epidermidis* and *S. aureus*. Studies by McCulley and Sciallis[45] on 43 patients with MGD found 42% positive for *S. epidermidis*. Thirty-seven percent grew *S. aureus*, 10% grew diphtheroids, and 22% grew *Propionibacterium acnes*.

McCulley and Dougherty[50] also reported that expression of the meibomian glands in patients with MGD always reflected the bacteria found along the anterior lid margin. However, the recovery rate of the glandular (meibum) bacteria was considerably less than the recovery rate from the anterior lid margin. Therefore, MGD may not represent a primary infectious disease but instead may reflect the contamination of meibomian secretion from the lid margins at the time of obtaining the cultures.

McCulley et al.[6] reported that meibum analysis has not revealed a qualitative abnormality in patients with MGD. However, preliminary gas-liquid chromatography data on the secretions suggest an increase in free fatty acids and a shift toward lipids with higher melting points. The free fatty acid could destabilize the tear film and cause epithelial abnormality as a result of direct toxicity to the cells. Lipids with higher melting points tend to stagnate the secretory flow, allowing greater access by bacterial lipolytic exoenzymes to the stagnant lipid pool that subsequently forms the lipid layer of the tear film. This could account for the fact that no single pathogen has been found in these patients, and it provides at least one possible mechanism by which bacteria contribute to the inflammatory disease process.

TREATMENT OF MEIBOMIAN GLAND DYSFUNCTION

Practitioners must explain to patients that chronic MGD is a condition that has no cure. It should be stressed that initial (and relatively vigorous) therapy is prescribed to bring the condition under control. After this acute phase of therapy, a minimal (variable) amount of chronic treatment is required to maintain control.[6]

Treatment of MGD should be directed toward relieving the obstruction of the ducts and orifices to allow normal flow of the meibomian gland secretions onto the precorneal tear film. This is best accomplished by the following measures:

- Treatment of anterior seborrheic or staphylococcal blepharitis (if present)
- Hot compresses two to four times a day
- Lid scrubs two to four times a day
- Forceful expression of the meibomian glands
- Topical antibiotics (if necessary)
- Tetracycline 250 mg by mouth four times a day (on an empty stomach) for 10–30 days

Expression of the meibomian glands should be performed professionally in the office at appropriate intervals. In addition, patients should be carefully instructed on home therapy, consisting of warm compresses, lid massage, and lid scrubs.

On initial examination of patients with MGD, it is often difficult to determine if antibiotic therapy is necessary. If evidence of staphylococcal blepharitis exists, a topical antibiotic ointment should be prescribed. The ointment should be applied to the lids after local hygienic maneuvers. Patients are instructed to place a small amount of ointment on a clean fingertip and rub the antibiotic into the lids and lashes. This is done two to four times a day, depending on the severity of the inflammatory process. If significant associated keratoconjunctivitis is present, an antibiotic drop can be prescribed four times a day.

McCulley and Sciallis[45] and Gutgesell et al.[31] have found only a minimal and inconsistent increase in inflammatory cells in the glands of patients with MGD. Therefore, corticosteroids and other anti-inflammatory agents are unlikely to modify the course of the condition and should be discouraged.

Studies have indicated that many patients with MGD respond well to oral tetracycline antibiotic therapy. The exact mechanism of this drug action is not known. Gutgesell et al.[31] suggest that the drug reduces the bacterial population and, thus, the quantity of lipolytic enzymes. This action may decrease the amount of free fatty acid in the meibomian glands.

Most patients with grade 3 or greater MGD should be started on oral tetracycline along with the local lid hygiene maneuvers. The initial dose is oral tetracycline 250 mg four times a day to be taken on an empty stomach and continued until the MGD is under control, after which time it can be slowly tapered. The majority of patients can be tapered from the tetracycline within 4–12 weeks, but an occasional patient requires low-dose oral tetracycline indefinitely to maintain control.

Intensive, acute therapy should be maintained until the condition is under control. This typically requires 2–6 weeks of vigorous therapy, after which the intensity of the therapy can be decreased. The goal should then be to determine the minimal amount of maintenance therapy required to maintain control. This frequently entails warm compresses and lid scrubs once or twice a day. An attempt should be made to avoid the chronic use of antimicrobial agents, either topically or systemically.

The use of preservative-free artificial tears for patients with concurrent keratoconjunctivitis sicca is also recommended.

MEIBOMIAN GLAND DYSFUNCTION AND CONTACT LENS INTOLERANCE

In contact lens wearers, the possibility of MGD is usually not investigated unless gross signs or significant symptoms are present. Therefore, it is common for apparently healthy eyes to have mild MGD, with patients experiencing only vague symptoms of contact lens intolerance.

It is clear that all prospective contact lens wearers should be screened for MGD. The screening process should include general observation of the lids and conjunctiva for gross anomalies. For example, a patient who presents with a pinguecula should be thoroughly evaluated for underlying lid margin disease as part of the spectrum of dryness and exposure disorders.

Korb and Henriquez[32] cite several mechanisms responsible for MGD-associated contact lens intolerance. Lens intolerance may occur secondary to mechanical obstruction of the meibomian glands by keratotic plugs, which results in alteration of their oil secretion. Intolerance may be related to the release of bacteria or their toxic by-products from the meibomian glands into the precorneal tear film.

Paugh et al.[51] studied the objective and subjective efficacy of meibomian gland therapy in contact lens wearers with recalcitrant MGD. Treatment of the condition with a 2-week course of unilateral lid margin hygiene improved symptoms of discomfort and dryness and increased the TBUT from 0.2 seconds in the control (untreated) eyes to 4 seconds in the treated eyes. It is therefore clear that the possibility of MGD should be investigated in all patients with unexplained contact lens intolerance.

Studies by Robin et al.[52] have shown that MGD may be associated with the development of soft contact lens deposits. They analyzed the meibomian gland structures of 28 patients who wore extended-wear hydrogel lenses for either myopia or aphakia. Fifteen of those patients repeatedly formed elevated nodular lipocalcium deposits on the anterior surface of their lenses. Thirteen patients

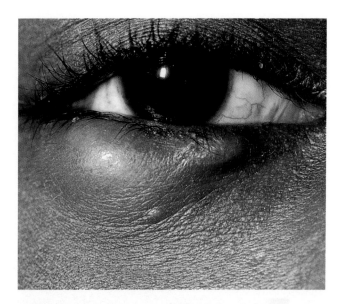

FIG. 9-20. *Internal hordeolum on a right lower lid, involving the meibomian glands. Note the localized swelling and loss of lashes.*

served as controls, with no history of deposit formation. Analysis consisted of meibomian transillumination biomicroscopy and infrared photography. The investigators found that all patients who formed deposits had moderate-to-severe structural abnormalities of their meibomian glands, and only two of the 13 control patients had any evidence of meibomian gland abnormalities.

Rapp and Broich[53] have noted that the lipid composition of soft contact lens deposits is similar to that of meibomian gland secretions. Patients with oily or greasy deposits on their lenses should be thoroughly evaluated for the presence of MGD, and appropriate therapy should be initiated.

HORDEOLUM

A hordeolum is a common infection characterized by acute localized swelling and tenderness of the glandular structures of the upper or lower lids. It is essentially an abscess with pustular formation in the lumen of the affected gland. When it affects the meibomian glands, it is relatively large and is referred to as an *internal hordeolum* (Fig. 9-20). A smaller, more superficial infection involves the glands of Moll and Zeis and is referred to as an *external hordeolum* or *stye* (Fig. 9-21).[54] Styes tend to occur in crops because the infecting organism spreads from one hair follicle to another, either directly or by transfer from the fingers.[55]

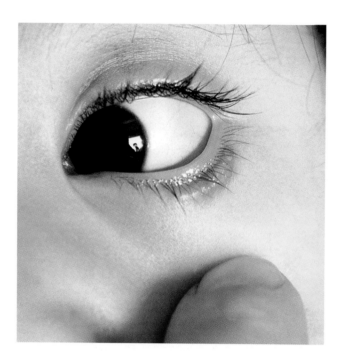

FIG. 9-21. *External hordeolum (styes) involving the glands of Moll and Zeis.*

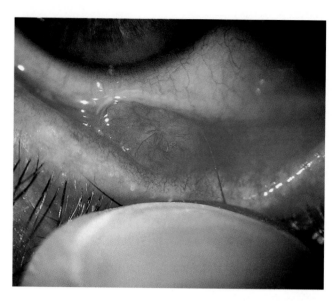

FIG. 9-22. *Chalazion pointed toward the conjunctival side of the eyelid.*

The causative organism is usually staphylococcal, although other organisms may play a role. The initial presenting symptom is tenderness of the lid, which may become quite marked as the condition progresses. The symptoms are usually in direct proportion to the amount of lid swelling. Internal hordeola are much more painful than external styes because the lesions are encased in fibrous tissue and also lie deeper within the lid.[56]

Treatment of internal and external hordeola consists of warm compresses for 5–10 minutes, three to four times a day. If warm compresses do not resolve a painful hordeolum within 48 hours, incision and drainage may be necessary. Frequently, a sulfuramide or an antibacterial ointment can be instilled into the conjunctival sac every 3 hours to prevent involvement of adjacent glands.

CHALAZION

Description

In contrast to a hordeolum, a chalazion is not associated with an inflammatory process but is a sterile granulomatous mass within the lid glands.[57] Chalazia have an obscure etiology and are characterized by a gradual painless swelling of the upper and lower lid. Unlike a hordeolum, which is located at the eyelid margin, a chalazion

usually lies deep in the tarsus (see Fig. 9-21). The tenderness is less severe than that of a hordeolum, and the mass develops slowly over a period of weeks. Palpation of the mass indicates a small, buckshotlike swelling in the substance of the lid, and this may be its only evidence.[25] The majority of chalazia points toward the conjunctival side of the lid (Fig. 9-22). When the lid is everted, the conjunctiva over the chalazion is seen to be injected and elevated (Fig. 9-23). If sufficiently large, a chalazion may press on the eyeball and induce regular or irregular astigmatism.

Pathologically, proliferation of the endothelium of the acinus and a granulomatous inflammatory response, including some Langhans-type giant cells, occur.

Treatment

The most common treatment for a chalazion is frequent hot compresses. Compresses are most effective when used soon after the onset of the chalazion. If the chalazion is large enough to distort vision or to be a cosmetic concern, excision may be indicated.

An alternative treatment involves steroid injection directly into the center of the chalazion. The suggested treatment is a 0.10–0.20 ml injection of Kenalog (triamcinolone). The steroid can be injected into the conjunctiva or the skin surface, depending on the location of the chalazion.[58,59] If chalazia occur repeatedly, have a solid appearance, or distort or contract the adjacent lid margin, biopsy should be performed to exclude metastatic

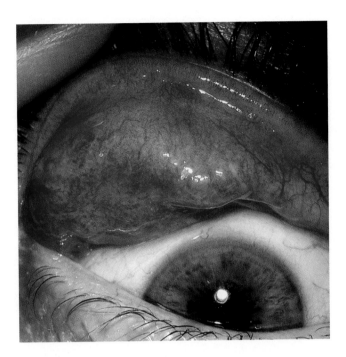

FIG. 9-23. *Chalazion on a patient's right upper lid.*

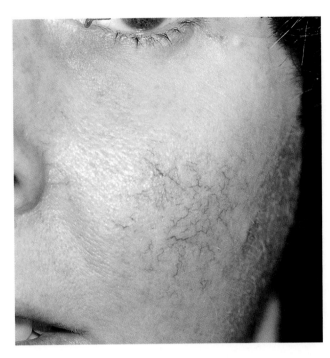

FIG. 9-24. *A 37-year-old woman with a history of dermatologic rosacea. Note the telangiectatic spots on the cheeks.*

sebaceous gland carcinoma (a rare but potentially life-threatening carcinoma).

ROSACEA BLEPHARITIS

Dermatologic Rosacea

Rosacea is a chronic skin disorder affecting the skin of the upper body and the eye. The dermatologic findings are usually limited to the sun-exposed areas of the face, the neck and the *V* of the chest.[60] The findings include blotchy or diffuse facial erythema, telangiectases, papules, pustules, and sebaceous gland hypertrophy. Rosacea is characterized by the appearance of the skin lesions on the central forehead, nose, cheeks, chin, and occasionally the neck and chest (Fig. 9-24). Initially, the hyperemia may be episodic, but within months or years, it becomes chronic, with the eventual development of telangiectases. The episodic flushing and lesions are frequently brought on by the consumption of alcohol, hot drinks, spicy foods, or exposure to ultraviolet light. Rhinophyma, an irregular lobulated thickening of the skin of the nose, with follicular dilation and a purplish red discoloration, may be a complication of long-standing involvement (Fig. 9-25).[61,62]

Although rosacea may begin as early as 2 years of age, it is most commonly seen between the ages of 30 and 60 years, with equal distribution between men and women.[63,64] A widespread clinical impression exists that rosacea affects mainly fair-skinned people of northern European or Celtic decent. However, studies have not substantiated this

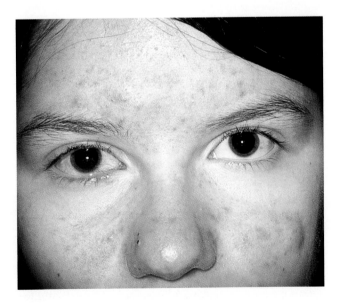

FIG. 9-25. *A 32-year-old woman with ocular rosacea in the right eye. Note the dilatated blood vessels in the skin of the nose, cheeks, and forehead.*

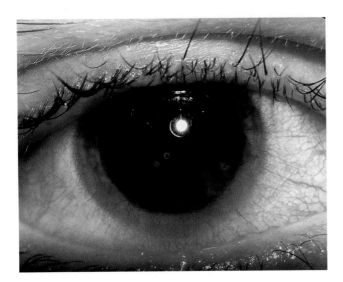

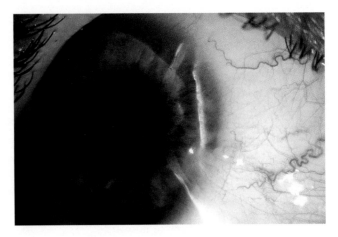

FIG. 9-27. *Marginal corneal thinning associated with ocular rosacea.*

FIG. 9-26. *Right eye of the patient in Fig. 9-25. Note the dilatated conjunctival vessels, mild blepharitis, 360-degree peripheral vascularization, and subepithelial infiltrates at 4 o'clock.*

assumption.[65] Acne rosacea and ocular rosacea have been documented in blacks, although the early skin lesions are frequently missed because of the increased skin pigmentation.[66] Although many theories have been advanced to explain the origin of rosacea, the etiology is still unknown. Dermatologic rosacea runs a chronic course punctuated by episodes of acute inflammation, with a mean duration between 9 and 13 years.[67]

Ocular Rosacea

Ocular rosacea is the term used to describe the spectrum of ocular findings associated with dermatologic rosacea. The ocular symptoms usually begin with a foreign-body sensation, pain, tearing, and burning. The ocular signs and symptoms may be unilateral, and rosacea patients may present with a unilateral red eye. The ocular manifestations of rosacea involve the lids, conjunctiva, and cornea and may include MGD, chronic staphylococcal blepharitis, keratitis, recurrent chalazia, dry eyes, peripheral corneal neovascularization, diffuse hyperemic conjunctivitis, marginal corneal infiltrates with and without ulceration, corneal thinning, episcleritis, and iritis (Fig. 9-26). The ocular manifestations may appear before the skin lesions on the face are noted. In one study, 20% of patients with rosacea presented first with ocular involvement, 53% developed skin lesions before any ocular findings, and 27% had simultaneous ocular and skin findings.[68] The dermatologic findings of ocular rosacea are easily overlooked by eye care professionals. Therefore, in suspected patients, all exami-

nations should be performed after the removal of facial makeup to enable the discovery of subtle skin changes.

One of the major ocular findings is that of dilated conjunctival blood vessels, which are dilated in a manner similar to that of blood vessels of the skin of the nose, face, and eyelids. The dilated blood vessels most often occur in the interpalpebral areas of the medial and lateral epibulbar conjunctivae. The vessels can be large and tortuous.[69]

Ocular remissions and exacerbations may occur independent of the skin anomalies. The most severe ocular complication of rosacea is keratitis with subsequent corneal thinning. This can result in considerable visual impairment. The keratitis typically involves the lower two-thirds of the cornea and begins as a peripheral vascularization of the cornea, followed by subepithelial infiltrates central to the vessels. Marginal corneal thinning occurs either by resolution of the infiltrates or by gross ulcerations (Fig. 9-27). The keratitis progresses by intermittent attacks that can result in corneal perforation, especially when steroid therapy has been introduced and injudiciously used.[70,71]

Etiology

Like dermatologic rosacea, the etiology of ocular rosacea is poorly understood. Numerous theories have been suggested, including *Demodex folliculorum* infestation, bacterial process, climatic exposure, autoimmune process, hypersensitivity reaction, and psychosis.[66]

Contact Lenses and Ocular Rosacea

Although patients with ocular rosacea can be successfully treated, they should be cautioned about the wearing of contact lenses. The underlying lid, conjunctival, and corneal complications associated with rosacea are a breeding ground for future complications. In moderate-to-severe ocular rosacea, the keratitis and vascularization represent an absolute contraindication to cosmetic contact lens wear.

Treatment

Topical dermatologic therapy for rosacea is generally less successful than systemic treatment. Topical metronidazole gel has been shown to be effective in substantially reducing the inflammatory skin lesions. Topical corticosteroids should be avoided because long-term therapy may cause atrophy, chronic vasodilatation, and telangiectasia.

The treatment of the ocular component of rosacea begins with advising the patient to avoid any stimuli that tend to exacerbate the condition (i.e., exposure to extreme heat and cold, excessive sunlight, alcohol consumption, and the ingestion of hot liquids and spicy foods).[60]

Many treatment modalities have been advocated, however, aggressive lid hygiene and systemic antibiotics remain the primary forms of therapy for ocular rosacea. Tetracycline and doxycycline have been found to be effective against the ocular and dermatologic manifestations of the disease. Tetracycline appears to alleviate the symptoms faster, whereas doxycycline has the advantage of easier compliance and less of a tendency for gastrointestinal side effects.[66]

The initial dose of tetracycline should be 250 mg orally four times a day for approximately 3–4 weeks followed by tapering based on clinical response. The dosage of doxycycline is generally 100 mg once a day for 6 weeks, with subsequent tapering to 50 mg daily for 1 month. Tetracycline or doxycycline should not be used in children under the age of 8 or until the enamel deposition on the maturing teeth is completed. Additionally, it should not be given to pregnant or lactating woman. Female patients should be warned that vaginal yeast infections may be a side effect of systemic tetracycline treatment. Patients who are intolerant to the tetracyclines may benefit from the use of erythromycin.[72,73] As with more severe MGD, some patients with rosacea may require chronic systemic maintenance therapy.

The importance of aggressive lid margin hygiene cannot be overemphasized. Warm compresses and lid scrubs are extremely helpful for managing the underlying blepharitis. Some practitioners recommend the use of a bacteriostatic ointment at bedtime after lid hygiene. The value of topical ointment in treating rosacea has not been verified in clinical studies. However, it does encourage patients to perform thorough lid hygiene in the morning to remove residual ointment.

General improvement is expected within the first 3 weeks. Irritation is usually diminished before the signs resolve. Many patients require some ongoing medication indefinitely. Abrupt tapering may cause recurrences, which can be difficult to re-treat.

Secondary infections should be treated with a topical antibiotic ointment. Steroid therapy can be useful in the severe inflammatory component of the blepharitis as well as for episcleritis, keratitis, and iritis. However, patients must be monitored closely for the length of therapy and the dose given because severe side effects have been reported, such as corneal melting and perforations.

PARASITIC BLEPHARITIS

Demodex Infestation

Demodectic or mite infestation is virtually ubiquitous in the human population, predominantly involving the eyelids, eyebrows, forehead, and nasal regions. Demodicosis is characterized by the presence of two distinct species living in the lash follicle and sebaceous glands of the eyelids, *Demodex folliculorum* and *Demodex brevis*.[74]

Demodex Folliculorum

D. folliculorum is a microscopic, eight-legged, transparent mite that inhabits the upper portion of the hair follicle, above the level of the sebaceous gland (Fig. 9-28). *Demodex* attach themselves to the hair follicle, with head down and feet facing the epithelial surface (Fig. 9-29).[75] *D. folliculorum* are colonial, with three or more organisms per follicle. The mite feeds on intact epithelial cells by puncturing the cell wall with its sharp mouth and extracting the cytoplasm. Later, its claws shred the cellular material and push it up, toward the epithelial surface (Fig. 9-30). This hyperkeratinized cellular debris combines with sebum and lipids to form a semiopaque, tubelike sleeve or collar that extends from the skin of the lid margin up the base of the lash (Fig. 9-31). These sleeves, also called *cuffs* or *collarettes*, are the best diagnostic sign of demodicosis. The folliculorum ova (eggs) are deposited

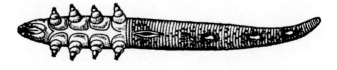

FIG. 9-28. *Illustration of the eight-legged* Demodex folliculorum *mite.*

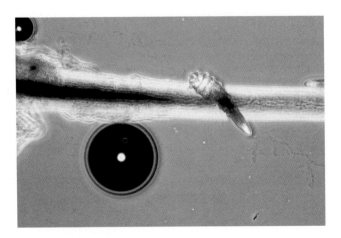

FIG. 9-29. *Light micrograph of the* Demodex folliculorum *mite on a human eyelash.*

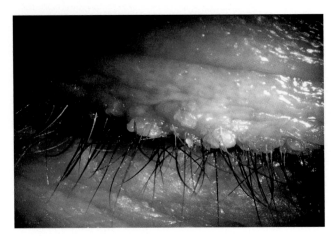

FIG. 9-31. *Severe* Demodex folliculorum *infestation resulting in debris at the base of the lash.*

and hatch within the hair or eyelash follicle. The organism has a limited life cycle of approximately 5–14 days.[76]

D. brevis is the smaller and stubbier of the two species, with the organisms being one-half the size of the folliculorum species.[77] *D. brevis* feeds on glandular cells of the sebaceous glands (Fig. 9-32). The obstruction and damage to the gland resulting from heavy infestation may affect the meibomian gland secretion, resulting in chalazion formation or compromises in tear-film integrity.[77,78]

The prevalence of *Demodex* species in humans appears to increase with the increasing age of the host. One study

reported a prevalence of 29% in people aged 0 to 25 years, 53% in people aged 26 to 50 years, and 67% in people aged 51 to 90 years.[79] Higher prevalence rates are commonly reported in the literature, often reaching estimates of 97–100% infestation in the elderly, thus supporting the ubiquitous nature of the mites.[80]

All stages in the *Demodex* life cycle are found in the hair follicle or sebaceous gland complex. However, a busy migration exists of mites of both species and both gen-

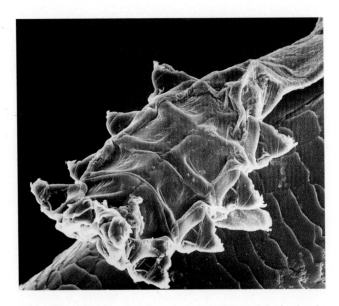

FIG. 9-30. *Scanning electron microscopy view of the body of a* Demodex folliculorum *mite resting on an eyelash.*

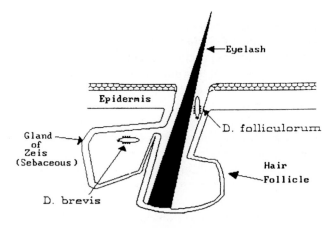

FIG. 9-32. *Schematic representation of the habitat of* Demodex folliculorum *and* Demodex brevis *in a pilosebaceous gland complex.* D. folliculorum *is usually found above the level of the sebaceous gland in the hair follicle, with its head downward and its opisthosoma toward (and in some cases protruding from) the follicle opening.* D. brevis *is usually found in the sebaceous gland of the complex. (Courtesy of Drs. William Edmondson and Michael Christensen.)*

ders across the lid margins, from one follicle to another. As the population of mites increases, an increase occurs in the keratinization of the outer layers of the epithelium surrounding the follicle. Histologic studies indicate that this aggregation of debris can block the hair follicle, trapping the *Demodex* in the sebaceous complex. Increases in mite population lead to increased signs of madarosis, hyperplasia, erythema, cuffing of the lashes, and symptoms of burning and itching. The itching is episodic, possibly paralleling bouts of frenetic reproductive activity of the mites at the mouth of the hair follicle. Patients with heavy mite infestation frequently experience a swelling of the lid margins as well as chronic blepharitis. Because bacteria and fungi have been found on the bodies of the mites, it is possible that the mite serves as a vector for ocular infection.

Diagnosis

The diagnosis of demodicosis is suggested by the presence of symptoms and signs of elongated tubelike collarettes, which can be found around the base of the lash. In general, *D. folliculorum* are difficult to see during a slit-lamp examination because the organisms are typically translucent and considerably narrower than the width of a human hair. Additionally, the mites recess back into the follicle under bright lights.

In practice, the diagnosis of demodicosis is best made by epilating the lash and suspending it in a viscous fluid (i.e., glycerin or peanut oil). Light microscopy examination of the base of the lash reveals mites clinging to the lash. A practical clinical guideline, suggested by Fulk and Clifford,[81] is that when one or more mites are found for every two epilated lashes, the mite population is abnormally high and symptoms are likely to occur.

Treatment

The goal of demodicosis treatment is to reduce and control the mite population to a level in which the pathologic effects are limited and the patient asymptomatic. Owing to the ubiquitous nature of the organisms, it is impossible to completely eliminate the species.

The general management of demodicosis begins by alleviating the patient's concerns related to acaraphobia (fear of mites). Mite infestation can be quite disconcerting for many patients. Therefore, the appropriate choice of words by the practitioner can go a long way toward improving the patient's understanding of the condition and acceptance of the therapy.

The treatment of choice is to topically anesthetize the lids and carefully clean the infested lid with a cotton-tipped applicator saturated with a contact lens clean-

ing solution. Patient maintenance begins with lid scrubs twice a day, followed by the application of an ophthalmic ointment (sulfacetamide or neomycin, polymyxin B, or bacitracin ointment) to the lid margins. This reduces concomitant bacterial infection. The viscous ointment is also thought to trap or possibly even smother the mites that emerge from the follicle, thereby reducing breeding and migration. The life cycle of the mites is approximately 5–14 days; therefore, it is necessary to maintain aggressive treatment for 2–3 weeks. Patients should be informed that it is impossible to totally eradicate the mites. Therefore, chronic lid margin hygiene is encouraged to control mite population and avoid recurrence of the heavy infestation.

PEDICULOSIS AND PHTHIRIASIS

Pediculosis (Body and Head Lice)

Pediculosis refers to the infestation by *Pediculus corporis* (body lice) and *Pediculus capitis* (head lice). These lice are morphologically similar to one another and interbreed freely.[82,83] Pediculus organisms are 1–3 mm in length and have long slender legs that allow them to move freely between the hair follicles of the head and body. The head louse primarily restricts itself to the scalp, particularly the occipital region, whereas the body louse primarily inhabits the seams of clothing, from where it feeds on the skin of the patient. The louse attaches its eggs to the seams of cloth and not to the host, as do other parasites. Head lice are much more common than body lice. It is estimated that in the United States between 3–10 million school children are infested each year.[84,85]

The lice are typically passed from person to person by close contact either with another infested person or with contaminated clothing, bedding, towels, hairbrush, and so on. Infestation of the eyebrows or eyelashes with body or head lice is extremely rare.[86]

Phthiriasis (Pubic Lice)

Phthiriasis refers to infestation by *Phthirus pubis* (pubic lice). Surprisingly, it is usually the pubic louse rather than the head louse that infests the eyebrows and eyelashes. *Phthirus pubis*, also called *crab louse*, has a broad shield-like body with two pairs of strong grasping claws on the central and hind legs, allowing it to hold onto eyelashes with considerable tenacity (Figs. 9-33 and 9-34). The lice are approximately 1.0–1.5 mm long, with an anatomic grasping span of 2 mm. *P. pubis* prefers to inhabit sites where the distance between adjacent hairs is similar to its

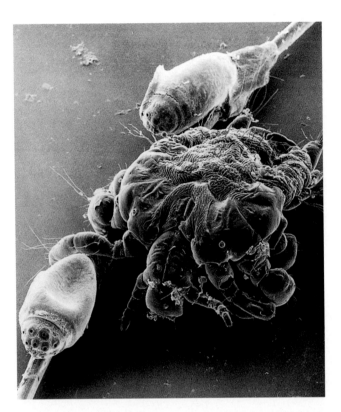

FIG. 9-33. *Electron micrograph of a pubic louse* Phthirus pubis, *with two nits (eggs) on a human eyelash.*

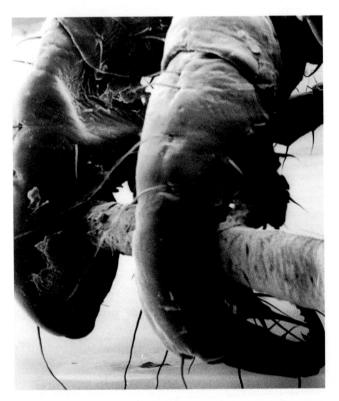

FIG. 9-34. *The crablike claw and opposing tibial thumb of* Phthirus pubis *allow it to hold onto the eyelashes with considerable tenacity.*

grasping span. These environments are found in the pubic region, chest, beard, and eyelashes. Conversely, the average spacing between neighboring hairs on the head is significantly more dense, approximately 1 mm.

P. pubis feeds off the host tissue fluid and blood. It does so by anchoring mouth hooklets to the host skin and then extending a long hollow tube directly into the dermis. Salivary material is injected into the host, which can cause a toxic immunologic reaction (Fig. 9-35).[75]

Pubic lice are primarily sexually transmitted in teenagers and young adults; however, infestation is possible from contaminated bedding, towels, and so on.[87] The eyelashes of children may be infested through eye-to-eye contact or direct contact with chest hairs of parents harboring the lice. *P. pubis* also accounts for approximately 1% of lice infestation on the scalp hair.[88]

Pubic lice lay their eggs (nits) on the hair shaft approximately 1–2 mm from the base. The eggs are firmly attached to the hair by cement secreted by the louse, which resists mechanical and chemical removal (Fig. 9-36). Adult lice lay seven to 10 eggs per day and the eggs hatch after 7–8 days. The average life cycle of the various species is approximately 17–28 days.[86] The lice die of starvation if away from a body for more than 10 days.[89]

Ocular Findings

Lice infestation of the eyelashes is almost always related to the pubic or crab louse. Early in the course of the infestation, the patient may be asymptomatic; this is especially true during the initial incubation period of approximately 30 days. After this period, the ocular symptoms may include moderate-to-severe itching and irritation of the eyelids, burning, erythema, and marked conjunctival injection. The patient's history may include exposure to known carriers.[90]

Close examination of the lid margins and lashes is essential to detect the presence of the parasites. For clinicians, the most obvious sign is the oval grayish-white nit cases attached to the superior and inferior lashes. Gross observation of the lids usually reveals a crusty appearance of the eyelid margins with reddish-brown discoloration. The dark red crusting is a mixture of blood from the host and feces from the parasite (Fig. 9-37). Lid erythema of infested

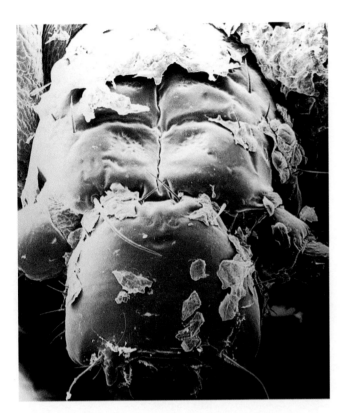

FIG. 9-35. *Electron micrograph of the head of* Phthirus pubis *with mouth hooklets, which anchor the lice to host skin. A long hollow tube extends directly into the dermis, and salivary material is injected into the host, causing a toxic reaction.*

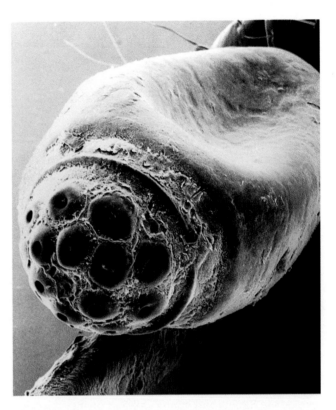

FIG. 9-36. *Electron micrograph of pubic lice nits (eggs) firmly attached to an eyelash by a cementlike substance secreted by the louse.*

patients is caused by a hypersensitivity reaction to the louse fecal deposits or the anticlotting components of the louse saliva introduced into the lid by the louse during feeding.

Pubic lice are brownish-gray and somewhat translucent. The actual organisms can be difficult to detect because they are normally nestled along the lid margin at the base of the lashes and are often partially covered by scaly skin shed by the host (Fig. 9-38). The louse can be seen firmly adhering to the lashes of the eyelid with its crablike claw and opposing tibial thumb.

In more severe infestation, shallow ulcerations may develop along the lid margin as well as mild keratoconjunctivitis secondary to the toxic excreta, saliva, and digestive juices of the organism.

Treatment

General Infestation

Effective management of lice infestation requires deinfestation of all affected areas of the body. In the case of pubic lice, other sexually transmitted diseases might be

suspected and the patient should be referred appropriately. Sexual partners and family members should be examined for eyelash infestation and counseled about the possibility of concurrent infestation of pubic hair. Additionally, the home environment should be sanitized, with heat being the most effective action. Lice are killed on bedding, clothing, and towels if they are washed at a temperature of 120°C for 30 minutes. Other items, such as combs or brushes, should be decontaminated in boiling water for 10 minutes or discarded.

The treatment plan must address any concomitant pelvic or head infestation. Over-the-counter pediculicide shampoos are usually recommended for head lice. These include pyrethrin (A-200, Lice-Enz, Pronto, and Rid) and permethrin (Nix). Lindane (Kwell 1% shampoo) is the treatment of choice for pubic lice and is available by prescription only. A single application to the pelvic region is usually sufficient. However, the shampooing may need to be repeated in 7 days because it is less effective against nits. Lindane shampoo should only be applied to nonocular areas of the body: It is too toxic for use on the lids,

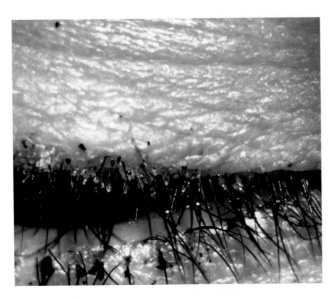

FIG. 9-37. *Eyelid appearance in louse infestation. Note the dark red crusts, which are a mixture of blood from the host and feces from the parasite.*

lashes, and eyes. Additionally, the shampoo should be avoided in infants and young children owing to reports of seizures and aplastic anemia with misuse of the product. Lindane should be avoided during pregnancy.

Ocular Infestation

None of the pediculicides can be safely used on or around the eyes or eyebrows because they may cause significant ocular irritation, including corneal toxicity. Ocular treatment should include manual removal of the nits and lice

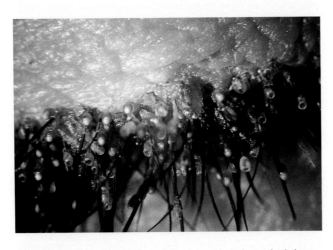

FIG. 9-38. *A single translucent louse nestled along the lid margin at the base of the lashes. Numerous nits are seen firmly attached to the eyelashes.*

with forceps. Although this sounds easy, the lice are difficult to see. In addition, they grasp onto the lash so tenaciously that removal can be quite tedious. Alternative methods include physically destroying the nits and lice using either cryotherapy or argon laser phototherapy. It has also been reported that a single application of 20% fluorescein immediately kills lice and nits. This method apparently is not only nontoxic to patients but produces no discomfort on application.

Often, the treatment of choice is to suffocate the organisms by applying a thick layer of ophthalmic ointment to the base of the lashes two to three times a day. Because petrolatum is ineffective against the nits, the applications must be continued for 10 days to 2 weeks to eradicate hatching lice.[86] Patients should be warned that symptoms may persist beyond effective eradication of the lice owing to residual lice-induced hypersensitivity reactions.

The patient should be followed weekly until parasitic infestation has been eliminated. If the nits persist, confirm patient compliance with instructions, and treat for an additional week.

REFERENCES

1. Fox BJ, Odom RB: Papulosquamous disease: A review. J Am Acad Dermatol 12:597, 1985
2. Mathers WD, Stone MS: Seborrheic dermatitis and seborrheic blepharitis. In Mannis MJ, Mascai MS, Huntley AC (eds): Eye and Skin Disease. Lippincott–Raven, Philadelphia, 1996
3. Rebora A, Ronbgiolett F: The red face: seborrheic dermatitis. Clin Dermatol 11:243, 1993
4. Mathes BM, Douglass MC: Seborrheic dermatitis in patients with acquired immunodeficiency syndrome. J Am Acad Dermatol 13:947, 1985
5. Soeprono FF, Schinella RA, Cockerall CJ, Comite SL: Seborrheic-like dermatitis of acquired immunodeficiency syndrome: a clinicopathologic study. J Am Acad Dermatol 14:242, 1986
6. McCulley JP, Dougherty JM, Deneau DG: Classification of chronic blepharitis. Ophthalmology 89:1173, 1982
7. Bownan RW, Dougherty JM, McCulley JP: Chronic blepharitis and dry eyes. Int Ophthalmol Clin 27:27, 1987
8. Trevor-Roper PD: Diseases of the eyelids. Int Ophthalmol Clin 14:362, 1974
9. Halsted M, McCulley JP: Seborrheic blepharitis. In Fraundelder FT, Roy FH (eds): Current Ocular Therapy. Saunders, Philadelphia, 1995
10. Thygeson P: Complications of *Staphylococcus* blepharitis. Am J Ophthalmol 68:446, 1969
11. Leibowitz HM, Capino D: Treatment of chronic blepharitis. Arch Ophthalmol 106:720, 1988

12. Dougherty JM, McCulley JP: Bacterial lipases and chronic blepharitis. Invest Ophthalmol Vis Sci 27:486, 1986

13. Dougherty JM, McCullley JP: Comparative bacteriology of chronic blepharitis. Br J Ophthalmol 68:524, 1984

14. Dougherty JM, McCulley JP: Analysis of free fatty acid component of meibomian secretions in chronic blepharitis. Invest Ophthalmol Vis Sci 27:52, 1986

15. White G: Dermatologic complications. In Silbert J (ed): Anterior Segment Complications of Contact Lens Wear. 1st ed. Churchill Livingstone, New York, 1994

16. Thygeson P: Complication of Staphylococcal blepharitis. Am J Ophthalmol 68:446, 1969

17. Brown DD, McCulley JP: Staphylococcal and mixed staphylococcal/seborrheic blepharoconjunctivitis. In Fraunfelder FT, Roy FH (eds): Current Ocular Therapy. Saunders, Philadelphia, 1995

18. Grayson M: Blepharitis. In: Diseases of the Cornea. 2nd ed. Mosby, St. Louis, 1983

19. Mudd S, Shayegani M: Delayed type hypersensitivity: *S. Aureus* and its uses. Ann N Y Acad Sci 236:244, 1974

20. Smolin G, Okumoto M: Staphylococcal blepharitis. Arch Ophthalmol 95:812, 1977

21. Ostler HB: Blepharitis. In Tasman W, Jaeger EA (eds): Duane's Clinical Ophthalmology. Vol. 4. Lippincott, Philadelphia, 1993

22. Reidy JJ: Angular blepharoconjunctivitis and perioral dermatitis. In Mannis MJ, Macsai MS, AC Huntley (eds): Eye and Skin Diseases. Lippincott–Raven, Philadelphia, 1996

23. Eyre JW: A clinical and bacteriological study of diplo-bacillary conjunctivitis. J Pathol Bacteriol 6:1, 1990

24. Duke-Elder S: Inflammations of the conjunctiva and associated inflammations of the cornea. In Systems of Ophthalmology. Vol. 8, Part I: Diseases of the Outer Eye. Mosby, St. Louis, 1965

25. Thygeson P. Etiology and treatment of blepharitis. A study in military personnel. Arch Ophthalmol 36:445, 1946

26. Baum J, Fedukowiccz HB, Jordan A. A survey of *Moraxella* corneal ulcers in a derelict population. Am J Ophthalmol 90:476, 1980

27. Cobo LM, Coster DJ, Peacock J: *Moraxella* keratitis in a nonalcoholic population. Br J Ophthalmol 65:683, 1981

28. Kowalski RP, Harwick JC: Incidence of *Moraxella* conjunctival infection. Am J Ophthalmol 101:437, 1986

29. Davis CE, Baer H: *Moraxella, Klingella* and *Acinetobacter*. In Braude AI, Davis CE, Fierer J (eds): Infectious Diseases and Medical Microbiology. 2nd ed. Saunders, Philadelphia, 1986

30. Robin J, Jester J, Nobe J, et al: In vivo transillumination biomicroscopy and photography of meibomian gland dysfunction. Ophthalmology 92:1423, 1985

31. Gutgesell VJ, Stern GA, Hood CI: Histopathology of meibomian gland dysfunction. Am J Ophthalmol 94:383, 1982

32. Korb D, Henriquez A: Meibomian gland dysfunction and contact lens intolerance. J Am Optom Assoc 51:243, 1980

33. Tripathi R, Tripathi B: The role of the lids in soft lens spoilage. CLAO J 7:234, 1981

34. Duke-Elder S, Wybar K: The anatomy of the visual system.

In Duke-Elder S (ed): System of Ophthalmology. Mosby, St Louis, 1961

35. Wolff E: Anatomy of the Eye and Orbit. HK Lewis, London, 1933

36. Henriquez A, Korb D: Meibomian gland and contact lens wear. Br J Ophthalmol 65:108, 1981

37. Andrews JS: The meibomian secretion, the preocular tear film and dry eye syndromes. Int Ophthalmol Clin 13:23, 1973

38. Tiffany JM: Individual variation in human meibomian lipid composition. Exp Eye Res 27:289, 1978

39. Keith CG: Seborrheic blepharo-keratoconjunctivitis. Trans Ophthalmol Soc UK 87:85, 1967

40. Nicolaides N: Skin lipids II: lipid class composition of samples from various species and anatomical sites. J Am Oil Chem Soc 42:691, 1965

41. Jester J, Nicolaides N, Smith R: Meibomian gland studies: histologic and ultrastructural investigations. Invest Ophthalmol Vis Sci 20:537, 1981

42. Knutson DD: Ultrastructural observations in acne vulgaris: the normal sebaceous follicle and acne lesions. J Invest Dermatol 62:288, 1974

43. Nicolaides N, Santos EC, Robin J, et al: Meibum lipids in rosacea blepharitis. Invest Ophthalmol Vis Sci 22(suppl):78, 1983

44. Molinari J: Color photography of meibomian glands. Am J Optom Physiol Opt 59:758, 1982

45. McCulley JP, Sciallis GF: Meibomian keratoconjunctivitis oculo-dermal correlates. CLAO J 9:130, 1983

46. Korb DR, Herman JP: Corneal staining subsequent to sequential fluorescein instillations. J Am Optom Assoc 50:361, 1978

47. McDonald JE: Surface phenomena of tear film. Am J Ophthalmol 67:56, 1969

48. Larke JR: The Eye in Contact Lens Wear. Butterworth, London, 1985

49. Norn M, Meibomiam orifices and Marx's line — studied by triple vital staining. Acta Ophthalmol 63;698:1985.

50. McCulley JP, Dougherty JM: Blepharitis associated with acne rosacea and seborrheic dermatitis. Int Ophthalmol Clin 25:159, 1985

51. Paugh JR, Knapp LL, Martinson JR, et al: Meibomian therapy in problematic contact lens wear. Optom Vis Sci 67:803, 1990

52. Robin JB, Nobe JR, Suarez E: Meibomian gland evaluation in patients with extended wear soft contact lens deposits. CLAO J 12:95, 1986

53. Rapp J, Broich IR: Lipid deposition on worn soft contact lenses. CLAO J 10:235, 1984

54. Vaughan D, Asbury T: General Ophthalmology. 8th ed. Lange Medical Publications, Los Altos, CA, 1977

55. Newell FW, Ernest JT: Ophthalmology Principles and Concepts. Mosby, St. Louis, 1974

56. Scheie JG, Albert DM: Textbook of Ophthalmology, 9th ed. Saunders, Philadelphia, 1977

57. Grayson M: Diseases of the Cornea. Mosby, St. Louis, 1979

58. Pizzarello LD, Jakobiec FA, Mofeldt AJ, et al: Intralesional corticosteroid therapy of chalazia. Am J Ophthalmol 85:88, 1978

59. Fanell JL: A better way to treat chalazia. Rev Optom 127:103, 1990

60. Brown SI, Shahinlan L: Diagnosis and treatment of ocular rosacea. Opthalmology 85:779, 1978

61. Frucht-Pery J, Brown SI: Ocular rosacea. In Fraunfelder FT, Roy FH (eds): Current Ocular Therapy. Saunders, Philadelphia, 1995

62. Stevens G, Lemp M: Acne rosacea. In Weingeist T, Gould D (eds): The Eye in Systemic Disease. Lippincott, Philadelphia, 1990

63. Jenkin MS, Brown SI, Lempert SL, Weinberg RJ: Ocular rosacea. In Srinivasan BD (ed): Ocular Therapeutics. Masson, New York, 1980

64. Savin J, Alexander S, Marks R: A rosacea-like eruption of children. Br J Dermatol 87:425, 1972

65. Marks R: Rosacea, flushing and perioral dermatitis. In Champion RH, Burton JL, Floling FJ (eds): Textbook of Dermatology. Blackwell Scientific, London, 1993

66. Brauner GJ: Cutaneous disease in black races. In Moschella SL, Hurley HJ (eds): Dermatology. Saunders, Philadelphia, 1987

67. Borrie P: Rosacea with special reference to its ocular manifestation. Br J Ophthalmol 65:458, 1953

68. Macsai MS, Mannis MJ, Huntley AC: Acne rosacea. In Mannis MJ, Macsai MS, Huntley AC (eds): Eye and Skin Disease. Lippincott–Raven, Philadelphia, 1996

69. Brown SI, Shahinlan L: Diagnosis and treatment of ocular rosacea. Ophthalmology 85:779, 1978

70. Browning DJ, Proia AD: Ocular rosacea. Surv Ophthalmol 31:145, 1986

71. Jenkins MA, Brown SI, Lempert, et al. Ocular rosacea. Am J Ophthalmol 88:618, 1979

72. Frucht-Pery J, et al: The effect of doxycycline on ocular rosacea. Am J Ophthalmol 107:434, 1989

73. Sneddon I: A clinical trial of tetracycline in rosacea. Br J Dermatol 78:649, 1966

74. English FP: Demodicosis. In Fraunfelder FT, Roy FH (eds): Current Ocular Therapy. Saunders, Philadelphia, 1995

75. Edmondson W, Christensen MT: Lid parasites. In Onofrey B (ed): Clinical Optometric Pharmacology and Therapeutics. Lippincott–Raven, Philadelphia, 1992

76. Heacock CE: Clinical manifestations of demodicosis. J Am Optom Assoc 57:914, 1986

77. English FP, Nutting WB: Demodicosis of ophthalmic concern. Am J Ophthalmol 91:362, 1981

78. Sengbusch HG, Hauswifth JW: Prevalence of hair follicle mites: *Demodex folliculorum* and *D. brevis* in a selected human population in western New York. J Med Entomol 23:384, 1986

79. Nutting WD, Beerman H: Demodicosis and symbiophobia: status, terminology, and treatments. Int J Dermatol 22:13, 1983

80. Desch C, Nutting WB: *Demodex folliculorum* and *D. brevis* of man: redescription and re-evaluation. J Parasitol 58:169, 1972

81. Fulk GW, Clifford C: A case report of demodicosis. J Am Optom Assoc 61:637, 1990

82. Couch JM, Green WR, Hirst LW, et al: Diagnosing and treating *Phthirus pubis palpebrum.* Surv Ophthalmol 26:219, 1982

83. Taplin D, Meinking T: Head lice infestation: biology, diagnosis, and management. pp. 1–31. Materia Medica/Creative Annex, New York, 1987

84. Hurwitz S: Insect bites and parasitic infestations. pp. 416. In Clinical Pediatric Dermatology: A Textbook of Skin Disorders of Childhood and Adolescence. Saunders, Philadelphia, 1993

85. Billstein SA, Mattaliano VJ: The "nuisance" sexually transmitted diseases: molluscum contagiosum, scabies, and crab lice. Med Clin North Am 74:1487, 1990

86. Satterfield D: Pediculosis. In Mannis MJ, Macsai MS, Huntley AC (eds): Eye and Skin Disease. Lippincott–Raven: Philadelphia, 1966

87. Efron N: Contact lens–associated eyelash disorders. Optician 216:5658, 1998

88. Kairys DJ, Webster HJ, Terry JE: Pediatric ocular phthiriasis infestation. J Am Optom Assoc 59:128, 1988

89. Elgart ML. Pediculosis. Dermatol Clin 8:219, 1990

90. Caroline,PJ, Kame RT, Hayashida JK, et al: Pediculosis: parasitic infestation in a contact lens wearer. Clin Eye Vision Care 3:82, 1991

10

Keratoconjunctivitis Sicca and Ocular Surface Disease

Leo P. Semes

GRAND ROUNDS CASE REPORT 1

Subjective:
A 52-year-old woman presents for relief of dry eye symptoms. Tear supplements had been used over the past 8–10 years, including drops and ointments. Diagnosis of Sjögren's syndrome was made 4 years ago, with concomitant rheumatoid arthritis. Current symptoms involve constant dryness from time of awakening until bedtime, when symptoms are the worst. The patient currently is using Tears Naturale II and Viva-Drops (Vision Pharmaceuticals, Inc., Mitchell, SD) eight times daily. There was no prior use of contact lenses, and the personal and medical family histories were otherwise unremarkable.

Objective:
- Best acuity: $^{20}/_{30}$ each eye (OU), distance and near.
- Biomicroscopy: corneal desiccation inferiorly, with scantly marginal tear strip. Mild conjunctival hyperemia, along with tear breakup time (TBUT) less than 2 seconds OU. Mild-to-moderate fluorescein staining of the entire bulbar conjunctiva right eye (OD) and mild staining of inferior bulbar conjunctiva left eye (OS); rose bengal staining moderate to severe OU across bulbar conjunctiva and inferiorly on cornea OU.
- Schirmer's test (no. 1) with anesthetic revealed no wetting after 5 minutes.

Assessment:
Keratoconjunctivitis sicca (KCS) with Sjögren's syndrome.

Plan:
Excess use of tear supplements may be contributing to a preservative toxicity effect or medicamentosa. A 2-week course of preservative-free lubricant was prescribed, with follow-up visit scheduled.

Follow-up:
TBUT and rose bengal staining unchanged, but fluorescein staining of conjunctiva is significantly reduced. Schirmer's test with anesthesia was 3 mm in 5 minutes OD and 0 mm in 5 minutes OS.

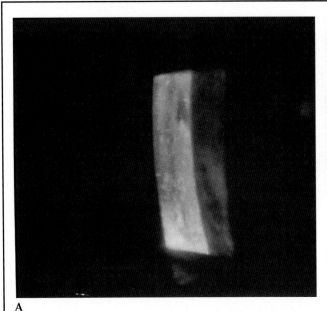

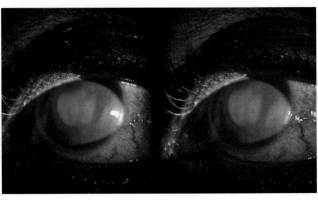

B

FIG. 10-1. *Grand Rounds Case 1.* **A:** *Demonstration of corneal fluorescein staining (erosions) in ocular surface disease secondary to keratoconjunctivitis sicca in a patient with Sjögren's syndrome.* **B:** *Rose bengal staining of exposed bulbar conjunctival surface. (Courtesy of Dr. Joel A. Silbert.)*

A

Comment:
This is a classic case of aqueous deficiency secondary to Sjögren's syndrome. Alternatives to consider in treatment include hypotonic tear supplements, ointment, or possibly saline drops. A regimen of frequent application of nonpreserved tear supplements was chosen for palliative relief and to reduce the medicamentosa effect of solution preservatives (Fig. 10-1).

Keratoconjunctivitis sicca (KCS), or dry eye, may be the most ill defined of all ocular disorders. Some authorities focus on ocular signs to support the diagnosis,[1] and others emphasize patient symptoms.[2-4] In the presence of symptoms, an algorithm to distinguish aqueous tear deficiency from meibomian gland disease has been developed.[5] Ocular surface disease (OSD) may represent a point on the dry eye spectrum combining significant symptoms and distinct ocular signs. A workshop has sought to categorize dry eye based on a consensus classification.[6]

The compartmental concept of tear film layers and concomitant evaluation and management options based on this artificial construct sometimes obscure the dynamic interaction between tear film layers. One theory about OSD begins with decreased osmolarity, leading to surface epithelial cell changes before overt clinical signs become evident.[7] Although specific diagnoses of tear film deficiencies exist and lead the way for management, clinicians may be confronted with patient symptoms in the absence of objective signs.

Not to be overlooked in tear film disorders and complications of contact lens wear are systemic conditions.

Perhaps no single entity figures more prominently than Sjögren's syndrome. This discussion focuses on KCS and ocular surface problems secondary to or masquerading as Sjögren's syndrome.

PRECORNEAL TEAR FILM

The structure, function, and composition of the tear film as well as pertinent diagnostic techniques are discussed in Chapter 1.

TEAR FILM DYNAMICS

During each blink, the lipid layer is compressed and increases its thickness by a factor of 1,000. The classic description of the lipid layer is a monomolecular layer that spreads over the aqueous layer on eyelid opening. Excess lipid disperses, and motion within the lipid layer equilibrates within 1 second of the completed blink.[8]

The aqueous layer remains continuous atop the adsorbed mucin layer and acts to cushion the globe from the lids. Aqueous deficiency, a signature of (but not exclusive to) Sjögren's syndrome, is the most common tear film abnormality when blepharitis (secondary lipid deficiency) is excluded. Although rapid TBUT is consistently observed, it has been suggested that a bare aqueous surface, even in the presence of vital dye staining, is never present.[8]

The implications for KCS can be summarized as follows:

- In mild forms, the mucin layer remains intact, but aqueous or lipid-contaminated aqueous diffracts light, which reduces contrast sensitivity[9] and may decrease visual acuity.
- When mucin is stripped from the surface, nerve endings are exposed and symptoms of discomfort are present commensurate with the area of involvement.
- Contact lens wear can aggravate this ocular surface problem, leading to clinical signs of OSD.
- Lipid-layer polarity alterations, generally associated with chronic blepharitis, may lead to evaporative tear loss and later to nonevaporative KCS.[10]
- Because elevated plasmin levels have been observed in tear deficiencies, some suggest that this increased proteolytic activity may accelerate ocular surface changes.[11]

SJÖGREN'S SYNDROME

Sjögren's syndrome is an autoimmune disease characterized histopathologically by lymphocytic infiltration of glands. Its prevalence worldwide varies between 0.1% and 5% because of inconsistent diagnostic criteria. Females are predominantly affected (up to 9 to 1), and a bimodal onset peak exists between the ages of 20 and 40 and again at approximately 60 years of age.[12] Ocular symptoms are familiar to the clinician and include generalized ocular irritation, contact lens intolerance, mucoid discharge, intolerance of light and smoke, and frequent but futile tear supplement use. Systemic effects include difficulty in swallowing, liquid supplementation required during eating, and fatigue. Clinical signs include arthralgias, enlarged salivary glands, recurrent oral fungal infections, dry mouth, and skin rashes. *Primary Sjögren's syndrome* is the term applied to manifestations of dry eye (KCS) and dry mouth (xerostomia).

Systemic involvement concomitant with this sicca complex has been classified as *secondary Sjögren's syndrome.* The most commonly associated systemic disorder is rheumatoid arthritis, but others implicated include systemic lupus erythematosus, polymyositis, scleroderma,

and biliary cirrhosis. Because of selective lacrimal and salivary gland involvement, the term *autoimmune exocrinopathy* has been suggested as a synonym for Sjögren's syndrome.[13] Reviews have addressed the spectrum as well as the disparity of the disorder.[12-17]

KERATOCONJUNCTIVITIS SICCA

Owing to reduced aqueous volume and concomitant decrease in defensive proteins (lactoferrin, lysozyme, and certain immunoglobulins), the correlation between coexisting lid infection among aqueous-deficient patients and the marked prevalence of blepharitis or conjunctivitis may be causally related. McGill and associates,[18] however, were unable to document any increase in the aqueous levels of lactoferrin or lysozyme in the presence of supervening infection. This finding suggests that the KCS patient is unresponsive or under-responsive to such infection.

Because KCS patients are at greater risk for infection, the patient must be vigilant for signs and symptoms of infection. Management should be aimed at re-establishing normal tear volume and ridding the lids of potential sources of infection. Although such lid disease may be considered *sterile* (the typically cultured organism is *Staphylococcus epidermidis* type IV),[18] treatment measures should be pursued aggressively. Lid margin hygiene consisting of warm compresses and lid scrubs is recommended as a primary measure. When meibomianitis supervenes, as manifested by frothy discharge, systemic tetracycline (250 mg by mouth four times a day) should be considered.[18] Alternatives to the traditional tetracycline regimen include doxycycline (100 mg by mouth twice a day) and erythromycin (50–100 mg by mouth twice a day). The ocular surface should be completely rehabilitated before considering contact lens application.

Among 109 cases of clinically confirmed KCS, there was a statistically significant association between corneal ulceration and the presence of rheumatoid arthritis.[19] This report implicated systemic complications rather than local ocular conditions for the ulcerations. As with any corneal ulcer, immediate and aggressive management is indicated.

TEAR FILM INSTABILITY

Dohlman[20] and Lamberts[21] describe the initiation of the cascade of complications in ocular surface disorders as *tear film instability.* Whether the microepithelial defects begin from an insufficient tear film or vice versa is open to discussion.[8,19] In any case, decreased aqueous volume, as demonstrated clinically by Schirmer's basic secretion test or by more sophisticated means, correlates with reduced ocular surface defenses and increased susceptibility to irritation, allergy, and infection.[21-23] One major consequence of reduced aqueous volume is reduced antibacterial function, as performed normally by lactoferrin and lysozyme.[24]

Smolin and Okumoto[25] have suggested that punctate inferior corneal staining is secondary to toxins produced by staphylococcal organisms. However, McGill and associates[18] were unable to demonstrate an increase in bacterial population among either blepharitis or dry eye patients with infection. This finding led them to conclude that squamous blepharitis is a sterile condition and that the inferior staining pattern evolves from an alteration of the lid–tear film interface. Tears are not retained, the tear volume drops, and intrapalpebral desiccation occurs.[18] This concept is supported by the presence of sicca symptoms with observation of a normal tear film.

Because instability of the tear film may be the keystone for developing ocular surface disorders, management plans may include volume enhancement through tear supplementation. Benzalkonium chloride (BAK) is an effective preservative for many ophthalmic solutions. BAK in commercial concentrations, however, may reduce TBUT.[26] For this reason, clinicians may wish to remind patients with KCS or even marginal dry eye who self-select ophthalmic solutions that BAK should be an acronym for *buy another kind.* Although most clinicians would favor the use of unpreserved lubricating solutions for their dry eye patients, such solutions have been shown to be detrimental to the corneal surface in some animal studies.[27,28]

A more significant consequence associated with an unstable tear film may be manifested as *persistent dry spots.* Brown[26] believes that repeated blinking may alleviate such drying. He also observed that persistent dry spots are associated with abnormalities of the distribution system or reduced tear flow.

SQUAMOUS METAPLASIA

Squamous metaplasia of the conjunctiva may occur secondary to changes in the ocular surface and may be related to environmental exposure.[29] Impression cytology studies suggest abnormal conjunctival epithelium as well as goblet cell alteration[29-31] in OSD. Tseng[31] proposes two possible mechanisms: loss of vascularization, which prevents normal epithelial differentiation, and inflammatory changes that induce epithelial alteration. Mechanical factors in aqueous deficiency among patients with Sjögren's syndrome may set the inflammatory stage for epithelial changes. Elevated cytokines have been demonstrated in

these cases.[32] Barton and associates[33] have reported similar observations in patients with ocular rosacea but did not demonstrate parallel changes in severe atrophic meibomian gland disorders or severe ocular irritation. A typical case of OSD in Sjögren's syndrome is illustrated in Figure 10-1.

MANAGEMENT STRATEGIES FOR KERATOCONJUNCTIVITIS SICCA

Traditional approaches to the effects of ocular surface drying consist of volume-enhancing or contact-enhancing agents. Few, if any, consistent strategies have emerged to guide the clinician in the management of patients with KCS. Individualized treatment programs are often proposed based on the clinician's observations and judgment. One staging system for KCS, based on severity measured by four diagnostic tests, advocates tear supplements up to four times daily and lubricating ointments at bedtime (grade I). Moderate (grade II) KCS would require the addition of sustained-release tear inserts or mucolytic agents. Severe (grade III) disease may be managed with punctal occlusion, bandage contact lenses, estrogen supplementation, or moisture chambers.[34] Contemporary recommendations for grades II and III may include the use of unpreserved cellulose-based polymers. The introduction of transiently preserved tear supplements has added an economic benefit.

Alternative classification schemes have been proposed without specific treatment recommendations.[5,6] Although diagnostic testing or staging schemes can quantify ocular surface disorders, clinicians may remain perplexed when confronted with refractory cases. The following two sections are intended as a menu of treatment options for KCS with the objective of ocular surface rehabilitation.

Tear Conservation

Conservation strategies may include punctal occlusion. Freeman[35] introduced a removable silicone punctum plug in 1974. He reported a 50–75% success rate based on improvement in patients' symptoms. No controls were included in this unmasked clinical trial. Willis and associates[36] objectively evaluated 18 dry eye patients with at least 8 months of follow-up after placing a plug. Decreases in rose bengal and fluorescein staining were observed along with enhanced Schirmer's test values. Significantly, at the 6-week evaluation, no changes in conjunctival impression cytology were observed from baseline. Other studies have shown enhanced hydration or reduced symptoms among contact lens wearers.[37-40] This effect may be short-lived and may not offer relief of cellular level changes.[41]

Benson and associates[42] studied the efficacy of laser occlusion among 22 patients whose puncta were sealed by argon laser an average of 16 months previously. They discovered that 19 of 22 (86%) had become patent, as determined by the primary dye test. Their conclusion was that this method is not effective for long-term punctal occlusion. Local humidity chambers (spectacle lenses with sealing side shields) have been proposed as a conservation measure as well.

Nontraditional Treatment for Keratoconjunctivitis Sicca

Methods other than traditional tear supplementation and conservation have been described. LaMotte and associates[43] found no difference in TBUT between a tear-supplement regimen and continuously supplied hydroxypropyl cellulose (Lacrisert, Merck, Inc., West Point, PA). Leibowitz and associates[44] reported improvement in objective signs (tear prism, fluorescein staining) as well as decreased symptoms in response to a long-lasting gel formulation. Based on a pathogenetic cascade that begins with aqueous evaporation (measured as increased tear osmolarity), Gilbard[45] identifies goblet cell loss, epithelial desquamation, and tear-ocular surface instability. In preclinical studies, TheraTears Advanced Tear Formulation (Advanced Vision Research, Woburn, MA) has been shown to restore conjunctival goblet cells. Experimental formulations, such as 3-isobutyl-1-methylxanthine, may actually stimulate tear production.[45]

Gilbard and Kenyon[46] instilled hypotonic saline solutions to determine their effect on lowering tear osmolarity. The hypo-osmolar effect lasted a maximum of 40 minutes after instillation, but rose bengal staining scores improved.

Subjective and objective improvement have been reported in response to extemporaneously prepared viscoelastic materials.[47-50] These formulations have yet to make their commercial debut.

The promise of systemic agents to enhance tearing has been reported. Bromhexine has been shown to decrease symptoms and to improve objective dry eye signs in the treatment of Sjögren's syndrome.[51,52] Oral cholinergic agents have been applied for tear stimulation. Oral pilocarpine (Salagen, 5-mg tablets) three times a day may be an alternative for patients with Sjögren's syndrome.[53] Excessive sweating is the most annoying and prevalent side effect.

Since the initial reports of a retinoid ointment in managing severe ocular surface disorders, much attention has been focused on the use of vitamin A and its structural relatives in the treatment of dry eye states. Tseng and

associates[54] studied 22 selected patients with severe dry eyes. They administered 0.01% or 0.1% all-*trans* retinoic acid in ointment form and observed clinical improvement in symptoms, visual acuity, rose bengal staining, and Schirmer's tests. In addition, reversal of squamous metaplasia was documented by impression cytology studies. They hailed their results as the first nonsurgical attempt to reverse diseased ocular surface epithelium. The postulated mechanism was increased circulation at the conjunctival level.

Soong and associates[55] found reversal of conjunctival keratinization using similar compounds but reported little benefit in KCS. Gilbard and associates[56] confirmed these results by determining that 0.01% vitamin A ointment was no more effective than placebo in increasing tear secretion, as indicated by Schirmer's test (basic secretion test); tear osmolarity; or in decreasing OSD (as shown by no changes in rose bengal score). Significantly, of the 11 patients followed, seven preferred placebo treatment, two expressed a preference for vitamin A ointment, and the remaining two offered no preference. In another study, refractory dry eye patients showed increased goblet cell counts in response to topical retinol palmitate over a 4-week dosing period.[57]

An immunologic approach to lacrimal gland dysfunction has been suggested from animal studies. Topical cyclosporine enhanced tear flow among a group of beagles serving as the animal model for KCS.[58] The therapeutic risk-benefit ratio was promising enough to initiate clinical trials on humans. Cyclosporine (0.1%) ophthalmic emulsion showed objective improvement in a group of 133 patients who completed a 12-week, placebo-controlled treatment trial.[59]

Topical fibronectin, an adhesive glycoprotein, was evaluated with artificial tears for the treatment of KCS. A controlled, double-masked clinical trial, comprising 272 patients who were followed for more than 2 months, did not demonstrate any statistically significant differences in improvement compared with placebo as measured by self-evaluation of symptoms, rose bengal and fluorescein staining, TBUT, Schirmer's testing, and conjunctival impression cytology.[60]

A gastric mucosa protectant, sodium sucrose sulfate (sucralfate), was tried on a group of 22 patients with primary Sjögren's syndrome. Over a 6-month treatment period, statistically significant improvement in rose bengal scores was demonstrated.[61] Although no controls were used in this study, sucralfate may show promise as a new adsorptive agent for the compromised ocular surface.

An exciting frontier in the treatment of severe KCS is limbal stem-cell transplantation. Allografts appear to have advantages over limbal autografts in presumed (i.e., acquired) stem-cell deficiency.[62] Guidelines for application of this surgical technique continue to evolve.[63] Any discussion of KCS necessarily focuses on aqueous deficiency. So often, however, the term *KCS* is tangentially applied to generalized tear film disorders. Brief mention must be made of significant deficiencies of other tear film components before discussion of contact lens complications arising from these ocular surface disorders.

MUCIN DEFICIENCY

True mucin deficiency is rare; one report estimates prevalence at 1:20,000.[64] Loss of goblet cells is a complication associated with inflammatory injuries to the conjunctiva or a side effect of prolonged topical therapies.[65,66]

In ocular cicatricial pemphigoid (OCP), erythema multiforme, and the Stevens-Johnson syndrome, goblet cell loss results from an autoimmune response that deposits immunoglobulins and complement at the basement membrane zone of the conjunctiva.[67] The progressive clinical picture includes bullae at the subepithelial level, conjunctival shortening, and symblepharon formation.[68] OCP that was initially treated as KCS is illustrated in Grand Rounds Case Report 2.

Drug-induced OCP can be potentiated by protracted use of topical antiglaucoma medication, such as echothiophate iodide, pilocarpine, epinephrine,[66] or timolol.[65,66] It is speculated that these patients may be predisposed to OCP and that these topical ophthalmic antiglaucoma medications merely hasten the cicatrizing process.[65] Milder forms of mucin deficiency may result in an unstable tear film or, as Lemp theorizes, mucin deficiency may be the basis for dellen formation.[69,70] In disorders of the mucous membranes with conjunctival shortening secondary to cicatrization, topical steroids may be beneficial.[65] Mondino[68] cites the potential for recurrent corneal erosion among patients with OCP. As with other erosive disorders, soft contact lenses may be used judiciously in the management of recurrent corneal erosion.[68,71] Conversely, large-diameter soft contact lenses may not be accommodated within scarred conjunctival fornices. Development

---

GRAND ROUNDS CASE REPORT 2

Subjective:
A 74-year-old man presented for routine examination. The patient admitted to no medications other than oral vitamins. There was a history of allergies to mold, dust, mildew, and tobacco. The remainder of the personal medical and familial history was unremarkable.

Objective:
- Best corrected acuity: OD 20/20-2 and OS 20/25+2
- TBUT more than 10 seconds OU
- Biomicroscopy: mild nuclear sclerosis
- Dilated funduscopy unremarkable OU

Assessment:
Healthy ocular status

Plan:
1. Prescription written for bifocals
2. Re-evaluation in 18 months

Follow-up:
At this visit, the patient complained of slight reduction in distance acuity and a nonspecific ocular itching, with watery discharge and mattering on awakening. Acuity was now 20/25 OU; TBUT was 5 seconds OU. No fluorescein staining OU. Balance of examination unchanged.

Assessment: Symptomatic dry eye

Plan: Palliative therapy of Duratears (Alcon Laboratories, Inc., Fort Worth, TX) ointment, and Tears Naturale II (Alcon Laboratories, Inc., Fort Worth, TX) during the day as needed. Reassess in 2 weeks.

At second follow-up, itching and redness associated with administration of eye drops; morning mattering continued. TBUT 2 seconds OD, 10 seconds OS. Moderate conjunctival hyperemia OU.

Assessment: Dry eye syndrome with possible allergic response to preservative in tear supplement.

Plan: Continue ointment, use nonpreserved tear supplement as needed.

Three months later, the patient returned with a unilateral red right eye with mucous discharge and mattering on awakening. Acuity was now OD $^{20}/_{40}$, OS $^{20}/_{30}$, TBUT 5 seconds OU. In addition, symblepharon formation was observed and was refractory to manipulation.

Assessment: Based on history of dry eye and presence of symblepharon, tentative diagnosis of early OCP was made.

Plan: A regimen of vitamin A drops was applied every 2 hours along with an oral supplement of vitamin A (10,000 IU by mouth).

Over the next 3 months, the patient's condition appeared to remain stationary. Conjunctival injection diminished. Based on immunofluorescent studies, the diagnosis of pemphigoid was confirmed. The patient was started on a regimen of 5 mg prednisone on alternate days.

During the next 2 months, the condition remained stable, with TBUT 5–6 seconds OU and some fluorescein corneal staining observed OD inferiorly. The patient remained on the vitamin A regimen (oral and topical) along with the prednisone. A trial of collagen plugs decreased symptoms, and silicone plugs were implanted into each inferior punctum.

During the next year, the patient was treated elsewhere for pemphigoid with an immunosuppressant agent. This trial produced fever, requiring hospitalization.

At his most recent follow-up visit, the patient complained of decreased vision OD. Dry eye symptoms remained under control using the regimen described. Visual acuity was OD $^{20}/_{200}$, OS $^{20}/_{40}$. Applanation tensions were 15 mm Hg OU. Nuclear sclerosis and posterior subcapsular cataracts were observed and were consistent with the reduced vision. Laser interferometry demonstrated the capability of $^{20}/_{40}$ OU. The patient was asked to continue his medication regimen and was sent to consultation for cataract surgery (Fig. 10-2).

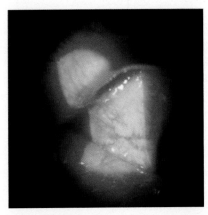

FIG. 10-2. *Grand Rounds Case 2. Symblepharon formation in a patient with ocular pemphigoid.*

Anterior Segment Complications of Contact Lens Wear

of highly oxygen-permeable scleral contact lenses may offer still another option for severe cases of KCS secondary to mucin deficiency.[72-75] Because of the increased risk of infection, mucosal scarring disorders may respond better to limited and indicated use of topical antibiotics rather than prophylaxis.[71]

Sullivan and associates[76] offered two cases that illustrate the return of goblet cells after vitamin A therapy. Both alcoholic patients in this series were placed on a 3-week daily regimen of 25,000 IU of oral vitamin A (form not reported). Improvement in goblet cell count, conjunctival appearance, and decreased keratinization were observed.

Tseng and associates[54,77] have advocated the topical application of a vitamin A analog (tretinoin) for treatment of advanced dry eye conditions, including severe xerosis and squamous metaplasia. Singer et al.[78] reported a single case of regeneration of goblet cells after 3 months of vitamin A therapy (45,000 IU/day, by mouth) in a 9-year-old boy with Stevens-Johnson syndrome. A larger series of refractory patients has been reported to respond to topical application of retinol palmitate with increased goblet cell counts.[57] The role of vitamin A in treating abnormalities of the ocular surface offers intriguing possibilities. Severe forms of OSD may respond to 0.1% topical retinoid ointment.[54] Clinical methodologies have not been reproduced and do not have control groups.[54-57] The varying dosage forms of vitamin A (ointment, drops, and oral supplementation), however, complicates any comparison. Oral supplementation may eventually constitute the treatment of choice.

Although no specific treatment seems to exist for the conjunctival consequences of mucin deficiencies, aside from palliative treatment, the response to immunosuppressive therapy appears promising.[66,67,76] Contact lens wear has a guarded prognosis among these patients.

LIPID DEFICIENCY

Isolated lipid deficiency is even less prevalent than mucin deficiency. Yet, when initiated by blepharitis or meibomian gland dysfunction, lipid deficiency may produce symptoms or clinical signs at the ocular surface that are indistinguishable from aqueous-induced KCS. Complete absence of meibomian secretions has been described in congenital ectodermal dysplasia.[8] Such patients are extremely poor candidates for contact lenses.

The altered polarity of cutaneous sebum disrupts the oily layer of the tear film and prematurely contaminates the aqueous layer.[8] This reduces TBUT and may initiate dry eye symptoms in chronic blepharitis.[79,80] Others

propose a dermatologic classification of blepharitis without focus on the ocular surface complications.[81] Management often requires a multifocal approach and should be considered before proceeding with or resuming contact lens wear.[81,82]

RELATIONSHIP OF KERATOCONJUNCTIVITIS SICCA TO CONTACT LENS WEAR

Evidence has been mounting for more than two decades that tear deficiencies may produce cellular changes of the ocular surface. Specifically, aqueous tear deficiency, as seen in Sjögren's syndrome, may lead to stratification of conjunctival epithelial cells.[4,31,45] The term applied to cellular level changes and the concomitant clinical observation of superficial epithelial punctate erosion is *OSD*. More advanced cases may manifest coarse mucus plaques or corneal alterations, such as the presence of filaments.[83] The exposed ocular surface and the palpebral conjunctiva are susceptible to tear deficiencies.

Because of their dynamic interaction with and dependence on the tear film, ocular surface cells (epithelial cells of the palpebral and bulbar conjunctiva as well as the cornea) may experience adverse effects in tear-deficiency states. As a corollary to aqueous deficiency in KCS, Lemp and colleagues[84] demonstrated a statistically significant association between ocular rosacea and deficient tearing. The presence of rosacea is a potential contraindication to successful contact lens wear.

To achieve patient comfort and to improve the success rate among soft contact lens wearers with mild KCS, Lemp[83] mandates tear supplementation. Although symptomatic relief in such patients may be achieved subjectively, the mechanism and the objective improvement in clinical signs remain obscure.[85] In another study, the investigators determined that TBUT could be prolonged with the use of rewetting drops but that the effect persisted for fewer than 5 minutes.[86] Fitting contact lenses in patients with significant ocular surface compromise should be approached cautiously.

Grand Rounds Case Report 3 illustrates a case in which temporary collagen and permanent silicone punctal implants were used in a hydrogel lens wearer with KCS. Punctal occlusion may play a supplemental role with other treatments in severe KCS cases.

Certain immunologic components of tears may influence the deposition of proteins on hydrogel contact lenses.[87-89] Deficiency of these components may accelerate protein deposition, which may occur as quickly as during the first minute of lens wear.[88] Because the ability

GRAND ROUNDS CASE REPORT 3

Subjective:

A 35-year-old man was successfully fitted with extended-wear soft lenses (weekly renewal) for myopia. He took no medication, admitted to no allergies, and had noncontributory medical and familial histories.

Objective:

- Best corrected acuities: $^{20}/_{20}$ OU, distance and near
- Biomicroscopy: Unremarkable during the fitting period and throughout the 3 months of postfitting follow-up

After 6 months of wear, the patient continued to observe a less comfortable right eye despite the use of enzymes, surfactants, and lubricating drops. No signs of corneal staining or diminished tear prism were observed. There were no signs of corneal hypoxia, although three to five epithelial microcysts were observed OU. The lenses were clean and demonstrated no defects.

Assessment:

Despite a good physiologic fit and good vision with extended-wear lenses, this patient described symptoms consistent with a dry eye. Although no specific form of tear film deficiency was shown, conservation of existing tears appeared to be an appropriate alternative for this minimal sicca case.

Plan:

A trial of dissolvable collagen implants inserted into the lower right punctum was performed. One week later, a removable silicone plug (Freeman type, Eagle Vision, Memphis, TN) was placed under topical anesthesia into the lower right punctum without incident. At a follow-up visit 1 week later, the plug remained in place and was well tolerated.

Follow-up:

The plug in the lower right punctum remained in place and was well tolerated for 2 years after initial placement. At that time, the patient described symptoms consistent with dry eye in the left eye. A second Freeman plug was placed into the lower left punctum.

Subsequently, the patient began monovision wear and now wears the lenses on a daily-wear basis. On his most recent follow-up visits (3 and 5 years after insertion of the silicone punctal plugs), the plugs are well tolerated and the patient remains asymptomatic (Fig. 10-3).

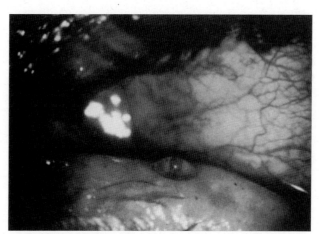

FIG. 10-3. *Grand Rounds Case 3. Freeman silicone punctal plug implanted in the inferior punctum.*

to measure these parameters eclipses our capacity to alter them, contact lens practitioners should be reminded that success rates are higher among patients with healthy and adequate tear films. An additional predictor of success among prospective contact lens wearers may be the pH of the ocular surface and tear film. Andres and associates[90] showed that ocular surface pH decreased with contact lens wear, was lower in environments acidified by SO_2, and was lower among patients with dry eye. In addition to other data gathered during the prefitting examination, these authors recommended a measurement of ocular surface pH. They further recommended the application of tear supplementation to counter any alteration in postfitting pH to enhance contact lens tolerance.

TABLE 10-1. *Concerns and Precautions in Contact Lens Fitting and Wear**

Tear film disorders
   Tear breakup time < 10 seconds
   Aqueous deficiency
   Lipid deficiency (as manifested by meibomian dysfunction
      or concomitant with blepharitis or ocular rosacea)
   Mucus deficiency
Ocular surface abnormalities
   Dellen, pterygia
   Conjunctival epithelial squamous metaplasia
   Blink or lid disorders
Nonocular factors
   Chronic use of preserved topical ocular medications
   Diagnosis of Sjögren's syndrome
   Certain systemic and topical medications (see text)

*Because not all factors may carry equal weight for each clinical situation, the practitioner is encouraged to exercise professional privilege in applying these guidelines.

Meibomian gland secretions contribute to the oily layer of the precorneal tear film. Henriquez and Korb[91] described a syndrome among contact lens wearers consisting of symptoms of ocular dryness, contact lens intolerance, and corneal fluorescein staining characterized by deficient or inadequate meibomian gland secretion. They and others have recommended hot compresses as initial treatment. Paugh and associates[92] demonstrated improved TBUT among 21 users of daily-wear soft contact lens using therapy consisting of hot compresses and lid scrubs. More severe cases require adjunctive antibiotic therapy.

More than 25 years ago, Mackie[93] identified abnormal blinking among rigid contact lens wearers as the major etiologic factor in ocular surface desiccation, with subsequent dellen and pterygium formation. Later, Farris[94] introduced evidence implicating contact lens wear as a cause of dry eye. He emphasized reduced tear osmolarity as the potential mechanism responsible for disruption of tear film (from any tear deficiency) and deposits on contact lenses. Recommendations for contact lens wearers with induced tear abnormalities, therefore, include humidity control, application of tear supplements, lid hygiene, and the use of nonpreserved ocular solutions.[94]

Prefitting Recommendations

A careful history is essential before any physical findings are collected. Questionnaires have proved useful for identifying KCS. Not to be overlooked is the influence of medications on the tear film. Systemic medications may unfavorably alter the delicate equilibrium of tear flow and tear film stability. The antimuscarinic effects of tropine

derivatives and antihistamines are well known to reduce tear flow. In addition, sedatives, nasal decongestants, antitussives, analgesics, antidiarrheals, β-adrenergic blockers, and tricyclic antidepressants have the potential to diminish tear flow.[95] Patients taking these medications should either be discouraged from contact lens wear or at least alerted to the drying effects and be prepared for frequent tear supplementation. Medications known to increase tear flow include those with cholinergic effects. Pilocarpine and the anticholinesterase group are most prominent.[95] Increased tear flow may influence the fit as well as hydration of contact lenses. (Table 10-1 lists the potential concerns when considering fitting contact lenses on patients with dry eye or OSD.)

Andres and associates[96] determined that a TBUT greater than 10 seconds was compatible with tolerable contact lens wear. This simple clinical test, perhaps combined with pH measurement, may be useful in predicting successful contact lens wear until more sophisticated techniques, such as tear osmolarity measurements and impression cytology, become routine office procedures.

A procedure for office practice that may have potential for early recognition of OSD among contact lens patients is conjunctival impression cytology.[29] One study investigated the conjunctival epithelial surface of established (greater than 5 years of wear) asymptomatic hydrogel lens wearers.[97] All 14 patients studied showed squamous metaplasia and abnormalities of epithelial nuclei. These surface and cell changes are similar to early changes in the ocular surface of dry eye patients. What appears to be unique to the contact lens group is that discontinuing lens wear reversed the conjunctival epithelial surface changes in selected cases. The mechanism of reversible surface changes appears to be chronic mechanical irritation produced by the hydrogel lens.[97] If one accepts the hypothesis of mechanical irritation, increased friction owing to tear film deficiency of any type may be an initial step in ocular surface changes at the cellular level.

Treatment of an unstable tear film before contact lens fitting may begin with tear supplementation. The major caveats against preserved tear supplements include disruption of tear film stability, increased corneal permeability, and epithelial cell cytotoxicity. Evidence favoring preservative-free tear supplements continues to mount.[27-30,98,99]

It is also important to consider whether dry eye contact lens wearers are at risk for further complications of the ocular surface. Although Finnemore[100] and Lemp[101] appear to disagree on the answer to this question, a common ground between them suggests identifying and treating prefitting problems and managing potential complications aggressively. In a worst-case

TABLE 10-2. *Potential Applications for Bandage Soft Contact Lenses in Abnormalities and Disorders of the Corneal Epithelium*

Filamentary keratitis in keratoconjunctivitis sicca
Selected mucin-deficient dry eye states
Mild degrees of exposure keratitis
Recurrent cornea erosion
Herpes simplex viral keratitis with persistent defects
Thygeson's keratitis
Corneal thinning
Endotheliopathies
Drug delivery

situation, dry eye states may represent a relative contraindication to contact lens wear.

Bandage lenses may prove useful in a number of clinical conditions affecting the ocular surface (Table 10-2). As expected, this management strategy is not without drawbacks.[83,102,103] The most common complication of bandage lenses in dry eye states is the development of surface deposits on the lenses; they are more prevalent among dry eye patients than in healthy subjects.[83] A more significant complication is the risk of infection. Stagnation of tears may lead to accumulation of metabolic waste products, with an avalanche of hypoxic changes of the corneal epithelial surface. When tear lysozyme or lactoferrin is reduced or when blepharitis is coincident, the risk of infection increases. A complication intermediate between these extremes is that of sterile infiltrates.[102] For these reasons, the regular frequent aggressive management strategy suggested by Finnemore[100] makes good clinical sense. See Chapter 21 for specifics on bandage lens therapy.

In patients with moderate-to-severe dry eyes, contemporary commercial tear supplements obviously have a role. Donshik and associates[104] have reported on the efficacy of a group of these products. Using outcome determinants of rose bengal staining scores and impression cytology, they concluded that all solutions tested improved patient comfort, with BION Tears (Alcon Laboratories, Inc., Fort Worth, TX) the greatest symptomatic relief. Solutions of Refresh Tears (Allergan, Inc., Irvine, CA) and BION Tears significantly reduced rose bengal staining scores and improved impression cytology. It should be kept in mind that the U.S. Food and Drug Administration has not approved any of these solutions specifically for application with contact lenses.

REFERENCES

1. Baum J: Clinical manifestations of dry eye states. Trans Ophthalmol Soc U K 104:415, 1995
2. McMonnies CW: Key questions in a dry eye history. J Am Optom Assoc 57:512, 1986
3. McMonnies CW: Responses to a dry eye questionnaire for a normal population. J Am Optom Assoc 58:588, 1987
4. Rubin MR: Egg white in the treatment of keratoconjunctivitis sicca. EENT Monthly 34:50, 1955
5. Pflugfelder SC, Tseng SCG, Sanabria O, et al: Evaluation of subjective assessments and objective diagnostic tests for diagnosing tear-film disorders known to cause ocular irritation. Cornea 17:38, 1998.
6. Lemp MA: Report of the National Eye Institute/industry workshop on clinical trials in dry eyes. CLAO J 21:221, 1995
7. Gilbard JP: Dry eye: pharmacological approaches, effects, and progress. CLAO J 22:141, 1996
8. Holly FJ: Tear film physiology. Int Ophthalmol Clin 27:2, 1987
9. Rolando M, Iester M, Macri A, Calabria G: Low spatial-contrast sensitivity in dry eyes. Cornea 17:376, 1998
10. Shine WD, McCulley JP: Keratoconjunctivitis sicca associated with meibomian secretion polar lipid abnormality. Arch Ophthalmol 116:848, 1998
11. Virtanen T, Konttinen Y, Honkanen N, et al: Tear fluid plasmin activity of dry eye patients with Sjögren's syndrome. Acta Ophthalmol Scand 75:137, 1997
12. Fox RI: Sjögren's syndrome. Controversies and progress. Clin Lab Med 17:431, 1997
13. Talal N: Overview of Sjögren's syndrome. J Dent Res (special issue)66:672, 1987
14. Roberts DK: Keratoconjunctivitis sicca. J Am Optom Assoc 62:187, 1991
15. Friedlaender MH: Ocular manifestations of Sjögren's syndrome: keratoconjunctivitis sicca. Rheum Dis Clin North Am 18:591, 1972
16. Fox RI: Systemic diseases associated with dry eye. Int Ophthalmol Clin 34:71, 1994
17. Fox RI: Clinical features, pathogenesis, and treatment of Sjögren's syndrome. Curr Opin Rheumatol 8:438, 1996
18. McGill J, Laikos G, Seal D, et al: Tear film changes in health and dry eye conditions. Trans Ophthalmol Soc U K 103:313, 1983
19. Hemady R, Chu W, Foster SC: Keratoconjunctivitis and corneal ulcers. Cornea 9:170, 1990
20. Dohlman CH: New concepts of ocular xerosis. Trans Ophthalmol Soc U K 41:105, 1971
21. Lamberts DW: Dry eye and tear deficiency. Int Ophthalmol Clin 23:123, 1983
22. Norn M: The effect of drops on tear flow. Trans Ophthalmol Soc U K 104:410, 1985
23. Thoft RA: Relationship of the dry eye to ocular surface disease. Trans Ophthalmol Soc U K 104:452, 1985
24. Bron AJ, Seal DV: The defences of the ocular surface. Trans Ophthalmol Soc U K 105:18, 1986
25. Smolin G, Okumoto M: Staphylococcus blepharitis. Arch Ophthalmol 95:812, 1977
26. Brown SI: Dry spots and corneal erosions. Int Ophthalmol Clin 13:149, 1973

27. Bernal DL, Ubels JL: Quantitative evaluation of the corneal epithelial barrier: effect of artificial tears and preservatives. Curr Eye Res 10:645, 1991

28. Adams J, Wilcox M, Trousdale MD, et al: Morphologic and physiologic effects of artificial tear formulations on corneal epithelial derived cells. Cornea 11:234, 1992

29. Nelson JD, Havener VR, Cameron JD: Cellulose acetate impressions of the ocular surface. Dry eye states. Arch Ophthalmol 101:1869, 1983

30. Nelson JD, Wright JC: Conjunctival goblet cell densities in ocular surface disease. Arch Ophthalmol 102:1049, 1984

31. Tseng SCG: Staging of conjunctival squamous metaplasia by impression cytology. Ophthalmology 92:728, 1985

32. Jones DT, Monroy D, Ji Z, Pflugfelder SC: Alterations of ocular surface gene expression in Sjogren's syndrome. Adv Exp Med Biol 438:533, 1998

33. Barton K, Nava A, Monroy DC, Pflugfelder SC: Cytokines and tear function in ocular surface disease. Adv Exp Med Biol 438:461, 1998

34. Lemp MA: General measures in management of the dry eye. Int Ophthalmol Clin 27:36, 1987

35. Freeman JM: The punctum plug: evaluation of a new treatment for dry eye. Trans Ophthalmol Soc U K 79:874, 1975

36. Willis RM, Folberg R, Krachmer JH, et al: The treatment of aqueous-deficient dry eye with removable punctal plugs. A clinical and impression-cytology study. Ophthalmology 94:514, 1987

37. Lowther GE, Semes L: Effect of absorbable intracanalicular collagen implants in hydrogel contact lens patients with the symptom of dryness. Int Contact Lens Clin 22(11,12):238, 1992

38. Pearce EI, Tomlinson A, Craig JP, Lowther GE: Tear protein levels following punctal plugging. p. 669. In WR Sullivan et al. (eds): Lacrimal Gland, Tear Film, and Dry Eye Syndromes 2. Plenum, New York, 1998

39. Tomlinson A, Craig JP, Lowther GE: The biophysical role in tear regulation. p. 381. In WR Sullivan et al. (eds): Lacrimal Gland, Tear Film, and Dry Eye Syndromes 2. Plenum, New York, 1998

40. Slusser TG, Lowther GE: Effect of lacrimal drainage occlusion with nondissolvable intracanalicular plugs on hydrogel contact lens wear. Optom Vis Sci 75:330, 1998

41. Virtanen T, Houtari K, Harkonen M, Tervo T: Lacrimal plugs as a therapy for contact lens intolerance. Eye 10:727, 1996

42. Benson DR, Hemady PB, Snyder RW: Efficacy of laser punctal occlusion. Ophthalmology 99:618, 1992

43. LaMotte J, Grossman E, Hersch J: The efficacy of cellulosic ophthalmic inserts for treatment of dry eye. J Am Optom Assoc 56:198, 1985

44. Leibowitz HM, Chang RK, Mandell AI: Gel tears. A new medication for the treatment of dry eyes. Ophthalmology 91:1204, 1984

45. Gilbard JP: Dry eye: pharmacological approaches, effects, and progress. CLAO J 22:141, 1996

46. Gilbard JP, Kenyon KR: Tear diluents in the treatment of keratoconjunctivitis sicca. Ophthalmology 92:646, 1985

47. DeLuise VP, Peterson WS: The use of topical Healon tears in the management of refractory dry-eye syndrome. Ann Ophthalmol 16:823, 1984

48. Limberg MB, McCaa C, Kissling GE, Kaufman HE: Topical application of hyaluronic acid and chondroitin sulfate in the treatment of dry eyes. Am J Ophthalmol 103:194, 1987

49. Nelson JD, Farris RL: Sodium hyaluronate and polyvinyl alcohol artificial tear preparations. A comparison in patients with keratoconjunctivitis sicca. Arch Ophthalmol 106:484, 1988

50. Sand BB, Marner K, Norn MS: Sodium hyaluronate in the treatment of keratoconjunctivitis sicca. Acta Ophthalmol 67:181, 1989

51. Avisar R, Savir H, Machtey I, et al: Clinical trial of bromhexine in Sjogren's syndrome. Ann Ophthalmol 13:971, 1981

52. Kriegbaum NJ, von Linstow M, Oxholm P, Prause JU: Keratoconjunctivitis sicca in patients with primary Sjogren's syndrome. A longitudinal study of ocular parameters. Acta Ophthalmol 66:481, 1988

53. Nelson JD, Friedlaender M, Yeatts RP, et al: Oral pilocarpine for symptomatic relief of keratoconjunctivitis sicca in patients with Sjogren's syndrome. p. 979. In WR Sullivan et al. (eds): Lacrimal Gland, Tear Film, and Dry Eye Syndromes 2. Plenum, New York, 1998

54. Tseng SCG, Maumenee AE, Stark WJ, et al: Topical retinoid treatment for various dry-eye disorders. Ophthalmology 92:717, 1995

55. Soong HK, Martin NF, Wagoner MD, et al: Topical retinoid therapy for squamous metaplasia of various ocular surface disorders. A multicenter, placebo-controlled double-masked study. Ophthalmology 95:1442, 1988

56. Gilbard JP, Huang AJ, Belldegrun R, et al: Open-label crossover study of vitamin A ointment as a treatment for keratoconjunctivitis sicca. Ophthalmology 96:244, 1989

57. Kobayashi TK, Tsubota K, Takamura E, et al: Effect of retinal palmitate as a treatment for dry eye: a cytological evaluation. Ophthalmologica 211:358, 1997

58. Kaswan RL, Salisbury M-A, Ward DA: Spontaneous canine keratoconjunctivitis sicca. A useful model for human keratoconjunctivitis sicca: treatment with cyclosporine eye drops. Arch Ophthalmol 107:1210, 1989

59. Tauber J: A dose-ranging clinical trial to assess the safety and efficacy of cyclosporine ophthalmic emulsion in patients with keratoconjunctivitis sicca. p. 969. In WR Sullivan et al. (eds): Lacrimal Gland, Tear Film, and Dry Eye Syndromes 2. Plenum, New York, 1998

60. Nelson JD, Gordon JF, the Chiron Keratoconjunctivitis Sicca Study Group: Topical fibronectin in the treatment of keratoconjunctivitis sicca. Am J Ophthalmol 114:441, 1992

61. Prause JU: Beneficial effect of sodium sucrose-sulfate on the ocular surface of patient with severe KCS in primary Sjogren's syndrome. Acta Ophthalmol 69:417,1991

62. Tan DT, Ficker LA, Buckley RJ: Limbal transplantation. Ophthalmology 103:29, 1996

63. Holland JE: Epithelial transplantation for the management of severe ocular surface disease. Trans Am Ophthalmol Soc 94:677, 1996

64. Beyer CK: The management of special problems associated with Stevens-Johnson syndrome and ocular pemphigoid. Trans Am Acad Ophthalmol Otolaryngol 83:701, 1977

65. Fiore PM, Jacobs IH, Goldberg DB: Drug induced pemphigoid. A spectrum of diseases. Arch Ophthalmol 105:1660, 1987

66. Pouliquen Y, Patey A, Foster CS, et al: Drug-induced cicatricial pemphigoid affecting the conjunctiva. Light and electron microscopic features. Ophthalmology 93:775, 1986

67. Chan LS, Soong HK, Foster CS, et al: Ocular cicatricial pemphigoid occurring as a sequela of Stevens-Johnson syndrome. JAMA 266:1543, 1991

68. Mondino B: Cicatricial pemphigoid and erythema multiforme. Ophthalmology 97:939, 1990

69. Lemp MA, Hammill JR: Factors affecting tear film breakup in normal eyes. Arch Ophthalmol 89:103, 1973

70. Lemp MA: The mucin-deficient dry eye. Int Ophthalmol Clin 13:195, 1973

71. Ormerod LD, Fong LP, Foster CS: Corneal infection in mucosal scarring disorders and Sjögren's syndrome. Am J Ophthalmol 105:512, 1988

72. Pullum KW, Buckley RJ: A study of 530 patients referred for rigid gas permeable scleral contact lens assessment. Cornea 16:612, 1997

73. Cotter JM, Rosenthal P: Scleral contact lenses. J Am Optom Assoc 69:33, 1998

74. Bennett HG, Hay J, Kiekness, et al: Antimicrobial management of presumed microbial keratitis: guidelines for treatment of central and peripheral ulcers. Br J Ophthalmol 82:137, 1998

75. Alongi S, Rolando M, Marci A, et.al. Bacterial load and protein deposits on 15-day versus 1-day disposable hydrophilic contact lenses. Cornea 17:146, 1998

76. Sullivan WR, McCulley JP, Dohlman CH: Return of goblet cells after vitamin A therapy in xerosis of the conjunctiva. Am J Ophthalmol 75:720, 1973

77. Tseng SCG: Topical tretinoin treatment for dry-eye disorders. Int Ophthalmol Clin 27:47, 1987

78. Singer L, Brook U, Romem M, Fried D: Vitamin A in Stevens-Johnson syndrome. Ann Ophthalmol 21:209, 1989

79. McCulley JP, Sciallis GF: Meibomian keratoconjunctivitis. Am J Ophthalmol 84:788, 1977

80. McCulley JP, Sciallis GF: Meibomian keratoconjunctivitis: oculodermal correlates. Contact Intraocul Lens Med J 9:130, 1983

81. Huber-Spitzy V, Baumgartner I, Bohler-Sommeregger K, Grabner G: Blepharitis—a diagnostic and therapeutic challenge. Graefes Arch Clin Exp Ophthalmol 229:224, 1991

82. Bowman RW, Dougherty JM, McCulley JP: Chronic blepharitis and dry eyes. Int Ophthalmol Clin 27:27, 1987

83. Lemp MA: Contact lenses and the dry-eye patient. Int Ophthalmol Clin 26:63, 1986

84. Lemp MA, Mahmood M, Weiler HH: The association of rosacea and keratoconjunctivitis sicca. Arch Ophthalmol 102:556, 1984

85. Efron N, Golding TR, Brennan NA: The effect of soft lens lubricants on symptoms and lens dehydration. CLAO J 17:114, 1991

86. Golding TR, Efron N, Brennan NA: Soft lens lubricants and prelens tear film stability. Optom Vis Sci 67:461, 1990

87. Boot N, Kok J, Kijlstra A: The role of tears in preventing protein deposition on contact lenses. Curr Eye Res 8:185, 1989

88. Leahy CD, Mandell RB, Lin ST: Initial *in vivo* tear protein deposition on individual hydrogel contact lenses. Optom Vis Sci 67:504, 1990

89. Lin ST, Mandell RB, Leahy CD, Newell JO: Protein accumulation on disposable extended wear lenses. CLAO J 17:44, 1991

90. Andres A, Garcia ML, Espina M, et al: Tear pH, air pollution, and contact lenses. Optom Vis Sci 65:627, 1988

91. Henriquez AS, Korb DR: Meibomian glands and contact lens wear. Br J Ophthalmol 65:108, 1981

92. Paugh JR, Knapp LL, Martinson JR, Hom MM: Meibomian therapy in problematic contact lens wear. Optom Vis Sci 67:803, 1990

93. Mackie IA: Localized corneal drying in association with dellen, pterygia and related lesions. Trans Ophthalmol Soc UK 41:129, 1971

94. Farris RL: The dry eye: its mechanisms and therapy, with evidence that contact lens is a cause. CLAO J 12:234, 1986

95. Farris RL: Tear analysis in contact lens wearers. Trans Am Ophthalmol Soc 83:501, 1985

96. Andres S, Henriquez A, Garcia ML, et al: Factors of the precorneal tear film break-up time (TBUT) and tolerance of contact lenses. Int Contact Lens Clin 14:103, 1987

97. Knop E, Brewitt H: Conjunctival cytology in asymptomatic wearers of soft contact lenses. Graefes Arch Clin Exp Ophthalmol 230:340, 1992

98. Caffery BE, Josephson JE: Is there a better "comfort drop"? J Am Optom Assoc 61:178, 1990

99. Ichijima H, Petroll WM, Jester JV, Cavanagh HD: Confocal microscopic studies of living rabbit cornea treated with benzalkonium chloride. Cornea 11:221, 1992

100. Finnemore VM: Is the dry eye contact lens wearer at risk? Not usually. Cornea (suppl. 1) 9:S51, 1990

101. Lemp MA: Is the dry eye contact lens wearer at risk? Yes. Cornea (suppl. 1) 9:S54, 1990

102. McDermott ML, Chandler JW: Therapeutic uses of contact lenses. Surv Ophthalmol 33:381, 1989

103. Dada VK, Karla VK, Angra SK: Role of soft contact lens in ocular surface problems. Indian J Ophthalmol 32:519, 1984

104. Donshik PC, Nelson JD, Abelson M, et al: Effectiveness of Bion Tears, Cellufresh, Aquasite, and Refresh Plus for moderate to severe dry eye. p. 753. In: WR Sullivan et al. (eds): Lacrimal Gland, Tear Film, and Dry Eye Syndromes 2. Plenum, New York, 1998

IV

Infection

11

Viral Infections and the Immunocompromised Patient

CONNIE L. CHRONISTER

GRAND ROUNDS CASE REPORT

Subjective:
A 45-year-old woman infected with human immunodeficiency virus (HIV) presents to the office wearing rigid gas-permeable contact lenses. She had been wearing rigid lenses all her lens-wearing life of 5 years. Her HIV infection was diagnosed 2 years ago. Her CD4 count was 540 cells/mm^3, and she has not had any acquired immunodeficiency syndrome (AIDS)–defining opportunistic infections. She has been healthy and has not needed any prophylactic anti–HIV medications or medications for opportunistic infections. Her chief complaint is lens discomfort with fluctuating vision. Her lenses are 3 years old, and she admits that she does not care for them very well and that she tends to overwear her lenses. She is highly myopic (8 D right eye [OD], 9 D left eye [OS]) and does not have any spectacles to wear when she is not wearing contact lenses.

Objective:
Slit-lamp examination revealed significant corneal superficial punctate keratitis (SPK), corneal epithelial edema, and an improperly fitting rigid lens (Fig. 11-1). Acuity is $^{20}/_{30}$ OD and $^{20}/_{40}$ OS, with no improvement after over-refraction. All other ocular health findings were unremarkable.

Assessment and Plan:
She is an example of a typical noncompliant rigid gas-permeable contact lens patient who happens to be HIV-positive. Some important considerations exist for HIV-infected patients. Most important, HIV-infected patients are more vulnerable to opportunistic infections and dry eye. First, this patient must be refracted and convinced to reduce her wearing time with contact lenses. As soon as the corneal staining and edema reduce to reasonable levels, spectacle refraction for eyeglasses should be provided so that the patient is not entirely dependent on her contact lenses. She must be educated on the importance of disinfection of her rigid lenses and the risks of opportunistic infections associated with her HIV-positive status. Her improperly fitting lenses must be replaced with more appropriately fitted gas-permeable lenses, and if she continues to exhibit corneal disease, contact lens wear should be changed to a different type of lens or discontinued altogether.

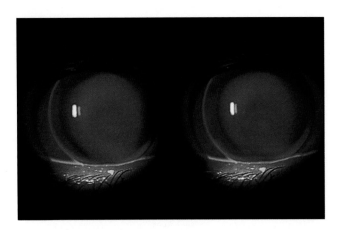

FIG. 11-1. *Improperly fitting rigid gas-permeable lens that is causing superficial punctate keratitis and corneal edema in a human immunodeficiency virus–infected patient.*

As an eye care professional, one must be aware of the many complications of viral diseases and their impact on contact lens patients. It is well established that ulcerative keratitis, although infrequent, is a very serious complication of contact lens wear. True visual morbidity can occur secondary to corneal ulceration. Most of the keratitis and conjunctivitis cases secondary to cosmetic contact lens wear result from bacteria, especially staphylococcus.[1-3] Viral disease can directly affect the cornea and thus have a profound effect on the ability to wear contact lenses.[3] However, viral corneal ulceration or keratoconjunctivitis has not been identified as a particular hazard of contact lens wear. Rather than being a contact lens complication, viral infections can affect a patient's ability to wear contact lenses and the transmission of viral infections.[3] Other viral diseases can have a direct effect on the immune system of the patient and thus can indirectly affect their ability to wear contact lenses. Additional concerns include when a patient can safely resume wearing contact lenses after a viral infection has resolved and preventing the transmission of viral infections. Thus, disinfection of lenses to guard against viral diseases is another important consideration for the patient and the eye care professional.

Patients that have active corneal viral disease should not wear contact lenses. Often, patients realize a problem exists and voluntarily remove their lenses before presenting to an eye care professional's office. The viral diseases that are notorious for causing a keratitis are herpes simplex and herpes zoster. Adenovirus and molluscum can also cause a keratitis, but other considerations are necessary for these viral infections. Another infection that is not viral but has viruslike properties (i.e., chlamy-

dia) can also have an effect on contact lens wear. HIV infection also has a multifaceted impact on a patient's ability to wear contact lenses.

VIRAL DISEASES THAT AFFECT THE ABILITY TO WEAR LENSES

Herpes Simplex Keratitis

Herpes simplex keratitis is a common viral infection found in young patients, many of whom may be contact lens wearers. It is the most common cause of corneal blindness in the developed countries.[4] Herpes simplex can be very devastating to the corneal surface and cause patients much discomfort. The difficulty with herpes simplex keratitis is that the virus is actively replicating on the corneal surface. In addition, the recurrent nature of the infection may be further detrimental to the cornea. Thus, contact lenses should never be worn during active infection.

Herpes simplex virus (HSV) is transmitted via direct contact with infected body fluids. It usually enters the host via mucous membrane exposure, breaks in mucous membranes, or percutaneous exposure. Two forms of herpes simplex exist: herpes simplex type I (HSV I) and herpes simplex type II (HSV II). HSV I usually causes infection in the ocular region or the facial labial cutaneous junction. HSV II is considered a sexually transmitted disease and usually causes infection in the genital area. Occasionally, HSV II can cause ocular infection, but the majority of HSV cases are caused by HSV I.

Once the virus enters the host, it causes a primary infection and travels to the cells in which it prefers to replicate. HSV replicates in tissues of ectodermal origin. Primary ocular herpes infection usually involves the eyelid skin in the form of vesicular eruptions. It can also cause corneal infections. After primary infection, the virus migrates up the ophthalmic division of the trigeminal nerve to remain latent in the ciliary or trigeminal ganglion. Reactivation of the virus causes it to migrate down the neuron to cause secondary ocular infection. The cornea is most commonly infected during reactivation. In fact, HSV I prefers to replicate in the cornea than in any other ocular tissue.

Active replication in the corneal epithelium causes the classic corneal dendrite (Fig. 11-2). The cornea may initially present with a punctate keratitis, which later develops into the true branching dendrite with end bulbs, or it may assume a geographic pattern of ulceration. The dendrite stains well with fluorescein, especially at the base, and rose bengal staining is notable at the lesion edges. Corneal sensitivity is often reduced in the involved eye. Corneal stromal disease secondary to HSV is usually related to the immunologic response to the infection rather than to direct replication of the virus. Stromal disease can occur in the form of necrotizing interstitial keratitis or diskiform keratitis. Conjunctivitis is also present during active infection. It classically produces diffuse conjunctival infection, follicles, and preauricular lymphadenopathy. HSV can cause infection of the corneal stroma and the endothelium.

Diagnosis of HSV is usually made based on the clinical presentation of the patient. If diagnosis is questionable, the virus can be cultured from the cornea, or an enzyme immunoassay test can be performed to detect HSV antigens.[4]

Herpes simplex keratitis can be a difficult management dilemma. The wearing of any contact lenses during active infection should be strongly discouraged. The lens can harbor the virus and interfere with the integrity of the damaged epithelium. Aggressive therapeutic treatment of HSV may include trifluridine ophthalmic drops (Viroptic) every 2 hours (or approximately 9 times a day), later tapered as the epithelial lesion improves.[1,2] Vidarabine (Vira A) ophthalmic ointment can be given at bedtime to protect the cornea while the patient sleeps. Vidarabine may also be used 5 times a day instead of trifluridine, but less visual disturbance occurs with solutions given during the day.[1,2] Antiviral toxicity can occur, and if necessary, acyclovir 200–400 mg by mouth four times a day can be used for 10–14 days.[1] The use of oral acyclovir, valacyclovir HCL, and other oral antivirals remains under therapeutic question and is under investigation. Contact lens wear is contraindicated with any of the aforementioned topical medications.

Patients are often anxious to resume contact lens wear. This can be a very difficult yet important decision by the practitioner. Little literature exists on HSV infection and contact lens wear. Clinical experience suggests that contact lenses should not be worn until complete resolution of the corneal lesion occurs and the eye is free of any viral infection (absence of any conjunctival hyperemia or any other signs of inflammation). Discard any lenses that may have been worn during active infection. Because these patients may be prone to recurrent infections, disposable lenses allow for a more compliant patient who is less likely to wear any contaminated lenses because they usually have an ample supply of lenses.

Disinfection against HSV can be very readily achieved by using hydrogen peroxide disinfection systems.[5] HSV has been selected by the U.S. Food and Drug Administration (FDA) as the lipid enveloped virus for the test of viricidal efficacy of contact lens disinfection systems.[3,5] The test virus is HSV I. Thus, cold chemical systems can also be used for disinfection of lenses, but the labeling

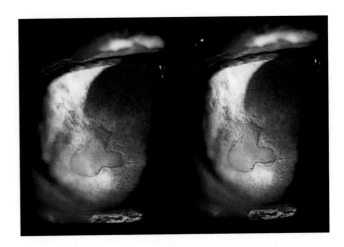

FIG. 11-2. *Herpes simplex virus corneal epithelial dendrite.*

should be checked to ensure that it deactivates HSV. The contact lens cases should also be properly disinfected with hydrogen peroxide or FDA-approved cold chemical disinfection systems. The case should be discarded, however, when contaminated with HSV.

Herpes Zoster Ophthalmicus

Herpes zoster virus (HZV) (also known as varicella-zoster virus), like herpes simplex, is a member of the herpesvirus family, but is a less common cause of keratitis. Primary herpes zoster *or* chickenpox typically occurs in young children. Recurrent infection of herpes zoster virus (shingles) usually occurs in the elderly or immunocompromised patients. Younger patients who may wear contact lenses and develop HZV infections include HIV-infected patients and other immunocompromised patients. Indeed, young patients manifesting herpes zoster should be screened for HIV. Secondary HZV infection in young patients (younger than age 40 years) is most likely to occur in immunocompromised patients secondary to HIV infection, cancer, chemotherapy, and organ transplantation.[4] When zoster is present in this population, the course may be much more severe with devastating sequelae, including dermatologic and corneal complications as well as retinal necrosis. Factors for reactivation have included trauma, emotional stress, immunosuppressive medications, irradiation, tuberculosis, malaria, and syphilis.[1] The infection is reactivated in relation to the immune suppression the patient is experiencing, although rare cases of secondary varicella zoster have occurred in young patients with healthy immune systems.

Primary HZV is transmitted via direct contact with an infected chicken pock or inhalation of infectious respiratory secretions. HZV causes disseminated infection, and young patients develop classic maculovesicular pox rash on the surface of the skin. Primary infection can cause keratitis, which can also be dendritic in appearance, and the conjunctiva may rarely develop vesicular lesions. Unlike herpes simplex, the pseudo-dendritic lesions do not typically stain well with fluorescein. The dendriform lesions of zoster do stain well with rose bengal. The immune system fights the virus and causes it to retreat and remain latent, most commonly in the dorsal root sensory ganglion. Ocular involvement can lead to dormancy in the trigeminal ganglion. Reactivation may occur months to years after the primary infection. In many adult patients, immunosuppression is the exogenous factor that reactivates HZV and causes herpes zoster.

Herpes zoster ophthalmicus (HZO) presents with vesicular eruptions that correspond to the ophthalmic division of the trigeminal nerve. Unlike HSV, the vesicular eruptions of HZO respect the forehead and scalp midline. If the tip of the nose is involved, this indicates nasociliary nerve involvement, and a higher likelihood exists of ocular involvement. Mucous plaques may form after the skin eruptions, associated with diffuse stromal haze and uveitis. A nummular form of zoster keratopathy may also threaten the cornea as an immune response to the virus antigen. In a very small percentage of zoster cases, diskiform keratitis may occur weeks to months later, leading to stromal edema and keratic precipitates.

Treatment of HZO includes systemic antivirals, such as 600–800 mg of oral acyclovir four times a day for 10 days.[1] Valacyclovir and famciclovir are newer forms of acyclovir that are now used to treat herpes zoster systemically.[2] Intravenous antiviral therapy is sometimes used in immunocompromised patients. Prednisolone acetate 1% can be used for uveitis or other ocular inflammations, such as stromal infiltrates or keratitis. The clinician must be sure that the diagnosis is herpes zoster and not herpes simplex before initiating any topical steroid treatment. Topical corticosteroids should be slowly tapered once the inflammatory condition subsides because recurrence is likely if treatment is abruptly discontinued. As with any use of topical corticosteroids, the patient's intraocular pressure should be monitored because steroid glaucoma may occur after steroid therapy in zoster cases.

Cycloplegic agents, such as homatropine or scopolamine, can be used to help with the ocular pain associated with inflammation. Any corneal lesion must be watched closely for secondary bacterial infection and treated with topical antibiotics if necessary. The vesicular skin lesions occur as a direct consequence of the presence of the virus. Starting as pustules, the lesions often become hemorrhagic, and, after a week to 10 days, they form crusts and scars when the virus is no longer active. The patient should keep the lesions clean with warm compresses and good hygiene. Topical antibiotic ointments and acyclovir ointment may be considered if necessary.[1] Early aggressive treatment with oral antivirals is often the most effective approach to prevent postherpetic pain, which may occur 1–3 months after resolution of the skin lesions and may last for months.

HIV-infected patients with herpes zoster may need more aggressive treatment with intravenous antivirals. Herpes zoster retinitis and acute retinal necrosis can also occur in these patients, and they must be very carefully monitored and comanaged with an infectious disease specialist.

Although corneal involvement is less common than with HSV, patients who develop HZO should immediately discontinue contact lens wear. The lenses should be discarded if worn during active infection. Disposable lenses should be considered if reinfection is likely to occur. Little information is available for HZV and contact lens wear. Clinical experience suggests that careful disinfection of lenses with commercially available hydrogen peroxide systems is effective (peroxide is effective against HSV). Contact lenses can be worn again after the infection has fully resolved, assuming that no staining, vascularization, or evidence of uveitis exists. Patient and practitioner must remember, however, that loss of corneal sensitivity often occurs during and after zoster infection of the cornea. As such, the risks of corneal involvement without the necessary protection of adequate sensation may mitigate against the regular use of contact lenses after zoster infection of the cornea. In addition, if the patient is immunocompromised, the risks of corneal suprainfection are also greater.

Adenovirus

Adenovirus is a common ocular infection that occurs in community and medical facility–based outbreaks. Most cases occur in patients 20–40 years of age, with no differentiation by gender, race, socioeconomic, or nutritional status.[4] Many contact lens patients are included in this age category. Therefore, adenovirus is a viral infection that should be considered in the contact lens population. Adenovirus causes minimal corneal disruption, particularly to the epithelium, and thus minimal potential for ulceration. Adenovirus causes a variety of eye syndromes, and many virus genomes and serotypes exist for this virus. Of the 41 serotypes, many are implicated in ocular infections. Adenovirus ocular infections include acute follicular conjunctivitis, epidemic keratoconjunctivitis (EKC), pharyngoconjunctival fever, and acute hemorrhagic conjunctivitis.

Adenovirus is a virulent organism, and transmission readily occurs via direct contact with the virus in secretions or on shared fomites (e.g., towels, linens, soap, eyeglasses).[4,6] Hand-to-eye transmission of adenovirus is also a common mode of transmission.[4] Crowding of infected patients in health facilities, schools, or other areas can enhance the spread of this infection. Eye care centers can be a mode of transmission through improper disinfection of eye-contact devices, such as tonometer tips.

The clinical presentation of EKC results from active replication of adenovirus in conjunctival epithelium and somewhat in the corneal epithelium.[4] This causes rapid onset of conjunctival hyperemia, folliculosis, and chemosis with occasional petechial hemorrhages and pseudomembrane formation. The eyelid is commonly swollen, and patients often exhibit preauricular lymph node swelling. The cornea can exhibit epithelial keratitis from viral replication, but the majority of corneal manifestations are delayed because of the immunologic response to the infection. After approximately 10–14 days into the course of the infection, an immunologic cell-mediated response to viral antigens at the level of Bowman's membrane occurs. This leads to subepithelial infiltrates, which can cause vision loss if they are located centrally along the visual axis.

Treatment of adenovirus remains a true clinical controversy. Some clinicians treat EKC with supportive therapy consisting of artificial tears, decongestants, and cold compresses.[1] Although discouraged by most authorities because of the consequences of misdiagnosis (herpes simplex, *Acanthamoeba*, or fungal infections), some clinicians aggressively treat patients with an antibiotic-steroid combination to reduce patient symptoms.[7] Topical nonsteroidal anti-inflammatory medications have been proposed as a safer method to reduce adenovirus symptoms.[7]

During all phases of active adenoviral infection, contact lenses must never be worn. Viruses can deposit in the lenses, and thus any lens worn during active infection must never be reused and should be immediately discarded.[8] The lens case should also be discarded. Contact lens wear could enhance the possibility of secondary infection from bacteria in a compromised, viral-infected cornea. Contact lens wear during the infiltrative phase of the infection is a clinical dilemma. The patient looks and feels better because, in this phase, the infection is resolving and the eye is usually white and quiet. On slit-lamp examination, subepithelial infiltrates can last for months. It is best to discontinue contact lens wear until no therapeutic treatment is required and the infiltrates disappear or appear fully inactive.

Adenovirus can survive for more than a week in a dried state on the surfaces of ophthalmic instruments.[6,9] Therefore, adenovirus is difficult to inactivate on instruments,

surfaces, and hands. Handwashing is not always effective for removing adenovirus.[10] Gloves should be worn when examining patients with EKC to help prevent transmission from patient to patient or from patient to practitioner.

Adenovirus requires vigorous adherence to disinfection protocols for trial contact lenses. Compared to HIV, HSV, and HZV, adenovirus is most resistant to disinfection and is known to be readily transmitted via tear film contamination.[8] Specific contact lens disinfection regimens have not been systematically tested for antiadenovirus activity, but 3% hydrogen peroxide has been shown to be effective.[5,11] Heat is the preferred disinfection method for adenovirus.[8] Thus, trial lenses should be disinfected with heat or hydrogen peroxide systems. Remember that high–water content lenses should not be disinfected with heat systems.

Molluscum Contagiosum

Molluscum contagiosum is a poxvirus that can cause wart-like lesions of the lids and lid margin. It can also cause a follicular conjunctivitis and superficial keratitis secondary to toxic reactions to molluscum contagiosum involving the eyelid margins. Contact lens patients can be affected by this condition because its peak occurrence in adults is in people 20–29 years of age. It is also common in young children, in whom it spreads by direct contact with lesions or through contaminated towels, toys, and so forth. Contaminated swimming pools can also be a source of infection. Molluscum is more severe in immunocompromised patients, including patients with AIDS.

Little information is available, but clinical experience suggests that contact lens wear should be discontinued and lenses discarded in patients with active molluscum contagiosum that includes conjunctival and corneal involvement. Minimal lid involvement with lesions that are not close to the lid margin may not require discontinuing contact lens wear. Daily disposable contact lenses may be a good option in these patients; it is up to the clinical judgment of the practitioner. Limited literature exists about contact lenses and molluscum contagiosum, so when in doubt, discontinue wear. Therapy of lid lesions should be done by a dermatologist. Therapies have included incision, cryotherapy, surgical excision, electrodessication, and caustic chemical applications.[4]

Chlamydial Infection

Although not considered a virus, *Chlamydia* is an organism with some viruslike qualities. *Chlamydia*, like viruses, is an intracellular parasite that is incapable of metabolic activities outside a living cell. To culture for *Chlamydia*,

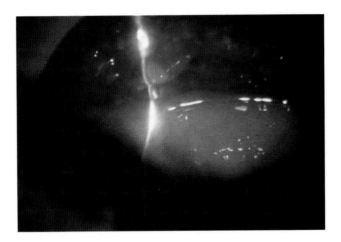

FIG. 11-3. *Chlamydial giant follicles seen on the everted upper lid.*

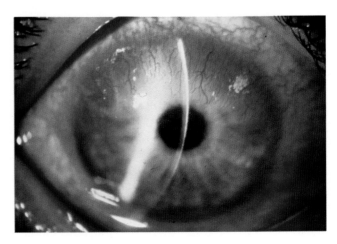

FIG. 11-4. *Chlamydial infiltrates and vascularization (note superior location).*

the specimen must be collected with a chlamydial collection swab and transported in a chlamydial culturette solution. The presence of inclusion bodies in the culture can be diagnostic.

In developed countries, *Chlamydia* is a common cause of adult inclusion keratoconjunctivitis in young sexually active patients, which can encompass a population that commonly wears contact lenses. Adult inclusion conjunctivitis is relatively uncommon and occurs in approximately 1 in 300 cases of genital chlamydial infection in the United Kingdom.[4] It is considered a sexually transmitted disease, and eye infection usually occurs through transfer from genital secretions during sexual activities. Adult inclusion conjunctivitis most commonly occurs in patients between the ages of 15 and 30 years.[4]

Like viral infections, adult inclusion conjunctivitis presents as an acute-onset follicular conjunctivitis with preauricular lymph node involvement. Follicles in chlamydia are typically quite large, and they may mimic the appearance of giant papillary conjunctivitis if the practitioner does not carefully examine the elevations (Fig. 11-3). Giant papillae tend to be more square, with flatter tops and a central vessel. Follicles are clearer and round, with vessels coursing over the elevations rather than through them. Unlike acute adenoviral keratoconjunctivitis, chlamydial infections may persist for many months if not properly treated. If a patient has a chronic conjunctivitis that resists traditional topical antibiotic treatment, chlamydia should be considered in the differential diagnosis. Corneal involvement includes limbal and corneal infiltrates most commonly seen superiorly (Fig. 11-4). Infiltrates can occur in the central cornea as well. Conjunctival scarring can occur in long-standing chronic

cases. This can cause additional corneal complications, such as pannus or corneal neovascularization, which also occurs superiorly.

Treatment of adult chlamydial keratoconjunctivitis includes a 3-week course of oral antibiotics (tetracycline 250 mg four times a day).[1] Semisynthetic tetracyclines, such as doxycycline or minocycline, can also be used.[1] Oral erythromycin is indicated for children or pregnant women. The patient's general physician should be consulted before initiating any oral antibiotics. Topical treatment with tetracycline ointment or erythromycin ointment can help the infection but should never be used instead of the oral antibiotic treatment. The treatment of infected sexual partners is also indicated to prevent reinfection.

Patients with active adult inclusion conjunctivitis should discontinue contact lens wear until the infection has resolved. Discard any worn lenses and used cases. Careful follow-up should occur if the cornea or conjunctiva has been damaged. Contact lens wear should continue with caution. Daily disposable lenses are a good option for healthy patients with a history of chlamydial infection.

Human Immunodeficiency Virus

General Considerations

HIV infection causes the eye care practitioner to consider several facets of the disease. One important consideration is the potential for opportunistic infection that is inherent to HIV infection. Another consideration is the effect HIV has on the ability of patients to wear and care for contact lenses. An additional concern is preventing transmission of the virus from patient to practitioner or from patient to patient.

HIV-infected patients that are still immunocompetent with adequate CD4$^+$ counts should be good candidates for contact lens wear. No established clinical criteria exist for when an HIV-infected patient should or should not wear contact lenses. The CD4$^+$ count in HIV-infected patients has become a standard for assessing the immunologic status of the patient as well as a way to predict the potential for certain opportunistic infections.[12] No studies have been done that allow the practitioner to use the patient's CD4$^+$ count as a predictor of successful contact lens wear in HIV-infected patients. Viral load, however, is a predictor of HIV infection. It is a measure of viral RNA via polymerase chain reaction testing that quantifies the amount of free virus in the patient's bloodstream. This can be another clinical tool for overall assessment of the patient. The optimal viral load is obviously no detectable virus. No standards have been established for contact lens wear in relation to viral load. Additional studies are certainly needed.

Physically healthy HIV-infected patients with no corneal problems can successfully wear contact lenses. As HIV infection progresses and the CD4$^+$ count declines and viral load increases, it is more likely that the patient may develop anterior segment problems that may interfere with contact lens wear. A study comparing the ocular flora of patients with AIDS to those of HIV-negative patients found little differences between the groups.[13]

One important complication is dry eye syndrome or keratoconjunctivitis sicca (KCS). Several reports have noted KCS and sicca complex in HIV-infected patients.[14-21] Approximately 17–20% of HIV-infected patients (determined by Schirmer testing) develop KCS during the course of their illness (Fig. 11-5).[13,14] This is greater than the incidence rate of less than 1% in the general population.[21] Dry eye certainly can be a complex problem for contact lens patients. Although no studies have been performed to correlate contact lens wear in HIV-infected patients with dry eye, several clinical problems could be surmised. The level of contact lens comfort could be diminished in these patients to the same level of discomfort experienced by non–HIV-infected patients with dry eye. In addition, patients with dry eye are particularly vulnerable to corneal epithelial defects from improper corneal wetting and from the reduction in lysozyme, lactoferrin, and immunoglobulins in the serous layer of the tear film. This could lead to secondary infections, which can occur in HIV-infected and non–HIV-infected patients who have epithelial defects and wear contact lenses. Although a study by Gritz et al.[13] reported the presence of KCS in AIDS patients, the level of immunosuppression did not appear to affect the ocular flora. HIV-infected patients who develop microbial keratitis can be more difficult to treat, and the potential for complications is greater than that seen in the

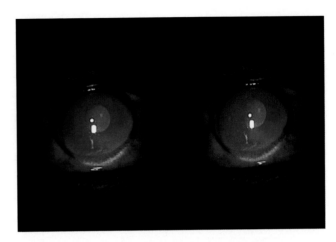

FIG. 11-5. *Dry eye in a human immunodeficiency virus–infected female. Note fluorescein staining along inferior cornea.*

non-HIV population.[22] Several studies have not reported an association of the presence of dry eye with the CD4$^+$ count or of the severity of HIV disease.[13-15]

HIV-infected contact lens wearers should be advised of the potential for dry eye problems. Proper lubrication is advised for lens-wearing and non–lens-wearing times. Punctal occlusion could be considered to enhance corneal wearing and possibly enhance contact lens tolerance. HIV-infected patients should be followed much more regularly than non–HIV-infected patients.

Opportunistic Infections in Patients Infected with Human Immunodeficiency Virus

Herpes Zoster Virus HIV-infected patients have a greater chance of developing herpes zoster infection than do uninfected people.[23] Approximately 5–15% of HIV-positive patients develop HZO.[24] As previously noted in the Herpes Zoster Ophthalmics section, this could affect their ability to wear contact lenses (Fig. 11-6). Studies suggest that HIV-infected patients with HZO may have a high rate of painful or sight-threatening complications.[25,26] One study reported a low incidence of stromal keratitis in HZO, but the zoster virus–associated infectious epithelial keratitis was particularly devastating and difficult to manage.[27] Engstrom and Holland[28] reported a case of zoster keratitis in a patient with AIDS that was very difficult to manage. Treatment for HIV-infected patients requires an intravenous dose of acyclovir followed by an oral maintenance regimen of acyclovir or famciclovir for the prevention of recurrence.[12]

The presence of HZO may be an indicator of a declining immune status. Use of contact lenses during active infection should be strongly discouraged, and continued

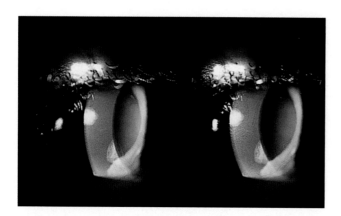

FIG. 11-6. *Herpes zoster virus corneal scar in a patient infected with human immunodeficiency virus.*

use after resolution of the herpes zoster infection should be closely monitored. HIV-infected immunocompetent patients with a history of HZO who continue to wear contact lenses should consider daily disposable lenses to eliminate disinfection concerns. This population also must be followed closely.

Herpes Simplex Virus   The incidence and clinical course of herpes simplex infection is little different for patients who are positive and negative for HIV.[23,29] HSV keratitis types 1 and 2 have been reported in HIV-infected patients.[30] The recurrence rate of HSV is greater in HIV-infected patients than in non–HIV-infected patients.[29] HSV keratitis in HIV-infected patients can be more resistant to treatment and often requires topical antiviral treatment with trifluridine along with oral acyclovir (400 mg 5 times a day or famciclovir 125–500 mg three times a day).[12] Long-term therapy of oral antivirals may be necessary to prevent recurrence of herpes simplex keratitis.

HIV-infected patients with herpes simplex keratitis must not wear contact lenses during any period of active infection. Because the recurrence rate of HSV keratitis is higher in HIV-infected patients than in non–HIV-infected patients, continued wear of contact lenses remains questionable. Suggestions include using daily disposable lenses in patients who have a history of HSV keratitis. Hydrogen peroxide disinfectants have proven to be effective against HSV and many other pathogens and are recommended for patients who can not wear daily disposable lenses. In addition, these patients should be followed very carefully and much more closely than non–HIV-infected patients with a history of HZV keratitis.

Microsporidia   Microsporidia are small, obligate, intracellular protozoal parasites that have been reported in HIV-infected patients.[31–34] Although microsporidia are

a rather infrequent cause of keratitis, microsporidial ocular infection may affect contact lens wear in an HIV-infected patient. Encephalitozoon has been isolated from conjunctival and corneal scrapings as the cause of keratitis in HIV-infected patients. It is most commonly seen in patients with decreased CD4$^+$ T lymphocyte counts.[33,35] One study reported a CD4$^+$ count of 2–50 cells/mm^3, indicating that ocular microsporidiosis occurs in patients with advanced AIDS.[33] Patients report foreign-body sensation, light sensitivity, conjunctival hyperemia, and tearing. The cornea exhibits diffuse, coarse, white infiltrates and erosions of the corneal epithelium. The lesions are variable in size and confined mostly to the epithelial layer.[35] The organism can be difficult to detect and requires special culturing and specimen collection via conjunctival and corneal scraping. Treatment options include oral itraconazole, topical fumagillin, and oral albendazole.[12,35,36]

Contact lens wear must be immediately discontinued in patients suspected of having microsporidial infection. All lenses and cases also must be discarded. Nothing has been written about contact lens wear in patients with a history of microsporidial infection. In light of the fact that microsporidial infections occur in patients with declining CD4$^+$ lymphocyte counts, the practitioner should be discouraged from allowing these patients to wear lenses. Daily disposable lenses can be used only after the microsporidial infection has fully resolved.

Molluscum Contagiosum   Molluscum contagiosum is more common, severe, and recurrent in HIV-infected patients than in non–HIV-infected people.[12,37,38] Eyelid infection occurs in up to 5% of HIV-infected patients.[39] Limited follicular conjunctivitis has been reported in HIV-infected patients versus noninfected patients. Treatment of molluscum includes cryotherapy, curettage, surgical excision, and incision.[12,37]

Conjunctival Microvasculopathy   Conjunctival microvasculopathy has been reported in 70–80% of HIV-positive patients.[12,40,41] HIV-infected patients with microvasculopathy are asymptomatic. Slit-lamp evidence of conjunctival microvasculopathy includes segmental vascular dilation and narrowing, comma-shaped vascular fragments, microaneurysm formation, and sludging of the blood column (Fig. 11-7).[12,40] The effect of the conjunctival microvasculopathy on contact lens wear has not been studied.[42] Because these patients remain asymptomatic and no treatment is indicated, contact lens wear is not contraindicated in patients who exhibit conjunctival microvasculopathy. The microvasculopathy appears to be noninfectious in nature.[41] No evidence exists to date that contact lens wear is detrimental in these patients, but further study is needed.

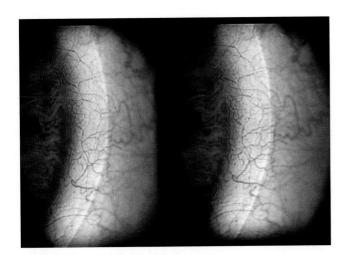

FIG. 11-7. *Conjunctival microvasculopathy in a human immunodeficiency virus–infected soft contact lens wearer.*

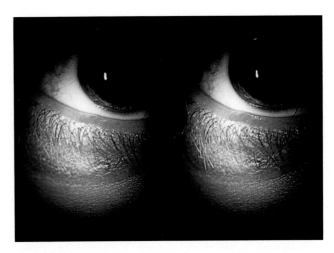

FIG. 11-8. *Kaposi's sarcoma lesion along the lower lid of a patient infected with human immunodeficiency virus.*

Kaposi's Sarcoma Kaposi's sarcoma (KS) is a vascularized malignancy that affects up to 25% of HIV-infected patients.[43] Ocular involvement occurs in 20% of HIV-infected patients with KS.[44] KS can be one of the early opportunistic malignancies found during the course of HIV infection and, thus, does not necessarily indicate significant HIV progression. KS is a painless lesion, and other than cosmetic concerns, many patients remain asymptomatic. KS ocular involvement may include loss of lashes and disruption of the lid margin (Fig. 11-8). Conjunctival lesions can also affect lid-globe congruity. If lid function or lid-globe congruity is affected, this could interfere with contact lens wear and physiologic tolerance. Thus, when these conditions present, contact lens wear should be considered contraindicated.[42,45] The literature on contact lens wear in KS is limited. Clinical experience compels the practitioner to discontinue contact lens wear in patients with KS that affects lid function or lid-globe congruity. There do not appear to be any special contact lens concerns in patients with mild lid lesions that are not affecting lid function in any way, although these patients should be followed closely for progression of KS. Without any other complications of HIV infection, patients with KS should be able to wear contact lenses. Additional research may reveal implications for KS patients and contact lens wear. Careful disinfection of contact lenses and cases as well as close follow-up of HIV-infected patients with KS is recommended.

Other Causes of Keratitis HIV-infected patients appear to have similar ocular flora to non–HIV-infected patients.[13] Corneal lesions occur in less than 5% of HIV-infected patients.[46] The majority of these corneal infections result from HSV and HZV. Bacterial and fungal corneal infections do not appear to be more common in HIV-positive people than in non–HIV-infected individuals.[46] The relative risk of developing bacterial or fungal infections secondary to contact lens wear in HIV-infected patients is not evident in the literature. Evidence exists that once an HIV-infected patient develops keratitis secondary to bacterial or fungal organisms, this can be very difficult to treat (Table 11-1).[47–52]

Nanda et al.[49] report pseudomonal infection occurring in an HIV-infected individual that was neutropenic and had external pseudomonal infection. The authors think that HIV-infected patients should not wear contact lenses. Maguen et al.[53] reported another case of a pseudomonal corneal ulcer associated with rigid gas-permeable daily-wear contact lenses in an HIV-infected patient. This infection progressed rapidly and required prompt intervention. These authors also caution against contact lens wear in HIV-positive patients with minimal signs of HIV infection.[53] Additional research is needed to determine the risks of contact lens wear in HIV-infected patients.

TABLE 11-1. *Organisms Causing Microbial Keratitis in Human Immunodeficiency Virus–Infected Patients*

Pseudomonas aeruginosa
Candida albicans
Staphylococcus aureus
Staphylococcus epidermidis
Bacillus spp.
α-Hemolytic *Streptococcus*
Micrococcus spp.
Capnocytophaga spp.

Intravenous drug abusers who are infected with HIV appear to have a greater risk of developing corneal ulceration. Candidal keratitis is more common in intravenous drug abusers compaired to nonintravenous drug abusers.[51,54] Contact lens wear in intravenous drug abusers should be carefully considered. Clinical evidence contraindicates lens wear in these patients, but research has not addressed this issue.

Additional Considerations for Contact Lens Wear in Patients Infected with Human Immunodeficiency Virus

Because corneal ulcerations, although somewhat rare, tend to be more severe and difficult to treat, HIV-infected patients who choose to wear contact lenses should strictly adhere to some precautions:

- Extended wear is contraindicated in HIV-infected patients. The risk of contact lens–induced keratitis resulting from extended wear is greater than for daily wear in the non–HIV-infected population.[55] Although the issue has not been researched, one would assume that the same applies to the HIV-infected population and may be worse, given the degree of immunocompromise in these patients.
- Daily-wear disposable lenses are a good alternative to allow for minimal exposure to possible pathogens. This also reduces the disinfection concerns.
- Careful disinfection of contact lenses is extremely important for HIV-infected patients.
- Contact lens cases should be kept clean and replaced frequently.
- HIV-infected patients require closer supervision and more numerous contact lens follow-up visits.
- Patients should be educated on the possibility of dry eye syndrome and other ocular pathogens.
- Under no circumstance should the patient share contact lenses with other individuals, even with careful disinfection.

IN-OFFICE INFECTION CONTROL PROCEDURES RECOMMENDED BY THE CENTERS FOR DISEASE CONTROL AND PREVENTION

Shortly after HIV was isolated in tears, the Centers for Disease Control and Prevention (CDC) published recommendations for the prevention of possible transmission of HIV from tears.[56–59] To date, the CDC has not updated their recommendations from 1986.[60,61] The Occupational Safety and Health Administration (OSHA) also uses these recommendations, and they should be adhered to whenever possible.

The following precautions are judged suitable to prevent the spread of HIV and other microbial pathogens that might be present in tears:

Handwashing. Practitioners should wash their hands before and after any patient encounter. If contact with tears occurs during a procedure, the hands should be washed immediately.[56]

Gloves. If the examiner is going to come into contact with bodily fluids that require universal precautions, such as blood, ear secretions, semen, and cerebrospinal fluid, gloves must always be worn. Tears are a bodily fluid that do not require universal precautions.[56] Thus, OSHA does not require gloves for contact with tear film. If the examiner has a break in the integrity of his or her skin and contact with tears is anticipated, gloves should be worn. Handwashing is necessary before gloving and after gloves are removed.

Instrument disinfection. Instruments that come into contact with the external surfaces of the eye or the tear film should be wiped clean and then disinfected by a 5- to 10-minute soak in one of the following:[56]

- 3% hydrogen peroxide
- Fresh solution containing 5,000 parts per million (mg/l) free available chlorine (a 1/10 dilution of household bleach [sodium hypochlorite])
- 70% ethanol
- 70% isopropyl alcohol

The device should be thoroughly rinsed and dried before use.

Further studies have shown that soaking in alcohol may damage tonometer tips and, thus, is not recommended for tonometer tips.[62] The manufacturer of the eye-contact devices should be consulted before using these CDC recommendations because damage to the devices can occur. Although not recommended by the CDC, many hospital-level disinfectants are available and effective against HIV.[5] These should be used with caution on eye-contact devices because any residual disinfectant left on the device could cause severe chemical ocular burns.

Contact lenses. Contact lenses used in trial fittings should be disinfected between each fitting by one of the following regimens:

- *Hard lenses.* Commercially available hydrogen peroxide contact lens disinfecting systems are currently approved for soft lenses. Alternately, most trial hard lenses can be treated with standard heat disinfection for soft lenses (78–80°C or 172–176°F) for 10 minutes. Practitioners should check with hard lens suppliers to ascertain which lenses can be safely heat treated.

- *Rigid gas-permeable lenses.* These trial lenses can be disinfected using commercially available hydrogen peroxide systems.[56] Rigid gas-permeable lenses warp if heat treated.
- *Soft contact lenses.* Soft trial-fitting lenses can be disinfected using commercially available hydrogen peroxide systems. Some soft lenses have also been approved for heat disinfection. Other than hydrogen peroxide, the chemical disinfectants used in standard contact lens solutions have not yet received FDA approval for deactivation of HIV.[3,60,61] Most cold chemical disinfectants do deactivate HSV, which is a larger-enveloped virus similar to HIV, but they have not yet been approved by the CDC.[5]

To date, there have been no reported cases of transmission of HIV via eye examination or contact lens fitting.[5]

REFERENCES

1. Bartlett JD, Jaanus SD, Ross RN: Clinical Ocular Pharmacology. 3rd ed. (Pocket Companion). Butterworth–Heinemann, Boston, 1997
2. Onofrey BE, Skorin L, Holdeman NR: Ocular Therapeutics Handbook: A Clinical Manual. Lippincott–Raven, Philadelphia, 1998
3. Levy SB, Cohen EJ: Methods of disinfecting contact lenses to avoid corneal disorders. Surv Ophthalmol 41:245, 1996
4. Pepose JS, Holland GN, Wilhelmus KR: Ocular Infection and Immunity. Mosby, St. Louis, 1996
5. Pepose JS: Contact lens disinfection to prevent transmission of viral disease. CLAO J 14:165, 1988
6. Nauheim RC, Romanowski EG, Araullo O, et al: Prolonged recovery of dessicated adenovirus type 19 from various surfaces. Ophthalmology 97:1450, 1990
7. Gordon YJ, Araullo-Cruz T, Romanowski EG: The effects of topical nonsteroidal anti-inflammatory drugs on adenoviral replication. Arch Ophthalmol 116:900, 1998
8. Balyeat HD, Bowman J, Rowsey JJ: Adenoviral keratoconjunctivitis associated with chemical disinfection of a flexible lens. Contact Intraocular Lens Med J 4:68, 1978
9. Warren D, Nelson KE, Farrar JA, et al: A large outbreak of epidemic keratoconjunctivitis: problems in controlling nosocomial spread. J Infect Dis 160:938, 1989
10. Jerrigan JA, Lowry BS, Hayden FG, et al: Adenovirus type 8 epidemic keratoconjunctivitis in an eye clinic: risk factors and control. J Infect Dis 167:1307, 1993
11. Craven ER, Butler SL, McCulley JP, et al: Applanation tonometer tip sterilization for adenovirus type 8. Ophthalmology 94:1538, 1987
12. Cunningham ET, Margolis TP: Ocular manifestations of HIV infection. N Engl J Med 339:236, 1998
13. Gritz DC, Scott TJ, Sedo SF, et al: Ocular flora of patients with AIDS compared with those of HIV-negative patients. Cornea 16:400, 1997
14. Lucca JA, Kung JS, Farris RL: Keratoconjunctivitis sicca in a female patient infected with human immunodeficiency virus. CLAO J 20:49, 1994
15. Lucca JA, Farris RL, Bielory L, Caputo AR: Keratoconjunctivitis sicca in male patients infected with human immunodeficiency virus type 1. Ophthalmology 97:1008, 1990
16. Chronister CL. Dry eye in an HIV-infected female. Clin Eye Vision Care 4:61, 1992
17. Kordossis T, Paikos S, Aroni K, et al: Prevalence of Sjogren's-like syndrome in a cohort of HIV-1 positive patients: descriptive pathology and immunopathology. Br J Rheumatol 37:691, 1998
18. Couderec LJ, D'Agay MF, Danon F, et al: Sicca complex and infection with human immunodeficiency virus. Arch Intern Med 147:898, 1987
19. Grier SA, Libera S, Klauss V, Goebel FD: Sicca syndrome in patients infected with the human immunodeficiency virus. Ophthalmology 102:1319, 1995
20. De Clerck LS, Couttenye MM, De Broe ME, Stevens WJ: Acquired immunodeficiency syndrome mimicking Sjogren's syndrome and systemic lupus erythematosus. Arthritis Rheum 31:272, 1988
21. Mody GM, Hill JC, Meyers OL: Keratoconjunctivitis sicca in rheumatoid arthritis. Clin Rheumatol 7:237, 1988
22. Hemandy RK: Microbial keratitis in patients infected with human immunodeficiency virus. Ophthalmology 102:1026, 1995
23. Hodge WG, Seiff SR, Margolis TP: Ocular opportunistic infection incidences among patients who are HIV positive compared to patients who are HIV negative. Ophthalmology 105:895, 1998
24. Jabs DA, Quinn TC: Acquired immunodeficiency syndrome. p. 289. In Pepose JS, Holland GN, Wilhelmus KR (eds): Ocular Infection and Immunity. Mosby–Year Book, St. Louis 1996
25. Kestelyn P, Stevens AM, Bakkers E, et al: Severe herpes zoster ophthalmicus in young African adults: a marker for HTLV III seropositivity. Br J Ophthalmol 71:806, 1987
26. Lewallen S: Herpes zoster ophthalmicus in Malawi. Ophthalmology 101:1801, 1994
27. Margolis TP, Milner MS, Shama A, et al: Herpes zoster ophthalmicus in patients with human immunodeficiency virus infection. Am J Ophthalmol 125:285, 1998
28. Engstrom RE, Holland GN: Chronic herpes zoster virus keratitis associated with the acquired immunodeficiency syndrome. Am J Ophthalmol 105:556, 1985
29. Hodge WG, Margolis TP: Herpes simplex virus keratitis among patients who are positive or negative for human immunodeficiency virus: an epidemiologic study. Ophthalmology 104:120, 1997
30. Rosenwasser GOD, Greene WH: Simultaneous herpes simplex types 1 and 2 keratitis in acquired immunodeficiency syndrome. (Letter) Am J Ophthalmol 113:102, 1992
31. Friedberg DN, Stenson SM, et al: Microsporidial keratoconjunctivitis in acquired immunodeficiency syndrome. Arch Ophthalmol 108:504, 1990

32. Metcalfe TW, Doran RML, Rowlands PL, et al: Microsporidial keratoconjunctivitis in a patient with AIDS. Br J Ophthalmol 76:177, 1992

33. Schwartz DA, Visvesvara GS, Diesenhouse MC, et al: Pathologic features and immunofluorescent antibody demonstration of ocular microsporidiosis (*Encephalitozoon hellem*) in seven patients with acquired immunodeficiency syndrome. Am J Ophthalmol 115:285, 1993

34. Bryan RT: Microsporidiosis: an AIDS-related opportunistic infection. Clin Infect Dis (suppl. 1) 21:S62, 1995

35. Diesenhouse MC, Wilson LA, Corrent GF, et al: Treatment of microsporidial keratoconjunctivitis with topical fumagillin. Am J Ophthalmol 115:293, 1993

36. Roseberger DF, Serdarevic ON, Erlandson RA, et al: Successful treatment of microsporidial keratoconjunctivitis with topical fumagillin in a patient with AIDS. Cornea 12:261, 1993

37. Robinson MR, Udell IJ, Garber PF, et al: Molluscum contagiosum of the eyelids in patients with acquired immune deficiency syndrome. Ophthalmology 99:1745, 1992

38. Kohn SR: Molluscum contagiosum in patients with acquired immunodeficiency syndrome. (Letter) Arch Ophthalmol 105:458, 1987

39. Bardenstein DS, Elmets C: Hyperfocal cryotherapy of multiple Molluscum contagiosum lesions in patients with the acquired immune deficiency syndrome. Ophthalmology 102:1031, 1995

40. Teich SA: Conjunctival microvascular changes in AIDS and AIDS-related complex. Am J Ophthalmol 103:332, 1987

41. Engstrom RE Jr, Holland GN, Hardy WD, Meiselman HJ: Hemorheologic abnormalities in patients with human immunodeficiency virus infection and ophthalmic microvasculopathy. Am J Ophthalmol 109:153, 1990

42. Wilson R: HIV and contact lens wear. J Am Optom Assoc 63:13, 1992

43. Tschachler E, Berbstresser PR, Stingl G: HIV-related skin diseases. Lancet 348:659, 1996

44. Dugel PU, Gill PS, Frangieh GT, Rao NA: Ocular adnexal Kaposi's sarcoma in acquired immunodeficiency syndrome. Am J Ophthalmol 110:500, 1990

45. Shuler JD, Holland GN, Miles SA, et al: Kaposi sarcoma of the conjunctiva and eyelids associated with the acquired immunodeficiency syndrome. Arch Ophthalmol 107:858, 1989

46. Akduman L, Pepose JS: Anterior segment manifestations of acquired immunodeficiency syndrome. Semin Ophthalmol 10:111, 1995

47. Parrish CM, O'Day DM, Hoyle TC: Spontaneous fungal corneal ulcer as an ocular manifestation of AIDS. (Letter). Am J Ophthalmol 104:302, 1987

48. Santos C, Parker J, Dawson C, Ostler B: Bilateral fungal corneal ulcers in a patient with AIDS-related complex. Am J Ophthalmol 102:118, 1986

49. Nanda M, Pflugfelder SC, Holland S: Fulminant pseudomonal keratitis and scleritis in human immunodeficiency virus-infected patients. Arch Ophthalmol 109:503, 1991

50. Lau RKW, Goh BT, Estreich S, et al: Adult gonococcal keratoconjunctivitis with AIDS. Br J Ophthalmol 74:52, 1990

51. Hemandy RK, Griffin N, Begona A: Recurrent corneal infections in a patient with the acquired immunodeficiency syndrome. Cornea 12:266, 1993

52. Chronister CL: Review of external ocular disease associated with AIDS and HIV infection. Optom Vis Sci 73:225, 1996

53. Maguen E, Salz JJ, Nesburn AB: Pseudomonas corneal ulcer associated with rigid, gas-permeable daily wear lenses in a patient infected with human immunodeficiency virus. Am J Ophthalmol 113:336, 1992

54. Arstimuno B, Nirankari VS, Hemandy RK, Rodrigues MM: Spontaneous ulcerative keratitis in immunocompromised patients. Am J Ophthalmol 115:202, 1993

55. Connor CG: Microbiological aspects of extended wear soft contact lenses. Optom Clin 1:79, 1991

56. Centers for Disease Control: Recommendations for prevention of possible transmission of human T-lymphocyte virus type III/lymphadenopathy-associated virus from tears. MMWR Morb Mortal Wkly Rep 34:533, 1985

57. Tervo T, Lahdevirta J, Vaheri A, et al: Recovery of HTLV III from contact lenses. Lancet 1:379, 1986

58. Ablashi DV, Sturzenegger S, Hunter EA, et al: Presence of HTLV-III in tears and cells from the eyes of AIDS patients. J Exp Pathol 3:693, 1987

59. Fujikawa LS, Salahuddin SZ, Ablashi D, et al: Human T-cell leukemia/lymphotropic virus type III in the conjunctival epithelium of a patient with AIDS. Am J Ophthalmol 100:507, 1985

60. Amin RM, Dean MT, Zaumetzer LE, Poiesz BJ: Virucidal efficacy of various lens cleaning and disinfecting solutions on HIV-1 contaminated contact lenses. AIDS Res Hum Retroviruses 7:403, 1991

61. Slonim CB: AIDS and the contact lens practice. CLAO J 21:233, 1995

62. Chronister CL, Russo P: Effects of disinfecting solutions on tonometer tips. Optom Vis Sci 67:818, 1990

12

Ulcerative Bacterial Keratitis*

BARRY A. WEISSMAN, MICHAEL J. GIESE,
AND BARTLY J. MONDINO

GRAND ROUNDS CASE REPORT

Subjective:
A 32-year-old woman presents for emergency care at 4:00 PM. She has worn disposable hydrogel contact lenses for correction of her modest myopia for 10 months on a 2-week flexible wear schedule (she usually sleeps with the lenses on her eyes 2 nights per week), but she ran out of sterile rinsing saline and has worn lenses for the last 4 consecutive nights. Because she obtained her last 3-month supply of contact lenses from a mail-order source, she is reluctant to contact her previous eye doctor.

Chief complaint: acute blurring in each eye (OU) (contact lenses in place) with increasing foreign-body sensation, photophobia, and lacrimation in the left eye (OS). The patient is in good general health and takes no medications besides birth control pills; her familial history, however, includes diabetes and cataract in her elderly mother.

Objective:
- Presenting visual acuities: $^{20}/_{30}$ right eye (OD) and OS with contact lenses, each improving with pinhole to $^{20}/_{25}$. Extra-ocular movements: full range and motility. Pupils: equal, round, and reactive to light and accommodation, with no afferent defects.
- Biomicroscopic examination: hydrogel lenses both centered, free moving, but mildly soiled (removed and placed in new case with unpreserved sterile saline).
- Slit-lamp examination reveals epithelial edema OD, and a 1-mm round staining corneal infiltrate at 8 o'clock surrounded by 1-mm area of epithelial edema, 3 mm from limbus, OS; mild conjunctival injection is seen in the sector adjacent to the infiltrate OS.
- The left upper lid is also hyperemic and swollen; no discharge, papillae, follicles, anterior chamber reaction, or rubeosis iridis are seen.
- Tonometry: OD 16 mm Hg (deferred OS).
- Ophthalmoscopy (undilated): normal OU.

Assessment:
1. Corneal edema OD, secondary to extended-wear hypoxia.
2. Presumptive active bacterial corneal ulcer OS. Must assume ulcer associated with *Pseudomonas aeruginosa* until proved otherwise because it is the most common and aggressive potential pathogen. Alternatives include

---

*Text adapted with permission from BA Weissman, BJ Mondino: Corneal infections secondary to contact lens wear. p. 255. In AJ Tomlinson (ed): Complications of Contact Lens Wear. Mosby–Year Book, St. Louis, 1992.

other gram-negative, or even gram-positive, bacterial infection. Given this setting, viral, fungal, and parasitic infections are unlikely.

Plan:
Either immediate referral for appropriate diagnostic and therapeutic management, or immediate initiation of same by:

- Obtaining cultures from the infiltrate (also lens and case if available) for immediate microscopic inspection of stained slides and laboratory investigations. Additional cultures of the lids and conjunctiva may be helpful.
- After cultures, initiating aggressive topical broad-spectrum (with good gram-negative coverage) antibiotic treatment (e.g., a loading dose of 1 drop/minute for 5 minutes, perhaps administered two times in the first hour, followed by one drop every 0.5–1.0 hour around the clock). Use dual therapy with fortified agents (e.g., tobramycin 13.6 mg/ml and cefazolin 50 mg/ml), or monotherapy with commercial-strength fluoroquinolones (e.g., ciprofloxacin 3 mg/ml or ofloxacin 3 mg/ml).
- Modifying treatment based on clinical course and results of specific culture and antibiotic sensitivities.
- Considering alternative diagnoses (e.g., *Acanthamoeba* keratitis) if ocular response to the treatment is not as expected.
- Providing close professional supervision until corneal epithelium heals and other signs and symptoms resolve. Patient re-education on care system compliance; periodic professional monitoring is advised before reconsideration of contact lens use. Extended wear should be discouraged, but resumption of daily wear can be permitted with appropriate patient education and professional supervision.

Most users of contact lenses rarely experience serious complications, although inconvenience, minor sequelae, and interruptions in lens wear are commonplace. The most common complications by far are those associated with lens care and solutions, and those directly or indirectly associated with lens soilage.[1] Physiologic complications, including changes in lid tissues, hyperemia of the bulbar conjunctiva, and corneal changes, including varieties of edema and superficial punctate staining (SPS), are common. More severe abrasions, stromal neovascularization, and corneal infiltrates may also occur. Usually, these are of short duration and limited tissue compromise if lens wear is improved or discontinued. The number of patients who have severe or permanent compromise of ocular tissues is quite small.

The surface of the cornea is most affected by the presence of a contact lens, probably owing to proximity. SPS and minor epithelial erosions are commonly seen and may be related to drying, allergic, and toxic effects of solutions (Fig. 12-1); mechanical problems with a lens fit; surface or edge problems; or a host of other potential insults.

A contact lens forms a potential barrier to corneal oxygen supply. Acute hypoxia induces metabolic changes in the epithelium, resulting in decreased glycogen stores, sensitivity, and epithelial adhesion. Epithelial edema may be seen in microcysts, microcystic edema, circular corneal clouding, and edematous corneal formations. Hypoxia also has been associated with vascularization (Fig. 12-2) of the cornea, acute stromal acidosis and swelling, chronic stromal thinning, and changes in endothelial cell morphology (acute blebs and chronic polymegethism). For detailed reviews of these topics, see Holden and associates[2] and Chapters 2, 3, and 14.

The most severe complication of contact lens wear (and a leading cause of vision loss[3]) is the subject of this discussion: direct microbial infection (Fig. 12-3). Although potential infectious microbes also include fungi, viruses, and protozoa, most corneal infections are associated with bacteria, which are the subject of this chapter. Other potential pathogens are considered in Chapters 11 and 13. Microbial infection is one of the less commonly encountered complications of contact lens wear.

DEFINITIONS

Corneal ulcer: The *Dictionary of Visual Sciences* defines a corneal ulcer as "pathological loss of substance of the surface of the cornea, due to progressive erosion and necrosis of the tissue."[4] Dohlman[5] similarly defines a corneal ulceration as an "epithelial defect that has become complicated by the disappearance of some underlying stro-

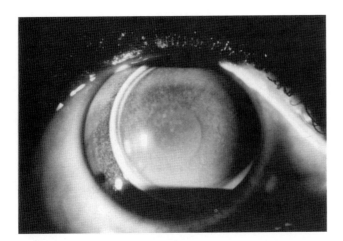

FIG. 12-1. *Fine pan-corneal superficial punctate staining associated with a reaction to a rigid contact lens solution. Patient is a 35-year-old hyperopic woman wearing rigid gas-permeable contact lenses with only minor subjective symptoms.*

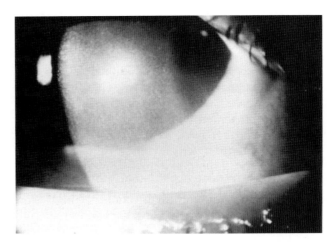

FIG. 12-3. *Corneal ulcer in contact lens wearer. Fluorescein staining shows an associated epithelial break. The patient complained of pain and photophobia in this eye for the 12 hours preceding presentation.*

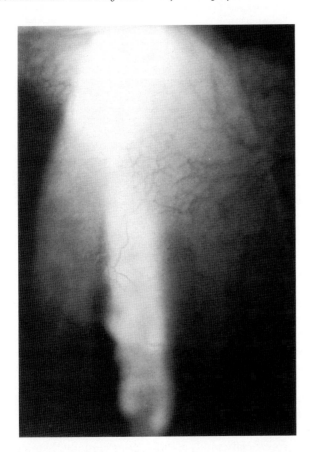

FIG. 12-2. *Superficial peripheral corneal vascularization in a highly myopic woman who has worn hydrogel contact lenses compliantly on a daily-wear basis for approximately a decade. Potential contributing factors include previous bilateral retinal detachment and repairs, acne rosacea, and contact lens–induced chronic peripheral corneal hypoxia.*

mal substance, usually following infection, chemical burns, trauma or desiccation." Corneal ulceration is therefore a nonspecific diagnosis; it implies excavation of the corneal tissues but does not provide information on the cause. Corneal ulceration need not be specifically infectious by definition; a Mooren's ulcer is an example of sterile corneal ulceration (Fig. 12-4).

Corneal signs of ulcerative keratitis include epithelial (and perhaps stromal) defect and associated corneal infiltrates (see definition later in this section) and edema. Conjunctival edema and injection often accompany severe keratitis, as does lid inflammation and an anterior chamber reaction (seen as flare and cells in the aqueous humor). Hypopyon may be associated with severe inflammation of the anterior segment. Subjective symptoms include ocular pain, photophobia, and decreased vision (owing to involvement of the corneal visual axis and cells in the anterior chamber).[6] Mild (or early) keratitis, however, may have minimal subjective symptoms. Neovascularization, scarring, and corneal thinning may result after episodes of acute or chronic keratitis (Fig. 12-5).

The pathophysiology of active corneal infection (ulcerative microbial keratitis) is not yet fully understood, but direct microbial invasion of the intact cornea is relatively rare in healthy individuals. In general, the process of infection is believed to depend on the mechanical, humoral, and cellular defense mechanisms of the host on one hand, and the inoculum size, pathogenicity, and virulence of the microorganisms on the other. Research using animal models has led to our current understanding of some mechanisms of corneal inflammation during bacterial keratitis (Fig. 12-6).

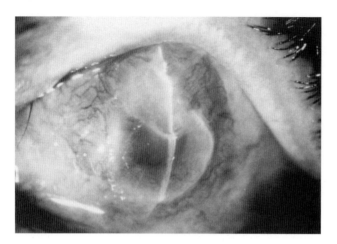

FIG. 12-4. *Severe Mooren's corneal ulcer. Full 360 degrees of the corneal periphery are involved, with marked inflammation, vascularization, and corneal thinning.*

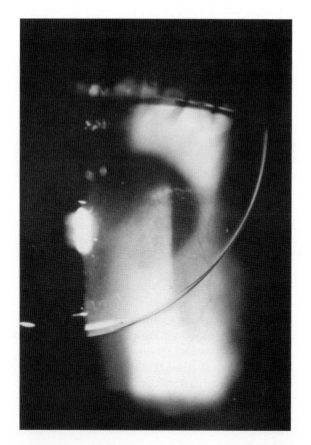

FIG. 12-5. *Healed corneal ulcer (presumably secondary to herpes simplex keratitis) in a young man. Rigid contact lens is now worn (as seen in photograph) to improve vision to $^{20}/_{20}$. Note vascularization of the corneal stroma and opacification or scarring. This area of the cornea is thinned, and the surface is irregular.*

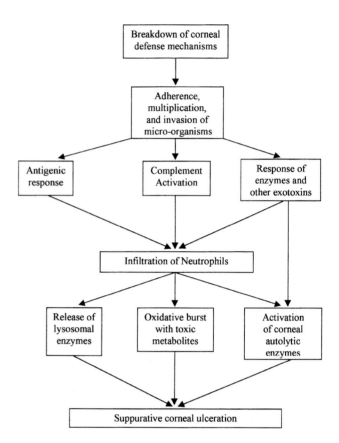

FIG. 12-6. *Pathogenic mechanisms of bacterial keratitis. (Modified, with permission, from KR Wilhelmus: Bacterial keratitis. p. 985. In JS Pepose, GH Holland, KR Wilhelmus [eds]: Ocular Infection and Immunity. Mosby–Yearbook, St. Louis, MO, 1996.)*

Corneal disease, trauma, surgery, and exposure (through eyelid disease or disorders of the ocular surface) are well-known factors contributing to microbial infections of the cornea. Contact lens wear has joined this list as a major potential predisposing factor, specifically for bacterial corneal infection (and occasionally amebic or fungal infection as well). Herpes simplex is a common viral cause of corneal ulceration, and although viral keratitis can be complicated by a secondary bacterial infection, it has not been specifically associated with contact lens wear (as a risk factor) and is not the subject of this discussion.

Keratitis is inflammation of the cornea and also does not specifically imply an infectious etiology. Noninfectious causes of keratitis include tear film abnormalities; exposure; immunologic reactions (perhaps to topical or systemic medications or contact lens solutions); denervation; dystrophies; and photic, mechanical, and chemical injuries.

Corneal infiltrates are a sign of keratitis. These are single or multiple transient discrete collections of gray or white material observed in the normally transparent corneal tissues, usually just beneath the epithelium (Fig. 12-7). Corneal infiltrates are inflammatory cells that have migrated through the cornea from the limbal vasculature or from the tears in response to chemotactic factors released from damaged local tissues. An infectious agent itself can form all (e.g., in infectious crystalline keratopathy) or part of the infiltrate. Inflammatory cells are believed to be primarily polymorphonuclear leukocytes (neutrophils) as well as macrophages and lymphocytes. Infiltration into the cornea is a complex and coordinated process (Fig. 12-8); research has focused on factors in the ocular tissues and tears, and their role in homeostasis and pathologic processes.

The small peripheral corneal infiltrates associated with blepharitis, for example, tend to be sterile, relatively benign and self-limited corneal lesions, immunologically associated with *Staphylococcus aureus* (specifically, with a hypersensitivity reaction to the ribitol teichoic acid of the bacteria cell wall) (Fig. 12-9).[7]

Sterile (noninfectious) and infectious corneal infiltrates have been associated with contact lens wear. Mondino and Groden[8] found that sterile central corneal infiltrates, similar in appearance to those encountered with adenovirus keratitis (epidemic keratoconjunctivitis) or chlamydial infections, could occur from exposure to contact lens solutions (specifically, the preservative thimerosal). Gordon and Kracher,[9] Bates et al.,[10] and Donshik et al.[11] described peripheral corneal infiltrates with contact lens wear, suggesting that such infiltrates were more common with extended-wear than daily-wear use of contact lenses. A new, perhaps inappropriate, term has been introduced into the literature specifically to identify sterile peripheral infiltrates associated with contact lens use: *contact lens–induced peripheral ulcers.*[12]

Distinguishing noninfectious sterile infiltrates from active corneal infection can be difficult. Stein and associates[6] provided additional information to help clinicians distinguish between sterile infiltrates and the infiltrates of active microbial corneal infection associated with contact lens wear. Fifty patients who presented with corneal infiltrates associated with contact lens wear were prospectively studied to determine which clinical signs and symptoms were most important in predicting the results of microbial culture. Twenty patients were found to have culture-positive corneal infections, 20 had sterile infiltrates, and the remaining 10 patients showed corneal infiltrates from which cultures were negative but which appeared clinically to be infectious in origin. Positive culture results were statistically associated with increased pain, discharge, epithelial staining, and anterior cham-

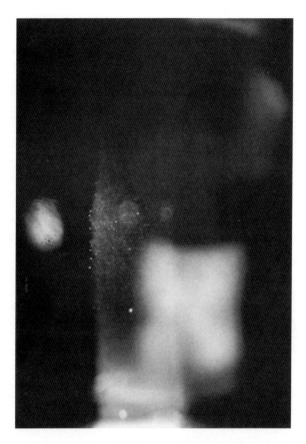

FIG. 12-7. *Two subepithelial corneal infiltrates (center of optic section) after one night of extended wear with a disposable hydrogel lens in a young man. These lesions did not show associated staining.*

ber reactions. Lesions that did not yield positive cultures (sterile infiltrates) were usually smaller (70% of these measured <1 mm in diameter), were multiple, showed minimal superficial punctate epithelial staining, and presented without substantial pain, discharge, or anterior chamber reaction.

We believe it important to emphasize that size and location should not be considered major distinguishing features with contact lens wear. All infections should begin as small infiltrates or epithelial defects, or both.[13] Mondino et al.[14] found that only 23 of 40 clinically diagnosed corneal infections associated with contact lens wear were central ulcers, whereas the remainder were peripheral.

Large studies of corneal infection always include substantial numbers of patients who clinically appear to have microbial keratitis and respond to treatment but who also have had negative culture results for any of a number of reasons (including previous antibiotic therapy and sampling error).[14,15] Considering the risk-benefit ratio of treating a sterile infiltrate versus not treating an

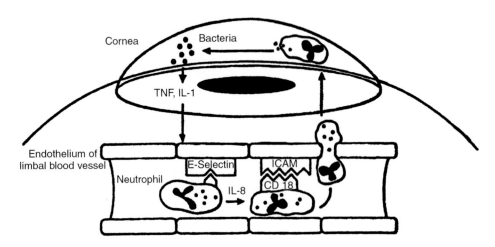

FIG. 12-8. *Inflammatory cell infiltration into the cornea is a complex and coordinated process. Bacteria enter the corneal stroma and multiply. This induces the production of proinflammatory cytokines and chemoattractants. These proteins activate endotherlial cells inducing the expression of adhesion molecules inducing rolling of the inflammatory cell. After this step, cells become activated and express integrins and endothelial cells express intercellular adhesion molecule-1. Binding of these two molecules allows for transmigration into the infected cite. (CD 18 = cluster designation 18; ICAM = intercellular adhesion molecule; IL-1 = interleukin-1; IL-8 = interleukin-8; TNF = tumor necrosis factor.) (Modified, with permission, from KR Wilhelmus: Bacterial keratitis. p. 992. In JS Pepose, GH Holland, KR Wilhelmus [eds]. Ocular Infection and Immunity. Mosby–Yearbook, St. Louis, MO, 1996.)*

infectious keratitis, it is probably better to overtreat rather than undertreat.

HISTORIC PERSPECTIVES

Before the widespread application of contact lenses over the last several decades, almost all cases of bacterial corneal ulceration occurred after trauma or were associated with systemic or concomitant ocular surface diseases.

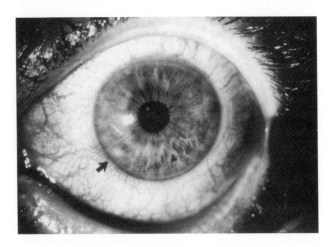

FIG. 12-9. *Hypersensitivity marginal corneal infiltrate* (Staphylococcus aureus) *at arrow. Patient does not wear contact lenses.*

Contact lens–associated corneal infection was itself also a relatively rare event until the introduction of extended wear. In 1966, only 14 cases of lost or blinded eyes could be documented by Dixon et al.[16] from almost 50,000 polymethylmethacrylate (PMMA) contact lens–wearing patients seen by a large ophthalmologic group during a single year. Eight of these patients had clear lapses in their lens care history. Several case reports in the late 1970s suggested that there might be more infections with the use of hydrogel contact lenses.[17,18] Ruben,[19] however, concluded (from his own experiences at Moorfields Eye Hospital in the United Kingdom) that the overall incidence of infection with use of hydrogel contact lenses was low when hygiene and lens care were good, although the rate might be somewhat greater than that found with PMMA lenses.

Wilson et al.[20] documented eight corneal ulcers in seven patients who were using hydrogel contact lenses with homemade saline for the care solution. They identified the same bacterial serotypes of *Pseudomonas* in the corneal ulcers as in the contact lens care systems used by four of their seven patients. It is important to note that all these patients used homemade saline inappropriately as a wetting agent, eye drop, or bath, after thermal disinfection of their contact lenses. Microbial contamination of care solutions was linked with microbial infection of the cornea by this study.

Cooper and Constable[21] also reported eight cases of infective keratitis in wearers of hydrogel contact lenses.

One patient wore the lens continuously (for therapeutic reasons), and three used their lenses daily or intermittently. Four of these eight patients, however, appeared to have no predisposing factors except that they were using their lenses for continuous or extended wear. Cooper and Constable's report[21] thus introduced the modern concerns about microbial infection in extended contact lens wear.

It is important to emphasize, however, that the use of all types of contact lenses, including refractive, cosmetic (soft, hard, hybrid, and gas permeable), and therapeutic, have been associated with corneal infection at one time or another.[22]

INCIDENCE

The first difficulty in determining the incidence of corneal infection with contact lens wear is to precisely define the disease to study. Many early reports did not clearly limit their discussions to corneal infection but may have grouped infectious and noninfectious infiltrates, ulcers, and keratitis. Here, only active corneal microbial infection are considered.

The second difficulty in studying this disease is that its presentation is a relatively rare event, especially when one restricts interest to any association with the daily wear of contact lenses. This is clearly documented by the results of Dixon et al.[16] Even the initial clinical studies of extended wear did not encounter many corneal infections. Only in analyzing the many studies since the 1970s does one observe the clearly changing trend.

Salz and Schlanger[23] presented perhaps the first modern report that attempted to determine an event rate for infectious keratitis associated with hydrogel extended wear. One hundred aphakic eyes (70 patients) using hydrogel contact lenses for extended wear were followed for 3 months to 7 years; five peripheral or paracentral ulcers were diagnosed and treated. Eichenbaum et al.[24] similarly studied a group of 100 aphakic eyes using hydrogel contact lenses for extended wear and found four infections in a year. Spoor et al.[25] studied 120 aphakic eyes using hydrogel contact lenses for extended wear and reported a 4.3% incidence of corneal infection in 3 years (if all infiltrates are counted, however, Spoor's incidence increases to perhaps 6%). These figures are from longitudinal studies, deal solely with aphakic eyes, and clearly appear fairly similar in results.

Weissman et al.[26] reported their experience at a referral center. Phakic and aphakic patients who used contact lenses for daily and extended wear were seen and treated for corneal infection associated with contact lens wear at a major university hospital (University of California at Los Angeles). These authors concluded that the risk of infection increased some six-fold with extended wear

compared with daily wear, and they found no difference in risk between phakic and aphakic eyes.

Chalupa et al.[27] reported a similar experience, observing corneal infection associated with contact lens wear over a 2-year period in a large population (estimated at 35,000–40,000) of contact lens wearers in Gothenberg, Sweden. They treated and studied 55 corneal infections in these patients during this period and found an incidence rate of approximately 1/15,000 for daily wear and 1/3,000 for extended wear of hydrogel lenses. Holden et al.[28] summarized this and their own data:

> The best estimate we can make is that in Western Australia in 1977, in Sweden in 1981–82, and in the U.S. currently [1986], about 1/100 patients will have a peripheral corneal erosion (ulcer) that heals without complications and about 1/1000–5000 will have a serious infection that adversely affects vision.

A large survey of the almost 3,000 members of the American Optometric Association's Contact Lens Section was conducted.[29] This study (440 responders) suggested that corneal infection occurred at an incidence rate of approximately 0.5% for daily wear and 3% for extended wear of cosmetic hydrogel contact lenses over 2-year blocks of time during 1980–1985.

MacRae et al.[30] summarized the experience collected from 48 U.S. Food and Drug Administration (FDA)–controlled studies of new contact lenses between 1980 and 1988. These data represented the experiences of 22,739 patients. The FDA received reports of 159 serious adverse reactions, and among these were 28 "corneal ulcers." From these data, MacRae calculated an infection rate of approximately 1/1,500 (events/patient-years) overall for daily wear of contact lenses, 1/244 for cosmetic hydrogel extended wear, and 1/185 for aphakic hydrogel extended wear. These data rely on reports, however, and not all adverse reactions or corneal infections may have been reported.

In late 1989, the *New England Journal of Medicine* published the Contact Lens Institute (CLI) studies of corneal infection with daily and extended cosmetic hydrogel lens wear. Two companion studies first estimated the relative risk of infection in a case-control study and then attempted to estimate the incidence of ulcerative keratitis for both modes of contact lens use. Schein et al.[31] identified 86 patients with corneal infections associated with contact lens wear and matched them with controls. Use of daily- or extended-wear hydrogel contact lenses under closed-eye (extended-wear) conditions resulted in a statistically significant increase in risk of infection (nine-fold for daily wear and 10- to 15-fold for extended wear). Moreover, the risk of infection appeared to increase with each additional night

TABLE 12-1. *Estimated Incidence of Corneal Infection Associated with Modes of Contact Lens Wear as Reported in Several Studies from 1966 to 1991*

Study (Year)	Estimated Incidence/10,000 Patient Years		
	Cosmetic Daily Wear	Cosmetic Extended Wear	Aphakic Extended Wear
Dixon (1996)[16]	2	—	—
Eichenbaum (1982)[24]	—	—	400
Spoor (1982)[25]	—	—	143
Holden (1986)[28]	—	7–100	—
Chalupa (1987)[27]	1	3	—
Weissman (1987)[26]	25	150	—
Contact Lens Institute (1989)[32]	4	21	—
MacRae (1991)[30]	7	41	54
Means	8	54	199
Approximate percentage	0.1	0.5	2

Source: Modified with permission from BA Weissman, BJ Mondino: Corneal infections secondary to contact lens wear. p. 255. In AJ Tomlinson (ed): Complications of Contact Lens Wear. Mosby–Year Book, St. Louis, 1992.

of contact lens wear. Poggio et al.[32] surveyed all practicing ophthalmologists in a five-state area (in New England) to identify all new cases of corneal infection with contact lens wear over a specific 4-month period. The denominator of the fraction was estimated from a telephone survey of 4,178 households in the same geographic area. The annualized incidence of corneal infection was 20.9/10,000 for extended wear and 4.1/10,000 for daily wear.

This large collection of data has been summarized (Table 12-1). Clearly, the risk of infection while wearing contact lenses is really quite low, but a substantial increase in risk occurs when the lenses are used on an extended-wear basis. Across the eight studies summarized here, covering 25 years of experience, the incidence of infection with cosmetic daily-wear contact lenses is only approximately 0.1%. The cosmetic use of extended wear increases this incidence to approximately 0.5%, and aphakic extended wear appears to be even more potentially hazardous, at approximately 2%.

OCULAR DEFENSE FACTORS

The blinking action of the lid and the flow of tears over the anterior segment of the eye mechanically remove micro-organisms. Tears are relatively cool and nutrient poor, and they contain various antibacterial substances, such as lysozyme, β-lysin, lactoferrin, and mucus, which may envelope micro-organisms. Tears also contain secretory immunoglobulin A as well as components of the alternative pathway of complement, which can trap and coat micro-organisms, suppress adhesion, and alter binding to the surface antigens of the microbe, resulting in lysis and enhanced phagocytosis. A more detailed discussion of these events can be found in Chapter 6.

The epithelium itself poses a formidable mechanical barrier to most microbes; only *Corynebacterium diphtheriae*, *Listeria* spp., *Neisseria gonorrhoeae*, and *Haemophilus aegyptius* (Koch-Weeks bacillus) are believed able to invade the intact corneal epithelium.[33,34]

It is thought that the normal ocular microbial flora of the conjunctiva and ocular adnexa exist in a stable balance between proliferation and control by the various indigenous antibacterial factors. *Staphylococci* and diphtheroids predominated in ocular cultures from 10,271 individuals aged 1–90 years.[35] These normal flora also protect the tissues from colonization by organisms of greater virulence and pathogenic potential.

RISK FACTORS

Certain risk factors are believed to encourage the infectious process. Several specific concerns have been raised about corneal infection with contact lens wear.

Extended Wear

The term *extended wear* derives from the concept that contact lens wear can be *extended* through one or more sleep cycles before cleaning and disinfection. The concept should be distinguished from *continuous wear*, which means that the lens is never removed for routine cleaning.

Patients (as opposed to clinicians) probably began the extension of contact lens wear. Anecdotal reports of the rare patient napping or sleeping with PMMA contact lenses still on the eye, perhaps parked on the sclera, were common 30 and 40 years ago.

Soon after hydrogel contact lenses were introduced for correction of refractive error, these devices were being used as bandages to treat diseases of the anterior segment, with the lenses often worn continuously.[36] Complications were common, but disasters were few. Dohlman et al.[37] found that 11 of 278 bandage soft lens patients developed corneal infiltrates. Four patients had definite infections, resulting in permanent damage to the eyes. These authors concluded, however, that the advantages of therapeutic soft lenses on a continuous basis in the treatment of eye disease far outweighed the risks.

Permalens (Cooper Vision, Fairport, NY) (perfilcon A) was developed in 1970 by DeCarle in England. This hydrogel contact lens appears to be the first produced solely for extended wear and was originally fitted very small in diameter and steep in relation to the corneal curvature. The FDA approved two hydrogel contact lens designs for aphakic extended-wear use in this country in June 1979 (Permalens and Hydrocurve [Wesley-Jessen, Inc., Chicago, IL]); other materials and designs for aphakic and phakic (original FDA approval in January 1981) patients followed over the next several years.[38]

Early clinical reports of the U.S. experience suggested that this form of contact lens wear was a success.[39-41] Complications occurred, but the risks appeared similar to those encountered with daily wear of contact lenses. The benefit of patient convenience led to much satisfaction for phakic and aphakic patients, perhaps justifying small risks.

Another clinical trial in the United Kingdom also concluded that continual wear of a particular soft contact lens (Sauflon 85) for 20 weeks was innocuous for 20 subjects.[42,43] Although several corneal functions were monitored, these authors found only a decrease in corneal sensitivity and an increase in lens deposits. No significant corneal swelling, infections, or other complications were noted.

Cooper and Constable's report[21] was perhaps the first indication of a problem. Zantos and Holden[44] (also in Australia) then reported on their study of 35 patients who wore a variety of contact lenses on a continuous-wear basis for up to 2 years. Originally intending to enroll 100 patients in a trial of this mode of contact lens wear, they observed multiple physiologic complications, including corneal edema, neovascularization, microcysts, 12 instances of acute red-eye reactions, and several infections. Three patients had small marginal ulcers and one developed multiple small central epithelial lesions, which later coalesced into a large central ulcer. Every patient who attempted continuous wear experienced some difficulty that resulted in an interruption of lens wear, and the study, therefore, was not extended beyond the first 35 patients.

Another report detailed the disastrous experience (multiple episodes of severe keratitis) of patients in Germany and Japan fitted with early silicone elastomer lenses for extended wear.[45]

As extended wear proliferated throughout North America in the early 1980s, the original glowing reports faded and the reality predicted by the observations of Cooper and Constable[21] and Zantos and Holden[44] became clear. Several reports in the early 1980s provided strong evidence that extended wear was associated with a higher rate of corneal infection in aphakic and phakic patients.[14,15,23-27,46,47]

Mondino and associates[14] studied 40 patients with corneal infections associated with contact lens wear over a 21-month period. Eleven of these patients wore lenses intended for daily wear, and all were found to be noncompliant with good contact lens care (e.g., eight patients reported occasionally sleeping with their lenses). Twenty-nine patients used extended-wear hydrogels (wearing their lenses from 3 days to 30 months), and 12 patients were considered compliant with the contemporary lens care guidelines. Of the noncompliant 17, the most common defect in compliance was microbial contamination of their care systems. This study highlights the conclusion that must be reached from the literature reviewed in this section: Specific risk factors for corneal infection during contact lens wear include sleeping with contact lenses on the eyes and noncompliance with contact lens care and hygiene.

Because approximately 30 million people in this country (perhaps 60 million throughout the world) now wear contact lenses,[48] often for extended wear, it is not surprising that many believe that contact lens–related microbial keratitis has the potential of becoming an important worldwide public health problem. Approximately 30% of all corneal ulcers treated at three centers were found to be related to contact lens wear: 196/658 between October 1982 and June 1986 seen at the Bascom-Palmer Eye Institute (Florida);[49] 60/191 between July 1983 and December 1984 seen at the Wills Eye Hospital (Pennsylvania);[50] and 136/397 between June 1982 and December 1985 seen at the Massachusetts Eye and Ear Infirmary.[51] Furthermore, extended wear of hydrogel contact lenses was associated with the majority of these infections at all centers.

Wilhelmus[22] suggested that the incidence of contact lens–associated microbial keratitis was increasing. A follow-up study at the Wills Eye Hospital indeed found that more than 40% of corneal ulcers treated in 1988 and 1989 were associated with contact lens wear.[52] Of those using contact lenses for cosmesis, 21/44 (48%) used their lenses for extended wear in this study.

Such concerns eventually led the CLI, an organization of the senior administrators of the major contact lens manufacturers in the United States, to sponsor two major epidemiologic studies of corneal infection and contact lens wear. These studies confirmed that extended wear of hydrogel contact lenses significantly increases the risk of corneal infection.[31,32]

Oxygen

Oxygen tension (in mm Hg) is found by multiplying the percentage of oxygen in the air by the barometric pressure (water vapor only slightly contaminates this calculation). As oxygen accounts for approximately 21% of the atmosphere and sea level pressure is given as 760 mm Hg, normal sea-level oxygen tension is approximately 155 mm Hg.

Polse and Mandell[53] proposed that there was a *critical oxygen tension* (COT) for the anterior corneal surface, below which corneal metabolism is compromised. By use of a goggle through which they passed gases of specified oxygen concentrations and observation of subsequent corneal swelling, these authors suggested that the COT was 11–19 mm Hg. Polse and Mandell's COT represents approximately 2% of the oxygen tension at sea level. Later human goggle studies, with better controls and additional subjects, increased the COT to 40–70 mm Hg (5–10% O_2).[54,55]

Alternative corneal functions, however, can be used to define other values for the COT. Millodot and O'Leary[56] found that a depression exists in human corneal sensitivity if anterior oxygen tension falls below 60 mm Hg. In rabbits, Uniacke et al.[57] found that epithelial glycogen was mobilized when the anterior oxygen tension was less than 40 mm Hg. Hamano et al.[58] found an increase in the production of lactate and a decrease in epithelial mitosis if the oxygen tension was less than 100 mm Hg. Masters[59] found changes in the epithelial mitochondria redox state less than 75 mm Hg.

Holden and Mertz[60] used contact lenses of known oxygen transmissibilities (Dk/t) (on a limited number of subjects) to determine the critical Dk/t. They suggested that human corneal swelling could be precluded by use of contact lenses with Dk/t values of 24×10^{-11} cm ml O_2/second ml mm Hg for daily-wear conditions or 87×10^{-11} cm ml O_2/second ml mm Hg for extended wear. Either situation presumably permits an oxygen tension of 40–70 mm Hg or more under the contact lenses. No hydrogel contact lens comes even close to the Holden-Mertz extended-wear critical Dk/t value, however, and few meet the daily-wear criterion. Silicone elastomers provide Dk/t values that surpass these criteria,[61,62] but these contact lenses are no longer generally available. New silicone hydrogels should, however, provide Dk/t values that approach these criteria.[63]

It is valuable to note that human corneal oxygen use[64] and oxygenation of the palpebral conjunctiva[65] vary substantially from individual to individual, thus limiting the precision of such predictions for specific patients.

Does hypoxia at the corneal surface result in compromise of the epithelium, which then secondarily becomes less able to resist microbial infection?[66] Although hypoxia causes all sorts of metabolic problems for the cornea, resulting in multiple changes in the epithelium, stroma, and endothelium, the link between these problems and infection per se has yet to be established.[67,68] It is also clear, however, that all extended wear, from a wearing schedule of 28 nights to only four nights in a row, causes ocular complications. No severe infections were encountered in one study, but epithelial microcysts, red-eye reactions, SPS, and other changes occurred at similar rates in several wearing schedules.[69]

Compliance

Another identified risk factor is that of noncompliance with contact lens care techniques. Mondino et al.[14] provided a definition of compliance with regard to contact lens wear. A compliant patient:

- Washes hands before any contact lens manipulations
- Appropriately uses an FDA-approved contact lens care system in a manner in agreement with the manufacturer's published guidelines and good hygiene
- Adheres to the recommended contact lens–wearing schedule for either daily or extended wear
- Is found to have no microbial contamination of the contact lens solutions and cases

Wilson et al.[20] established the link between poor contact lens care and hygiene and corneal infection by demonstrating the same serotype of *Pseudomonas* in corneal ulcers and the contact lens care systems of their patients. Others have since confirmed these results.[15,70] Garwood presented data suggesting that the incidence of corneal infection increases more than 10-fold when cleaning and disinfection techniques are not employed with daily-wear use of disposable hydrogel contact lenses.[71]

Collins and Carney[72] and Chun and Weissman[73] studied compliance in contact lens wear. They found that 40–70% of contact lens wearers were noncompliant by history!

Several authors have studied microbial contamination of contact lens solutions and cases. Pitts and Krachmer[74] cultured the contact lens cases and conjunctiva of 29 patients and found that 10 (34%) had contaminated cases despite use of heat disinfection. Donzis et al.[75] cultured all elements of the contact lens care systems of 100 asymptomatic contact lens users, including 38 rigid lens users and 62 hydrogel users (50 for daily wear and 12 for extended wear). More than 50% of these patients had microbial contamination in some element of their care system; the microbes found by culture included potential pathogenic bacteria, such as gram-negative *Pseudomonas* and *Serratia*, gram-positive *Staphylococcus* and *Bacillus*, as well as two cultures of the protozoan *Acanthamoeba*.

Campbell and Caroline[76] believe that even patients who use care regimens compliantly may not be able to eliminate microbes from their care systems. They suggest that care systems that are effective during manufacturer studies may later become ineffective in the home environment because the bacteria encountered are more resistant, through development of bacterial biofilm. Thirty-nine of 45 patients studied used their disinfection techniques correctly, but 29% of the patients using heat disinfection, 50% of those using peroxide disinfection, and 75% of those using chemical disinfection had bacteria recovered from their contact lens cases.

Microbes adhere to contact lens surfaces, most likely by formation of biofilms. This raises the issue of the lens acting as a vector, transferring pathogenic agents from the contaminated case or solutions directly to the ocular surface. *Pseudomonas* appears to be responsible for one-half to two-thirds of culture-positive corneal infections in contact lens wearers. Therefore, investigators have studied the ability of several subtypes of this particular microorganism to attach to corneas as well as to new and worn, rigid and hydrogel, high– and low–water content, and ionic and nonionic contact lenses. However, the exact role of bacterial adherence in the pathogenesis of corneal infection has yet to be clearly described.[77] It seems unlikely that bacteria themselves stuck in a biofilm on a lens surface might infect an eye, but their progeny might do so.

Rauschi and Rogers[78] suggested that hydrogel contact lens wear itself did not appear to substantially change the ocular flora, and Gopinathan et al.[79] concluded that extended wear also does not change the microbiological contamination of worn contact lenses. Høvding,[80] however, found that the conjunctival presence of gram-negative bacteria appeared to increase during contact lens wear.

The source of these microbes is still unclear. Bacteria cultured from the healthy (non–lens-wearing) eye are usually those found also on the skin and in the upper respiratory tract (i.e., staphylococci and diphtheroids), and these have indeed been associated with corneal infection. Schein et al.,[51] however, point out that the relative paucity of corneal infections involving enteric bacteria (such as *Escherichia coli*, *Proteus*, and *Klebsiella*) argues against fecal contamination. However, wet areas in the bath and kitchen, such as faucets and sinks, are often contaminated with gram-negative bacteria (specifically *Pseudomonas*) and packaged meat may harbor *Serratia*; these may be the reservoirs for such bacteria. Wilcox et al.[81] presented data that suggests that gram-negative bacteria indeed derive from the domestic water supply, whereas other bacteria most likely have the lid margins as their source. *Acanthamoeba*, on the other hand, is ubiquitous.

Despite the common nature of noncompliance across all forms of contact lens care (suggested by history and documented by contamination of care systems), the reported incidence figures suggest that corneal infection is rare, at least until lenses are used for extended wear.

Blepharitis

Patients presenting for initial or continued contact lens care who show signs of blepharitis or dacryocystis are believed to be at greater risk of infection. This is because they clearly have a load of pathogenic microbes in close proximity to the ocular surface, which is presumed to be already laboring under the mechanical and physiologic stress of contact lens wear. Signs of acute blepharitis include inflammation of the lid margins with yellow or frothy exudates or dry flaky debris on the eyelashes. Chronic blepharitis also shows meibomian gland inspissation, with telangiectatic and dilated blood vessels, and perhaps small irregularities in the lid margin (Fig. 12-10). The tear film is abnormal. The bulbar conjunctiva may be white and quiet, or inflamed; the cornea may be clear or may exhibit SPS. Small, marginal limbal sterile ulcers or phlyctenules may present, and some patients have recurrent styes and chalazia. Some patients are symptomatic, especially those who have marginal ulcers, phlyctenules, or chalazia, but others may have no specific complaints.

Although corneal phlyctenules and peripheral infiltrates may initially be sterile, it is presumed that any epithelial defect increases the risk of a secondary direct infection, especially when bandaged by a contact lens and considering the proximity of available microbes. In addition, the tear film is often compromised in blepharitis. This is partially owing to interference with the normal production of sebum from the meibomian glands and the rain of bacterial toxins and metabolic waste products falling into the palpebral aperture, but may also be related to mechanical irregularities in the apposition of the diseased lid margins to the globe.

Staphylococcus spp. are known to be important agents in blepharitis, but many other microbes may be involved, including other bacteria and even arthropods such as lice or *Demodex folliculorum*.

Patients who have acne rosacea are particularly at risk for blepharitis (usually associated with *S. aureus*), show corneal neovascularization, and are also more at risk for corneal ulceration and infection even when no contact lenses are worn.

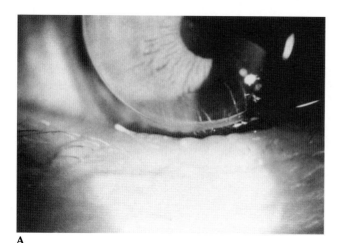

A

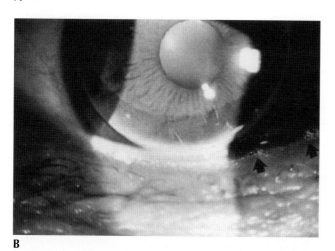

B

FIG. 12-10. *Mild blepharitis at the lower eyelid margin of a male rigid gas-permeable cosmetic contact lens wearer. **(A)** Notching (chronic) and **(B)** frothing (acute) (arrows) aspects of blepharitis are seen with **(A)** white and **(B)** colbalt blue illuminations.*

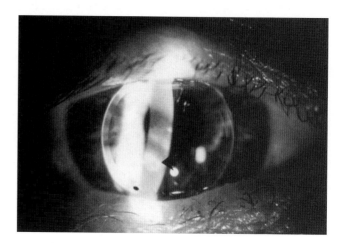

FIG. 12-11. *Apparently full-thickness epithelial layer break or abrasion (arrow) in the inferior cornea of a woman wearing rigid gas-permeable contact lenses for daily-wear correction of severe keratoconus. Patient reported only mild foreign-body sensation. No infiltration was seen, and this lesion healed almost totally with antibiotic coverage in 24 hours.*

Diabetes Mellitus

Diabetes mellitus has been suggested as a risk factor for corneal infection, specifically when contact lenses are used for extended wear. Eichenbaum et al.[24] studied 100 aphakic patients who wore hydrogel contact lenses on an extended-wear basis, and all three patients who were diabetic developed infections. A fourth patient, who also had cancer of the colon, also developed a corneal infection. None of 135 control patients wearing spectacles (including eight diabetics) developed corneal infections. Spoor et al.[25] found that their data agreed with this conclusion.

Diabetic patients have systemic metabolic abnormalities that place them at greater risk for microbial infections. Millodot and O'Leary[82] determined that contact lens wear and diabetes specifically result in abnormal fragility of the corneal epithelial layer.

Epithelial Trauma

Epithelial trauma that occurs while wearing (Fig. 12-11), removing, or inserting a contact lens may play a role in subsequent corneal infection. As noted in the Ocular Defense Factors section, the intact corneal epithelium presents a substantial barrier to infection. Before a microbe can establish itself as a colony, it must adhere to its target. Experimental bacterial inoculation of linear abrasions has been effective in first increasing adherence of *P. aeruginosa* to the cornea and then producing corneal ulceration.[83–85] Stern et al.[86] showed that *Pseudomonas* adheres better to injured or exposed basal epithelial cells than to an intact epithelial surface or even to exposed bare corneal stroma.

Direct damage may not be necessary. An electron microscopy study of primate corneal epithelia after use of excessively thick hydrogels for daily or extended wear showed epithelial thinning (loss of superficial cells and flattening of the remaining ones), edema, and degenerative cytoplasmic changes.[87]

Adams et al.[46] found that five of six patients presenting with corneal infections associated with extended wear of hydrogel lenses reported recent manipulations of their lenses. These authors speculated that the manipulation might have led to epithelial defects that predisposed these patients to the infectious process. Mondino et al.,[14] however, could not support this particular hypothesis with data from their series.

Minor epithelial erosion (see Fig. 12-11) undoubtedly is a common occurrence in any contact lens practice.[88] What is not clear, however, is why such lesions appear to be clinically relatively innocuous when contact lenses are used on a daily-wear basis and if, or how, the role of such lesions changes during extended wear. Some believe that treatment of minor epithelial staining with prophylactic topical antibiotics represents cautious practice, whereas others think that this practice risks encouraging resistance among local bacteria and hence eventual superinfection, and that the toxicity of some antibiotics may actually prolong the healing process.

Steroid Use

Topical corticosteroid use is generally recognized as a predisposing factor for corneal microbial infection,[37,89] particularly with herpes, *Pseudomonas*, and fungi. These drugs suppress immunologic defense mechanisms and inflammatory reactions (as well as increasing the risks of collateral glaucoma and cataract formation), and by doing so may also mask the severity of an infection. Chalupa et al.[27] identified inappropriate steroid therapy as a major factor contributing to the severity of corneal infection after contact lens wear.

Therapeutic or Bandage Use of Hydrogel Contact Lenses

Therapeutic hydrogel contact lenses are used to protect the corneal surface, facilitate healing, and relieve pain in patients with ocular surface disease. Conditions often managed with hydrogel bandage lenses include symptomatic relief of filamentary keratitis or bullous keratopathy, persistent nonhealing epithelial defects (including those found after refractive surgery procedures), exposed sutures (e.g., after keratoplasty), neurotrophic or exposure keratitis, keratitis sicca, and ocular pemphigoid. All these situations involve disruption of the epithelial surface barrier. Many patients are elderly, some are diabetic, and often they are using topical corticosteroids. The combination of known risk factors places these patients at particular risk, and it is not surprising that infection is a major concern in this group of patients.[37,90]

For example, six corneal ulcers (bacterial and fungal by culture) developed in 38 eyes treated with therapeutic hydrogel contact lenses for severe epithelial diseases, including Stevens-Johnson and Sjögren's syndromes, ocular pemphigoid, neurotrophic keratitis, herpes simplex keratitis, and ocular burns.[91] Several factors were thought to contribute to these infections, including concurrent dry eye, use of antibiotics and steroids, and microbial contamination of a bottle of sodium chloride drops in one

case. See Chapter 21 for an in-depth discussion of therapeutic or bandage lenses.

Smoking

The CLI study of corneal infection associated with contact lens wear investigated a number of potential risk factors. These included age, gender, and race of the contact lens user; age of the contact lens and type of fit (initial or replacement); length of time since last professional evaluation; and identification of providing professional. The only factor that appeared to have some statistical relation to corneal infection was smoking, which was statistically significant for extended-wear use of contact lenses and almost significant for daily-wear use of lenses.[31] The later data of Cutter et al.[92] supported this observation about occurrence of noninfectious corneal infiltrates in association with hydrogel lens wear. The mechanism remains unclear.

Other Potential Risk Factors

Some clinical reports have suggested additional risk factors, such as travel and warm weather,[27,93] but these have not been scientifically verified.

Micro-Organisms

Humans live, and mostly thrive, among a large collection of microbiological life. Some forms of these micro-organisms are symbiotic, aiding humans in such processes as the digestion of food and producing vitamins as by-products of their own development. Others ignore human life, invisible to their existence. Some microbes are well known as human pathogens; many do not usually cause difficulties but are capable of inducing human disease if given the appropriate opportunity.

Studies of the normal flora of the ocular surface suggest a predominance of staphylococci and diphtheroids.[35] Species of greater potential virulence are only rarely encountered.

Neisser was perhaps the first to isolate and describe a bacterial ocular pathogen, the gonococcus, in 1879. Koch observed the second such microbe a few years later while studying the etiology of cholera in Egypt, and Weeks later isolated this bacterium, now known as the Koch-Weeks bacillus or *Haemophilus aegyptius*. Morax then isolated a diplobacillus from a case of subacute angular conjunctivitis in 1897; this bacterium was independently identified by Axenfeld and is known as *Moraxella lacunata*.[94]

Many bacteria have since been identified as potential corneal pathogens; those now particularly associated with corneal infection after contact lens wear are discussed in the following Bacteria section.

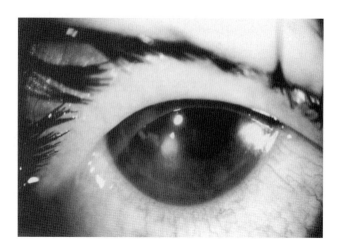

FIG. 12-12. *Small corneal ulcer in eye of woman who wore hydrogel contact lenses for cosmetic extended wear. Although this lesion appears clinically consistent with a gram-positive bacterial infection, in culture it was positive for* Pseudomonas aeruginosa.

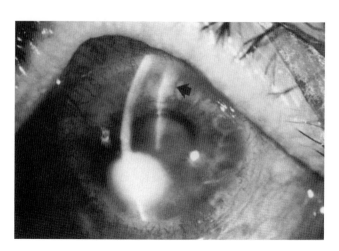

FIG. 12-13. *Large corneal ulcer culture-positive for* Staphylococcus aureus. *This elderly patient did not wear contact lenses but may have been diabetic (note iris rubeosis, arrow).*

Bacteria

Bacteria have been classically grouped according to their morphology (rod, spiral, or coccus); their reaction to Gram's, Giemsa, and other stains; and other aspects of their biochemistry (e.g., coagulase-negative, fastidious nutrition). Modern microbiology has only begun to organize its taxonomy around information retrieved from genetic studies.

It is not possible to make a specific and reliable, etiologic diagnosis based solely on the clinical appearance of a corneal ulcer (Fig. 12-12). Corneal ulcers associated with gram-positive bacteria, however, are usually smaller, more localized and distinct, and less purulent and aggressive than those associated with gram-negative bacteria. Nevertheless, with no or improper therapy, perforation may occur within several days even when gram-positive bacteria are involved.
Gram-Positive Bacteria *Staphylococcus epidermidis* and *S. aureus* are very common gram-positive inhabitants of healthy human skin and, in particular, the eyelid. *S. aureus* causes a wide variety of pyogenic (pus-forming) infections and is a common cause of food poisoning. *S. aureus* is also well established as a cause of conjunctivitis and blepharitis, and has been associated with corneal marginal infiltrates and phlyctenules.[7] Both *Staphylococcus* species have also been frequently cultured from corneal infections, with and without contact lens wear (Fig. 12-13).

Streptococcus pneumoniae and *S. pyogenes* are two other gram-positive bacteria commonly cultured from corneal ulcers. *S. pneumoniae* (the pneumococcus), in particular, exists as part of the flora of the upper respiratory tract in the healthy adult population, and this can serve as a reservoir for pneumonia as well as ear and eye infections. *S. pneumoniae* was first identified as a cause of

human keratitis in 1893,[95] and this bacterium has long been considered a common cause of central corneal infections. *Streptococcus* spp. corneal infections commonly produce hypopyon and are thought to be more aggressive than *S. aureus*, which is, in turn, more aggressive than *S. epidermidis*. Under certain conditions (e.g., topical steroid treatment), *Streptococcus viridans* (another common normal inhabitant of the upper respiratory tract) may multiply under an intact epithelium to assume an arborizing crystalline appearance.[96,97] (One clinically similar case has been reported after application of topical steroids and a therapeutic hydrogel lens to treat complications of penetrating keratoplasty; culture was positive, however, for gram-negative *Haemophilus aphrophilus*.[98]) A study of more than 3,500 corneal ulcer cultures (from 1938 to 1968) seen in New York suggested that 85% were associated with either *Staphylococcus* or *Streptococcus* spp. (only 194 positive cultures [5%] of *P. aeruginosa* were found).[35]

Another gram-positive bacterium, *Bacillus* spp., occasionally causes corneal infection and severe endophthalmitis (*Bacillus cereus,* in particular, has emerged as a potentially virulent intraocular pathogen).[22,70,99] *Bacillus* has also been found in the contact lens care systems of approximately 5% of asymptomatic patients,[75] and it forms spores that are resistant to heat and many forms of chemical disinfectants. Heat of 121°C for 15 minutes, or 5 hours of exposure to 3% hydrogen peroxide, however, may eliminate viable forms of this bacteria.[70]
Gram-Negative Bacteria *Pseudomonas* (principally *aeruginosa*) is a gram-negative, slender, rod-shaped bacterium capable of producing devastating corneal infections. *Pseudomonas* is a ubiquitous micro-organism in

nature, distributed widely in soil, water, plants, the mammalian gut, and sewage. In the home, *P. aeruginosa* is often found in and around sinks and other wet areas. It can use many different organic compounds (including atmospheric carbon dioxide) as a source of carbon and energy and is able to contaminate fluorescein solutions, eye cosmetics, saline, and distilled water. *Pseudomonas* rarely causes systemic infections in healthy individuals but can become a major pathogen when the opportunity presents, causing pneumonia in myelosuppressed cancer patients and sepsis after burns. It is a common cause of death in victims of cystic fibrosis.

It has been thought that *Pseudomonas* spp. are not able to invade the intact epithelium but aggressively destroy corneal tissues once a wound has allowed adhesion by a sufficient load of these bacteria.[84,85] (Other research contests this view, suggesting that at least some strains are more toxic than others and can invade intact epithelium.[100]) *Pseudomonas* liberates endotoxin, exotoxins, and proteolytic enzymes (proteases) and, thus, can lead to a rapidly progressive corneal ulcer characterized by melting and purulence. Patients with *Pseudomonas* corneal infections often present with large epithelial defects, dense anterior stromal infiltrates, severe stromal edema, and mucoid material clinging to the lesion (Fig. 12-14). Ring infiltrates also may be seen (Fig. 12-15). The host immunoreaction to the stromal infection may be partially responsible for the rapid, massive, and persistent destruction of corneal structure in this disease. Although the organism is resistant to many antibiotics, prompt use of fortified aminoglycosides or commercial-strength fluoroquinolones have proved helpful in treatment of *Pseudomonas* infections.

Serratia marcescens is another gram-negative rod also capable of liberating endotoxin, but corneal infections are generally not as serious as those associated with *Pseudomonas*. *Serratia*, however, can develop resistance to certain preservatives often used in contact lens care systems, such as benzalkonium chloride and chlorhexidine.[101]

The endotoxin released by gram-negative bacteria, such as *Pseudomonas* and *Serratia*, is heat resistant and, therefore, may not be eliminated from contact lens care systems even after thermal disinfection has killed all bacteria. Endotoxin is itself immunogenic and, even in the absence of viable bacteria, has been shown to cause corneal ring infiltrates.[102]

Moraxella (gram-negative diplobacilli) (principally *Moraxella lacunata*) is well known as an ocular pathogen but is usually associated with corneal infection in debilitated individuals, such as chronic alcoholics, and have only occasionally been identified in corneal infection associated with contact lens wear. *Moraxella* spp. often cause angular blepharitis in children.

Other Bacteria Although the usual bacterial pathogens detailed in the previous Gram-Positive Bacteria and Gram-

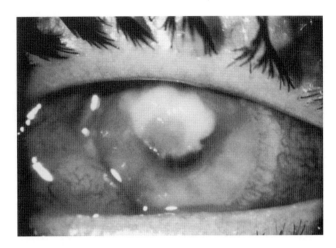

FIG. 12-14. *Large corneal ulcer (culture positive for* Pseudomonas aeruginosa*) in the eye of a patient who used disposable hydrogel contact lenses for extended wear. Note characteristic gelatinous material clinging to the lesion.*

Negative Bacteria sections are well known and are recovered from the vast majority of corneal infections, the clinician must always be on guard for the rare contaminant. Several other bacteria have occasionally been cultured from contact lens care systems and corneal infections. *Propionibacterium acnes* is an example of a gram-positive bacterium occasionally cultured from corneal infections after contact lens wear. Similarly, gram-negative organisms occasionally found by culture include the enteric bacteria *Klebsiella* and *Proteus*. Occasionally, corneal infections give mixed (Fig. 12-16) or negative (Fig. 12-17) culture results.

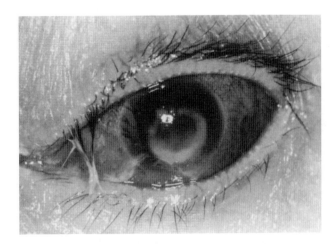

FIG. 12-15. *Large culture-positive* Pseudomonas aeruginosa *infection of the central cornea, showing a ring infiltrate. Patient was aphakic and used a hydrogel contact lens for extended wear.*

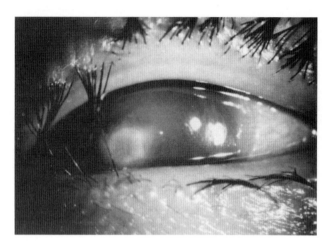

FIG. 12-16. *Corneal ulcer that yielded mixed culture results* (Staphylococcus aureus *and* Pseudomonas aeruginosa) *from a woman wearing hydrogel contact lenses. This patient was not compliant with good contact lens care.*

Fungi

Although several authors have reported fungal deposits in hydrogel contact lenses, corneal infection has been very rare. Wilson and Ahearn[103] reported 11 instances of fungal lens contamination in 450 patients using hydrogel contact lenses for extended wear during a clinical experience of 5 years. These authors found only two instances of associated corneal fungal infection, but the same organism was found in the lens growths and eye lesions in both these events. One fungus was *Fusarium verticilloides* and the other *Curvularia lunata*. Several additional patients

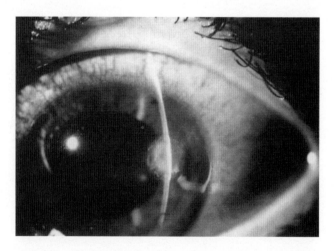

FIG. 12-17. *Corneal ulcer in the eye of a patient who used hydrogel lenses for cosmetic daily wear. Cultures were negative. One should suspect microbial etiology and treat such lesions aggressively even in the absence of positive cultures.*

experienced ocular injection, SPS, and irritation while wearing these contaminated lenses, and the authors thought it likely that liberated fungal toxins were involved. Other fungi commonly identified in human corneal ulcers, but not specific to contact lens wear, are *Candida* (a yeast) and *Aspergillus*. Penley et al.[104] suggested that either heat disinfection or at least 45 minutes of soaking in 3% hydrogen peroxide eliminates viable fungi from contaminated hydrogel contact lenses.

Fungal ulcers can clinically appear chronic and indolent or acute and severe, depending on the exact organism and the host status. They are often difficult to diagnose clinically because cultures are frequently negative. Biopsy can be helpful. Fungal corneal infections may demonstrate feathery borders (hyphate edges), raised infiltrates, endothelial plaque, and satellite lesions by biomicroscopy.

Several antifungal agents are available, including a commercial ophthalmic preparation of natamycin, and specially prepared amphotericin B or miconazole ophthalmic solutions. Treatment is often difficult, and results are unpredictable.

Viruses

Neither herpetic nor adenoviral corneal infections are common occurrences in ophthalmic practice. Herpetic corneal infection is considered a major cause of blindness. Herpes simplex is known as the *great imitator* of corneal infection and should be considered in the differential diagnosis of most corneal diseases (see Fig. 12-5), especially when a dendritic lesion or loss of corneal sensitivity is present. Corneal disease related to adenoviral infection, whether explosive epidemic keratoconjunctivitis or milder varieties, is self-limiting. Although transient subepithelial infiltrates and punctate subepithelial scars are common sequelae, this infection rarely leads to severe permanent vision loss. Both viral infections are occasionally encountered in patients concomitantly wearing contact lenses and could be spread through poor disinfection of diagnostic contact lenses (B. Christensen, personal communication, 1991), but neither has been etiologically linked to any form of contact lens wear.

The human immunodeficiency virus has been isolated from the tears, conjunctiva, and corneas of infected individuals,[105] but there have been no documented cases suggesting that this disease can be transmitted through any form of ocular contact or contact lens wear. It is mandatory, however, to disinfect all office instruments and diagnostic contact lenses between patients and to follow Centers for Disease Control and Prevention guidelines for all patient care activities.

It is intuitively likely, moreover, that patients with human immunodeficiency virus infection (as well as other immunodeficient states) are at some increased risk for microbial keratitis while wearing contact lenses, and if such infection develops, the initiation of the disease and its course may be potentiated by immune system compromise.[106] See Chapter 11 for additional information on viral infections and contact lens wear.

Amoebae

Acanthamoebae are a group of free-living protozoa found ubiquitously in soil, water, and air across a broad range of climate and environmental conditions. They exist in two forms, mobile trophozoites and cysts. Cysts have a double wall, which is responsible for this micro-organism's impressive resistance.

Corneal infection associated with *Acanthamoeba* was first reported in 1974.[107] Although only a small number were reported through 1981, a dramatic increase was seen in the middle of that decade, particularly in contact lens wearers. The observation that *Acanthamoeba* keratitis occurs in patients who had previously healthy eyes but used homemade saline as part of their contact lens care was made in 1985.[108]

Although the assertion has been contested,[109] infection is attributed to exposure to nonsterile water sources during contact lens use or swimming, including tap water, well water, water from a home purification kit, saline intended for intravenous use, and even saliva. Daily wear of hydrogel contact lenses appears to be the primary predisposing mode of lens use, but several other types of contact lens wear have also been associated with this infection, including extended wear of hydrogel lenses, rigid gas-permeable lenses, and hard lenses, and the SoftPerm (Wesley-Jessen, Inc., Chicago, IL) hybrid lens.[110,111]

Stehr-Green et al.[112] suggest that merely rinsing a rigid gas-permeable contact lens in tap water before insertion is a risk factor for this disease. They reviewed the epidemiology of more than a decade of *Acanthamoeba* keratitis in the United States. They studied 208 case reports, of which 189 provided information on suspected risk factors. Contact lenses of all types were worn by 85% of these patients, and 64% of the wearers had a history of use of salt tablet–prepared saline. In this series, patients aged 50 years and more commonly had a concomitant history of ocular trauma.

The clinical features of *Acanthamoeba* infection include a long, progressive history of severe pain and photophobia, central or paracentral infiltrates (early in the disease course), and ring infiltrates (similar in clinical appearance to the ring infiltrates seen in *P. aeruginosa* infection) late in the disease course. Additional signs include a dendriform epithelial lesion (often clinically suggestive of herpetic keratitis), recurrent epithelial breakdown, radial keratoneuritis, and chemosis. An anterior chamber reaction usually occurs, whereas sclerokeratitis occasionally occurs. Initial cultures and smears are often negative unless special techniques (i.e., calcofluor white stain or culturing on nonnutrient agar with an *E. coli* overlay) and deeper biopsy are used. A more detailed discussion of fungal and *Acanthamoeba* keratitis can be found in Chapter 13.

DISTRIBUTION OF MICROBIAL KERATITIS

Patterns of microbial keratitis have been reported from various referral centers in North America and Europe, describing the distribution of culture results from corneal infections in the general population (not restricted to contact lens wearers). Gram-positive bacteria dominate the overall culture results of these studies (Table 12-2); but the

TABLE 12-2. *Comparison of Microbial Keratitis Culture Results 1938–1983* *

	New York Locatcher-Khorazo[94] (1938–1968) 3,535	California Ostler[136] (1947–1976) 134	New York Asbell[137] (1950–1976) 494	Florida Liesegang[138] (1969–1977) 371	Texas Jones[139] (1972–1979) 232	California Ormerod[113] (1972–1983) 186	Total Number (%)
Staphylococcus	1,755	27	239	70	79	95	2,265 (48)
Other gram-positive bacteria	1,341	57	30	70	136	64	1,689 (36)
Pseudomonas	200	18	40	74	57	37	246 (5)
Other gram-negative bacteria	59	22	104	39	46	46	316 (7)
Fungus	2	—	5	134	40	20	201 (4)

*Not specifically contact lens–wearing populations. Column headings list state, study (year), and number of positive cultures. These numbers of positive cultures in the table are the best possible values found in the various cited studies, but some inconsistencies and inaccuracies may exist, probably related to conversion of data from numbers to percentage and back, and to instances of mixed culture results.
Source: Modified with permission from BA Weissman, BJ Mondino: Corneal infections secondary to contact lens wear. p. 255. In AJ Tomlinson (ed): Complications of Contact Lens Wear. Mosby–Year Book, St. Louis 1992.

prevalence of pseudomonal and fungal infections appears to increase in warmer southern latitudes, and staphylococcal and streptococcal infections predominate in cooler northern climates.[113] Systemic associations include alcoholism, diabetes, psychological disturbances, and coma or stupor, both of which lead to corneal exposure. Specific ocular predisposing factors include trauma, corneal surgery, previous herpetic corneal infection, use of topical steroids, dry eye, and exposure keratitis and, of course, contact lens use (most particularly extended wear).

On the other hand, *Pseudomonas* has been noted to account for 50–75% of corneal ulcers (when cultures are positive) across a broad range of studies of cosmetic contact lens wearers in various localities (Table 12-3). It appears that contact lens wear may selectively alter the susceptibility of the normally resistant healthy cornea to infection by this gram-negative bacterium.[114,115] *Staphylococcus* spp. bacteria are the second most common group. Other bacteria, fungi, and protozoa are less commonly encountered but must always be considered in the differential diagnosis.

Several authors have noted that infections associated with the extended or continuous use of *therapeutic* hydrogel *bandage* lenses for treatment of epithelial corneal surface disease appear to be more associated with cultures of gram-positive bacteria (e.g., *Streptococcus* spp.) and unusual micro-organisms (e.g., fungi)[51,90] than with *Pseudomonas* (Table 12-4).

MANAGEMENT

Management of corneal infection with contact lens wear includes prevention, rapid diagnosis, and appropriate treatment.

Prevention

The two principal risk factors identified for corneal infection associated with cosmetic contact lens wear are extended-wear use of contact lenses and poor contact lens care techniques. The therapeutic use of hydrogel contact lenses (as bandages for some corneal diseases) is also considered a third major risk factor, but this risk is often unavoidable. Prevention consists of minimizing the risk to patients by avoiding the use of contact lenses in an extended-wear mode as much as possible. In cases in which such use is necessary (e.g., sometimes in the management of pediatric aphakia or the use of hydrogel lenses as bandages), patients (or their guardians) should provide informed consent and, as alerted to these risks, should present without delay if any signs or symptoms of infec-

tion occur. The number of successive nights of cosmetic extended wear should be also reduced to six or less, if at all possible, in agreement with current FDA guidelines.

Rigid gas-permeable lenses and disposable hydrogel lenses have been proposed for extended wear, with the implied suggestion that these offer improved physiologic results and thus reduce the rate of infection. Experience suggests otherwise.[116–118] Grant and Holden[119] report a persistent incidence of 1% peripheral corneal ulcers with extended-wear use of disposable hydrogel contact lenses. In addition, study of the material properties of three disposable hydrogel contact lens materials indicates that their oxygen permeabilities are identical to those of reusable materials of the same water content.[120]

Compliant and hygienic use of contact lens care regimens and elimination of exposure to nonsterile water (e.g., swimming with contact lenses on the eyes) or any homemade solutions are also important measures in decreasing the risk of infection (particularly by *Acanthamoeba*). Contact lens wear should be discontinued during illness (colds and flu), episodes of ocular irritation, and in the face of ipsilateral or contralateral ocular or adnexal infection.

A third additional preventative measure is routine professional care and supervision. Immunosuppressed or diabetic patients and patients who present with severely compromised tear films, acne rosacea, chronic blepharitis, poor personal hygiene, or use of topical ophthalmic steroids (e.g., to control uveitis) should probably be discouraged from cosmetic contact lens wear. When lenses must be worn for some overriding benefit (e.g., aphakia), these patient populations should restrict their use of contact lenses to daily wear, if at all possible. It is believed that contact lens patients should obtain professional evaluations at scheduled intervals of 6–9 months under normal conditions, and more frequently (e.g., perhaps every 2–4 months) if any increased risk is suspected (e.g., in instances of therapeutic use, after corneal grafts, or with extended wear).

Early Recognition and Diagnosis

Patients must participate actively in their own care. Every contact lens wearer, particularly those who occasionally or regularly sleep with their lenses on, should know the signs and symptoms of corneal infection: ocular pain, photophobia, conjunctival injection, lid edema, tearing, and perhaps discharge or decreased vision. Should any of these occur, the contact lenses should immediately be removed. Because these signs and symptoms can also be associated with many relatively benign complications, some of which may have nothing to do with lens wear

TABLE 12-3. *Distribution of Bacterial Keratitis Among Contact Lens Wearers*

	California Weissman[15] (1984) 13/18	Pennsylvania Galentine[140] (1984) 29/56	Texas Patrinely[141] (1985) 14/14	California Ormerod[113] (1986) 36/42	Florida Alfonso[142] (1986) 64/118	California Mondino[14] (1986) 29/40	Pennsylvania Donnenfeld[50] (1986) 53/136	Sweden Chalupa[27] (1987) 28/25	Florida Koidou-Tsiligianni[49] (1989) 103/196	Massachusetts Schein[31] (1989) 34/60	Pennsylvania Cohen[52] (1991) 44/51	Total Number (%)
Staphylococcus	2	11	6	12	5	14	4	1	16	17	9	97 (22)
Other gram-positive bacteria	1	0	2	8	4	5	13	0	5	5	3	46 (10)
Pseudomonas	9	13	6	17	40	12	20	27	63	15	20	242 (54)
Other gram-negative bacteria	1	0	0	6	10	3	5	0	16	6	4	51 (11)
Fungus	0	1	0	2	2	0	0	0	0	1	3	9 (2)
Amoebae	0	0	0	1	0	0	0	0	0	2	2	5 (1)

Column headings list state, study (year), and number of positive cultures per number of infections. Because of differences in methods of reporting among the several studies and because cultures may yield more than one positive result, the numbers in these tables do not always add to the numbers of total positive cultures.

Source: Modified with permission from BA Weissman, BJ Mondino: Corneal infections secondary to contact lens wear. p. 255. In AJ Tomlinson (ed): Complications of Contact Lens Wear. Mosby–Year Book, St. Louis 1992.

TABLE 12-4. *Gram Stain Classification of Microbes Commonly Associated with Corneal Infection in Contact Lens Wear*

Bacteria
  Gram-negative
    Cocci
      Neisseria gonorrhoeae
      Moraxella spp.
    Bacilli (rods)
      Pseudomonas aeruginosa[a]
      Other *Pseudomonas* spp.
      Serratia marcescens[a]
      Proteus spp.
      Klebsiella spp.
      Escherichia coli
      Enterobacter aerogenes
      Morganella morgagnii
  Gram-positive
    Cocci
      Staphylococcus aureus[a]
      Staphylococcus epidermidis[a]
      Staphylococcus pneumonia[a]
      Streptococcus viridans
      Streptococcus pyogenes
      Enterococcus
      Micrococcus spp.
    Bacilli
      Bacillus spp.
      Propionibacterium acnes
      Corynebacterium spp.
      Mycobacterium spp.
Fungi
  Fusarium[a]
  Aspergillus
  Penicillium
  Curvularia
  Candida (yeast)
Protozoa
  Acanthamoeba spp.
Viruses
  Herpes simplex
  Herpes zoster
  Adenovirus spp.
  Human immunodeficiency virus

[a]Microbes of particular concern.
Source: Modified with permission from BA Weissman, BJ Mondino. Corneal infections secondary to contact lens wear. p. 255. In AJ Tomlinson (ed): Complications of Contact Lens Wear. Mosby–Year Book, St. Louis, 1992.

specifically, patients should be aware that if such changes persist or worsen after lenses have been removed, they should immediately report to an ophthalmic professional.

The ophthalmic clinician must be able to identify an early or potential corneal infection. Any acutely inflamed and painful eye in a patient wearing a contact lens must be considered a medical emergency and the patient should be examined as soon as possible. The observation of an epithelial defect with associated infiltrate, pain, and per-

haps discharge should immediately suggest infectious keratitis. All contact lens wear should be discontinued (both eyes) to minimize risk of the infection becoming bilateral, and the patient managed appropriately.

Treatment

For many years, academic corneal specialists taught that initial management of suspected microbial corneal infection includes corneal scrapings for stains and cultures to do the following:

- Identify the offending pathogen
- Determine its sensitivities to various antibiotics

Immediate microscopic examination of stained slides often assists in early identification. Treatment with antibiotics before culturing is known to decrease the potential information gathered from such laboratory investigations. This could complicate later care should the corneal infection worsen despite initial treatment. Culture media should include blood and chocolate agars, as well as Sabouraud's and thioglycolate media. Jones advocated initiation of antibiotic treatment of bacterial keratitis based on the immediate Gram's stain results, whereas Baum suggested a broad-spectrum, shotgun approach based initially on clinical appearance while awaiting results of laboratory investigations to assist in refinement of the treatment if needed.[121]

Although most academic corneal specialists still agree that cultures should be obtained before initiating medical therapy, some have questioned the need for laboratory investigations (smears, stains, cultures, and antibiotic sensitivity testing) before initiating treatment, especially for small infiltrates or even less-severe ulcers off the visual axis.[122-125]

After cultures have been taken, immediate broad-spectrum antibiotic therapy should be initiated. All contact lens–associated corneal infections should be considered the result of *Pseudomonas aeruginosa* until proved otherwise because of the prevalence of this bacterium in positive cultures and because of its potential catastrophic course without appropriate intervention. The use of topical steroids and patching, therefore, should not be considered for initial management for any contact lens–associated epithelial defect.[27,126] Both appear to worsen the course of any infectious process, especially those of *Pseudomonas* spp., herpes, and fungi.

Presumed bacterial corneal infections usually have been initially treated with broad-spectrum antibiotics (with good gram-negative and gram-positive bacterial coverage), typically combinations of cephalosporins and aminoglycosides, often in fortified form. Specially prepared ophthalmic formulations of vancomycin are used to treat resistant gram-positive bacterial infections. New ophthalmic commercial-strength fluoroquinolone preparations have shown excellent in vitro activity against many common corneal pathogens and have proved effective in treating keratitis as monotherapy with few adverse reactions (Table 12-5).[127–130] Resistance is emerging, however, leading in some instances to treatment failures.[131,132] Clinicians may need to reconsider the use of dual therapy in the near future.

Other newly emerging antibiotics may be more potent (i.e., not requiring fortification), show more broad-spectrum activity, and be less subject to the induction of either toxic host reactions or resistant bacterial subpopulations.

Initial treatment is often modified by the clinical course and by the identification and sensitivity of causative microbes isolated by culture and stain results. Some patients, especially those with severe infections and those who are suspected of being potentially noncompliant, should be hospitalized. Persistent and refractory corneal infections may require these measures[133]:

- Subconjunctival depot antibiotics (in which the medicine slowly leaks back out through the needle tract to bathe the anterior segment of the eye)
- Use of collagen shields presoaked in antibiotics
- Iontophoresis
- Systemic treatment
- Tectonic corneal transplantation to remove the large reservoir of microbial colonization (and thereby improve the effectiveness of medical management)
- Positioning of a conjunctival flap to encourage healing of a sterilized but persistent epithelial defect

More detailed discussions of the treatment of active bacterial infections and of viral, fungal, and protozoan corneal infections are beyond the scope of this chapter. Chapters 11 and 13, and other texts should be consulted.

New Strategies

During bacterial diseases, bacteria release enzymes that can cause tissue damage. New treatment strategies under development are directed at eliminating the effects of these enzymes and the secondary host response (which can lead to additional damage). Such agents include several classes of metalloproteinase inhibitors, inhibitors of leukocyte substances, inhibitors of bacterial substances, and inhibitors of inflammatory mediators.

Healing and Recovery

Bacteria are eliminated from corneal tissue by pharmacologic and host-defense mechanisms. A general optimal duration of antibiotic therapy has not been established

TABLE 12-5. *Fluoroquinolone Antibiotics*[143,144]

Ciprofloxacin 0.3%
Ofloxacin 0.3%
Norfloxacin 0.3%
Lomefloxacin 0.3%

and may indeed differ with different bacterial strains and individual patient immunologic responses. All viable bacteria are usually killed with 1 week of topical therapy; *S. epidermidis* infections may even heal in 5 days. It should be emphasized, however, that *Pseudomonas* corneal ulcers may take up to 22 days to heal.[134] Bacterial components and undigested bacteria may remain at the infection site and inside neutrophils to stimulate continued host response long after all viable micro-organisms have been killed.

Patients who respond well to antimicrobial treatment are usually considered healed when the epithelial defect closes and other signs and symptoms decline. When damaged, Bowman's membrane is replaced by fibrovascular pannus and necrotic tissue is sloughed. Complete re-epithelialization may be followed by partial regression of any neovascularization. An opaque scar may form, composed primarily of disorganized collagen fibrils that gradually remodel over the following months.

Refitting of contact lenses may be reconsidered and may even be indicated for vision rehabilitation perhaps 6 weeks after the eye is stable and quiet after an infection. The practitioner should re-evaluate current contact lens design, prescribing modality (e.g., extended wear) and lens care regimen to reduce the risks of recurrence.

SUMMARY

Corneal infection is a rare but potentially serious complication of contact lens wear. Contact lens wear, especially extended wear, has become an important risk factor in corneal infection. Bacteria (particularly *Pseudomonas* spp. and *Staphylococcus* spp.) are the most common microbes isolated from corneal infections after cosmetic contact lens wear, followed by fungi and protozoa. Therapeutic (bandage) lens use is also particularly hazardous, and the clinician who follows such patients must be particularly alert for potential fungal or gram-positive infections. Viral corneal infections may also occur concomitant with contact lens wear, but there does not appear to be any etiologic linkage. Clinically, observation of a corneal epithelial defect and associated infiltrate in a setting of pain and discharge and with a history of contact lens wear must be presumed to be a microbial corneal infection until proved otherwise. Such an event must be treated as a medical emergency. Management consists initially of prevention, but in the event that signs or symptoms appear, immediate response, rapid diagnosis, and appropriate therapeutic actions are necessary.

REFERENCES

1. Herman J: Clinical management of GPC. Contact Lens Spectrum 2:24, 1987

2. Holden BA, Brennan NA, Efron N, Swarbrick H: The contact lens: physiological considerations. p. 1. In Aquavella JV, Rao GN (eds): Contact Lenses. Lippincott, Philadelphia, 1987

3. Wilhelmus KR. Bacterial keratitis. p. 970. In Pepose JS, Holland GH, Wilhelmus KR (eds): Ocular Infection and Immunity. Mosby–Year Book, St. Louis, 1996

4. Cline D, Hofstetter HW, Griffins JR: Dictionary of Visual Sciences. 3rd ed. Chilton, Radnor, PA, 1980. p. 684

5. Dohlman CH: The function of the corneal epithelium in health and disease. The Jonas S. Friedenwald Memorial Lecture. Invest Ophthalmol 10:383, 1971

6. Stein RM, Clinch TE, Cohen EJ, et al: Infected vs sterile corneal infiltrates in contact lens wearers. Am J Ophthalmol 105:632, 1988

7. Mondino BJ, Dethlefs B: Occurrence of phlyctenules after immunization with ribitol teichoic acid of *Staphylococcus aureus*. Arch Ophthalmol 102:461, 1984

8. Mondino BJ, Groden LR: Conjunctival hyperemia and corneal infiltrates with chemically disinfected soft contact lenses. Arch Ophthalmol 98:1767, 1980

9. Gordon A, Kracher GP: Corneal infiltrates and extended-wear contact lenses. J Am Optom Assoc 56:198, 1985

10. Bates AK, Morris RJ, Stapleton F, et al: "Sterile" corneal infiltrates in contact lens wearers. Eye 3:803, 1989

11. Donshik PC, Suchecki JK, Ehlers WH: Peripheral corneal infiltrates associated with contact lens wear. Trans Am Ophthalmol Soc 93:49, 1995

12. Grant T, Chong MS, Vajdic C, et al: Contact lens induced peripheral ulcers during hydrogel contact lens wear. CLAO J 24:145, 1998

13. Jones DB: Early diagnosis and therapy of bacterial corneal ulcers. Int Ophthalmol Clin 13:1, 1973

14. Mondino BJ, Weissman BA, Farb MD, Pettit TH: Corneal ulcers associated with daily-wear and extended-wear contact lenses. Am J Ophthalmol 102:58, 1986

15. Weissman BA, Mondino BJ, Pettit TH, Hofbauer JD: Corneal ulcers associated with extended-wear soft contact lenses. Am J Ophthalmol 97:476, 1984

16. Dixon JM, Young CA, Baldone JA, et al: Complications associated with the wearing of contact lenses. JAMA 195:901, 1966

17. Freedman H, Sugar J: *Pseudomonas* keratitis following cosmetic soft contact lens wear. Contact Lens J 10:21, 1976

18. Krachmer JH, Purcell JJ Jr: Bacterial corneal ulcers in cosmetic soft contact lens wearers. Arch Ophthalmol 96:57, 1978

19. Ruben M: Acute eye disease secondary to contact lens wear. Lancet 7951:138, 1976

20. Wilson LA, Schlitzer RL, Ahearn DG: *Pseudomonas* corneal ulcers associated with soft contact-lens wear. Am J Ophthalmol 92:546, 1981

21. Cooper RL, Constable IJ: Infective keratitis in soft contact lens wearers. Br J Ophthalmol 61:250, 1977

22. Wilhelmus KR: Review of clinical experience with microbial keratitis associated with contact lenses. CLAO J 13:211, 1987

23. Salz JJ, Schlanger JL: Complications of aphakic extended wear lenses encountered during a seven-year period in 100 eyes. CLAO J 9:241, 1983

24. Eichenbaum JW, Feldstein M, Podos SM: Extended-wear aphakic soft contact lenses and corneal ulcers. Br J Ophthalmol 66:663, 1982

25. Spoor TC, Hartel WC, Wynn P, Spoor DK: Complications of continuous-wear soft contact lenses in a nonreferral population. Arch Ophthalmol 102:1312, 1984

26. Weissman BA, Donzis PB, Hoft RH: Keratitis and contact lens wear: a review. J Am Optom Assoc 58:799, 1987

27. Chalupa E, Swarbrick HA, Holden BA, Sjöstrand J: Severe corneal infections associated with contact lens wear. Ophthalmology 94:17, 1987

28. Holden BA, Kotow M, Grant T, et al: The CCLRU position on hydrogel extended wear. CCLRU, School of Optometry, University of New South Wales, Australia. March 4, 1986

29. Weissman BA, Remba MJ, Fugedy E: Results of the extended wear contact lens survey of the Contact Lens Section of the American Optometric Association. J Am Optom Assoc 58:166, 1987

30. MacRae S, Herman C, Stulting RD, et al: Corneal ulcer and adverse reaction rates in premarket contact lens studies. Am J Ophthalmol 111:457, 1991

31. Schein OD, Glynn RJ, Poggio EC, et al: The relative risk of ulcerative keratitis among users of daily-wear and extended-wear soft contact lenses. A case control study. Microbial Keratitis Study Group. N Engl J Med 321:773, 1989

32. Poggio EC, Glynn RJ, Schein OD, et al: The incidence of ulcerative keratitis among users of daily-wear and extended-wear soft contact lenses. N Engl J Med 321:779, 1989

33. Jones DB: Pathogenesis of bacterial and fungal keratitis. Trans Ophthalmol Soc UK 98:367, 1978

34. Ogawa GSH, Hyndiuk RK: Bacterial keratitis and conjunctivitis: clinical disease. p. 125. In Smolin G, Thoft RA (eds): The Cornea. 3rd ed. Little, Brown and Company, Boston, 1994

35. Locatcher-Khorazo D, Seegal BC, Gutierrez EH: The bacterial flora of the healthy eye. pp.13–23. In Locatcher-Khorazo D, Seegal BC (eds): Microbiology of the Eye. Mosby, St. Louis, 1972

36. Binder PS: The extended wear of soft contact lenses. J Clin Exp Ophthalmol 15:15, 1974

37. Dohlman CH, Boruchoff A, Mobilia EF: Complications in use of soft contact lenses in corneal disease. Arch Ophthalmol 90:367, 1973

38. Hartstein J (ed): Extended Wear Contact Lenses for Aphakia and Myopia. Mosby, St. Louis, 1982

39. Stark WJ, Kracher GP, Cowen CL, et al: Extended-wear contact lenses and intraocular lenses for aphakic correction. Am J Ophthalmol 88:535, 1979

40. Binder PS, Woodward C: Extended-wear Hydrocurve and Sauflon contact lenses. Am J Ophthalmol 90:309, 1980

41. Stark WJ, Martin NF: Extended-wear contact lenses for myopic correction. Arch Ophthalmol 99:1963, 1981

42. Hirji NK, Larke JR: Corneal thickness in extended wear of soft contact lenses. Br J Ophthalmol 63:274, 1979

43. Larke JR, Hirji NK: Some clinically observed phenomena in extended contact lens wear. Br J Ophthalmol 63:475, 1979

44. Zantos SD, Holden BA: Ocular changes associated with continuous wear of contact lenses. Aust J Optom 61:418, 1978

45. Roth HW, Iwasaki W, Takayama M, Wada C: Complications caused by silicon elastomer lenses in West Germany and Japan. Contacto 19:28, 1980

46. Adams CP, Cohen EJ, Laibson PR, et al: Corneal ulcers in patients with cosmetic extended-wear contact lenses. Am J Ophthalmol 96:705, 1983

47. Hassman G, Sugar J: *Pseudomonas* corneal ulcer with extended-wear soft contact lenses for myopia. Arch Ophthalmol 101:1549, 1983

48. Barr J: The 1997 report on contact lenses. Contact Lens Spectrum 1:23, 1998

49. Koidou-Tsiligianni A, Alfonso E, Forster RK: Ulcerative keratitis associated with contact lens wear. Am J Ophthalmol 108:64, 1989

50. Donnenfeld ED, Cohen EJ, Arentsen JJ, et al: Changing trends in contact lens associated corneal ulcers; an overview of 116 cases. CLAO J 12:145, 1986

51. Schein OD, Ormerod LD, Barraquer E, et al: Microbiology of contact lens–related keratitis. Cornea 8:281, 1989

52. Cohen EJ, Gonzalez C, Leavitt KG, et al: Corneal ulcers associated with contact lenses including experience with disposable lenses. CLAO J 17:173, 1991

53. Polse KA, Mandell RB: Critical oxygen tension at the corneal surface. Arch Ophthalmol 84:505, 1970

54. Mandell RB, Farrell R: Corneal swelling at low atmospheric oxygen pressures. Invest Ophthalmol Vis Sci 19:697, 1980

55. Holden BA, Sweeney DF, Sanderson G: The minimum precorneal oxygen tension to avoid corneal edema. Invest Ophthalmol Vis Sci 25:476, 1984

56. Millodot M, O'Leary DJ: Effect of oxygen deprivation on corneal sensitivity. Acta Ophthalmol 58:434, 1980

57. Uniacke CA, Hill RM, Greenberg M, Seward S: Physiological tests for new contact lens materials. 1. Quantitative effects of selected oxygen atmospheres on glycogen storage, LDH concentration and thickness of the corneal epithelium. Am J Optom Arch Am Acad Optom 49:329, 1972

58. Hamano H, Hori M, Hamano T, et al: Effects of contact lens wear on mitosis of corneal epithelium and lactate content in aqueous humor of rabbits. Jpn J Ophthalmol 27:451, 1983

59. Masters BR: Oxygen tensions of rabbit corneal epithelium measured by non-invasive redox fluorometry. Invest Ophthalmol Vis Sci 25:S102 (abstract 63), 1984

60. Holden BA, Mertz GW: Critical oxygen levels to avoid corneal edema for daily and extended wear contact lenses. Invest Ophthalmol Vis Sci 25:1161, 1984

61. Jones DP, Fitzgerald JK: Silicon lens: new oxygen performance correlations. Contacto 22:18, 1978

62. Weissman BA, Fatt I, Pham C: Polarographic oxygen permeability measurement of silicon elastomer contact lens material. J Am Optom Assoc 63:187, 1992

63. Alvord L, Court J, Davis T, et al: Oxygen permeability of a new type of high Dk soft contact lens material. Optom Vis Sci 75:30, 1998

64. Larke JR, Parrish ST, Wigham CG: Apparent human corneal oxygen uptake rate. Am J Optom Physiol Opt 58:803, 1981

65. Isenberg SJ, Green BF: Changes in conjunctival oxygen tension and temperature with advancing age. Crit Care Med 13:683, 1985

66. Imayasu M, Petroll WM, Jester JV, et al: The relation between contact lens oxygen transmissibility and binding of *Pseudomonas aeruginosa* to the cornea after overnight wear. Ophthalmology 101:371, 1994

67. Weissman BA, Mondino BJ: Is daily wear better than extended wear? Arguments in favor of daily wear. Cornea (suppl.)9:S25, 1990

68. Harding AS, Lakkis C, Brennan NA: The effects of short term contact lens wear on adherence of *Pseudomonas aeruginosa* to human corneal cells. J Am Optom Assoc 66:775, 1995

69. Kenyon E, Polse KA, Seger RG: Influence of wearing schedule on extended-wear complications. Ophthalmology 93:231, 1986

70. Donzis PB, Mondino BJ, Weissman BA: Bacillus keratitis associated with contaminated contact lens care systems. Am J Ophthalmol 105:195, 1988

71. Garwood PC: Complications with daily wear disposable contact lenses. Contact Lens J 19:137, 1991

72. Collins MJ, Carney LG: Patient compliance and its influence on contact lens wearing problems. Am J Optom Physiol Opt 63:952, 1986

73. Chun MW, Weissman BA: Compliance in contact lens care. Am J Optom Physiol Opt 64:274, 1987

74. Pitts RE, Krachmer JH: Evaluation of soft contact lens disinfection in the home environment. Arch Ophthalmol 97:470, 1979

75. Donzis PB, Mondino BJ, Weissman BA, Bruckner DA: Microbial contamination of contact lens care systems. Am J Ophthalmol 104:325, 1987

76. Campbell RC, Caroline PJ: Inefficacy of soft contact lens disinfection techniques in the home environment. Contact Lens Forum 15:17, 1990

77. Baum JL, Panjwani N: Adherence of *Pseudomonas* to soft contact lenses and cornea: mechanisms and prophylaxis. p. 301. In Cavanagh H (ed): The Cornea: Transactions of the World Congress on the Cornea III. Raven, New York, 1988

78. Rauschi RT, Rogers JJ: The effect of hydrophilic contact lens wear on the bacterial flora of the human conjunctiva. Int Contact Lens Clin 5:56, 1978

79. Gopinathan U, Stapleton F, Sharma S, et al: Microbial contamination of hydrogel contact lenses. J Appl Microbiol 82:653, 1997

80. Høvding G: The conjunctival and contact lens bacterial flora during lens wear. Acta Ophthalmol 59:387, 1981

81. Wilcox MD, Power KN, Stapleton F, et al: Potential sources of bacteria that are isolated from contact lenses during wear. Optom Vis Sci 74:1030, 1997

82. O'Leary DJ, Millodot M: Abnormal epithelial fragility in diabetes and contact lens wear. Acta Ophthalmol 59:827, 1981

83. Ramphal R, McNiece MT, Polack FM: Adherence of *Pseudomonas aeruginosa* to the injured cornea: a step in the pathogenesis of corneal infections. Ann Ophthalmol 13:421, 1981

84. Hyndiuk RA: Experimental *Pseudomonas* keratitis. Trans Am Ophthalmol Soc 79:540, 1981

85. Stern GA, Lubniewski A, Allen C: The interaction between *Pseudomonas aeruginosa* and the corneal epithelium. An electron microscopic study. Arch Ophthalmol 103:1221, 1985

86. Stern GA, Weitzenkorn D, Valenti J: Adherence of *Pseudomonas aeruginosa* to the mouse cornea. Epithelial v stromal adherence. Arch Ophthalmol 100:1956, 1982

87. Bergmanson JP, Ruben CM, Chu LW: Epithelial morphological response to soft hydrogel contact lenses. Br J Ophthalmol 69:373, 1985

88. Weissman BA, Chun MW, Barnhart LA: Corneal abrasion associated with correction of keratoconus—a retrospective study. Optom Vis Sci 71:677, 1994

89. Jones DB. Decision-making in the management of microbial keratitis. Ophthalmology 88:814, 1981

90. Kent HD, Cohen EJ, Laibson PR, Arentsen JJ: Microbial keratitis and corneal ulceration associated with therapeutic soft contact lenses. CLAO J 16:49, 1990

91. Brown SI, Bloomfield S, Pearce DB, Tragakis M: Infections with the therapeutic soft lens. Arch Ophthalmol 91:275, 1974

92. Cutter GR, Chalmers RL, Roseman M: The clinical presentation, prevalence, and risk factors of focal corneal infiltrates in soft contact lens wearers. CLAO J 22:30, 1996

93. Donzis PB: Corneal ulcers from contact lenses during travel to remote areas (letter). N Engl J Med 338:1629, 1998

94. Locatcher-Khorazo D, Seegal BC, Gutierrez EH: Bacterial infections of the eye. p. 63. In Locatcher-Khorazo D, Seegal BC (eds): Microbiology of the Eye. Mosby, St Louis, 1972

95. Gasparrini E: Il diplocco di Frankel in patologia oculare: studio sperimentale e clinico. Ann Ottol 22:131, 1893

96. Meisler DM, Langston RH, Naab TJ, et al: Infectious crystalline keratopathy. Am J Ophthalmol 97:337, 1984

97. Reiss GR, Campbell RJ, Bourne WM: Infectious crystalline keratopathy. Surv Ophthalmol 31:69, 1986

98. Groden LR, Pascucci SE, Brinser JH: *Haemophilus aphrophilus* as a cause of crystalline keratopathy. Am J Ophthalmol 104:89, 1987

99. Ormerod LD, Smith RE: Contact lens–associated microbial keratitis. Arch Ophthalmol 104:79, 1986

100. Fleiszig SM, Lee EJ, Wu C, et al: Cytotoxic strains of *Pseudomonas aeruginosa* can damage the intact corneal surface in vitro. CLAO J 24:41, 1998

101. Farris RL: Is your office safe? No. Cornea (suppl.)9:S47, 1990

102. Belmont JB, Ostler HB, Dawson CR, et al: Non-infectious ring-shaped keratitis associated with *Pseudomonas aeruginosa*. Am J Ophthalmol 93:338, 1982

103. Wilson LA, Ahearn DG: Association of fungi with extended-wear soft contact lenses. Am J Ophthalmol 101:434, 1986

104. Penley CA, Llabrés C, Wilson LA, Ahearn DG: Efficacy of hydrogen peroxide disinfection systems for soft contact lenses contaminated with fungi. CLAO J 11:65, 1985

105. Fujikawa LS, Salahuddin SZ, Ablashi D, et al: HTLV-III in the tears of AIDS patients. Ophthalmology 93:1479, 1986

106. Nanda M, Pflugfelder SC, Holland S: Fulminant pseudomonal keratitis and scleritis in human immunodeficiency virus-infected patients. Arch Ophthalmol 109:503, 1991

107. Naginton J, Watson PG, Playfair TJ, et al: Amoebic infection of the eye. Lancet 7896:1537, 1974

108. Moore MB, McCulley JP, Luckenbach M, et al: *Acanthamoeba* keratitis associated with soft contact lenses. Am J Ophthalmol 100:396, 1985

109. Chynn EW, Talamo JH, Seligman MS: *Acanthamoeba* keratitis: Is water exposure a true risk factor? CLAO J 23:55, 1997

110. Koenig SB, Solomon JM, Hyndiuk RA, et al: *Acanthamoeba* keratitis associated with gas-permeable contact lens wear. Am J Ophthalmol 103:832, 1987

111. Moore MB, McCulley JP, Newton C, et al: *Acanthamoeba* keratitis. A growing problem in soft and hard contact lens wearers. Ophthalmology 94:1654, 1987

112. Stehr-Green JK, Bailey TM, Visvesvara GS: The epidemiology of *Acanthamoeba* keratitis in the United States. Am J Ophthalmol 107:331, 1988

113. Ormerod LD, Hertzmark E, Gomez DS, et al: Epidemiology of microbial keratitis in southern California. A multivariant analysis. Ophthalmology 94:1322, 1987

114. Fleiszig SMJ: The Pathogenesis of Contact Lens Related Infectious Keratitis (Thesis, 1990). Melbourne, Australia, University of Melbourne

115. Klotz SA, Misra RP, Butrus SI: Contact lens wear enhances adherence of Pseudomonas aeruginosa and binding of lectins to the cornea. Cornea 9:266, 1990

116. Dunn JP, Mondino BJ, Weissman BA, et al: Corneal ulcers associated with disposable hydrogel contact lenses. Am J Ophthalmol 108:113, 1989

117. Mertz PH, Bouchard CS, Mathers WD, et al: Corneal infiltrates associated with disposable extended wear soft contact lenses: a report of nine cases. CLAO J 16:269, 1990

118. Ehrlich M, Weissman BA, Mondino BJ: *Pseudomonas* corneal ulcer after use of extended-wear rigid gas-permeable contact lens. Cornea 8:225, 1989

119. Grant T, Holden BA: The clinical performance of disposable (58%) extended wear lenses. J Br Contact Lens Assoc (suppl., Transactions of the British Contact Lens Association International Contact Lens Centenary Congress)11:63, 1988

120. Weissman BA, Schwartz SD, Gottschalk-Katsev N, Lee DA: Oxygen permeability of disposable soft contact lenses. Am J Ophthalmol 110:269, 1990

121. Jones DB, Baum JL: Initial therapy of suspected microbial corneal ulcers. I. Broad antibiotic therapy based on prevalence of organisms. Surv Ophthalmol 24:97, 1979

122. McDonnell PJ, Nobe J, Gauderman WJ, et al: Community care of corneal ulcers. Am J Ophthalmol 114:531, 1992

123. McLeod SD, Kolahdouz-Isfahani A, Rostamian K, et al: The role of smears, cultures and antibiotic sensitivity testing in the management of suspected infectious keratitis. Ophthalmology 103:23, 1996

124. McLeod SD, DeBacker CM, Viana MA: Differential care of corneal ulcers in the community based on apparent severity. Ophthalmology 103:479, 1996

125. Rodman RC, Spisak S, Sugar A, et al: The utility of culturing corneal ulcers in a tertiary referral center versus a general ophthalmology clinic. Ophthalmology 104:1897, 1997

126. Clemons CS, Cohen EJ, Arentsen JJ, et al: *Pseudomonas* ulcers following patching of corneal abrasions associated with contact lens wear. CLAO J 13:161, 1987

127. Steinert RF: Current therapy for bacterial keratitis and bacterial conjunctivitis. Am J Ophthalmol (suppl.)112:10S, 1991

128. Leibowitz HM: Clinical evaluation of ciprofloxacin 0.3% ophthalmic solution for treatment of bacterial keratitis. Am J Ophthlamol 112:34S, 1991

129. O'Brien TP, Maguire MG, Fink NE, et al: Efficacy of ofloxacin vs cefazolin and tobramycin in the therapy for bacterial keratitis. Report from the Bacterial Keratitis Study Research Group. Arch Ophthalmol 113:1257, 1995

130. The Ofloxacin Study Group. Ofloxacin monotherapy for the primary treatment of microbial keratitis: a double-masked, randomized, controlled trial with conventional therapy. Ophthalmology 104:1902, 1997

131. Knauf HP, Silvany R, Southern PM Jr, et al: Susceptibility of corneal and conjunctival pathogens to ciprofloxacin. Cornea 15:66, 1996

132. Blanton CL, Rapuano CJ, Cohen EJ, et al: Initial treatment of microbial keratitis. CLAO J 22:136, 1996

133. Dunn JP, Mondino BJ, Weissman BA: Infectious keratitis in contact lens wearers. p. 64.1. In Bennett ES, Weissman BA (eds): Clinical Contact Lens Practice. Lippincott, Philadelphia, 1991

134. Groden LR, Brinser JH: Outpatient treatment of microbial corneal ulcers. Arch Ophthalmol 104:84, 1986

135. Weissman BA, Mondino BJ: Corneal infections secondary to contact lens wear. p. 255. In Tomlinson AJ (ed): Complications of Contact Lens Wear. Mosby–Year Book, St. Louis, 1992

136. Ostler HB, Okumoto M, Wiley C: The changing pattern of the etiology of central bacterial corneal (hypopyon) ulcer. Trans Pac Coast Otolaryngol Ophthalmol Soc 57:235, 1976

137. Asbell P, Stenson S: Ulcerative keratitis. Survey of 30 years' laboratory experience. Arch Ophthalmol 100:77, 1982

138. Liesegang TJ, Forster RK: Spectrum of microbial keratitis in South Florida. Am J Ophthalmol 90:38, 1980

139. Jones DB: Strategy for initial management of suspected microbial keratitis. pp. 86–119. In Barraquer JI, Binder PS, Buxton JN, et al (eds): Symposium on Medical and Surgical Diseases of the Cornea. Trans New Orleans Acad Ophthalmol. Mosby, St. Louis, 1980

140. Galentine PG, Cohen EJ, Laibson PR, et al: Corneal ulcers associated with contact lens wear. Arch Ophthalmol 102:891, 1984

141. Patrinely JR, Wilhelmus KR, Rubin JM, Key JE: Bacterial keratitis associated with extended wear soft contact lenses. CLAO J 11:234, 1985

142. Alfonso E, Mandelbaum S, Fox MJ, Forster RK: Ulcerative keratitis associated with contact lens wear. Am J Ophthalmol 101:429, 1986

143. Jauch A, Fsadni M, Gamba G. Meta-analysis of six clinical phase III studies comparing lomefloxacin 0.3% eye drops twice daily to five standard antibiotics in patients with acute bacterial conjunctivitis. Graefe's Arch Clin Exp Opthalmol 237:705, 1999

144. Vajpayee RB, Gupta SK, Angra SK, Munjal A: Topical norfloxacin therapy in Pseudomonas corneal ulceration. Cornea 10:268, 1991

13

Protozoan and Fungal Keratitis in Contact Lens Wear

JAMES V. AQUAVELLA, JOSEPH P. SHOVLIN,
AND MICHAEL D. DEPAOLIS

GRAND ROUNDS CASE REPORT

Subjective:
A 23-year-old construction worker presented with a red, irritated right eye. Prior history of working with insulation 2 days earlier. History of soft lens wear for myopia for 5 years, with saline made from salt tablets and distilled water. Patient attributed contact lens irritation to insulation fibers.

Objective:
- Best acuity with pinhole: right eye (OD) $^{20}/_{40}$, left eye (OS) $^{20}/_{20}$
- Biomicroscopy: OS normal findings, OD bulbar conjunctiva 1+ injected, with multiple areas of punctate epithelial keratitis, and no anterior chamber reaction
- All other ocular findings normal each eye (OU)

Assessment:
Insulation keratitis OD

Plan:
1. Cultures
2. Fornices swabbed (no fibers found)
3. Irrigation
4. Tobramycin drops q3h for 24 hours, then four times a day for 1 week
5. Follow up in 1 week or sooner if signs or symptoms warrant

Other:
The patient returned 2 days later with symptoms of increased irritation and blurred vision. Epithelial involvement of dendriform appearance without ulceration is now present, with mild flare of the anterior chamber. All other findings are normal.

Plan:
1. Scopolamine 0.25% twice a day OD
2. Continue tobramycin four times a day OD

3.   Lids and fornices swabbed again (no evidence of insulation fibers or other foreign body)
   The patient was seen 2 days later with no improvement in symptoms or visual acuity. Cornea and anterior chamber unchanged, except for faint midstromal infiltrates with radial, linear, and branching pattern. Patient now thought to have an atypical herpes simplex infection.

Plan: Trifluridine drops (Viroptic, Glaxo Wellcome Inc., Research Triangle Park, NC) q2h OD

The patient was seen 1 day later. Condition unchanged, with exception of mild perineural edema of stroma and increased pain. Results from initial cultures were negative for bacteria and viruses. Contact lens case was not available for culture.

Plan: Sulfacetamide sodium-prednisolne sodium phospahte (Vasocidin) drops three times a day added to trifluridine drops q2h. Because of unusual radial pattern of infiltrates along the corneal nerves, a consultation with an anterior segment specialist was obtained 10 days later.

Diagnosis: Persistent insulation keratitis. Herpes simplex keratitis believed unlikely because of poor response to trifluridine for 12 days, negative history of herpetic disease, and absence of corneal hypoesthesia.

Plan: Trifluridine tapered. Add prednisolone (Pred Forte) four times a day with erythromycin (Ilotycin) ointment three times a day.

The patient was seen 1 week later with visual acuity OD $^{20}/_{100}$. Epithelium intact with less stromal edema and infiltration, but endothelial keratic precipitates noted. Medications were tapered.

Two weeks later, cornea unchanged. Cultures negative for bacteria, viruses, and fungi. Second consultation arranged. At time of this consultation, the patient had developed a ring-shaped infiltrate with a partial epithelial defect. Giemsa smear taken after vigorous corneal scraping.

Results: *Acanthamoeba* cysts

Plan: Immediately placed on neomycin and polymyxin sulfates and gramicidin ophthalmic solution (Neosporin), propamidine isethionate (Brolene), topical miconazole (Monistat), oral ketoconazole (Nizoral), prednisolone, and atropine 1% OD.

Over 2 months, ring infiltrate partially resolved, with residual haze. After an indolent and inexorable course and a short period of quiescence, a penetrating keratoplasty was performed for visual restoration.

Three months postoperatively, graft is clear and a rigid contact lens for optic rehabilitation is anticipated.

ACANTHAMOEBA

Acanthamoebae are small, free-living, facultative protozoa found in soil, water, and air.[1-4] Certain species have even been cultured from the human nasopharynx in healthy individuals. The life cycle has only two stages, the trophozoite, or slowly motile form, and the sessile cystic form (Fig. 13-1). The latter has a double wall, which is responsible for its impressive resistance to most medications. This protozoan is classified in the phylum *Sarcomastigophora*.

Identifications are based primarily on morphology, nuclear divisions, temperature tolerance, isoenzyme analysis, and pathogenicity.[2] Restriction enzyme analysis of either mitochondrial DNA or cellular DNA was applied to differentiate species.[5] As more precise biochemical and genetic identification tools become available, periodic revisions of the classification of this group of protozoans will probably become necessary.[2]

Clinicians and microbiologists regard *Acanthamoeba* as an exotic organism encountered in rare infections, such as meningoencephalitis and keratitis.[2] However, 22 species

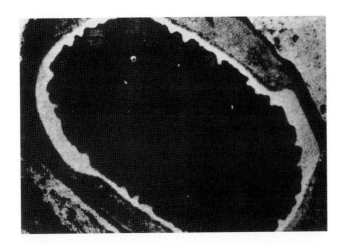

FIG. 13-1. *An* Acanthamoeba *cyst shows an ectolayer that is less electron dense than the endolayer. (Reprinted with permission from LS Hirst, WR Green, W Merz, et al: Management of* Acanthamoeba *keratitis: a case report and review of the literature. Ophthalmology 91:1105, 1984.)*

TABLE 13-1. *Organisms Isolated from Human Ocular Infections*

Acanthamoeba castellani
Acanthamoeba culbertsoni
Acanthamoeba hatchetti
Acanthamoeba polyphaga
Acanthamoeba rhisodes

have been identified as systemic pathogens, and at least five, perhaps up to seven, of these are potential ocular parasites (Table 13-1).[1,6]

Life Cycle

The trophozoite is characterized by a single nucleus and a large karyosome or endosome.[2] Acanthamoebae are sluggish; the trophozoite moves in a relatively straight line and often forms tracks on agar. Tracks on blood agar led to the discovery of *Acanthamoeba* in an earlier case of keratitis. The acanthamoeba trophozoite encysts in an unfavorable environment (i.e., in a culture plate when the food supply is exhausted, when cell crowding occurs, and low pH exists).[3]

Cysts usually have wrinkled ectocystic walls. The size of the cysts varies among species, ranging from the smallest (*A. polyphaga* and *A. hatchetti*, 13.1 μm) to the largest (*A. tubeashi* and *A. comandoni*, 19.1 μm).[2] Some species have distinct wrinkled ectocysts; others are round or triangular. Pores (osteoles) are visible at certain intervals in the cyst wall where the ectocyst makes contact with the endocyst. Precysts contain many food particles but no longer have a functioning contractile vacuole. The number of osteoles varies in different species, which may help to account for a differing resistance to antiparasitics, although no apparent species-related variability exists in corneal virulence.[3] Cysts are resistant to dryness, cold, and various antimicrobial agents.

Acanthamoeba Keratitis

Acanthamoebae can directly infect the cornea (usually after trauma or contact lens wear), causing a serious and relentless keratitis, owing to high resistance of the organism to therapy.[2] Over the last 20 years, *Acanthamoeba* keratitis, formerly a relatively unknown entity, has now been recognized as a distinct, although still uncommon, entity.[2,6,7] *Acanthamoeba* keratitis was first reported in 1973; only a small number of cases were reported until 1981, none in contact lens wearers. The association of *Acanthamoeba* keratitis in healthy soft contact lens wearers who used homemade saline was first reported in 1985.[1,6,7]

Acanthamoeba keratitis often causes marked visual impairment and even loss of the eye.[3,4] Up to July of 1989, 250 cases had been reported to the Centers for Disease Control and Prevention.[2] It is believed that the incidence of this infection is greater than the number of cases reported.

The presumed cause of infection is amebic contamination of the lens during cleaning and storage, or contact with water. Epithelial trauma may also be involved, but some patients with superficial punctate keratopathy, corneal abrasions, and *Acanthamoeba* contamination of contact lenses and cases do not develop clinical infection.[6] The development of infection may depend on several factors, including the size and virulence of the inoculum, the frequency of contact with the cornea, and the host response.[1,3,6] It is important to recognize that acanthamoeba contamination of lens care systems generally occurs when bacterial or, in many cases, fungal contamination is also present.

The epidemiology of *Acanthamoeba* keratitis in the United States has been reviewed.[1,8-10] Of 208 cases identified, 189 had information concerning risk factors (history of corneal trauma, exposure to contaminated water, or contact lens wear). The majority of cases were in four states (California, New York, Pennsylvania, and Texas), which suggests a geographic predisposition. Contact lenses were worn by 85%; 64% of the contact lens wearers also gave a history of using saline prepared from distilled water and salt tablets. Patients aged 50 years and older were

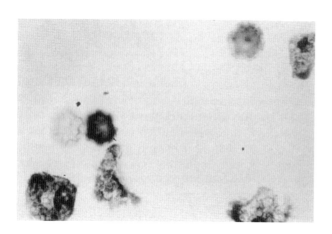

FIG. 13-2. *This differential stain shows various trophozoites and cysts (smaller object).*

more likely to have had a history of trauma than younger patients; 49% of the cases occurred in males, although nationwide, only 28% of soft contact lens wearers are male. The authors suggested that this might be owing to the higher incidence of trauma in males.[10]

Detection

The diagnosis of *Acanthamoeba* keratitis is difficult and, in many cases, is made only after no response to treatment for suspected bacterial, fungal, or viral infections, especially herpes simplex. In one report, 90% of early cases were at first presumed to be herpes simplex keratitis.[3,6,7]

Not considering the diagnosis has important implications because a better prognosis clearly exists when the disease is treated early in its course.[3,6,11,12] In many cases, it remains difficult to diagnose *Acanthamoeba* by clinical examination alone. A high index of suspicion, especially in contact lens wearers, is essential because several good laboratory tests are available for identifying the organism.[13,14]

Symptoms include decreased vision, mucous discharge, foreign-body sensation, epiphora, photophobia, and blepharospasm. Severe or moderate ocular pain disproportionate to the degree of anterior segment inflammation is very characteristic.

Laboratory tests to aid in diagnosis include impression cytology, indirect and direct fluorescence antibody testing and staining techniques,[15] polymerase chain reaction (PCR) analysis, and cell cultures.[16] Corneal biopsy may be required to obtain adequate tissue if scrapings do not yield pathogens.[14] It should also be noted that, as in the case of fungal keratitis, the epithelium can remain intact[2,3] during the infection. Specular and confocal microscopy

have been used to identify cysts in the stroma and may obviate the need for biopsy in some cases.[1] Confocal microscopy provides real-time evaluation at the cellular level, with greater axial and lateral spatial resolution compared to specular microscopy.[5]

The use of transport media is not recommended, but when it is necessary to use this system, Page's saline for amoeba in a sterile glass vial, pretreated with a siliconizing agent, provides an adequate transport medium. The specimen should be kept at room temperature, never frozen or refrigerated.[1,10]

Because microbial keratitis may be caused by bacteria (including the mycobacteria species that grow rapidly), fungi, and viruses, it is imperative to collect specimens for simultaneous testing so that findings can be interpreted for definitive diagnosis.[2] Co-infection from various microbial vectors is possible. If epithelial involvement occurs, a greater likelihood exists of obtaining a positive culture or smear (Fig. 13-2 and Table 13-2).

A simple technique described by Johns and coworkers[17] allows practitioners to examine hydrogel lenses suspected of containing cysts or trophozoites by simple light microscopy. Their study found that trophozoites were likely to adhere to lenses with a greater affinity than do cysts.[17]

Detection of *Acanthamoeba* by Culture

Acanthamoeba grows rapidly on non-nutrient agar layered with enteric bacteria (usually gram-negative) (Fig. 13-3). If a cyst is present in the specimen, it excysts in a favorable environment with bacteria as nutrients. As the amoeba engulfs the bacteria, it moves to the periphery of the area of the bacterial growth, usually within 2 or 3 days of incubation. Within 2–3 more days, when the supply of bacteria is exhausted, cyst formation begins. When all the trophozoites are encysted in an older culture, they are often arranged in a cluster. To an inexperienced observer under low magnification, the trophozoites look like crystals. The way to identify the trophozoite is to observe only one suspected trophozoite for the presence of a contractile vacuole, which disappears and reappears after a few seconds, differentiating the trophozoite from artifact. Because more than one species of *Acanthamoeba* is usually found in every case of keratitis, sensitivity testing is important.

An activated charcoal-yeast extract serves as a cost-effective medium for effective detection. Inadvertent inoculation with the extract should be avoided.[2]

Immunodiagnosis and Species Identification

Serologic tests are generally not considered useful. Isoenzyme analysis allows species identification. Cysts and trophozoites can be stained for species identification or subcultured on fresh plates.[5]

TABLE 13-2. *Procedures Routinely Used for Specimen Preparation, Collection, Transport, and Identification*

Microbiological preparation
1. Three sides previously washed and cleaned with soap and water and placed on slide folders.
2. The following materials are obtained: one Coplin jar of methanol (fixative for Hemacolor and modified acid-fast stain); one Coplin jar of Schaudinn's fixative for trichrome stain; one blood agar plate; one chocolate agar plate; one thioglycolate broth; one Sabouraud agar slant for yeast or mold; and one viral transport media for viral culture.

Specimen collection and transport
After anesthetic is placed in the eye, examination of the cornea under the slit lamp locates the ulcer or lesion to be scraped. The scalpel retrieves the scraping taken for preparation and direct culture medium inoculation.
1. *Slide preparation.* It is important to prepare a thin smear because cysts are probably buried in a thick smear and may not be visible. Fix the slide immediately in methanol for Hemacolor and acid-fast stain and in Schaudinn's stain for trichrome stain. Hemacolor reveals cell reactions, trophozoites, and cysts. Trichrome reveals trophozoites and cysts more easily because it is a differential stain (see Fig. 13-2). The number of scrapings desirable from suspected infectious keratitis cases is limited by the need to avoid undue damage to the cornea. On the other hand, a rapid diagnosis can be made from a good smear preparation while the culture report is pending.
2. *Culture inoculation.* In cases in which the smear may be negative, the culture may be positive, and vice versa. The procedure for *Acanthamoeba* differs from that used to culture other micro-organisms. The specimen is simply brought into contact without streaking out into the agar, or gram-negative bacteria, usually *Escherichia coli*, are added. (Heat-killed *E. coli* may be necessary so as not to overwhelm the *Acanthamoeba* organism.) The plates are sealed with adhesive tape to prevent dehydration. All inoculated media should be incubated for at least 2 weeks before results are reported as negative. Clinically, there may be concomitant infections, especially with streptococci.

Detection of Acanthamoeba *by smear*
Acanthamoeba trophozoites are more difficult to detect than cysts in smears because trophozoites resemble leukocytes.
1. *Giemsa-Wright of Hemacolor (<1 min)* is the most rapid method for detection of amoebae. The smear can be examined with a low-power objective. Hemacolor is not a differential stain, and cells and cysts are stained purple. The mature cyst is polygonal, with a double wall (wrinkled ectocyst or round endocyst).
2. *Wheatley trichrome (75 min)*, a differential stain, is helpful in the detection of cysts. The cyst wall stains green, the cytoplasm stains green-purple, and the karyosome stains red. Polymorphonuclear cells and macrophage can be differentiated from cysts by morphology.
3. *Calcofluor white with methylene blue (5 min)* is used for detection of fungi. It stains *Acanthamoeba* cysts green and trophozoites or young cysts orange. Examination requires a fluorescence microscope, and no permanent smear can be saved for future examination.
4. *Fluorescein-conjugated lectin (2 hrs)* is the latest method reported for staining trophozoites and cysts.
5. *Gomori methenamine-silver (rapid or overnight method)* results are not easy to interpret if the preparation is not skillfully done.
6. *Periodic acid–Schiff (overnight preparation)* stains cyst walls red.
7. *Immunofluorescent antibody (2 hrs)* stains trophozoites and cysts with the use of rabbit antiserum to *Acanthamoeba*.
8. *Electron microscopy (a few days)* can detect cysts and microcysts in biopsy specimens.

Source: Adapted with permission from P Ma, GS Visvesvera, AJ Martinez, et al: *Naegleria* and *Acanthamoeba* infections: review. Rev Infect Dis 12:490, 1990.

Indirect immunofluorescence and immunoperoxidase techniques are commonly used to identify amoebae in formalin-fixed, paraffin-embedded tissue sections. The usefulness of either technique depends on the preservation of the morphologic integrity and antigenic activity of the amoebae in fixed tissues, and on the specificity of the antiserum used for typing of the amoebae.

Polymerase Chain Reaction Analysis PCR analysis may be a more sensitive test than cultures as a diagnostic test. PCR testing includes analysis of tears and epithelium, and appears to be very effective in detecting early disease.

Electron Microscopy Electron microscopy is an effective method of detecting parasites in corneal tissue.[5]

Confocal Microscopy Tandem confocal microscopy has been used to make a diagnosis and to manage treatment of *Acanthamoeba* keratitis because of its ability to detect the organism in the cornea in vivo. Bacterial contaminants and artifacts are possible and may result in overreporting of this disease.[18]

Pathology Acanthamoebae have been isolated from human throats, nasal mucosa, bone graft, skin nodules, stool, and even dust in the air. There has been a sudden increase in the incidence of *Acanthamoeba* keratitis, primarily in contact lens wearers. High morbidity and even mortality may be reduced with rapid diagnosis and early intervention. One death was reported from ocular infection via a hematogenous route.[3]

Pathologic studies of an involved cornea in an early case showed destruction of the anterior cornea, with infiltration of acute inflammatory cells into the stroma. Infil-

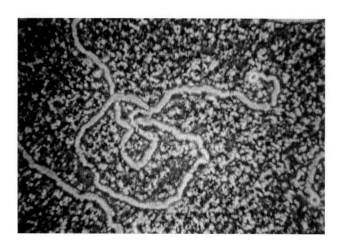

FIG. 13-3. *Culture plate shows* Acanthamoeba *tracking after 4 days. (Courtesy of Dr. D. Lamberts.)*

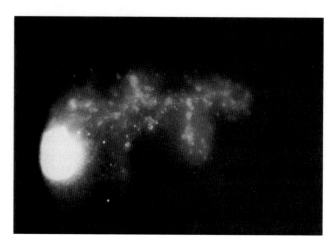

FIG. 13-4. *Raised epithelial lines of the cornea forming a dendritiform pattern. (Courtesy of Dr. B. Christensen.)*

trating amebic organisms between lamellae of the stroma are readily apparent at medium-power magnification.[2] When penetrating keratoplasty is performed at a later stage in the disease process, considerable loss of corneal substance occurs, often followed by ulceration, descemetocele, and eventually perforation of the cornea.[2] Finding amoebae at the surgical margins of removed corneal buttons usually enables practitioners to correctly predict recrudescence after initial successful keratoplasty.

Clinical Presentation

The onset of corneal infection in *Acanthamoeba* keratitis occurs in various ways and with variable intensity. In almost every case, one or both of two factors, trauma and contaminated water, appear to be incriminated. Most cases related to contact lens wear certainly appear to be the combined result of microscopic epithelial trauma and contamination of contact lens solutions, such as homemade saline.[6,7]

When trauma is severe enough to cause a full-thickness epithelial defect, a more rapid process usually develops, with corneal ulceration, increasing infiltration and clouding of the cornea, nongranulomatous uveitis, and often scleritis, resulting in severe pain, hypopyon, hyphema, and vision loss.[2,6,7,14] When the condition occurs in contact lens wearers, symptoms usually begin more subtly but progress just as inexorably.[2,3] When no obvious trauma has occurred, the early clinical findings may be nonspecific or may suggest and treat herpes simplex keratitis. In addition, decreased corneal sensitivity has been reported as an early sign in *Acanthamoeba* keratitis, thereby increasing the chance of diagnostic confusion between

Acanthamoeba and herpes simplex keratitis.[5] It is believed that a significant epithelial break may not be needed to cause clinical infection. Variation in epithelial receptor sites may account for the degrees of response and may determine whether infection will occur.[7]

A wide variety of epithelial defects has been reported,[1] including superficial punctate keratopathy, dendriform and pseudo-dendriform lesions, and scattered epithelial and subepithelial opacities.[11,16,18–20] These defects may wax and wane throughout the course of the infection, whether the disease is effectively treated.[5]

Elevated corneal lines of the epithelium are another significant clinical sign of *Acanthamoeba* keratitis (Fig. 13-4). These lines were initially misinterpreted as epithelial rejection lines in one patient after successful grafting, and as healing epithelium or dystrophic changes in another individual.[2] When scraping was performed, the lines were found to represent acanthamoebae, primarily trophozoites.

Stromal findings include a radial keratoneuritis,[18–20] which is often helpful in distinguishing *Acanthamoeba* keratitis from herpes simplex and fungal keratitis (Fig. 13-5). Unlike herpes simplex and other similar presentations, usually minimal vascularization exists with *Acanthamoeba* infections.[3] John et al. described a bull's-eye pattern lesion in patients with *Acanthamoeba* keratitis.[17,19] The appearance in some cases of *Acanthamoeba* keratitis of satellite lesions causes confusion because of the suspicion of fungal infection.

Additional clinical findings include a preauricular adenopathy, pseudomembrane formation, severe chemosis, follicular reaction, fluctuating epithelial defects in addition to the raised epithelial lines, and early and late

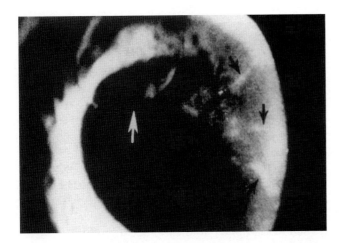

FIG. 13-5. *White arrow points to biopsy site and black arrows point to radial infiltrates in* Acanthamoeba *keratitis. (Reprinted with permission from MB Moore, JP McCulley, C Newton, et al:* Acanthamoeba *keratitis: a growing problem in soft and hard contact lens wearers. Ophthalmology 94:1654, 1987.)*

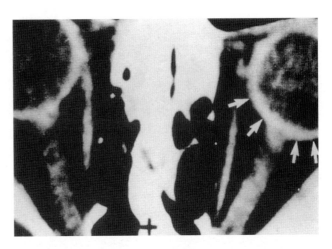

FIG. 13-6. *Scleral thickening and dense edema* (white arrows) *on computed tomographic scan of patient with an ocular* Acanthamoeba *infection. (Reprinted with permission from MJ Mannis, R Tamaru, AM Roth, et al:* Acanthamoeba *sclerokeratitis: determining diagnostic criteria. Arch Ophthalmol 104:1313, 1986.)*

decreased corneal sensitivity. Late reduced sensitivity is probably related to perineural edema and steroid therapy.[3] Common lid abnormalities include lid edema and reactive pseudoptosis.[5]

In some patients, the condition waxes and wanes[3,4,7] and may apparently clear completely, only to reappear as a rapidly progressive abscess characterized by a ring-shaped infiltrate of definite diagnostic importance,[2] although it is not pathognomonic (Fig. 13-6). The infiltration forms a 360-degree annular paracentral ring with a clear or relatively clear center before progressing to more extensive and deeper corneal invasion, destruction, descemetocele, and occasionally even frank corneal perforation.[2] Ring infiltrates may appear as partial or complete, double or concentric.[3,13] An annular ring or radial nerve infiltrate should alert the practitioner to the possibility of amebic infection, especially in cases of resistant, puzzling keratitis.[2] Such suspicion leads to simple, readily available diagnostic studies that usually confirm the diagnosis.

Optic disk edema with a contiguous scleritis has been noted in several cases,[10] which helps to account for the intense pain that invariably accompanies this disease (Fig. 13-7). One study has actually found peripheral corneal hyperesthesia and central corneal hypoesthesia[9] owing to late perineural edema and steroid usage.

In a large series of *Acanthamoeba* cases reviewed,[21] the following diagnostic findings were observed: scleritis, 14%; hypopyon, 39%; ring infiltrate, 57%; epithelial defect, 93%; and suppuration (eventual), 100%.

Contact Lens–Related Factors: Minimizing Risks

Acanthamoebae have been found in air, soil, salt water, fresh water, chlorinated water, hot tubs,[8] and in water in frozen lakes.[1,6] Because of the wide distribution of acanthamoebae, human exposure is thought to be frequent. At present, the great majority of acanthamoeba infections occurs in wearers of contact lenses.[1,10]

Because of the difficulty of treatment and the increased incidence and awareness, prevention of *Acanthamoeba* infection is critical.[1,3] Because amoebae have been cultured from all types of lenses[1,2,3,7,9,12,17] and most solutions,[2,3] good hygienic care is important. The role of

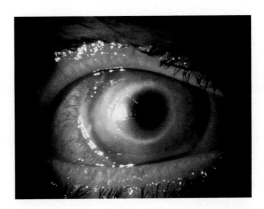

FIG. 13-7. *Ring infiltrate in patient with* Acanthamoeba *keratitis.*

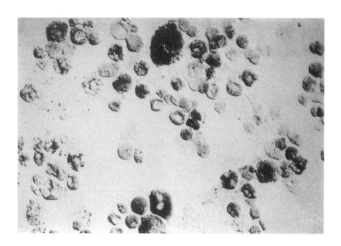

FIG. 13-8. Acanthamoeba *cysts and trophozoites adhering to an extended-wear soft lens. (Reprinted with permission from KJ Johns, WS Head, CM Parrish, et al: Examination of hydrophilic contact lenses with light microscopy to aid in the diagnosis of* Acanthamoeba *keratitis. Am J Ophthalmol 108:329, 1989.)*

extended wear in this disease is unclear, but increased contact time may predispose the patient to increased risk of infection, as in bacterial keratitis.

By one estimate, more than 90% of contact lens–related cases might be avoided by eliminating the use of homemade saline solutions and tap water rinsing.[6] The use of tap water rinses with rigid lenses has been debated. Most authorities recommend not using tap water rinses after lenses have been soaked in the disinfecting solution. *Acanthamoeba* cysts are apparently resistant to chlorine in levels up to 10 parts per million, an important consideration in that certain municipal water supplies (especially on the East Coast) generally demonstrate low levels of chlorine.[3] The same point applies to swimming pools.

Spray salines seem to work best for rigid lenses. Sterile saline should be used for all enzyme soaks for rigid and soft contact lenses because complete eradication by sterilization is probably not needed to avoid infection. Regular cleaning and thorough rinsing are most likely sufficient for removing the bulk of organisms[22] because trophozoites and cysts do not adhere as tenaciously as bacteria to the surface of various lenses (Fig. 13-8). They essentially lack a glycocalyx, which most bacteria and fungi produce.

One study[23] found hydrogen peroxide ineffective against *A. castellani* and *A. polyphaga*,[1,2,8] although another study found hydrogen peroxide without a catalyst effective against *A. castellani*.[1]

Other forms of cold disinfection appear variably effective. A conditioning solution for rigid lenses preserved with polyaminopropyl biguanide is effective against several species.[22] Chlorhexidine-thimerosal and chlorhexidine-edetate have been shown effective against *A. castellani* but not *A. polyphaga*.[23] Alkyltriethanol ammonium chloride-thimerosal has been effective against both.[23] Sorbic acid, potassium sorbate, and edetate disodium-thimerosal are ineffective against *A. castellani*.[23] Thermal disinfection, on the other hand, has consistently been amebicidal and cysticidal.[1,3,24] In one study, after exposure to a nonamebicidal or noncysticidal disinfecting agent, *Acanthamoeba* did not encyst for 21 days.[22] This attests to the organism's ability to survive for long periods.

Several recommendations based on epidemiologic studies and susceptibility studies[10,24] seem prudent.

- Contact lens wearers should not wear their lenses in or around hot tubs,[8] swimming pools,[14] and brackish water.[3]
- Patients should be cautioned against the use of tap water as a rinsing or storing solution.
- Exposure of contact lenses to saliva, and ocular or lens contact with soil, distilled water, hospital saline,[1] or homemade saline[3,6,7] should also be avoided. Another possible source of lens contamination is water held in storage tanks, such as those often found on trains and airplanes.[3]
- Patients should always wash their hands and avoid contamination of bottle tips.
- Small bottles of sterile, commercially available saline should be changed frequently.
- When enzyme products are used, tap water or distilled water should never be used as a diluent.
- Cases should be cleaned frequently, air-dried daily, and replaced on a regular basis.
- In-office disinfection of lenses should include an initial cleaning with an amebicidal alcohol-based cleaner[22] and heat disinfection whenever possible. For lenses that do not withstand heat, a chemical disinfection system approved by the U.S. Food and Drug Administration suffices. Storage solutions should be changed every 3 months.
- Before inserting trial lenses on a prospective patient, additional cleaning and rinsing with sterile saline seems prudent.

Therapy

The treatment of *Acanthamoeba* keratitis can be medical or surgical, or both.[1] Specific treatment is frequently unsatisfactory. Major reliance is placed on antiparasitic or antifungal drugs, cycloplegics, neomycin, and corticosteroids.[2,24–29] Many cases require eventual or emergency keratoplasty, often repeated. Approximately 30% of cases recur after successful initial grafting.[3] With epithelial disease, early débridement may prove helpful in debulking the infectious load, and it allows better penetration of medications.[1,11]

Acanthamoeba infections are highly resistant to chemotherapeutic agents.[1,3,22,23] Initial reports of medical therapy demonstrated abysmal results[1,3,14] because most commercially available antimicrobial agents are ineffective in concentrations tolerated by the cornea. In addition, many chemotherapeutic agents seem to provide temporary improvement, yet in reality, they cause the organism to encyst. Several investigators have performed susceptibility tests against various strains isolated, with conflicting findings.[2] More than one antimicrobial agent has frequently been used at the same time, often in conjunction with corticosteroids and surgical intervention. This has created difficulty in attempting to specify which agents have antiamebic effects. Topical and oral agents should be chosen from two or more of the following categories: antibiotics or aminoglycosides (inhibit protein synthesis), antifungals (destabilizes cell walls), antiparasitics or aromatic diamidine (inhibit DNA synthesis), and cationic antiseptics or biocides (inhibits membrane function). Topical antifungals may have good penetration characteristics but may actually be less effective in imparting a clinical cure when used alone. Biocides, such as Bacquacil and Cosmocil, seem to be the mainstay in initial topical agent selection. To minimize significant medicamentosa, an agent from each of several categories can be rotated on a daily basis. The first medical cure was reported in 1985, with propamidine isethionate (Brolene), a pre–sulfa era, over-the-counter drug available in the United Kingdom that was made available in this country under orphan drug status. Propamidine 0.1% is an antibiotic, antiparasitic, and antifungal agent that appears to be amebicidal and cysticidal in in vitro studies.[29] An analog ointment, dibromopropamidine, 0.15%, has also been successful.[2] Shovlin et al.[3] have reported recurrent epithelial defects with this drug, which may mimic a recurrence. Except in a few cases, however, such treatment has not eliminated the need for ultimate keratoplasty.[20]

A combination of neomycin, polymyxin-B, gramicidin, and miconazole nitrate also has shown positive results.[6,15,25] Miconazole is amebicidal and cysticidal at levels reached by topical application, although in vitro studies indicate that the effect of neomycin and polymyxin-B is only inhibitory. Fortified aminoglycosides have shown limited success in inhibiting this pathogen. Most antibiotics have shown little, if any, antiparasitic effect. Fluorocytosine was found to be amebicidal in one study but not in several others.[2]

The antifungal agent clotrimazole 1% has been reported effective in several patients, two of whom had developed recurrences while on propamidine, miconazole, and neosporin solution.[28] Although relatively toxic, clotrimazole is usually better tolerated than miconazole. It is available commercially as a cream or as a 1% suspension formulated in artificial tears.

The role of topical steroids remains controversial. Some authorities believe that steroids have been shown to inhibit metamorphogenesis and promote re-epithelialization in this disease, resulting in improved outcome. Clinical deterioration can occur and adverse effects can develop while on steroid therapy. The current trend seems to be to avoid their use because of the blunting or suppression of the host response,[1,7] and they may allow deeper penetration of the organism until other chemotherapeutics have made an impact on the infection. Of course, when keratoplasty is performed, steroids must play an integral part of postoperative therapy.

Consultation with a pain management clinic can be helpful because pain is a major problem in the management of these patients. Narcotics are often ineffective and pose the risk of addiction when used for the typically lengthy course of the disease. Clinoril (Sulindac) may provide more relief than other nonsteroidal medications or mild narcotic-analgesic combinations.[1,9] In a few cases, a retrobulbar alcohol nerve block has been used after intravenous sedation.[3,7,25]

Attempted surgical intervention has included conjunctival flaps, cryotherapy, and full-thickness grafting. Applying heat (40°C) to the affected cornea may provide therapeutic benefit in the management of *Acanthamoeba* keratitis.[30] It should be noted that conjunctival flaps, which are sometimes helpful in treating resistant fungal infections, have been dismal failures in *Acanthamoeba* keratitis because of retraction and erosion through the flaps.[3,23]

Cryotherapy has usually been ineffective;[27] the cysts are not killed and the infected eyes do not tolerate the procedure well.[4,26] Another report[25] was more encouraging, showing that cryotherapy may render the cysts more susceptible to medical therapy.[26,27] Cryotherapy has been used at the time of penetrating keratoplasty to destroy any remaining parasites before transplantation.[5]

In cases of medical failure, penetrating keratoplasty is often required. Although early grafting was at one time advocated to remove the bulk of infected tissue,[24] graft rejection or failure occurs approximately 50% of the time when the transplant is done in the face of an active, progressive, and unresponsive infection[1] (Fig. 13-9). Recurrence in the graft is not uncommon (approximately 30%) and may be complicated by uncontrolled glaucoma, cataracts, wound leak and dehiscence, persistent epithelial defects, stromal melting, and phthisis.[7,14] Penetrating keratoplasty should be reserved for impending perforation or for visual rehabilitation when the infection has cleared and accompanying inflammation has cleared. The

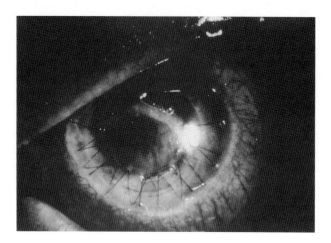

FIG. 13-9. *A discouraging sign (ring infiltrate) after grafting for* Acanthamoeba keratitis. *(Courtesy of Dr. K. Zadnik.)*

use of wide margins is suggested as an additional method of debulking organisms. Confocal microscopy can aid in evaluating the peripheral cornea.

The chance for a successful graft is increased if medical treatment can be maintained for 1 year before surgery.[1,3] Medical management must be aggressive to saturate the cornea with appropriate chemotherapeutics. Some have suggested that antiamebic therapy should be continued through the time of and for several months after surgery to reduce recrudescence.[1,4]

Antisense therapy is being investigated as a viable treatment method. Various strategies for blocking the life cycle seem to hold promise in the fight to impart timely clinical cure. An attempt is made to block encystment using an oligonucleotide strategy.[3]

Additional Protozoans

Other protozoans have reportedly caused ocular infection. Additional amoebae that have been implicated include *Naegleria*, *Hartmannella*, and *Vahlkampfia*. A nonamebic protozoan, *Microsporidia*, has gained some attention. It is an obligate intracellular protozoan found on corneal scrapings of patients infected with human immunodeficiency virus from nasopharyngeal or urinary colonization.[31] Other nonocular sites of infection include the bowel, biliary tract, lower respiratory tract, kidney, and skeletal muscle. Generally, microsporidiosis presents as a superficial punctate keratitis or multifocal keratitis (may be confined to the superficial cornea for months) in immunoincompetent patients. The genus *Encephalitozoon* is responsible. A stromal keratitis is possible after trauma, especially

in immunocompetent patients, and the genus *Nosema* is often the causal agent. Bee stings are a common vector because the protozoan can accompany the inoculation.

Diagnosis is made by Gram's stain, cytology with chromotrope-based stain, electron microscopy, or confocal microscopy.

Treatment regimens can vary in their effectiveness. A slight improvement has been noted with trimethoprim-sulfisoxazole. Itraconazole, propamidine isethionate, albendazole, and especially topical fumagillin bicyclohexylammonium salt (Fumadil B) have shown promise in imparting a clinical cure.[31]

Summary

It should be noted that most cases of *Acanthamoeba* keratitis have occurred in relatively young and healthy individuals. The ubiquitous presence of acanthamoebae in the environment and the relative rarity of infections suggest that opportunistic involvement might be expected in immunosuppressed individuals, but this has not been the case with keratitis associated with this pathogen.

Acanthamoeba infections should be suspected in a healthy contact lens wearer who develops radial nerve infiltrates, elevated epithelial lines, bull's-eye–like keratopathy, or annular infiltrates, especially after a history of trauma. A higher index of suspicion should accompany any patient who develops a protracted keratitis with disparate pain and who has a history of using unpreserved saline, especially homemade saline made from salt tablets and distilled water. Therapeutic results may depend on timely diagnosis, the virulence of the organism, and the eventual acquisition of resistance by the organism.

Prevention should always be an integral part of management with every contact lens patient to avoid this relentless pathogen. Contact lens wearers must be scrupulous in handling, cleaning, and disinfecting their lenses. Lenses must not be immersed in distilled or tap water after the disinfecting process for rigid, soft, or hybrid lenses and before the lens is inserted.

FUNGAL KERATITIS

Fungal keratitis (keratomycosis) is an uncommon complication of contact lens wear in most of the United States and is often overlooked as a possible cause of suppurative keratitis.[1,32–36] Too often, it is considered a disease limited to the Southern and Southwestern states.[33,36] The frequency of fungal keratitis has increased during the 1980s and 1990s in the contact lens–wearing population, especially with the increasing use of topical corticosteroids, which enhances the growth of fungi while suppressing the host immune response.[36] The increasing use of broad-spectrum antibiotics may provide an uncompetitive environment in which to grow.[36]

Clinical awareness by the contact lens practitioner, as well as proper laboratory methodology for identification of fungal keratitis, aids in the correct diagnosis and provides the best possible outcome.

Classification

Fungi are primitive, nonmotile, plantlike organisms that may grow as unicellular organisms called *yeasts* or as multicellular filamentous structures called *molds*.[33] It is noteworthy that yeasts are the most commonly found fungal organisms in conjunctival cultures of healthy subjects and can be part of the normal external ocular flora.[32,37,38] Fungi are divided into four major classes: *Zygomycetes, Ascomycetes, Basidiomycetes,* and *Deuteromycetes* (Fungi Imperfecti). The class *Zygomycetes* consists of nonseptate filamentous fungi, which are rare corneal pathogens.[34] The class *Ascomycetes* includes fungi with separate hyphae and spores contained in sacsorasci.[33] Corneal pathogens representing this group include the genera *Aspergillus* and *Penicillium.*

Fungi of the class Basidiomycetes have separate hyphae and spores. Mushrooms and plant rusts are members of this group.[33] The class of *Deuteromycetes* contains most of the human pathogens.

Of the more than 40 genera of fungi known to cause keratomycosis, most are saprophytic. These cause opportunistic corneal infection in traumatized and immunologically compromised or suppressed eyes (Table 13-3).[1,32,36] *Candida albicans* is the most important species of yeast responsible for fungal infection, comprising between 5% and 7% of cases in a series from the southern United States and from 32–43% in a larger series from the northern corridor.[37] *Fusarium*, the most common genus of filamentous fungi, has an incidence in major clinical series ranging between 45% and 61%.[33,34] Other important fungal pathogens include *Aspergillus, Cephalosporium, Curvularia,* and *Alternaria* species. Among the ocular pathogens, *Fusarium* is generally considered the most virulent. *Aspergillus* remains the most common causative organism of fungal infection worldwide.[38]

Detection

A proper history should record onset and duration of symptoms, prior treatment if any (especially steroids), clinical response, and a careful review of the patient's con-

TABLE 13-3. *Reported Causes of Keratomycosis*

Absidia
Acremonium
Acrostalagmus
Acrothesium
Allescheria
Alternaria
Aspergillus
Beauveria
Blastomyces
Botrytis
Candida
Cephalosporium
Cryptococcus
Curvularia
Fusarium
Fusidium
Gibberella
Glenospora
Helminthosporium
Hormodendrum
Lasiodiplodia
Microsporum
Monosporium
Mucor
Oospora
Paecilomyces
Penicillium
Periconia
Phialophora
Phycomycetes
Rhizomucor
Rhizopus
Rhodotorula
Scopulariopsis
Sporothrix
Sporotrichum
Sterigmatocystis
Tetrapoloa
Trichoderma
Trichophyton
Trichosporon
Tritirachium
Ustilago
Verticillium

Source: Reprinted with permission from SB Koenig: Fungal keratitis. In KF Tabbara, RA Hyndiuk (eds): Infections of the Eye. Little, Brown and Company, Boston, 1986.

tact lens wear and solution regimen. The diagnosis of keratomycosis must be confirmed by laboratory investigation. With any keratitis suspected of being infectious, adequate scrapings must be taken from the cornea for culture and cytologic study. The initial management of microbial keratitis depends on the corneal smear. Because fungi may be present only in the deep stroma,[33] it may be necessary to perform a limited keratectomy biopsy, espe-

TABLE 13-4. *Procedures Routinely Used for Specimen Preparation and Identification*

Slide preparation. Corneal smears are prepared on five pre-cleaned glass slides and immediately fixed in methanol for 5 minutes. Corneal biopsy specimens are fixed in 10% formalin solution. One slide is held in reserve while others are processed with Gram's, Giemsa, Grocott-Gomori silver, and periodic acid–Schiff (PAS) reagent.

Culture inoculation. Multiple corneal scrapings of material from the bed and leading edge of the ulcer are inoculated on laboratory media by a streak technique. The c-streak method of direct plating is helpful in determining if the fungal colony is a contaminant or a true inoculum from the spatula. Media selected for the culture should enable recovery of the fungi as well as rare aerobic and anaerobic bacteria. Standard media include blood, chocolate, and Sabouraud's agar, as well as thioglycolate broth,[1,33] but Sabouraud's medium, a peptone and dextrose mixture, is the most popular medium for fungal recovery. The agar should contain 50 mg/ml gentamicin without cycloheximide, which has a tendency to inhibit saprophytic fungi. Cycloheximide is present in some commercial media. Cultures should be held for 2–3 weeks to avoid true-negative readings, although growth usually occurs in the first week. Growth beyond 1 week is unusual and may be a contaminant.[33] Transport of media or a delay in inoculation often gives poor results. Cultures should be checked daily for evidence of growth.

Detection of fungi by smear. Corneal scrapings can be processed with Giemsa and Gram's stains, which selectively stain fungal protoplasm[33]; cell walls are not stained.[41] However, proteinaceous debris and thick smears may reduce the contrast between fungal elements and the background, which may interfere with proper identification.[33,41,58] Giemsa stain colors hyphal elements purple-blue and may be slightly more sensitive for demonstrating fungi. In one series, fungi were detected in 75% of corneal scrapings with either Gram's or Giemsa stain.[32,33] (see Fig. 13-10). The Grocott-Gomori methenamine-silver stain is the most selective method for identifying fungal elements in tissue. One study showed an 86% identification rate in a series of culture-proven cases of fungal infection.[36] The technique depends on the reduction of silver by oxidized carbohydrate components of the cell wall to stain the fungus black. Forster and coworkers[41] have described a modified technique for corneal scrapings with methenamine silver that allows rapid cytoplasmic diagnosis. Corneal scrapings stained with Gram's and Giemsa stains can be re-examined by this technique. At times, only one fungal element is seen on an entire slide, but this finding is enough to make a diagnosis.[33] The PAS reagent is useful for identifying fungal elements in tissue and cytoplasmic preparations.[38,39] Carbohydrates in the fungal cell wall that react with periodic acid stain magenta.[33] Potentially more reliable are calcofluor and ink–potassium hydroxide preparations.[40]

Source: Reprinted with permission from SB Koenig: Fungal keratitis. In KF Tabbara, RA Hyndiuk (eds): Infections of the Eye. Little, Brown and Company, Boston, 1986.

cially when initial cultures are negative. Anterior chamber paracentesis for smear and culture has been recommended if surface scrapings and biopsies are negative when the invasion is deep and mycotic endophthalmitis is suspected, because filamentous fungi have the ability to penetrate an intact Descemet's membrane. It is not performed in routine evaluation of fungal keratitis.

Because it is often difficult to establish a diagnosis of fungal keratitis, the use of smears and cultures is extremely important.[35] Gram's and Giemsa stains (see Fig. 13-10) are the most commonly used stains for rapid diagnosis. Initial studies report the detection of hyphal elements of filamentous fungi, blastospores, or pseudohyphae of yeast in 78% of smears of fungal keratitis.[35] Reports suggest a much lower yield, perhaps as low as 30%.[39] Culture media for suspected fungal keratitis should include the same culture media used for a general workup of any case of microbial keratitis. These include sheep's blood agar, chocolate agar, Sabouraud's dextrose agar, and thioglycolate broth. Positive growth should be expected in approximately 90% of cases of fungal keratitis.[35] Initial growth can occur within 72 hours in 83% of cultures and within 1 week in 97% of cases. Increasing the humidity of the medium by placing the plates in plastic bags has been recommended to enhance the chance of growth. Methods of detection, although not widely available, include immunofluorescence staining, electron microscopy, PCR, and confocal microscopy. Confocal microscopy is not overly effective in yeast-related keratitis but is extremely useful in filamentous keratitis.

Fungi have been recovered in patients at the initial visit from topically applied medications, cosmetics, contact lenses, storage cases, and contact lens solutions. Cultures and smears can be obtained to increase the chances of identifying causative organisms.[35] Fungal sensitivities are available from some laboratories but are of limited value in light of the paucity of antifungal medications. This information may include minimal inhibitory concentration data as well as synergy studies, which allow a choice of the best single or combination antifungal agent. These specialized tests are important, especially when initial therapy is unsuccessful (Table 13-4).

Histopathology

In keratomycosis, fungi may be identified histologically throughout all levels of the cornea and may extend beyond boundaries of clinically recognized infection.[40] The histopathologic findings in keratomycosis include the loss of corneal epithelium, Bowman's layer, and variable amounts of stroma. The secretion of enzymes, such as phospholipase, protease, and pseudocollagenase, causes

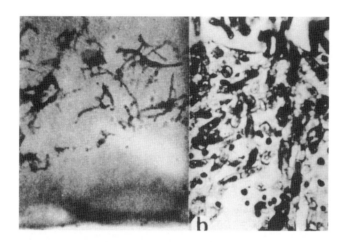

FIG. 13-10. *Fungal smears, Gram's (left) and Giemsa (right), showing hyphal elements in filamentous fungi.*

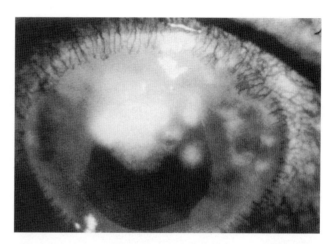

FIG. 13-11. *Feathery infiltrates with satellite lesions in fungal keratitis.*

coagulative necrosis, with loss of keratocytes and disruption of collagen lamellae.[33,40] The surrounding inflammatory cell infiltrate is typically a granulomatous reaction, although chronic nongranulomatous and purulent inflammatory reaction may occur.[41] As in other forms of microbial keratitis, fungal infection of the cornea commonly stimulates an outpouring of inflammatory cells into the anterior chamber, causing a sterile hypopyon.[33] Certain filamentous fungi can penetrate an intact Descemet's membrane, which usually acts as a relative barrier to limit fungal invasion.[40] Hyphal elements are commonly arranged parallel to collagen lamellae; perpendicular orientation may imply increased virulence or suggest steroid usage.

Corneal microabscesses located peripherally to the main ulcer are common histologic findings in fungal infection and correspond to the satellite lesions noted clinically.[33] Peripheral corneal ring abscesses are characteristic of fungal keratitis and are composed of collections of polymorphonuclear leukocytes, plasma cells, and eosinophils around invading hyphae.[33,40] The abscess formation probably represents a host immune response to fungal antigen and corresponds to the immune ring described.[40,42,43]

Clinical Presentation

Early diagnosis of fungal infection is aided by a high index of suspicion based on the patient's history and the presence of slit-lamp findings suggestive of fungal disease. The symptoms of fungal keratitis may not present acutely as with other forms of microbial keratitis, especially bacterial. Patients may present with an initial foreign-body sensation for several days with a slow onset of increasing pain.[35]

The clinical appearance of fungal keratitis varies with the infectious agent and with the stage of the disease.[1,42] A history of trauma,[32] especially with vegetative matter, or contact lens wear[1,33] is common. Fungal keratitis continues to be a disease most commonly encountered in the rural setting.[35]

The time interval from trauma to clinical findings can range from 24–48 hours to as long as 10–21 days. This depends on the organism and its virulence, the size of the inoculum, and the host resistance.

Clinical features vary, and none seem to be pathognomonic,[33] allowing keratomycosis to be easily confused with other forms of microbial keratitis. Filamentous fungal ulcers can present with a whitish or grayish surface involving any part of the cornea, which may be rough and raised above the corneal plane in one area. The edges are crenellated and irregular, often with feathery extensions under an intact epithelium, and satellite lesions are seen occasionally.[33] However, post-traumatic fungal keratitis may initially present as a discrete stromal abscess or plaque without an overlying defect (Fig. 13-11).[33] The ulcer base may actually have a dry texture. An immune ring may be present where fungal antigen and host antibody meet. Corneal endothelial white plaque and hypopyon are associated findings commonly found even with small ulcers. These have no diagnostic value even though the signs are disproportionate. Progressive infection may lead to perforation and fungal endophthalmitis.[42]

Fungal ulcers in patients with pre-existing corneal disease most commonly occur in areas of exposure. Secondary fungal keratitis develops in patients who are

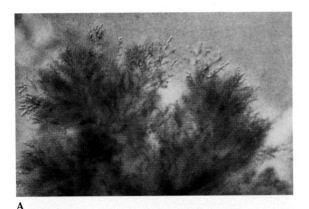

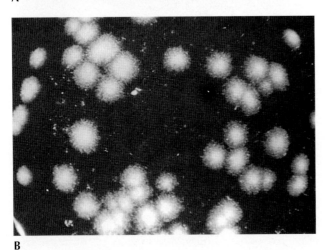

FIG. 13-12. *(A) Filamentous fungi infiltrating a soft contact lens. (B) Yeast contamination of a soft contact lens. (Courtesy of Dr. R. Weisbarth.)*

immunologically suppressed or compromised systemically or locally in the eye. Evidence of keratitis sicca, neurotrophic keratitis, or herpetic keratitis should be sought.[32,33,42] Prolonged steroid use is often a significant factor. Fungal invasion should be suspected if a chronic ulceration appears indolent and worsens despite seemingly adequate therapy. *Candida* is a more common pathogen in this group of patients. Fungal keratitis caused by yeast (i.e., *Candida* spp.) is usually associated with an overlying epithelial defect. The infiltrate usually appears more discrete and suppurative,[42] lacking the hyphate margins seen in filamentous fungal keratitis. Progressive corneal ulceration caused by yeast may occur very slowly. *Candida* is often a secondary invader.

Fungal ulceration can simulate herpetic, bacterial, and *Acanthamoeba* keratitis. The confusion is understand-

able because of the presence of necrosis and hypopyon, especially in advanced disease.

Contact Lens–Related Factors: Minimizing Risks

Fungi are not part of the normal ocular flora,[38] even in contact lens wearers, but they do frequently contaminate contact lens paraphernalia.[8,44-51] Dunn and associates[1] found fungal contamination in 3% of hard lens cases and in up to 50% of homemade saline solutions.

The contact lens itself can harbor fungi.[32] Wilson and Ahearn[46] estimate that 2–5% of worn extended-wear lenses are contaminated with fungi. Other studies have found fungal spoliation rates of 8–41%.[32]

Wilhelmus and associates,[32] reviewing a large series of culture-proven ulcerative keratitis, found that 4% of patients wearing cosmetic or aphakic lenses and 27% of those wearing therapeutic soft contact lenses had a keratomycosis. The spectrum of responsible fungi in contact lens–related keratitis includes hyphal molds and yeasts.[32,33] Filamentous fungi, such as *Fusarium*, account for most corneal infections associated with wearing refractive or cosmetic soft contact lenses, whereas yeast (i.e., *Candida*) causes most fungal ulcers in patients wearing therapeutic or bandage contact lenses.[32] How different contact lenses influence the development of fungal infection remains unclear.[45] Geographic considerations may play a role in the extent of contamination because a higher incidence of certain fungal disease clearly exists in non–contact lens wearers in the southeastern United States compared with those in the more northern regions.[1,36,37]

Studies have shown that certain fungi can adhere to and penetrate soft contact lens materials, especially extended-wear lenses (Fig. 13-12).[1,32,52] In addition, older or damaged lenses with surface irregularities and deposits permit fungal attachment and growth.[32,44,46] Tear components, such as lysozyme, lactoferrin, and albumin, further enhance the adherence of *Candida* to hard and soft lenses.[53] After adherence, fungal enzymes appear able to degrade hydrophilic polymers, permitting invasion and proliferation within the lens matrix.[32]

Heat disinfection is usually the most dependable method for preventing fungal contamination of soft contact lenses.[1,32,49,51] Even so, bacterial and fungal spores can survive the temperature cycle of thermal disinfection.[28] Cold disinfection, even a 10-minute hydrogen peroxide soak, may not be enough to render certain fungi inactive.[2,51] Penley and associates[51] recommend that the soaking time for lenses should exceed 45–60 minutes in 3% hydrogen peroxide. The recommendation poses problems with most available systems. Additional developments in new disinfecting techniques that reliably kill fungi and innovative ways to limit fungal adherence to contact lens surfaces require further investigation.[32]

Predisposing factors appear to be improper lens care in refractive or cosmetic wearers and chronic epithelial defects and topical corticosteroid use in therapeutic lens wearers.

Several recommendations seem prudent in minimizing the risk of developing keratomycosis or other forms of microbial keratitis while wearing contact lenses:

- Avoid wearing lenses in moldy environments.
- Wash hands before each lens manipulation.
- Do not reuse solutions or use homemade saline or distilled water for rinsing lenses or as an enzyme diluent.
- Clean and disinfect lenses daily with a system approved by the U.S. Food and Drug Administration; use enzyme weekly.
- Maintain an appropriate wearing time for specific lenses.

Awareness and recognition of fungal contamination of contact lenses are necessary to decide when to replace lenses and when to reinstruct patients in proper lens care. Any lens suspected of containing fungi should be replaced rather than attempting a cleaning and disinfecting cycle or disinfection with an antifungal medication or other solution.[32,50] Even though certain patients wear lenses with grossly visible fungal spots without sequelae, the lenses of other patients who experienced pain, conjunctival hyphema, and corneal punctate staining yielded fungi on culture.[46] In most of these cases of ulceration, the keratoconjunctivitis cleared within a few days without treatment. It was theorized that the findings were the result of fungal toxins.[46]

Other Risk Factors

Trauma is the most common risk factor in fungal keratitis, and it most commonly occurs outdoors and involves plant matter. Gardeners and patients using motorized lawn equipment are especially predisposed. Additional risk factors include the use of corticosteroids (topical and systemic) and chronic use of antibiotics, neurotrophic ulcers (varicella zoster and herpes simplex), and penetrating keratoplasty. Predisposing risks for fungal keratitis in grafted patients include suture problems, topical steroid and antibiotic usage, contact lens wear, graft failure, and persistent epithelial defects.

Some systemic risk factors may include diabetes mellitus and patients who are hospitalized or chronically ill,

and any disease with accompanying immunosuppression or incompetence.[35]

Therapy

The initial management of suspected microbial keratitis, including keratomycosis, depends on the history, clinical impression, and results of corneal scrapings.[32] Regardless of the ulcer's appearance, antifungal therapy is usually not introduced until a definitive diagnosis (specifically, laboratory confirmation) is made. The presence of hyphae, pseudohyphae, or yeast in a smear prepared from a corneal lesion dictates antifungal therapy.[32,38,42]

The ideal antifungal agent is characterized by broad-spectrum activity, absence of de novo and induced fungal resistance, solubility in water or organic solvents, stability in aqueous preparations, adequate ocular penetration, absence of local and systemic toxicity, and availability for topical, subconjunctival, or systemic administration. No such agent exists.[32] A variety of agents have been used clinically for fungal infection, including thimerosal, gentian violet, zinc, silver nitrate, copper sulfate, boric acid, and halogens. These agents are far from ideal, however, because of ocular toxicity, generally poor ocular penetration, or inadequate activity.

Several broad classes of newer antifungal agents are available, ranging from antibiotics to antiseptics. These antifungals are divided into three major groups: polyene antibiotics, imidazoles, and pyrimidines. They are far from ideal but are relatively safe.

The mainstay of therapy has been the polyene antibiotics. A broad-spectrum antibiotic in the first stages of fungal infection may be recommended in case of comorbidity. The polyene antibiotics are produced from a variety of *Streptomyces* species. They work by binding to the sterol groups in the fungal cell membranes, rendering them permeable.[32] This leads to lethal imbalance in cell contents. In addition to their antifungal action, some of the polyenes have antitumor and immunopotentiating effects.

Single drug use with natamycin 5% (commercially available) is recommended as the initial medical therapy for fungal keratitis. If a worsening of keratitis occurs, topical amphotericin B 0.15% is substituted with or without flucytosine 1%. Natamycin is a broad-spectrum antifungal agent that has been used effectively in the treatment of fungal keratitis caused by *Fusarium*, *Cephalosporium*, *Aspergillus*, and *Candida* species.[32,54] It is bland and demonstrates little, if any, corneal or conjunctival toxicity after topical administration. Despite prolonged contact with the cornea, natamycin (5%) achieves poor ocular penetration and is not beneficial in deep infections. Sub-conjunctival injections may cause conjunctival necrosis and granulomatous inflammation and produce low drug levels in the cornea and anterior chamber.[32,42,54]

Hourly topical natamycin (5%) around the clock is the best initial treatment for filamentous fungal keratitis. Intensive topical antifungal therapy for at least 6 weeks is continued until signs of resolution include the rounding up of the ulcer margin, decreased intensity of the infiltrate, diminished corneal edema, and resolution of the overlying epithelial defect.[33,54] The degree of intraocular inflammation and size of hypopyon is not a useful parameter in assessing resolution or progression of microbial keratitis.[33] As in other causes of microbial keratitis, the absence of progression implies clinical improvement. Occasionally, a fungal ulcer may worsen after initial therapy, exhibiting an increase in intraocular inflammation, increased hypopyon, and marked stromal edema.[32,54] As the fungal ulcer resolves, the frequency of antifungal administration is gradually decreased generally after 4 weeks of therapy.

Amphotericin B, another polyene antifungal agent, was used for many years as the major antifungal therapy, especially if *Candida* was the causal organism.[16] It is very effective, especially for yeast infections, but irritating to the cornea in the concentration prescribed and must be prepared extemporaneously. Today, a diluted concentration (0.15%) is less irritating and is used primarily topically, while natamycin, which is sometimes difficult to obtain, is procured or when sensitivity studies show it to be more effective than natamycin. Initial therapy may include topical administration every 30–60 minutes. Drops are prepared from a commercial intravenous preparation (Fungezone) using sterile water.[55] This concentration is nephrotoxic; therefore, serum creatinine needs to be followed. Subconjunctival injection is extremely painful and may cause yellowing of the conjunctiva and nodule formation. Intravenous administration of amphotericin B may be complicated by nephrotoxicity, hypokalemia, and thrombocytopenia and is rarely indicated for the treatment of keratomycosis.[32]

Nystatin is a tetraene polyene antifungal agent that was used in the past for the treatment of superficial keratomycosis caused by *Candida albicans*. It penetrates the cornea poorly and has limited activity against other fungal pathogens.[54] The dermatologic preparation is well tolerated when applied topically every 4–6 hours.[32]

Imidazole compounds are a relatively new class of drugs with remarkably broad antifungal activity and less ocular toxicity than most of the polyene antibiotics. These agents possess antifungal, antiprotozoan, and antibacterial activity against several species of fungi, amoebae, and

bacteria.[32] In contrast to polyenes, they are relatively resistant to light, hydrolysis, and pH changes and are soluble in organic substances.[33] Imidazoles reported in the treatment of ocular fungal disease include clotrimazole, miconazole, econazole, ketoconazole, and thiabendazole. Their antimycotic activity, like that of the polyenes, includes an effect on cell membranes and their permeability to various cell constituents.

In addition to inducing biochemical and morphologic changes, imidazoles appear to limit fungi by acting in synergy with host defense cells. These compounds have been advocated for treatment of filamentous keratomycosis associated with deep infiltration, impending perforation of the cornea, or scleral abscess.[54] Miconazole has been used successfully in the treatment of corneal ulcers caused by *Alternaria, Rhodotorula, Penicillium, Aspergillus, Fusarium,* and *Candida* species.[54,56] *Candida* infection usually responds to topical medication alone. The drug demonstrates good ocular penetration after topical or subconjunctival administration and is associated with no significant ocular toxicity.[33,55] Initial therapy may include hourly administration of topical miconazole (10 mg/ml) and daily subconjunctival injection (10 mg). With clinical improvement, injections may be discontinued and the frequency of topical administration gradually tapered over a 6- to 12-week period.[33,38,56]

Ketoconazole is a relatively new water-soluble compound that is structurally related to miconazole.[33] It has broad-spectrum activity as an antifungal, with a typical dosage (approximately 300 mg/day) showing encouraging results in the treatment of keratomycosis in humans.

Clotrimazole has a wide spectrum of activity but poor activity against gram-positive bacteria and *Fusarium* species. Topical clotrimazole in 1% solution of araches oil is reported to be well tolerated. It can be given hourly until clinical response occurs, then tapered to four times a day for 8–12 weeks.[53] Oral clotrimazole may soon be available in this country. Jones[54] has successfully treated two cases of *Aspergillus fumigatus* keratitis with oral clotrimazole that had not responded to systemic amphotericin B. Children tolerate oral administration better than adults and may be given up to 150 mg/kg per day.[33] Systemic levels after oral administration are low and may not reach mean inhibitory concentrations of infecting fungi.

The halogenated pyrimidine 5-fluorocytosine is active by deamination by a fungal enzyme and may be used as an adjunct in the treatment of keratomycosis caused by *Candida* species and certain strains of *Aspergillus*.[33] Therapeutic levels have been found in the aqueous humor after oral administration of 200 mg/kg per day. The drug can be applied topically or given orally. Its effectiveness is limited because it penetrates cell walls poorly.

Several topical antifungal agents may act synergistically against a particular fungal organism.[35] Amphotericin B 0.15% and subconjunctival injections of rifampin were found to be more effective than amphotericin alone. Amphotericin B and flucytosine also have a synergistic effect. Resistance to an antifungal is rare except in the case of flucytosine, in which systemic resistance has been documented.[35]

Medicamentosa is extremely common with topical medications and results in eyelid margin irritation, persistent conjunctivitis, and nonhealing epithelial defects. This problem is likely to occur after several weeks of therapy and responds to tapering of medications. In a large south Florida series of fungal cases, the average treatment duration was 38 days. Ninety-one percent of the cases were treated with natamycin 5%.[36]

Susceptibility and synergy studies are beneficial guides for therapy. No place exists for steroid therapy in fungal corneal disease, except in the later stages of a healing fungal ulcer after clear clinical evidence of control of the keratitis. Steroid therapy, when used, must be used in conjunction with topical antifungal medications. If steroid therapy has been initiated before a definitive diagnosis of fungal infection, it should never be stopped abruptly but tapered gradually.

Adjunct therapy includes topical cycloplegia with homatropine or cyclopentolate, which allows some movement of the pupil, prevents the development of posterior central synechiae, and reduces the possibility of pupillary block glaucoma.[33] Elevated tension caused by intraocular inflammation is best managed by a topical beta blocker or a carbonic anhydrase inhibitor.

Parasympathomimetic agents may cause increased intraocular inflammation or induce relative pupillary block and should be avoided if possible. Secondary bacterial infection should always be considered if the ulcer worsens.

Pre-existing ocular surface disease and eyelid abnormalities must be identified and corrected.[33] Lubricants, bandage contact lenses, or partial tarsorrhaphy may promote re-epithelialization after the fungus has been eradicated.

Surgical management includes initial corneal scrapings taken at the slit lamp during initial diagnostic evaluation. This procedure serves as surgical débridement; necrotic tissue is excised, leaving a clean base for better penetration of antifungal agents because the epithelium is a barrier to most effective agents.[33,54,56] Deep corneal curettage may enhance resolution of the ulcer by removing a large portion of the fungal inoculum.

Donnenfeld described success in applying heat to the cornea in fungal keratitis. This is believed to affect the barrier function of these organisms. Heat less than 41°C is required to avoid collagen destruction.[57]

Conjunctival flaps may be indicated for treatment of fungal infections that do not respond to medical therapy.[33,42,53] Large central ulcers are best treated with a total conjunctival flap; peripheral lesions may be managed by partial flaps. Flaps offer little, if any, tectonic support. If possible, a partial flap should be oriented vertically, with a visual axis that is spared.[33] Flaps should not be used in cases of impending corneal perforation because perforation may occur beneath the flap.[58] Grafting can be performed at a later date, after resolution of the infection and intraocular inflammation. Tissue adhesives may have therapeutic value and have been shown to be fungistatic.[59]

With impending perforation, acute penetrating keratoplasty may be indicated. Although penetrating keratoplasty may be successful in eliminating residual infection and restoring the architectural integrity of the globe,[33] the prognosis for visual recovery may be poor. Antifungal medication should be continued after grafting if significant residual infection at the wound margin is suspected.[59] Recurrence weeks after surgery is possible. Postoperative complications include peripheral anterior synechiae, secondary angle-closure glaucoma, cataract formation, and graft failure.[33,54,55] If the infection is allowed to progress until it involves the limbus or sclera, unfavorable outcomes secondary to scleritis, endophthalmitis, and recurrences are more common. The size of trephination should leave a 1- to 1.5-mm clear zone of clinically uninvolved cornea to reduce the possibility of residual fungal organisms peripheral to trephination. Confocal microscopy may aid in making a definitive assessment of a clear margin. The role of topical steroids in the immediate postoperative course is controversial. The effects of other immunosuppressive agents, such as cyclosporin A, on fungal growth has not been well documented clinically.[35,60] Lamellar keratoplasty and excimer ablation are contraindicated in the treatment of active or deep fungal ulcers. Fungi may be present within deep corneal stroma, regardless of the appearance. Therapeutic keratectomy using the 193-μm excimer laser may be used for corneal smoothing after resolution of the fungal ulceration when significant scarring and corneal irregularity limit vision.

Summary

Jones[54] estimates that 300 cases of fungal keratitis occur each year. This represents a dramatic increase in incidences during the 1970s, 1980s, and 1990s, and many of these occur in contact lens wearers.[32] Although it is unrealistic to believe that all contact lens–related infections, including fungal keratitis, can be prevented, good reason exists to believe that the incidence can be substantially reduced. Apart from strict adherence to the principles of lens hygiene, regular professional examinations should be performed.

It is essential that patients recognize the early manifestations of corneal infections, discontinue lens wear, and seek immediate attention. At the same time, practitioners must manage patients with infections aggressively to reduce ocular morbidity.

REFERENCES

1. Dunn JP, Mondino BJ, Weissman BA: Infectious keratitis in contact lens wearers. p. 5. In Bennett ES, Weissman BA (eds): Clinical Contact Lens Practice. Lippincott, Philadelphia, 1991

2. Ma P, Visvesvera GS, Martinez AJ, et al: *Naegleria* and *Acanthamoeba* infections: review. Rev Infect Dis 12:490, 1990

3. Shovlin JP, Depaolis MD, Edmonds SE, et al: *Acanthamoeba* keratitis: contact lenses as a risk factor. Int Contact Lens Clin 14:349, 1987

4. Auran JD, Starr MB, Jakobiec FA: *Acanthamoeba* keratitis: a review of the literature. Cornea 6:2, 1987

5. Alizadeh H, Niederkorn JY, McCulley JP: *Acanthamoeba* keratitis. p. 1267. In Krachmer JH, Mannis MJ, Holland EJ (eds): Cornea. Mosby, St. Louis, 1997

6. Moore MB, McCulley JP, Luckenbach M, et al: *Acanthamoeba* keratitis associated with soft contact lens wear. Am J Ophthalmol 100:396, 1985

7. Moore MB, McCulley JP, Newton C, et al: *Acanthamoeba* keratitis: a growing problem in soft and hard contact lens wearers. Ophthalmology 94:1654, 1987

8. Samples JR, Binder PS, Luibel FJ, et al: *Acanthamoeba* keratitis possibly acquired from a hot tub. Arch Ophthalmol 102:707, 1984

9. Koenig SB, Solomon JM, Hyndriuk RA, et al: *Acanthamoeba* keratitis associated with gas permeable contact lens wear. Am J Ophthalmol 103:832, 1987

10. Stehr-Green JK, Bailey TM, Visvesvera CS: The epidemiology of *Acanthamoeba* keratitis in the United States. Am J Ophthalmol 107:331, 1989

11. Holland GN, Donzis PB: Rapid resolution of early *Acanthamoeba* keratitis after epithelial débridement. Am J Ophthalmol 104:87, 1987

12. Ficker L, Hunter P, Seal D, et al: *Acanthamoeba* keratitis occurring with disposable lens wear. Am J Ophthalmol 100:453, 1989

13. Theodore FH, Jakobiec FA, Juechter KB, et al: The diagnostic value of ring infiltrate in *Acanthamoeba* keratitis. Ophthalmology 92:1471, 1985

14. Cohen EJ, Buchanan HW, Laughrea PA, et al: Diagnosis and management of *Acanthamoeba* keratitis. Am J Ophthalmol 100:389, 1985

15. Marines HM, Osatao MS, Font RL: The value of calcofluor white in the diagnosis of mycotic and *Acanthamoeba* infections of the eye and the ocular adnexa. Ophthalmology 94:23, 1987

16. Epstein RJ, Wilson LA, Visvesvera GS, et al: Rapid diagnosis of *Acanthamoeba* keratitis from corneal scrapings using indirect fluorescent antibody staining. Arch Ophthalmol 104:1318, 1986

17. Johns KJ, Head WS, Parrish CM, et al: Examination of hydrophilic contact lenses with light microscopy to aid in the diagnosis of *Acanthamoeba* keratitis. Am J Ophthalmol 108:329, 1989

18. Pfister DR, Cameron JD, Krachmer JH, et al: Confocal microscopy findings of *Acanthamoeba* keratitis. Am J Ophthalmol 121:119, 1996

19. Florakis GJ, Folberg R, Krachmer JH, et al: Elevated corneal epithelial lines in *Acanthamoeba* keratitis. Arch Ophthalmol 106:1202, 1988

20. Moore MB, McCulley JP, Kaufman HE, et al: Radial keratoneuritis as a presenting sign in *Acanthamoeba* keratitis. Ophthalmology 93:1310, 1986

21. Mannis MJ, Tamaru R, Roth AM, et al: *Acanthamoeba* sclerokeratitis: determining diagnostic criteria. Arch Ophthalmol 104:1313, 1986

22. Penley CA, Willis SW, Sicker SG: Comparative antimicrobial efficacy of soft and rigid gas permeable contact lens solutions against *Acanthamoeba*. CLAO J 15:257, 1989

23. Ludwig IH, Meisler DM, Rutherford I, et al: Susceptibility of *Acanthamoeba* to soft contact lens disinfection systems. Invest Ophthalmol Vis Sci 27:626, 1986

24. Hirst LS, Green WR, Merz W, et al: Management of *Acanthamoeba* keratitis: a case report and review of the literature. Ophthalmology 91:1105, 1984

25. Berger ST, Mondino BJ, Hoft RH, et al: Successful medical management of *Acanthamoeba* keratitis. Am J Ophthalmol 110:395, 1990

26. Binder PS: Cryotherapy for medically unresponsive *Acanthamoeba* keratitis. Cornea 8:106, 1989

27. Matoba AY, Pare PD, Le TD, et al: The effects of freezing and antibiotics on the viability of *Acanthamoeba* cysts. Arch Ophthalmol 107:439, 1989

28. Driebe WT, Stern GA, Epstein RJ, et al: *Acanthamoeba* keratitis: potential role for topical clotrimazole in combination chemotherapy. Arch Ophthalmol 106:1196, 1988

29. Wright P, Warhurst D, Jones BR: *Acanthamoeba* keratitis successfully treated medically. Br J Ophthalmol 69:778, 1985

30. Perry, HD, Donnenfeld ED, Foulks GN, et al: Decreased corneal sensation as an initial feature of *Acanthamoeba* keratitis. Ophthalmol 102:1567, 1995

31. Davis RM, Font RL, Keisler MS, et al: Corneal microsporidiosis: a case report including ultrastructural observations. Ophthalmol 97:954, 1990

32. Wilhelmus KR, Robinson NM, Font RA, et al: Fungal keratitis in contact lens wearers. Am J Ophthalmol 106:708, 1988

33. Koenig SB: Fungal keratitis. In Tabbara KF, Hyndiuk RA (eds): Infections of the Eye. Little, Brown, Boston, 1986

34. Schwartz LK, Loignon LM, Webster RG: Post-traumatic phycomycosis of the anterior segment. Arch Ophthalmol 96:860, 1978

35. Alfonso EC, Rosa RH: Fungal keratitis. p. 1253. In Krachmer JH, Mannus MJ, Holland EJ (eds): Cornea. Mosby, St. Louis, 1997

36. Liesegang TJ, Forster RK: Spectrum of microbial keratitis in south Florida. Am J Ophthalmol 90:38, 1980

37. Chin GN, Hyndiuk RA, Kwasny GP, Schultz RO: Keratomycosis in Wisconsin. Am J Ophthalmol 79:121, 1975

38. Ando N, Takatori: Fungal flora of the conjunctival sac. Am J Ophthalmol 94:67, 1982

39. Jones DB, Wilson L, Sexton R, Rebell G: Early diagnosis of mycotic keratitis. Trans Ophthalmol Soc UK 89:805, 1970

40. Naumann G, Green WR, Zimmerman LE: Mycotic keratitis. A histopathologic study of 73 cases. Am J Ophthalmol 64:668, 1967

41. Forster RK, Wirta MG, Solis M, Rebell G: Methenamine silver stained corneal scrapings in keratomycosis. Am J Ophthalmol 82:261, 1976

42. Feder RS: Diagnosis and treatment of fungal keratitis. Arch Ophthalmol 108:1224, 1990

43. Brown SI, Bloomfield S, Pierce DB, Tragakis M: Infections with the therapeutic soft lens. Arch Ophthalmol 91:275, 1974

44. Yamamoto GK, Pavan-Langston D, Stowe GC, Albert DM: Fungal invasion of a therapeutic soft contact lens and cornea. Ann Ophthalmol 11:1731, 1979

45. Chusner R, Cunningham RD: Fungal contaminated soft contact lenses. Ann Ophthalmol 15:724, 1983

46. Wilson LA, Ahearn DG: Association of fungi with soft contact lenses. Am J Ophthalmol 101:434, 1986

47. Sagan W: Fungal invasion of a soft contact lens. Arch Ophthalmol 94:168, 1976

48. Gasset AR, Mattingly TP, Hood I: Source of fungus contamination of hydrophilic soft contact lenses. Ann Ophthalmol 11:1295, 1979

49. Charles AM, Callender M, Grosvenor T: Efficacy of chemical aseptizing system for soft contact lenses. Am J Ophthalmol 50:777, 1973

50. Gasset AR, Ramer RM, Katzen D: Hydrogen peroxide sterilization of hydrophilic contact lenses. Arch Ophthalmol 93:412, 1975

51. Penley GA, Llabres C, Wilson LA, Ahearn DG: Efficacy of hydrogen peroxide disinfection systems for soft contact lenses contaminated with fungi. CLAO J 11:65, 1985

52. Yamaguchi T, Hubbard A, Fukushima A, et al: Fungus growth on soft contact lenses with different water contents. CLAO J 10:166, 1984

53. Butrus S, Klotz SA: Blocking *Candida* adherence to contact lenses. Curr Eye Res 5:745, 1986

54. Jones DB: Decision making in management of fungal keratitis. Ophthalmology 88:814, 1981

55. Wood TO, Williford W: Treatment of keratomycosis with amphotericin B 0.15%. Am J Ophthalmol 81:847, 1976

56. Foster CS: Miconazole therapy for keratomycosis. Am J Ophthalmol 91:622, 1981

57. Donnenfeld E: Treating difficult infections of the cornea. Presentation at the Southern Educational Congress of Optometrists, Atlanta, February, 1998

58. Sanders N: Penetrating keratoplasty in the treatment of fungal keratitis. Am J Ophthalmol 70:24, 1970

59. Rao GN, Reddy MK, Vagh MM, et al: Results of cyanoacrylate tissue adhesive application in active filamentous fungal keratitis. Presentation at the Castroviejo Cornea Society, San Francisco, October 29, 1994

60. Johns KJ, O'Day DM: Pharmacologic management of keratomycosis. Surv Ophthalmol 33:178, 1988

V

Complications of Extended-Wear Lenses

14

Complications of Hydrogel Extended-Wear Lenses

HELEN A. SWARBRICK AND BRIEN A. HOLDEN

GRAND ROUNDS CASE REPORT

Subjective:

A 35-year-old architect was seen at the Cornea and Contact Lens Research Unit (CCLRU) clinic in January 1987 for screening before enrollment in a long-term clinical study of disposable hydrogel extended-wear lenses. He was wearing hydrogel contact lenses on a flexible extended-wear basis (2 or 3 nights per week). The patient was in good health, took no medications, and had an unremarkable personal and familial ocular history.

Objective:

- Spectacle prescription: right eye (OD) –1.75/–0.50 × 120 (6/6⁺), left eye (OS) –1.75/–0.50 × 50 (6/6⁺)
- K readings: OD 43.25/43.75, OS 43.25/43.87
- Tear breakup time < 10 seconds; partial blinker. Upper eyelid: hyperemia grade 1 each eye (OU), papillae grade 0.5 OU. Slight (grade 0.5) punctate epithelial stipple staining OU. Otherwise, no abnormalities detected.

The patient was enrolled in the study and was dispensed disposable lenses (Etafilcon A, Johnson & Johnson, Jacksonville, FL) on February 17, 1987. Lenses were –2.00 D OU (base curve 8.7 mm, lens diameter 14 mm). Visual acuity with the lenses at dispensing was 6/4.8 OU. The patient began a 13-night extended wearing schedule immediately, with lens disposal every 2 weeks. He was issued sterile, unpreserved aerosol saline for lens rinsing as necessary, and thimerosal-free in-eye lubricating drops for insertion morning and evening or as necessary.

The patient adapted to lens wear rapidly. Aftercare examinations conducted after 3 days; 1 and 2 weeks; 1, 2, and 3 months of wear; and then at 3-month intervals revealed no problems. The patient continued lens wear for 27 months without incident. A fluctuating microcyst and vacuole response was recorded during this period, with a peak at 24 months (microcysts OD 50, OS 60; vacuoles OU 10). Visual acuity with the contact lenses deteriorated slightly over time, and a change in lens prescription (OU –2.25 D) was made at 27 months.

Event 1:

At the 27-month scheduled visit (April 10, 1989), two small asymptomatic epithelial infiltrates were noted near the inferior limbus in the right eye; there was no associated epithelial staining. No action was taken, although the patient was reminded of his obligation to notify the clinic immediately of any unusual symptoms, such as redness, irritation, or blurred vision, particularly in one eye only.

Event 2:

On the morning of July 6, 1989 (29 months of wear), the patient contacted the clinic and was seen at 10:40 AM. He had awakened at 6:00 AM with extreme irritation, photophobia, and lacrimation, particularly in the left eye. He bathed his eyes in saline but this had not relieved the symptoms. His current lenses had been worn consecutively for 18 nights.

Slit-lamp examination revealed the following:

- Bulbar hyperemia OD grade 2, OS grade 3.5
- OS, subepithelial infiltrates at the superior and inferior corneal periphery, with slight overlying staining
- Microcysts OD 40, OS 60
- Vacuoles OD 10, OS 30

Assessment and Plan:

The lenses were removed, and the patient was advised to return the following day. A diagnosis of contact lens–induced acute red eye (CLARE) (Fig. 14-1) was made on the basis of patient symptoms and clinical findings. The following day, the patient reported significant regression of symptoms, although he was still slightly photophobic. Subepithelial infiltrates were still present at the superior limbus, but there was no staining. Bulbar conjunctival hyperemia had also subsided (OD grade 1.5, OS grade 2.5). Slight endothelial bedewing was noted in the left eye.

The patient was seen again 7 and 14 days after the episode. The signs and symptoms continued to clear. Two weeks after the CLARE episode, the infiltrates and endothelial bedewing had resolved. Microcysts and vacuoles were noted breaking through the epithelial surface. Bulbar hyperemia had reduced to grade 1 OU. The patient was advised to return to lens wear gradually, with daily wear for 3 days, building up to 1 week and then 2 weeks of extended wear if no problems occurred. The importance of strict compliance with the prescribed wearing and disposal schedule was emphasized. At the next scheduled visit (33 months), the patient had successfully resumed his original wearing schedule and no unusual corneal signs were present.

Event 3:

Lens wear continued without incident over the next 21 months. On July 11, 1991, the patient contacted the clinic. The previous afternoon he had noted a foreign-body sensation in the right eye, which had gradually worsened. He removed the lenses in the evening and reinserted them the following morning, but the right eye became increasingly irritated. The lenses had been worn for 5 consecutive nights at the time of the episode.

Slit-lamp examination of the right eye revealed slight hyperemia (grade 1.5) and a small circular corneal epithelial ulcer at 11 o'clock, approximately 0.4 mm in diameter and 1.5 mm from the limbus (Fig. 14-2). The lesion stained intensely with fluorescein and was surrounded by stromal infiltration and haze (grade 3). A large microcyst response (>100 OD) was also noted. Endothelial bedewing was observed, but there was no anterior chamber flare or ocular discharge.

Assessment and Plan:

On the basis of presenting symptoms and clinical signs, a contact lens–induced peripheral ulcer (CLPU) was diagnosed. The patient's lenses, solutions, and lens case were retained for microbiologic evaluation, and the patient was advised to discontinue lens wear and return the following day.

One day later, the symptoms had resolved completely and the epithelial ulcer was healing well. No epithelial staining was seen, although the epithelium appeared disrupted and showed poor wetting over the lesion. Bedewing, infiltrates, and haze had regressed slightly, and the microcyst response was also slightly reduced. One week later, a small cluster of epithelial infiltrates remained, surrounding a circular epithelial scar at the location of the lesion (Fig. 14-3). Microcyst numbers had reduced to 26, and epithelial staining, endothelial bedewing, and stromal haze were absent.

The laboratory report of cultures from the patient's lenses revealed significant growth of gram-negative bacteria, including *Pseudomonas* spp. and *Enterobacteria* spp. Cultures of lens solutions and lens case were negative. The patient was counseled on hygiene practices and lens care. After all signs of corneal inflammation had resolved, the patient was advised to resume lens wear on a daily-wear basis. Resumption of extended wear was subsequently introduced but limited to no more than 1 week (6 nights) between overnight lens removals.

Event 4:
Lens wear continued without incident for a further 18 months. On January 19, 1993, the patient again presented with a CLPU in the right eye at a routine scheduled appointment. The patient reported only minor symptoms of irritation and redness. The CLPU was smaller than 1 mm in diameter and was positioned at 12 o'clock, approximately 2 mm from the limbus. A small infiltrate was also noted at 11 o'clock, and grade 2.5 bulbar and limbal hyperemia were recorded. One week later, the infiltrate had resolved, and a circular scar remained at the site of the CLPU. Extended wear was resumed on a 6-night-per-week basis.

Event 5:
Two years later, after an uneventful lens-wearing period, the patient contacted the clinic to report that he had gotten sawdust in his eyes during house renovations. When seen later that day (March 15, 1995), a subconjunctival hemorrhage was noted OD, and focal infiltrates (3 OD, 1 OS) were also seen. Resolution was followed over a 2-month period, during which daily lens wear was cautiously resumed at 3 weeks and extended wear at 8 weeks. A second foreign-body episode 1 month later, which triggered a recurrence of infiltrates, was managed in a similar fashion. Over the following 2.5 years, the patient presented on a number of occasions with asymptomatic infiltrates but successfully continued with a 6-night extended-wear regimen.

Event 6:
On January 23, 1998, the patient presented for an unscheduled appointment with copious discharge and ocular redness in the right eye only. There were no other significant symptoms, although he had influenza. The patient reported that he had reverted to daily wear 3 days previously and that the lenses were 1 day old. Severe bulbar and limbal hyperemia were noted, particularly in the right eye (OD grade 4, OS grade 2.5). Three small (0.1 mm in diameter) focal epithelial infiltrates were also noted OD, overlying a diffuse infiltration from 10 to 2 o'clock. High levels of *Haemophilus influenzae* were cultured from the right eyelid margin and lens vial solutions. A diagnosis of bacterial conjunctivitis with associated infiltrates was made. After a 4-day period with no lens wear, ocular and influenza symptoms and signs had resolved, apart from one faint epithelial infiltrate. Daily wear was resumed, and extended wear reintroduced 1 week later.

Event 7:
Soon after, on February 28, 1998, the patient awoke with a sore red right eye. Examination again revealed infiltrative keratitis OD (focal and diffuse infiltrates), but with cells and flare in the anterior chamber (cells grade 2, flare grade 0.5). The patient was referred for ophthalmologic assessment and treatment, which comprised antibiotic and steroid eye drops. The patient was monitored closely over the ensuing 3 weeks, during which medication was tapered and the infiltrates cleared. Because of the recurrent infiltrative episodes, however, the patient was advised to remain in daily lens wear.

Follow-up:
At regular aftercare examinations over the last year, the patient has admitted to occasional lapses in extended wear and has presented on occasions with asymptomatic faint infiltrates. At his most recent aftercare examination (December 21, 1998), almost 12 years after commencing participation in CCLRU hydrogel extended-wear lens studies, he remains a reasonably successful and satisfied flexible extended lens wearer (maximum 2 or 3 nights a week), without significant ocular signs or symptoms.

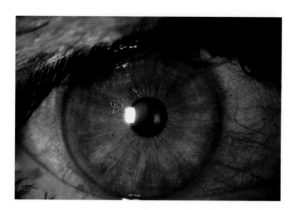

FIG. 14-1. *Contact lens–induced red eye reaction in a patient using hydrogel extended-wear lenses. The etiology of this acute inflammatory response is unclear. (Photograph by Timothy Grant.)*

Continuous wear is still the so-called Holy Grail of contact lenses. Promised to the profession and the public for over 25 years, the possibility that contact lenses could be left in the eye indefinitely is still the most sought-after and most revolutionary concept in the use of external devices for vision correction. In every survey conducted at the CCLRU, the mode of lens wear preferred by the vast majority of prospective and successful patients is continuous lens wear.[1] Contact lens wearers want safe, comfortable, permanent correction of vision through contact lenses, corneal onlays, or refractive surgery.

Experience with rigid gas-permeable (RGP) contact lenses has proved that extended wear (i.e., sleeping in lenses) can be safe and effective. Long-term clinical studies with a substantial number of patients (> 300 at the

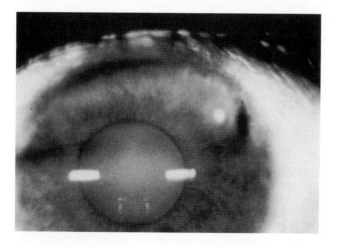

FIG. 14-2. *Contact lens–induced peripheral ulcer in a patient using hydrogel extended-wear lenses, showing intense uptake of fluorescein at the site of the lesion. (Photograph by Mee Sing Chong.)*

CCLRU) have established that lenses with truly high oxygen transmissibility [Dk/t (oxygen transmissibility) $> 100 \times 10^{-9}$ (cm $\times$ ml O_2)/(s $\times$ ml $\times$ mm Hg)] present no significant threat to corneal integrity or vision. Discontinuations from this mode of lens wear occur primarily owing to mechanical discomfort, eyelid irritation, and other problems related to persistent deposits and corneal staining. Because high-Dk/t RGP lenses are safe and effective for many patients, it is unfortunate that this type of lens was not the initial offering for extended wear.

Patient and practitioner preoccupation with immediate comfort has driven the extended-wear modality ever since deCarle first introduced the concept in the early 1970s.[2] As detailed in this chapter, the reality did not live up to the promise. A regular cycle of sensational antilens publicity ensued for 25 years as one media group or another discovered that hydrogel lens extended wear presents a significant threat to corneal health and integrity for many wearers. Misconceptions about the oxygen needs of the cornea, difficulties in defining the nature of soft contact lens extended-wear effects on corneal structure and function, and inadequate long-term data on the clinical performance of extended-wear soft contact lenses have bedeviled the field and led to occasional public skepticism about contact lenses in general. The major cycles of public and practitioner alarm associated with the safety of hydrogel extended wear occurred first in the United Kingdom[3] and Australia,[4,5] and then in Europe and the United States.[6]

Although reliable up-to-date figures are difficult to find, it is clear that extended hydrogel lens wear is still prescribed at moderate levels in the United States. In 1996, it was estimated that up to 22% of American contact lens wearers wore their lenses for extended periods.[7] This modality is now rarely used in many other countries, however, including the United Kingdom and Australia, where extended-wear usage has remained relatively steady at less than 1% of new fits per year.[8,9] The impact of disposable lenses, which now comprise the majority of new fittings worldwide,[10,11] has done little to increase the popularity of the extended-wear modality in these countries. This may be explained in part by well-publicized reports in the literature indicating that the risks of severe corneal responses, such as microbial keratitis, are not significantly diminished by the use of disposable lenses for extended wear.[12,13] Major problems still occur, however, from the indiscriminate use of hydrogel extended-wear lenses in many less-developed countries, such as the Philippines and China (personal communication, Dr. Arthur Back, CCLRU).

The last major challenge for contact lenses remains the production of a high-Dk/t soft contact lens that promotes a healthy, resistant epithelium and is truly biocompatible. Such a lens could minimize the risk of infection during lens

FIG. 14-3. *Superficial circular scar that remains after resolution of a contact lens–induced peripheral ulcer. (Photograph by Timothy Grant.)*

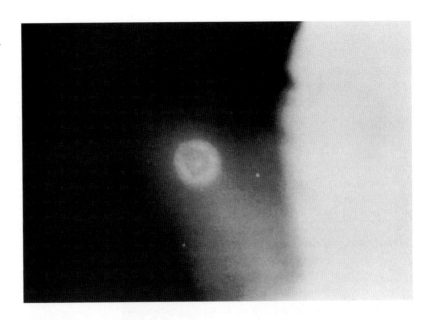

wear and would finally meet the needs and expectations of prospective contact lens wearers. Ideally, the truly safe high-Dk/t soft contact lens is capable of weeks to months of continuous wear before disposal or is durable enough to use for long-term daily wear in regions of the world, such as Asia, where millions of potential wearers would find a reusable contact lens economically feasible. The introduction of new high-Dk/t soft contact lenses, based on novel polymer formulations, promises a new era in extended wear, although the clinical performance of these new lenses has yet to be rigorously evaluated in the real world.

Hypoxia, inflammation, and infection remain major areas for concern with hydrogel lens extended wear. This chapter discusses adverse responses associated with hydrogel lens extended wear under these three headings. However, it should be borne in mind that many complications are multifactorial in etiology, and management of adverse responses frequently requires a broad approach to maintain ocular health and continue the patient successfully in lens wear.

CORNEAL HYPOXIA

Oxygen Supply

When the eye is open, the cornea receives its oxygen supply directly from the atmosphere (21% O_2).[14,15] This oxygen is used mainly in the epithelium to provide energy (via the Krebs cycle) for tissue replication, growth, and maintenance, through the metabolism of glucose, which is supplied principally from the aqueous,[16] and glycogen, which is stored in the epithelium.[17] Traditionally, the stroma has been regarded as having a low level of metabolic activity and, therefore, a relatively low requirement for oxygen.[18] However, research has suggested that the stroma is much more metabolically active than previously thought,[19] although the oxygen requirements of this tissue layer have yet to be defined. It is also not clear whether the corneal endothelium requires atmospheric oxygen to maintain normal metabolic functioning. Although this tissue layer has been shown to have a relatively high metabolic rate by volume,[18] a significant oxygen supply is available from the aqueous humor.[20,21]

When the eye closes, atmospheric oxygen no longer reaches the anterior corneal surface unless the eyelids form an imperfect seal.[22] Therefore, in most cases, the oxygen requirements of the cornea during eye closure must be met by diffusion of oxygen from the vascular capillary plexus of the upper palpebral conjunctiva.[23] Although significant individual differences exist in the levels of oxygen available from this source, it is generally agreed that oxygen availability is reduced from 21% to approximately 8% O_2 during prolonged eye closure.[22,24]

Contact lenses can also reduce the level of oxygen that reaches the anterior corneal surface. During open-eye lens wear, oxygen availability at the corneal surface under the contact lens depends on the circulation of oxygenated tears behind the contact lens and also on the Dk/t of the contact lens itself. Therefore, the fitting and movement characteristics of the lens on the eye, the permeability (Dk) of the contact lens polymer, and the thickness profile of the contact lens all have a significant influence on the level of oxygen available to the cornea for maintenance of normal metabolic activity.

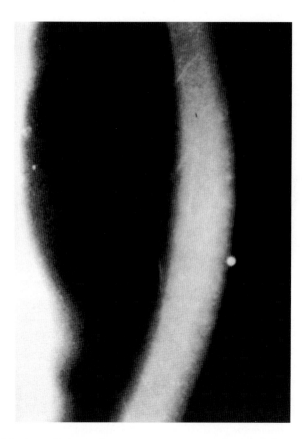

FIG. 14-4. *Striae in the posterior stroma, associated with more than 6% corneal edema. (Reprinted with permission from SG Zantos, BA Holden: Ocular changes associated with continuous wear of contact lenses. Aust J Optom 61:418, 1978.)*

If oxygen availability at the lens front surface is reduced, oxygen levels behind the lens also decrease. Therefore, the oxygen supply to the anterior corneal surface during contact lens wear is further restricted during the closed-eye phase of extended lens wear. Because the level of oxygen supplied from the capillary plexus of the palpebral conjunctiva is reduced relative to atmospheric oxygen levels,[22,24] the barrier presented by the contact lens achieves greater significance than during open-eye wear. Furthermore, the contribution to corneal oxygenation of tear circulation behind the lens is significantly reduced, if not abolished.[25] Therefore, the level of oxygen that reaches the cornea during closed-eye lens wear depends on the amount of oxygen that permeates from the palpebral conjunctival blood vessels and on the Dk/t of the contact lens. Oxygen availability to the cornea can be increased under these circumstances either by increasing the Dk of the contact lens polymer or by reducing lens thickness (L).

Because oxygen is a primary requirement for the maintenance of normal corneal metabolic activity, a reduc-

tion in oxygen availability (hypoxia) has acute and chronic effects on corneal structure and function. The most dramatic, and the most easily observed in a clinical situation, is corneal swelling or edema.[17] A reduction in oxygen levels in the epithelium leads to an alteration in metabolism; the rate of aerobic metabolism (through the Krebs cycle) is reduced, and the rate of anaerobic metabolism increases to provide energy for cellular processes. As a result of this alteration in the balance of metabolic activity, excess lactate or lactic acid is generated.[23,26] According to the theory of Klyce,[27] this by-product of anaerobic metabolism accumulates in the stroma and induces an osmotically driven influx of water into the tissue, resulting in stromal swelling.

Corneal Edema

Corneal swelling or edema represents a rapid and easily quantifiable response to anterior corneal hypoxia. Many studies have used this response as an index of hypoxia, and it is clearly established that a direct correlation exists between oxygen levels at the anterior corneal surface and the average corneal swelling response.[28] It is also clear that significant individual differences exist in the corneal edema response to hypoxia.[28] This is important to keep in mind when individual patient responses during contact lens wear are assessed.

The corneal edema response is most accurately quantified by using a pachometer to measure corneal thickness before and after application of a hypoxic stress. This approach is used routinely in research on contact lens effects, in which accuracy is desirable. Such instruments are not yet regarded as standard equipment in contact lens practices. However, the corneal swelling response can be estimated with reasonable accuracy by assessing the posterior corneal appearance with a slit-lamp biomicroscope. At corneal edema levels of approximately 6%, striae, which appear as thin white or silvery lines, can be observed at the level of the posterior stroma and Descemet's membrane (Fig. 14-4).[29,30] At higher levels of corneal swelling (10–15%), more defined stromal folds can be seen.[31] La Hood and Grant[32] have suggested that the percentage of corneal swelling can be estimated by counting the number of striae and folds seen. In their study, the presence of one stria correlated with a mean swelling response of 5%, five striae with 8% swelling, and 10 striae with an 11% swelling response. The presence of one fold correlated with a mean edema response of 8%, five folds with 11% edema, and 10 folds with 14% edema. This approach provides the contact lens practitioner with an easy method for evaluating the individual corneal edema response by quantification of the striae and folds response.

The cornea can tolerate some reduction in oxygen availability before corneal swelling occurs. Holden and coworkers[28] have shown that, on average, corneal edema can be avoided if oxygen levels remain more than 10% (Fig. 14-5). At this oxygen level, however, other, more subtle changes in corneal physiology can be detected. For example, lactate begins to accumulate in the anterior chamber and epithelial cell mitosis is reduced at oxygen levels below 13%.[33] An endothelial bleb response is obtained below 15% oxygen.[34] Other subtle acute and chronic changes in corneal structure and function that occur in response to corneal hypoxia are discussed later in the Effects of Hypoxia on Corneal Structure and Function section.

Overnight wear of contact lenses represents the most stressful situation encountered by the contact lens–wearing cornea in terms of hypoxia. Therefore, it is not surprising that the cornea typically exhibits a significant overnight swelling response when lenses are worn during sleep. The amount of overnight swelling is directly related to the Dk/t of the lens worn[35] and can range from as high as 20% with thick, low–water content hydrogel lenses to as low as 3–4% (equivalent to that experienced with no lens on the cornea)[36–38] for RGP lenses with extremely high Dk/t.[38]

Once the eye opens after sleep, the cornea begins to deswell as an increased oxygen supply becomes available from the atmosphere. This deswelling is enhanced by the resumption of circulation of oxygenated tears behind the lens, driven by blink-activated lens movement. Although rigid and soft lenses of comparable Dk/t induce similar levels of overnight swelling, the rate of deswelling on eye opening is typically more rapid with rigid than with soft lenses[39,40] because of their greater on-eye movement and tear exchange. It has been estimated that tear exchange of approximately 10–20% occurs with each blink with rigid lenses (depending on lens fitting characteristics)[41,42] compared with 1–2% with soft lenses.[43]

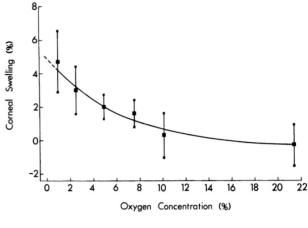

FIG. 14-5. *Mean corneal edema response in eight unadapted subjects after 8 hours of exposure to different oxygen concentrations, delivered to the eyes through sealed goggles. The error bars represent ± 1 standard deviation. (Reprinted with permission from BA Holden, DF Sweeney, G Sanderson: The minimum precorneal oxygen tension to avoid corneal edema. Invest Ophthalmol Vis Sci 25:476, 1984.)*

In an important early study, Holden et al.[44] monitored the corneal edema response in a group of subjects who wore various types of hydrogel lenses continuously for 7 days. Their findings are important in understanding the chronic effects of hypoxia on the cornea. The lenses worn in this study were found to induce 10–15% overnight edema. The level of edema depended on the water content of the lens material and the average lens thickness. Compared to low-minus lenses of comparable center thickness, high-minus lenses with greater peripheral thickness induced greater amounts of overnight corneal swelling (Fig. 14-6).

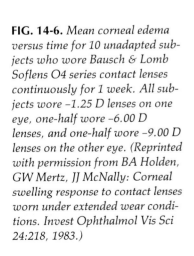 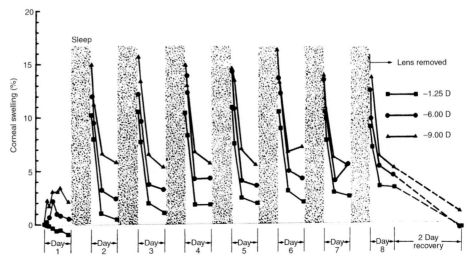

FIG. 14-6. *Mean corneal edema versus time for 10 unadapted subjects who wore Bausch & Lomb Soflens O4 series contact lenses continuously for 1 week. All subjects wore –1.25 D lenses on one eye, one-half wore –6.00 D lenses, and one-half wore –9.00 D lenses on the other eye. (Reprinted with permission from BA Holden, GW Mertz, JJ McNally: Corneal swelling response to contact lenses worn under extended wear conditions. Invest Ophthalmol Vis Sci 24:218, 1983.)*

TABLE 14-1. *Overnight Corneal Edema Responses (Mean ± Standard Deviation) with Hydrogel Lenses*[a]

Lens Type	Material	Tc (μm)[b]	n[c]	Overnight Edema Response (%)
Permalens[d]	Perfilcon A	204	31	12.3 ± 2.1
Hydrocurve II[e]	Bufilcon A	56	15	11.8 ± 3.4
SeeQuence[f]	Polymacon	37	14	11.7 ± 2.7
Bausch & Lomb 70[f]	Lidofilcon A	149	12	11.5 ± 1.8
Vantage Thin[d]	Tetrafilcon A	32	19	11.0 ± 2.4
DuraSoft 3[e]	Phemfilcon A	47	10	10.9 ± 3.3
Permaflex Naturals[d]	Surfilcon A	144	44	10.5 ± 2.4
ACUVUE[g]	Etafilcon A	69	24	10.4 ± 3.2
NewVues[h]	Vifilcon A	81	10	10.3 ± 3.0
Cibathin[h]	Tefilcon	35	5	10.2 ± 2.1

[a]All lenses were –3.00 D back vertex power.
[b]Measured lens center thickness (mean).
[c]Number of subjects.
[d]Manufactured by Coopervision Inc., Fairport, NY.
[e]Manufactured by Wesley-Jessen, Des Plaines, IL.
[f]Manufactured by Bausch & Lomb, Inc., Rochester, NY.
[g]Manufactured by Vistakon, Jacksonville, FL.
[h]Manufactured by CIBA Vision, Duluth, GA.
Source: Data from D La Hood, DF Sweeney, BA Holden: Overnight corneal edema with hydrogel, rigid gas-permeable and silicone elastomer contact lenses. Int Contact Lens Clin 15:149, 1988; and unpublished Cornea and Contact Lens Research Unit studies.

In addition, Holden and coworkers found that the cornea can eliminate on average 8% edema during the open-eye phase of hydrogel lens extended wear. This means that at the end of the day after a 24-hour cycle of hydrogel lens wear, the cornea still typically shows some residual edema (see Fig. 14-6). They concluded that the cornea experiences chronic corneal edema during hydrogel lens extended wear and that the cornea, therefore, is in a state of chronic low-grade hypoxic stress. This conclusion has important implications for the long-term health of the cornea and has been an essential factor driving research and development of contact lenses in the 1980s and 1990s.

Critical Oxygen Transmissibility to Avoid Edema

Holden and Mertz[35] used these findings and other data to derive the critical lens Dk/t required to limit overnight corneal edema to 4%, the level reported (at that time) to occur during sleep without a lens on the eye.[36,37] They found that a Dk/t of 87×10^{-9} (cm × ml O_2)/(s × ml × mm Hg) is required to meet this criterion, a level not achievable with purely hydrogel-based technology. To limit overnight edema to 3.2%, the mean level of no-lens overnight edema reported since by La Hood and coworkers for a group of 41 subjects,[38] a Dk/t of at least 125×10^{-9} (cm × ml O_2)/(s × ml × mm Hg) is required.

According to Holden and Mertz, a lens causing 8% overnight edema, which should allow the cornea to recover completely from overnight edema, requires a Dk/t of 34×10^{-9} (cm × ml O_2)/(s × ml × mm Hg). Although this compromise Dk/t value is theoretically achievable with extremely thin high–water content hydrogel lenses, such lenses are impractical because of their fragility, and have been shown to cause other problems, such as dehydration staining owing to pervaporation of water through the lens from the epithelium.[45,46] The conclusion from this research is that soft contact lenses that rely solely on water in the polymer to achieve oxygen permeability cannot provide sufficient oxygen to the cornea during eye closure to avoid chronic hypoxic stress during extended wear.

In the 1980s and 1990s, significant advances were made in developing RGP polymers, which can deliver considerably higher levels of oxygen to the cornea than is possible with hydrogel lenses. Because of the increased Dk of some RGP polymers, coupled with the more rapid deswelling of the cornea with rigid lenses after overnight lens wear,[39,40] it is possible to avoid chronic hypoxic stress during extended wear of RGP lenses. Tables 14-1 and 14-2 illustrate the average overnight edema responses with a range of hydrogel and RGP lenses typically used for extended wear. It is clear from the tables that hydrogel lenses cause levels of overnight swelling greater than 8%, thus, inevitably inducing some residual edema during the open-eye phase of extended wear. However,

TABLE 14-2. *Overnight Corneal Edema Responses (Mean $\pm$ Standard Deviation) with Rigid Gas-Permeable and Other Lenses*[a]

Lens Type	Material	Tc (μm)[b]	n[c]	Overnight Edema Response (%)
Rigid gas-permeable lenses				
Boston IV[d]	Pasifocon A	145	16	12.9 $\pm$ 3.5
Paraperm EW[e]	Pasifocon C	145	23	11.0 $\pm$ 2.8
Alberta[f]	Sulfocon A	150	8	10.4 $\pm$ 3.4
Equalens[d]	Itafluorofocon A	158	20	10.2 $\pm$ 2.8
Quantum[g]	FSA[h]	154	16	10.1 $\pm$ 2.5
Fluoroperm 92[d]	FSA	146	8	7.6 $\pm$ 2.5
Advent[i]	Fluorofocon A	203	22	6.0 $\pm$ 2.7
Menicon SF-P[j]	Melafocon A	160	10	5.0 $\pm$ 2.8
Other lens types				
Silsoft[g]	Elastofilcon A	110	11	2.0 $\pm$ 1.9
High-Dk soft 1[k]	—	72	10	3.8 $\pm$ 1.8
High-Dk soft 2[k]	—	75	9	3.9 $\pm$ 1.3
High-Dk soft 3[k]	—	90	7	3.6 $\pm$ 2.3
No lens	—	—	41	3.2 $\pm$ 16

[a]All lenses were –3.00 D back vertex power.
[b]Measured lens center thickness (mean).
[c]Number of subjects.
[d]Manufactured by Polymer Technology, Rochester, NY.
[e]Manufactured by Paragon Vision Sciences, Mesa, AZ.
[f]Manufactured by Progressive Optical Research, Calgary, Alberta, Canada.
[g]Manufactured by Bausch & Lomb, Inc., Rochester, NY.
[h]Fluorosilicone acrylate.
[i]Manufactured by 3M Corporation, St. Paul, MN.
[j]Manufactured by Menicon USA, Clovis, CA.
[k]Prototype high-Dk soft lenses, formulation commercial in confidence.
Source: Data from D La Hood, DF Sweeney, BA Holden: Overnight corneal edema with hydrogel, rigid gas-permeable and silicone elastomer contact lenses. Int Contact Lens Clin 15:149, 1988; and unpublished Cornea and Contact Lens Research Unit studies.

some RGP materials induce levels of edema approaching the 4% ideal level of edema suggested by Holden and Mertz.[35]

Between 1995 and 2000, considerable research efforts have been directed toward developing high-Dk/t soft lenses, based on novel polymer formulations. These materials incorporate a highly oxygen-permeable silicone- or fluorosilicone-based polymeric phase that allows oxygen transmission through the polymer itself rather than relying on the water held in the polymer matrix for oxygen diffusion. Indeed, these polymers, which still contain some water (typically <30%), show reducing oxygen permeability as the water content increases.[47] The structure of the polymer matrix is also critical for optimizing oxygen performance. In the lotrafilcon material (CIBA Vision, Duluth, GA), which is a biphasic block-copolymer, continuous pathways of polymer are structured around lakes of water, allowing oxygen movement from lens front-to-back surface along these oxygen highways. Early studies of the overnight edema response with these new-generation soft lenses (such as reported by Dr. Deborah Sweeney at the European Research Symposium, Prague, 1998) (see Table 14-2) suggest overnight edema levels close to those obtained without a lens on the eye,[48,49]

confirming the high Dk values found with in vitro testing methods.[47]

Effects of Hypoxia on Corneal Structure and Function

Epithelium

In a hypoxic environment, such as during contact lens wear, epithelial metabolic activity alters, with a decrease in the rate of aerobic metabolism and a compensatory upregulation of anaerobic metabolism. However, because anaerobic glycolysis provides significantly less energy in the form of adenosine triphosphate compared with aerobic metabolism through the Krebs cycle, less energy is available for normal epithelial cellular processes. Consequently, hypoxia has a number of subtle acute and chronic effects on epithelial structure and function.

The change in metabolic activity is reflected immediately in reduced adenosine triphosphate levels in the epithelium[50] and in alterations in the epithelial mitochondrial redox state.[51,52] The concentrations of several metabolic enzymes, such as lactic dehydrogenase and succinic dehydrogenase, are also affected.[53–55] In addition, glycogen stores in the epithelium are mobilized to fuel anaerobic glycolysis.[17,50,56]

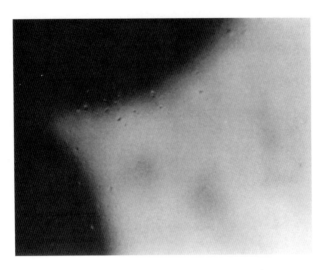

FIG. 14-7. *Slit-lamp photograph of corneal epithelial microcysts in a patient using hydrogel extended-wear lenses. Note that microcysts show reversed illumination (i.e., the distribution of light in the microcysts is opposite to that of the background). This suggests that microcysts comprise apoptotic cells or pockets of cell debris. (Photograph by Timothy Grant.)*

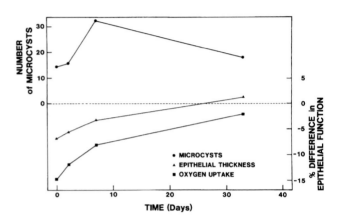

FIG. 14-8. *Mean changes in epithelial thickness, epithelial oxygen uptake rate, and epithelial microcyst numbers after cessation of long-term hydrogel lens extended wear. Data on day 0 were obtained within 2 hours of lens removal. (Reprinted with permission from BA Holden, DF Sweeney, A Vannas, et al: Effects of long-term extended contact lens wear on the human cornea. Invest Ophthalmol Vis Sci 26:1489, 1985.)*

Maintenance of epithelial structural and functional integrity is compromised as a result of the reduction in energy available for normal cellular processes. The rate of cell mitosis is dramatically reduced,[43] and other cell regulatory functions, such as synthesis of cellular components and waste removal, are similarly affected. This is evidenced by distortion of epithelial cells, degenerative intercellular changes, the formation of lipidlike bodies within cells, and the loosening of tight junctions between epithelial cells.[57–59] Inter- and intracellular fluid accumulation may also occur,[57,58] giving rise to epithelial edema. Also, a significant fall occurs in transcorneal potential,[59,60] owing in part to the loosening of intercellular junctions and in part to reduced energy availability for active cation pumping.[61]

These acute changes typically are not apparent clinically, although severe epithelial edema may be observed with the slit lamp. However, more chronic changes in epithelial integrity that occur in response to extended contact lens wear and the resultant chronic hypoxic environment are observable with the slit lamp. The most obvious of these chronic changes is the appearance of *epithelial microcysts* (Fig. 14-7).[5,62–64] These small inclusions, 15–50 μm in diameter, are usually distributed in an annulus in the corneal midperiphery and appear after approximately 3 months of extended lens wear.[63,64] The number of microcysts may fluctuate during lens wear,[64] in some cases reaching as many as several hundred.

The level of microcystic development has proved to be a useful clinical index of the degree of chronic hypoxic stress experienced by the cornea during extended wear.[64] Although their exact nature is unclear, epithelial microcysts are believed to comprise pockets of disorganized cellular materials[65] or apoptotic cells.[66] As such, the microcysts reflect the reduced efficiency of epithelial functioning under hypoxic conditions. After cessation of lens wear, the number of microcysts increases temporarily (Fig. 14-8)[64,67] owing to a resurgence in normal aerobic metabolic activity and an increased rate of elimination of cellular waste products. The fact that microcysts take several months to develop and to disappear after cessation of lens wear[62–64] suggests that they represent fundamental changes in tissue synthesis processes in the epithelium.

Other, more subtle, changes also occur in the epithelium in response to chronic hypoxic stress. The epithelium gradually adapts to the reduced oxygen availability in the long term by decreasing its oxygen use.[68] This is evidenced by a reduction in oxygen consumption rate after several months to years of extended-wear hydrogel lens use (see Fig. 14-8).[67] Although the exact mechanism for this change is not known, it may either represent a chronic reduction in the level of metabolic activity in individual epithelial cells or may result from an overall decrease in cell numbers.

Chronic hypoxia also results in thinning of the epithelium (see Fig. 14-8)[67] as a consequence of the overall decrease in epithelial cell mitotic rate and tissue synthesis. In addition, superficial epithelial cells tend to survive longer before sloughing off into the tear film.[69] This may represent a compensatory mechanism for reduced cell production and turnover, but, as a result, the vitality of the surface cells may be compromised. In particular, epithelial fragility is increased,[70] potentiating the risk of traumatic injury. This risk is compounded by a reduction in epithelial sensitivity,[71,72] a change believed to reflect a reduction in the concentration of the neurotransmitter acetylcholine in the epithelium.[73] The mechanism for this is unclear, although it appears to be related directly to hypoxic stress.[72]

The integrity of the epithelial barrier is also compromised at a more fundamental level. Long-term hypoxia results in a reduction in the density of hemidesmosomes, which anchor the basal cell layer of the epithelium to the underlying basement membrane,[74] resulting in a significant reduction in the strength of epithelial adhesion.[74,75] This subtle alteration in epithelial integrity significantly increases the risk of epithelial damage, and may lead to the spontaneous loss of large areas of epithelium (Fig. 14-9).[76,77] Subsequent to epithelial injury, wound healing may be impeded under hypoxic conditions induced by contact lens wear.[78] Taken together, these alterations in epithelial integrity render the epithelium more susceptible to damage or injury and almost certainly less resistant to microbial attack, which probably contributes to the substantially increased risk of corneal infection during use of extended-wear hydrogel lenses compared with daily wear. Imayasu and colleagues[79] have indeed demonstrated increased levels of subtle epithelial damage, and greater bacterial adherence to the cornea with low-Dk/t lenses compared to high-Dk/t lenses, confirming the role of oxygen in maintaining an effective epithelial barrier against infection.

Stroma

Contact lens–induced hypoxia appears to have little direct effect on the stroma. However, through its swelling response, the stroma provides one of the most accessible measures of acute hypoxic stress. As discussed earlier in the Corneal Hypoxia section, stromal edema arises because of an osmotically driven influx of water into the tissue. The increased osmotic pressure in the stroma results from an increase in the concentration in the tissue of lactate, which is produced by anaerobic epithelial metabolism. Therefore, this stromal response to hypoxia reflects changes in epithelial metabolic activity rather than a response of the stroma per se.

It has been suggested, however, that chronic stromal edema may cause a gradual leaching of ground substance or glycosaminoglycans from the stroma.[80] This may in part explain the stromal thinning that has been reported

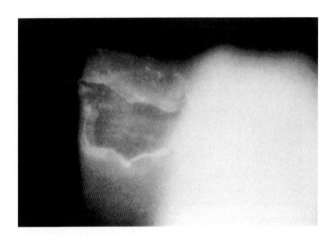

FIG. 14-9. *Spontaneous full-thickness loss of epithelium after mild abrasion in a patient with long-term use of extended-wear hydrogel lenses. It is likely that epithelial adhesion has been compromised owing to chronic hypoxia. (Reprinted with permission from Holden BA, Swarbrick HA: Extended wear: physiological considerations. p. 581. In ES Bennett, BA Weissman [eds]: Clinical Contact Lens Practice. Lippincott, Philadelphia, 1991.)*

after many years of hydrogel lens extended wear.[67,81] This stromal thinning may not be apparent clinically because of residual daytime edema; indeed, corneal thickness measured during the open-eye phase of extended wear may remain close to baseline values. Once residual edema has subsided, however, the stroma is slightly thinned relative to pre–lens-wearing baseline thickness.

Endothelium

The understanding of the effects of hypoxia on the endothelium has evolved significantly since the late 1970s. Traditionally, it was thought that the endothelium was resilient to changes in anterior corneal oxygen levels because it is immediately adjacent to the aqueous humor, which has a relatively high oxygen tension.[20,21] In 1978, Zantos and Holden[82] reported the appearance of small nonreflective areas scattered over the endothelial mosaic shortly after insertion of a contact lens. These *endothelial blebs* (Fig. 14-10) have since been reported in association with exposure to hypoxic or anoxic gas mixtures and eye closure, suggesting that they represent a response to reduced oxygen availability.

When endothelial bleb formation soon after contact lens insertion was first reported,[82] it was postulated that the endothelium was responding to reduced oxygen levels at the anterior corneal surface, which suggests that it did receive significant oxygen flux through the corneal tissue from the atmosphere. Indeed, evidence exists that oxygen tension in the anterior chamber is affected by reductions

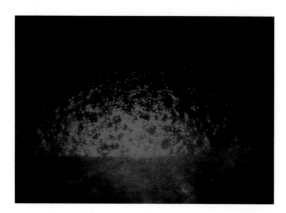

FIG. 14-10. *Endothelial blebs, observed within minutes after the insertion of a contact lens. Blebs are thought to represent an acute response to stromal acidosis. (Photograph by Steve Zantos and Brien Holden.)*

in oxygen availability at the anterior corneal surface.[83–85] Therefore, the endothelial bleb response was initially thought to represent a response to acute corneal hypoxia,[86] and, consequently, endothelial *polymegethism* (variation in cell size) and *pleomorphism* (variation in cell shape) in response to long-term contact lens wear were also attributed to the effects of chronic hypoxic stress. Further studies have established, however, that it is more likely that the endothelial bleb response is induced by changes in stromal pH,[87] or stromal acidosis because blebs are also produced by exposure of the cornea to nonhypoxic stimuli, such as carbon dioxide and oxygen gas mixtures.[87]

Corneal Acidosis

In the open eye, a carbon dioxide concentration gradient exists from the aqueous humor, where carbon dioxide tension is approximately 55 mm Hg, to the atmosphere, where carbon dioxide tension is close to zero.[88] When the eye is closed or when a contact lens is placed on the eye, the efflux of carbon dioxide from the cornea is impeded,[89] and carbon dioxide tension in the tissue increases. In the presence of water, carbon dioxide forms carbonic acid, causing an acidic shift in the tissue. The possible acute and chronic effects of this stromal acidosis on corneal structure and function have only recently received attention.

Bonanno and colleagues[90–93] demonstrated changes in stromal pH during eye closure and contact lens wear. Their careful work has established that the extent of stromal acidosis during open-eye contact lens wear is directly related to the Dk/t of the lenses worn. Lenses such as PMMA, which transmit no oxygen through the lens mate-

rial, cause more profound reductions in stromal pH than high-Dk/t RGP lenses.[92] Changes in stromal pH during hydrogel lens wear similarly reflect the lens Dk/t.[93] Eye closure also causes a significant reduction of stromal pH,[90] which is exacerbated by the presence of a lens on the eye.[92,93] These studies have implicated carbonic acid and lactic acid, a by-product of anaerobic epithelial metabolism, as the agents responsible for stromal acidosis.[91]

Subsequent research using intracellular fluorophotometric techniques in rabbits has confirmed that contact lens wear induces rapid acidification of the epithelium, endothelium, and aqueous humor.[94,95] The primary mechanism for posterior corneal acidosis appears to be carbon dioxide retention, whereas epithelial acidosis is augmented by hypoxia and the associated lactate accumulation. Cohen and coworkers showed that acute corneal acidosis can influence corneal recovery from induced edema.[96,97]

Despite these findings, the effects of chronic stromal acidosis on the corneal tissue are a matter for speculation at this time. However, considerable evidence exists that the endothelium is particularly susceptible to variations in ambient pH. Gross changes in endothelial morphology can be produced in vitro by exposure to relatively large shifts in pH.[98] In addition, endothelial barrier function,[99] fluid transport,[100,101] transendothelial potential,[100,102] and intracellular pH[103] decrease with decreasing ambient pH in vitro.

Endothelial Polymegethism and Pleomorphism

The demonstrated sensitivity of the endothelium to changes in pH has promoted speculation that more long-term changes in endothelial morphology associated with contact lens wear may represent a response to chronic corneal acidosis rather than hypoxia, as was originally hypothesized.[104] Schoessler and Woloschak[105] first reported increased endothelial polymegethism and pleomorphism after long-term PMMA lens wear (Fig. 14-11). This finding has since been confirmed by many investigators in response to long-term wear of daily- and extended-wear rigid and soft lenses.[67,106–112] Silicone elastomer lenses, with high transmissibility for oxygen and carbon dioxide, appear to cause minimal changes in endothelial morphology.[113] Moderate- to high-Dk RGP lenses worn for extended wear produce less marked and rapid endothelial changes than low-Dk RGP or hydrogel lenses.[114]

The relationship between the transient endothelial bleb response and more long-term changes in endothelial appearance is not clear. The endothelial bleb response is thought to represent localized cell edema, which disrupts the specular reflection from the endothelium.[115] The exact mechanism for this response has not been elucidated, however. It is interesting that the bleb response decreases during extended wear,[116] which suggests that lens wear may lead to a loss of the ability of endothelial cells to respond to local environmental changes. This reduction in cellular adaptability to chronic hypoxia or acidosis requires further investigation but may have considerable significance in terms of our understanding of chronic corneal changes during long-term extended wear.

The nature of endothelial polymegethous changes is not well understood. An associated reduction in cell density has not been demonstrated,[67,105,106] which suggests that cell loss is unlikely to explain the observed morphologic changes. Bergmanson[117] suggested that polymegethism may in fact be an artifact produced by distortions of the normally perpendicular endothelial cell walls, but with minimal changes in absolute cell volume. However, observations of clustering of small cells in grossly polymegethous endothelia[118] are difficult to reconcile with this theory. Further work is needed to clarify the understanding of this phenomenon.

The effects of chronic acidosis on endothelial structure show minimal recovery after cessation of lens wear. Indeed, the weight of evidence indicates that contact lens–induced endothelial polymegethism is irreversible,[110,119,120] although some slight recovery has been reported in the long term.[121] The relatively permanent nature of these changes is obviously cause for concern. However, conflicting evidence exists concerning the extent of functional compromise associated with these endothelial morphologic changes.

Rao and coworkers[122,123] reported that patients with high levels of preoperative polymegethism are more likely to experience complications after intraocular surgery. This suggests that endothelial morphologic changes compromise the functional reserve of the endothelium, making it more susceptible to added stresses, such as surgery. However, a later study by Bates and Cheng[124] did not substantiate Rao's findings.

Some support for a link between endothelial polymegethism and functional compromise comes from Sweeney,[125] who has described a *corneal exhaustion* syndrome in long-term wearers of low-Dk/t lenses. These apparently successful wearers demonstrated sudden reduced tolerance to lens wear, blurred or fluctuating vision, and an excessive open-eye edema response during lens wear. All patients described by Sweeney also showed moderate-to-severe endothelial changes. Sweeney hypothesized that after many years of chronic stress induced by wear of low-Dk/t lenses, the endothelium had functional compromise.

Although the endothelium is the primary site for fluid pumping from the edematous cornea, attempts to link

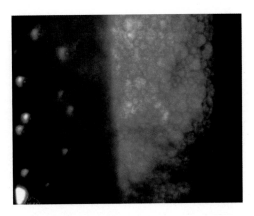

FIG. 14-11. *Endothelial polymegethism (changes in endothelial cell size) in a long-term contact lens wearer. The etiology and functional significance of these chronic changes in endothelial morphology are unclear. (Photograph by Steve Zantos and Brien Holden.)*

contact lens–induced endothelial polymegethism with slower corneal deswelling rates have yielded equivocal results.[126,127] Fluorometric studies have also shown that endothelial permeability is increased with long-term contact lens wear.[112,128] However, the nature of the structural changes that cause this increase in permeability has not been elucidated, and a direct link to endothelial morphologic changes has not been established.

It is clear from this discussion that the long-term consequences of endothelial changes in response to contact lens wear have yet to be clarified, and much research is still required to confirm the potential for functional compromise of the endothelium as a result of chronic stromal acidosis.

INFLAMMATION

Inflammation represents the body's response to a stimulus that is perceived as threatening to tissue integrity. The inflammatory response of a tissue or system typically involves vasodilation, increased permeability of the vasculature, and release of immunogenic mediators, antibodies, and inflammatory cells into the extravascular space. Characteristic symptoms associated with inflammation include hyperemia, edema, heat, and pain. The tissue response is aimed at interrupting, neutralizing, and eliminating the inflammatory stimulus and repairing the damaged tissue.[129]

Inflammatory ocular responses can be triggered by a wide range of stimuli of endogenous or exogenous origin, such as physical or toxic trauma, invasion of pathogens,

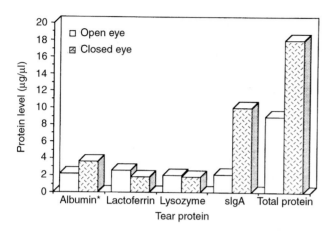

FIG. 14-12. *Differences in protein composition of the open-eye and closed-eye tear fluid. Together with increased plasmin activity, conversion of complement C3 to C3c, and the presence of large numbers of polymorphonuclear cells in the closed-eye tear film, these changes suggest that the closed eye may be in a state of subclinical inflammation. *Albumin includes pre-albumin; the levels of albumin are negligible in the open eye but comprise the dominant portion in the closed eye. (Data from RA Sack, KO Tan, A Tan: Diurnal tear cycle: evidence for a nocturnal inflammatory constitutive tear fluid. Invest Ophthalmol Vis Sci 33:626, 1992.)*

and allergenic stimuli. The presence of a contact lens on the eye thus provides many potential triggers for an inflammatory response. During extended wear, the continual presence of the lens and the physiologic compromise of the tissue owing to chronic hypoxic stress inevitably provide the opportunity for more frequent and severe inflammatory responses. A complex diversity of stimuli may trigger contact lens–related inflammatory episodes, including mechanical trauma, chemicals leaching from the lens substance, deposits on the lens surface, debris trapped behind the lens, or the presence of micro-organisms. Repeated or continuous contact of the tissue with chemicals or lens deposits may, for example, provoke a delayed hypersensitivity reaction, whereas debris behind a lens may induce an acute inflammatory response when the lens is worn overnight.

A number of inflammatory mediators have been demonstrated in the tear fluid, in the quiet eye and during inflammatory events, including immunoglobulins sIgA and IgG, plasmin,[130] complement proteins,[131] vitronectin,[132] histamine,[133,134] interleukins 8 and 6 (IL-8, IL-6), and the arachidonic acid metabolite leukotriene LTB$_4$.[133,135] The role of these substances in the inflammatory events in the corneal tissue is complex. It is clear that many of these substances serve to modulate or regulate the inflammatory response, and some also act chemotactically to recruit

polymorphonuclear leukocytes into the cornea or tear film during inflammatory episodes. Although some of these mediators are normally present in tear fluid, others appear only after the occurrence of injury or in the presence of antigens. Some inflammatory mediators (e.g., sIgA, IL-8) are produced locally by lacrimal gland, corneal, and other tissues, whereas others (e.g., vitronectin, complement proteins) derive from serum and reach the cornea via limbal and conjunctival blood vessels, which become engorged and leaky in the early phase of the inflammatory response.

Many of these tear-borne inflammatory mediators have been demonstrated to vary in concentration on a diurnal basis. It has been established that during eye closure, the nature and composition of the preocular tear film changes from a dynamic reflex tear-rich layer to a secretory IgA-rich layer, which is stagnant in nature.[136] This is accompanied by conversion of complement C3 to C3c[136] and activation of plasminogen,[130] followed by the recruitment of large numbers of polymorphonuclear leukocytes into the tear film.[137] In addition, a significant rise occurs in the concentration of albumin in the closed-eye tear fluid.[136] A range of other inflammatory mediators is also found in increased concentration in closed-eye tear fluid, including histamine, IL-8, LTB$_4$, and vitronectin.[132,133,135] Together, these changes in tear film composition during eye closure (Fig. 14-12) suggest that the closed eye is in a state of subclinical inflammation.[136] This state probably serves the purpose of protecting the vulnerable ocular surfaces from entrapped pathogenic micro-organisms, but it may also render the anterior ocular structures more susceptible to acute inflammatory reactions in response to inflammatory stimuli. Although it has been suggested that overnight lens wear may affect this normal homeostatic diurnal variation in tear film composition, thereby potentiating the risk of acute inflammation, Stapleton and colleagues were unable to demonstrate such an effect.[138]

Long-term extended hydrogel lens wear stimulates increased conjunctival and limbal hyperemia and limbal vessel penetration into the cornea beyond the translucent limbal zone (Fig. 14-13).[139] Although the hyperemic response subsides rapidly once the lens is removed, limbal vessel ingrowth does not regress; the new vessels usually empty, but they may refill rapidly if the precipitating stimulus is reapplied.[140] The chronic limbal vascular response is of clinical concern because the presence of an active vascular bed immediately adjacent to the corneal tissue increases the risk of rapid corneal infiltration or neovascularization if a more severe or acute inflammatory stimulus occurs.[139]

This low-grade chronic vascular response during hydrogel lens wear has long been thought to be inflammatory in nature, stimulated by the persistent presence of the contact lens and exacerbated by mild chronic peripheral corneal edema as well as pressure exerted by the lens on the limbal vasculature. Work by Papas and coworkers,[141] however, suggests that hypoxia may also play an important role. In a short-term study comparing conventional hydrogel and novel high-Dk/t soft lenses, they demonstrated a significantly reduced limbal vascular response with the high-Dk/t lenses. Clinical researchers from the University of Waterloo[48,142] have also reported reduced limbal and bulbar hyperemia and less corneal vascularization with similar high-Dk/t lenses compared to conventional hydrogel lenses worn in extended wear for up to 6 months. It is hoped that longer-term studies may confirm this clinically important finding.

Corneal infiltrates have been reported in association with hydrogel lens daily and extended wear,[143,144] although this acute inflammatory response is certainly more common during extended wear.[145,146] Corneal infiltrates (Fig. 14-14) may be subepithelial or stromal, the latter representing a more severe response, and are believed to comprise polymorphonuclear cells that have migrated from the limbal blood vessels in response to activated immunogenic substances in the corneal tissue or tear fluid.[135,143,147] In many cases, a precise cause for the inflammatory response is not apparent, and these cases of idiopathic corneal infiltration may represent an exacerbation of the mild inflammatory response of the limbal and conjunctival vasculature to the subtle stimuli associated with the chronic presence of a contact lens on the eye. Cessation of lens wear usually leads to resolution of the corneal infiltrates over time, but reapplication of the stimulus may cause a reactivation of the inflammatory reaction. Therefore, issuing fresh lenses and a critical evaluation of lens-wearing and lens-care regimens are indicated (see Grand Rounds Case Report).

The spectrum of corneal infiltrative conditions has been comprehensively categorized by clinical researchers at the CCLRU,[148] based on clinical manifestations, patient symptoms, and the course of events (this categorization system is due to be published as a CCLRU continuing education brochure, entitled "CCLRU-LVPEI Guide to Corneal Infiltrative Conditions Seen in Contact Lens Practice"). At the mild end of the spectrum, asymptomatic infiltrative responses may represent a normal corneal response as they can occur in the non–contact lens–wearing population.[149] In contact lens wearers, these asymptomatic infiltrative episodes are usually of only minor clinical concern, although the presence of a mild-to-moderate conjunctival hyperemic reaction may warrant temporary lens discontinuation until the infiltrates resolve. In the event of significant patient symptoms, however,

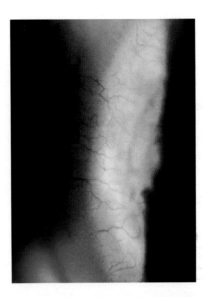

FIG. 14-13. *Limbal vessel proliferation and penetration beyond the translucent limbal zone in a hydrogel lens wearer. Such changes may predispose the cornea to acute neovascularization in the presence of a precipitating stimulus. (Photograph by Charles McMonnies.)*

clinical intervention is warranted, particularly if multiple focal infiltrates are observed or if any associated corneal staining exists. More severe infiltrative conditions, including CLARE, CLPU, and microbial kerati-

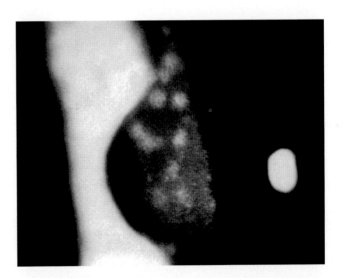

FIG. 14-14. *Focal stromal infiltrates, which are thought to consist of leukocytes or monocytes that have invaded the cornea during an acute inflammatory reaction. (Reprinted with permission from BA Holden, HA Swarbrick: Extended wear lenses. p. 566. In AJ Phillips, J Stone [eds]: Contact Lenses. 3rd ed. Butterworths, London, 1989.)*

tis are discussed in more detail below (see also Grand Rounds Case Report).

Contact Lens–Induced Acute Red Eye

The CLARE reaction is an acute inflammatory response that occurs only during extended wear.[5,150–152] Some confusion appeared to exist in the early literature on the nature and etiology of this characteristic response, and this confusion was mirrored in the variety of names given to the response, such as *tight lens syndrome* and *nonulcerative keratitis*. Experience suggests that the CLARE reaction is distinctive in its signs and symptoms. The reaction shows all the typical features of an acute inflammatory episode, including acute severe conjunctival and limbal hyperemia (see Fig. 14-1), corneal infiltration, and ocular pain. Typically, the contact lens–wearing patient awakens in the early morning with unilateral ocular discomfort or pain, accompanied by marked ocular redness, tearing, and photophobia. Clinical signs include conjunctival and limbal hyperemia and subepithelial infiltrates invading the cornea from the limbus.[151] If the patient has not removed the lens, lens movement may be minimal, with flakes of tear debris trapped between lens and cornea, although this is by no means a universal finding.[151] On lens removal, epithelial staining is usually minimal, although the pattern of the trapped tear debris may be seen imprinted on the cornea. Epithelial staining overlying the corneal infiltrates is rare.[151]

Clinical management involves cessation of lens wear until corneal infiltrates have resolved. This resolution usually occurs over a period of days to weeks without medical intervention, although the institution of prophylactic antibiotic therapy should be considered if epithelial staining overlies the infiltrates. Recommencement of lens wear on a daily basis, using a fresh lens, is usually successful, and extended wear can soon be resumed. However, patients who have experienced one CLARE reaction are more susceptible to repeated episodes during extended wear.[152]

The etiology of this interesting and characteristic extended-wear response has remained elusive for many years, although research has clarified many of its aspects. Early work by Zantos and Holden[150] implicated toxins released by the breakdown of contaminants trapped between the lens and cornea during closed-eye lens wear. The possibility that lens parameters may change in the closed-eye environment, resulting in steepening of the lens base curve and consequent lens tightening,[153] added some support to this theory, and the reaction was sometimes referred to as tight lens syndrome. However, not all CLARE reactions are associated with a tight lens; many CLARE patients examined at the CCLRU clinic have been wearing relatively flat lenses that displayed adequate lens move-

ment when observed soon after the episode. Crook[154] also found that CLARE reactions occurred with steep- and flat-fitting lenses. However, the recovery of large numbers of inflammatory cells, together with epithelial cell debris and mucus, from the post-lens tear pool of CLARE patients[155] added further weight to this early theory.

An understanding of the etiology of the CLARE response has been greatly advanced by elucidation of the role of bacterial lens contamination and colonization in triggering the inflammatory episode. Studies by Baleriola-Lucas and colleagues[156,157] have revealed that patients who experience CLARE reactions form a subgroup of extended-wear hydrogel lens wearers who show repeated high levels of gram-negative bacterial lens contamination. Holden and coworkers[158] reported an unusually high incidence of CLARE responses in an extended-wear study group who were subsequently found to have worn lenses that had been inadvertently contaminated with large numbers of gram-negative bacteria. Although the presence of bacteria on the lens did not cause frank corneal infection, they hypothesized that the release of endotoxins from breakdown of the polysaccharide cell walls of these bacteria during eye closure may play a role in triggering the acute inflammatory response.[158] Sankaridurg and coworkers have also linked bacterial lens contamination by *Haemophilus influenzae* to the production of CLARE responses in extended-wear users.[159]

Further work by Willcox and colleagues has revealed some of the subtleties of the response. They have established that inflammatory mediators in tear fluid recovered immediately after sleep, in particular, IL-8 and LTB_4,[133,135] are implicated in the chemotaxis of polymorphonuclear cells.[147] Gram-negative bacteria recovered from lenses worn by CLARE patients were also found to exhibit chemotaxis for polymorphonuclear cells.[147]

The particular bacterial strain contaminating the lens has also been shown to be significant. The existence of distinct strains of the gram-negative bacterium *Pseudomonas aeruginosa*, with different pathogenicity, has been convincingly demonstrated. Strains recovered from cases of microbial keratitis have been found to exhibit either cytotoxicity or the ability to invade epithelial cells.[160] However, bacteria recovered from CLARE patients were unable to infect corneal cells in a mouse model.[161,162] Thus, the less virulent inflammatory strains may be responsible for the limited nature of the CLARE response, compared to the potentially more destructive response associated with frank corneal infection.

Contact Lens–Induced Peripheral Ulcers

Another acute inflammatory response associated with hydrogel lens extended wear is CLPU. This response (see

Fig. 14-2) is characterized by small (<2-mm diameter), circular, full-thickness epithelial lesions in the paracentral or peripheral cornea associated with stromal infiltration. As reported by Grant and coworkers in CCLRU studies, these ulcers have occurred at a rate of between 2 and 3% per patient a year and have been observed almost exclusively during hydrogel lens extended wear.[163] Although differentiation from potential or early microbial keratitis may be difficult, these authors based their diagnosis of CLPU on the presence of a small circumscribed peripheral ulcer without raised edges, the absence of severe ocular pain, mucopurulent discharge, and anterior chamber reaction,[164] and when carried out, negative culture results. In all cases reported in detail by Grant and colleagues (11 cases), the ulcerative episode followed a benign course and resolved within 2 weeks without medical intervention.

Grant and coworkers believe that CLPU responses have been reported in the literature but have been categorized as either infiltrative keratitis or corneal ulceration, often of presumed microbial origin.[165–170] Although they emphasize a conservative approach to any cases of epithelial erosion associated with underlying stromal infiltration, they comment that an effort should be made to distinguish the relatively innocuous CLPU reaction from the much more serious condition of infectious corneal ulceration, particularly when adverse responses to contact lens wear are reported in the literature.

CLPUs often give rise to minimal patient symptoms; some patients may not contact their practitioner because of the mild nature of symptoms, and the occurrence of a CLPU episode may be detected only at routine aftercare visits on the basis of residual scarring, which takes the form of a small white circular opacity in the corneal periphery (see Fig. 14-3). More frequently, however, the patient experiences some ocular discomfort or foreign-body sensation associated with photophobia and excessive lacrimation. Clinical signs accompanying the ulcer include increased conjunctival and limbal hyperemia and subepithelial or stromal infiltrates underlying and surrounding the lesion. Large numbers of epithelial microcysts, endothelial bedewing, and corneal and conjunctival staining unassociated with the lesion were also noted in some patients.[163]

Resolution of symptoms is rapid once the lens is removed, and the lesion typically resolves completely within 2 weeks without medical intervention. Although this supports the inflammatory rather than infectious nature of this reaction, it is important to stress that a conservative approach to management is recommended, to avoid the risk of misdiagnosis or subsequent infectious keratitis. If medical intervention is not pursued, extreme care must be taken in diagnosis, and close patient follow-up is essential to monitor resolution of the lesion. According to Stein et al.,[164] the differential diagnosis of sterile versus infected corneal infiltrates hinges on the presence, size, and position of any epithelial lesion, the severity of patient symptoms, and the presence or absence of ocular discharge and anterior chamber reaction.

The etiology of CLPU is currently unclear. From the work of Willcox and colleagues at the CCLRU, in collaboration with the L. V. Prasad Eye Institute in Hyderabad, India, some evidence exists to suggest that patients with CLPU carry significant numbers of gram-positive bacteria on their lenses.[171] This suggests that CLPU may be related in some way to the staphylococcal marginal ulcers seen in association with chronic blepharitis.[172] These researchers have reported that colonization of contact lenses by *Streptococcus pneumoniae*, a gram-positive bacterium, can lead to the development of CLPU.[173] Bacteria implicated in the production of CLPU do not appear to infect the ulcer; scrapes taken from the ulcer bed have proved to be culture negative,[163] and histologic examination of the ulcers has shown a classic acute polymorphonuclear infiltrative response, with no evidence of micro-organisms.[174] Further work is clearly indicated to determine the etiology of this response, although its relatively low incidence among contact lens wearers continues to frustrate research in this area.

Contact Lens–Induced Papillary Conjunctivitis

Contact lens–induced papillary conjunctivitis (CLPC) is a chronic inflammatory response of the superior palpebral conjunctiva that can occur during daily and extended wear of hydrogel and RGP lenses.[175–178] In the early stages, clinical signs may be minimal compared to patient symptoms, which include increased mucus discharge after sleep and ocular itching. As the condition progresses, the patient reports increasing stringy mucus discharge and tearing during the day, blurring of vision owing to lens deposits or excess mucus, excessive lens movement and occasional lens displacement, and intense itching and lens awareness after a period of lens wear. These symptoms may become severe enough to limit wearing time and eventually lead to complete lens intolerance. Patients with CLPC seldom report pain; this may be related to the lower touch sensitivity of the palpebral conjunctiva compared to the corneal surface.[179]

Clinical signs of CLPC are subtle in the early stages of the condition and are often limited to slightly increased redness and mild edema of the palpebral conjunctival tissue. As the condition progresses, however, uniform small elevated papillae appear (Fig. 14-15), and these increase

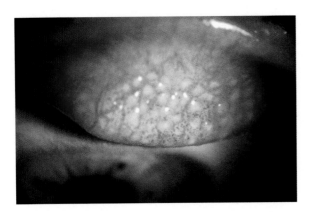

FIG. 14-15. *Contact lens–induced papillary conjunctivitis of the upper palpebral conjunctiva. This chronic inflammatory response has a complex etiology, which may include responses to mechanical and atopic stimuli. (Photograph by Geri Bergstein.)*

in size and number if clinical intervention does not occur. The characteristic rough appearance of the palpebral conjunctiva during CLPC can be visualized most clearly with the aid of sodium fluorescein dye and slit-lamp observation of the everted lid. If left untreated, the condition can progress to the more serious *giant papillary conjunctivitis* (Fig. 14-16), which is more resistant to treatment and frequently results in an inability to resume lens wear.

Allansmith and colleagues,[176] who first described this condition in detail, think that papillary conjunctivitis represents a cutaneous basophilic hypersensitivity reaction potentiated by antigens produced in response to lens deposits. Recovery of the condition after lens replacement[175,176] or with the use of a disposable lens regimen[180–182]

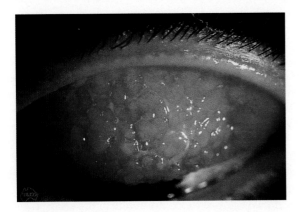

FIG. 14-16. *Giant papillary conjunctivitis, a more severe response that may develop if contact lens–induced papillary conjunctivitis is left untreated during hydrogel contact lens wear. (Photograph by Timothy Grant.)*

provides some support for this theory, as does the relatively low incidence of CLPC with rigid compared to hydrogel lenses.[183] However, individual patient susceptibility may also play a significant role. Fowler and colleagues[184] noted that surface deposits on soft lenses worn by patients with CLPC or GPC were indistinguishable from those on lenses worn by asymptomatic patients. In addition, papillary conjunctivitis can occur in response to chronic mechanical trauma, such as irritation from exposed suture ends after anterior segment surgery,[185,186] which suggests a mechanical component in the pathogenesis of this condition. Consequently, a multifactorial etiology has been proposed, which suggests that chronic irritation of the palpebral conjunctiva, as a result of repeated contact with lens surface deposits or a rough lens edge, allows access of the antigen to the mucous membrane, initiating a hypersensitivity reaction in susceptible individuals. Further work is needed to clarify the etiology of this particularly recalcitrant contact lens–related adverse response.

Early clinical intervention is the key to successful management of CLPC. As with other inflammatory reactions, reduction or removal of the triggering stimulus is the most effective option. Cessation of lens wear usually leads to rapid relief of symptoms within days, although clinical signs can persist for months and resumption of lens wear frequently precipitates a recurrence of symptoms. Dispensing a fresh lens,[175,176] instituting a regular lens replacement schedule,[187] or modifying the lens care regimen by introducing regular enzymatic protein removal[176,188] may allow resumption of lens wear in some cases, particularly in the early stages of the condition. Grant and coworkers[182] reported successful rehabilitation of patients with CLPC through the use of a daily-wear, daily-disposal regimen for 6 weeks, followed by the gradual resumption of extended wear with weekly lens disposal. These patients continued to show clinical signs of CLPC although symptoms were greatly alleviated, presumably because the degranulation of mast cells was inhibited. Others have reported the successful management of early CLPC by instituting a weekly disposal regimen while continuing with extended wear.[180,181]

In severe cases, suppression of the reaction using anti-inflammatory medications, or drugs such as cromolyn sodium ophthalmic solution, a mast cell stabilizer, may be required to provide relief of symptoms.[189–191] Loteprednol etabonate, a new corticosteroid based on the soft drug (site-specific) concept,[192,193] and suprofen, a nonsteroidal anti-inflammatory agent,[194] have also been shown to be effective in the management of CLPC. Vitamin A drops have been reported to alleviate the condition,[191] although convincing evidence of the benefit of this approach is still awaited.

A significant number of patients who develop severe CLPC or GPC are unable to resume lens wear at all despite intensive therapeutic measures. This emphasizes the importance of avoiding the development of this condition or, at the least, ensuring early detection of papillary changes.

CORNEAL INFECTION

Corneal infection is the most serious adverse response associated with contact lens wear. Before 1980, microbial keratitis was rarely seen in healthy eyes and was typically associated with trauma or corneal surface disease. However, early reports in the 1970s from the United Kingdom and Australia[3-5] warned of the potential danger of serious corneal infections with soft lens extended wear. With the increasing popularity of contact lens wear, the incidence of this complication has increased dramatically in the contact lens–wearing population, and it is now recognized that contact lens wear, and in particular hydrogel lens extended wear, is a significant risk factor in the development of corneal infection. Up to 66% of cases of corneal ulceration seen at major eye centers in the United States and the United Kingdom are now contact lens related.[12,195,196] It has been demonstrated convincingly that, compared with daily wear of rigid or hydrogel lenses, a significantly increased risk of corneal infection exists when hydrogel lenses are worn on an extended-wear basis[13,197-202] and that the risk is exacerbated as the number of consecutive nights of lens wear increases.[198,199]

The inflammatory process accompanying corneal infection follows a typical course. Hyperemia, tearing, and pain can progress rapidly to corneal infiltration, epithelial edema, and erosion, associated with a mucopurulent discharge. In many cases, a uveal response characterized by aqueous flare may be observed, and a severe infection may initiate a hypopyon. Vascularization of the cornea may also be stimulated. Tissue lysis occurs as a result of bacterial activity and also because of the release of lysosomal enzymes from inflammatory cells, and may progress to perforation of the cornea in extreme cases. Certainly, if the stroma is involved, scarring remains after resolution of the infectious process. If the scarring is centrally located, vision is reduced and surgical intervention may be required to restore useful vision.

Pseudomonas aeruginosa

Although a number of different pathogens have been reported to cause corneal infection, *P. aeruginosa* is the most common organism implicated in contact lens–related microbial infection.[196,203-206] *P. aeruginosa* is an oppor-

tunistic gram-negative organism commonly found in water, sewage, and soil and is known to contaminate basins, sludge areas, and toilets. Cytotoxic and invasive strains of this bacterium have been implicated in microbial keratitis,[160] whereas less-virulent strains are more likely to provoke inflammatory responses rather than frank infection.[161,162] Invasive strains of *P. aeruginosa* have been demonstrated to invade intact epithelial cells in vitro and in vivo,[207,208] suggesting that a break in the epithelium may not be required for the organism to gain entry to the tissue as has been proposed.[209,210] Cytotoxic strains, which appear to lack the ability to invade cells, nevertheless, may induce significant damage to intact surface epithelial cells,[211] thus potentiating the disease process. The infective course after inoculation can be extremely rapid, with the potential for severe stromal scarring or loss of the eye within as little as 24 hours.[212]

The mucus layer of the tear film may act as a significant barrier against infection by *P. aeruginosa* in the healthy cornea.[213] Hydrogel lens wear compromises the integrity of this layer, as evidenced by reduced tear breakup times immediately after lens removal.[214] Disruption of the normal eyelid-mediated cleaning and resurfacing processes of the eye resulting from the continual presence of the lens during hydrogel lens extended wear may therefore play a significant role in the pathogenesis of pseudomonal keratitis.

Acanthamoeba

Since the 1980s, amebic organisms of the genus *Acanthamoeba* have gained prominence as potential pathogens in contact lens–related corneal infection.[215,216] Infections with these organisms are less common than *Pseudomonas* and the clinical course is more prolonged. The disease, which is characterized by severe ocular pain, unilateral peripheral annular and central diskiform stromal infiltration, and recurrent overlying epithelial breakdown,[216] may evolve gradually over several months, frequently after a cyclical course of remission and recurrence.[215,216]

Differential diagnosis of *Acanthamoeba* keratitis may be difficult, particularly in the early stages of the disease. These infections also present a considerable challenge for management. The potential for eradication of the pathogen by pharmacologic intervention is moderate at best, and keratoplasty remains an important management option.[215,216] This is because *Acanthamoeba* can exist as either an active trophozoite or a dormant cyst within the corneal tissue, and, in its cystic state, the organism is particularly resistant to pharmacologic agents.[216] Although these infections are often associated with mild or moderate corneal trauma,[216] evidence exists to suggest that the organism can penetrate the intact corneal epithelium; the presence of a break in the epithelium may not be a necessary precondition for stromal invasion by the organism.[217]

Significant predisposing factors include soft contact lens wear in conjunction with the use of homemade saline or tap water rinses.[215] Because *Acanthamoeba* can use bacteria as a food source, bacterial contamination of contact lenses[218] or lens cases[219] may also act as a significant contributing factor in *Acanthamoeba* keratitis.

Infection Risk Factors

It must be borne in mind that contact lens–related ulcerative keratitis is rare; for cosmetic extended hydrogel lens wear, annualized incidences of approximately 0.2% have been reported from large-scale studies.[199,200] Case-control studies, however, have clearly demonstrated that hydrogel lens extended wear carries an increased risk of corneal infection compared with rigid and hydrogel lens daily wear. The risk associated with cosmetic hydrogel lens extended wear has been estimated at between two and 15 times greater than that of daily wear of hydrogel lenses.[12,198,201,202]

A number of factors may contribute to this increased risk in extended wear. It is likely that subtle compromise of the epithelial barrier function as a result of chronic hypoxic stress is a significant contributing factor. The increased fragility and reduced adhesion of the epithelium with chronic hypoxia[70,74] may potentiate the risk of subtle corneal trauma, allowing access of the pathogen to the tissue. Reduced wound healing has been demonstrated under hypoxic conditions,[78] and chronic hypoxia may also lead to a reduction in synthesis by epithelial cells of key elements of the normal cellular antimicrobial defense systems. Enhanced adhesion of *P. aeruginosa* to the corneal epithelium with short-term, low-Dk/t lens wear[79] and after extended hydrogel lens wear[220] may also play an important role.

Although contamination of lens care solutions may provide a source for the infecting organism, particularly in the case of *Acanthamoeba* infection,[215] the significance of this route is unclear. Although studies based on patient reports and case studies have implicated patient noncompliance as a contributing factor in individual cases of microbial keratitis,[169,221] case-control studies have not identified noncompliance with normal lens care as an obligatory risk factor.[12,198,202] Furthermore, it is expected that this route is more significant during daily lens wear, in which contact between lenses and contaminated solutions can occur more frequently. Similarly, contamination owing to lens handling is likely to be more common during daily wear. Indeed, it has been suggested that the

normal antimicrobial action of tear components, such as lysozyme and lactoferrin, may act to reduce the microbial load introduced by lens handling,[222] which suggests that this source of pathogens is likely to be less significant during extended wear than with daily wear. On the other hand, studies show that the closed-eye environment causes an increase in normal conjunctival microbiota.[223] Proliferation of entrapped pathogens during closed-eye lens wear may therefore play a role in extended-wear infections. Willcox and colleagues[224] suggested that the water supply may provide a significant source of lens contamination by gram-negative organisms, whereas gram-positive bacteria probably gain access to the eye from the surrounding skin, in particular from eyelid margins.

The anterior eye is rich in defense systems that normally protect the eye from invading organisms. In the non–lens-wearing eye, infection is rare in the absence of ocular trauma. The contact lens, however, provides a substrate to which bacteria can attach and subsequently proliferate in the nutrient-rich environment of the tear fluid.[225,226] Furthermore, *P. aeruginosa*, in common with other slime-producing bacteria, is known to elaborate a glycocalyx in this situation, which aids in adhesion of the bacteria to the lens surface and protects the proliferating organisms from the host defenses.[227,228] In the stagnant post-lens tear film environment that prevails during extended wear, bacteria probably have a greater chance to develop colonies in this fashion, thus providing a potent source of bacteria for corneal invasion.

Another factor proposed to explain the higher incidence of corneal infection with extended wear is the possibility that contact lens wear itself may alter the normal ocular microbiota, allowing growth of pathogenic organisms. Research findings in this area have been conflicting, with some studies showing little effect[229,230] and others reporting significant changes in the spectrum and levels of microbial contamination of external ocular sites, contact lens cases, or the contact lens itself with various modalities of lens wear[231,232] and even after cessation of lens wear.[233] Large-scale clinical studies indicate an increase in lid and conjunctival microbial colonization with long-term daily wear and an increase in the incidence of pathogenic organisms with extended hydrogel lens wear,[234] but little change in the incidence of lens contamination over time was found in either lens modality.[235]

An alternative hypothesis is that lens wear alters the subtle balance of tear film constituents, compromising the host defense system and potentiating infection in this way. Again, little evidence exists to support this suggestion. Indeed, despite considerable deposition of tear film components, in particular the antibacterial protein lysozyme, on contact lenses during wear, the eye seems to be able to replenish these components, resulting in no significant change in tear film composition during lens wear,[236] even in the overnight situation.[138] Cowell and colleagues[237] demonstrated that a relatively small change in sodium chloride concentration in the tear fluid significantly increases bacterial adhesion to contact lenses.

Several factors are known to exacerbate the severity of contact lens–related corneal infections. Delay in removing lenses and seeking treatment after onset of symptoms has been identified as a particularly significant predisposing factor.[4,238] Other factors that appear to increase the risk of a severe progression of corneal infection during extended wear include aphakia[239] and diabetes[240,241] (in which epithelial integrity is compromised by surgical intervention or an underlying abnormal condition), lens wear in warm climates,[242] and the initiation of inappropriate antibiotic[204] or corticosteroid[197] therapy.

Treatment and Patient Management

The clinical detection of corneal infection is usually initiated by patient symptoms, which can range from mild ocular discomfort and foreign-body sensation to severe ocular pain, redness, and heavy discharge. Any epithelial erosion overlying corneal infiltrates should be considered a potential corneal infection. Immediate lens removal and prompt diagnosis and treatment are imperative because of the frequent presence of highly virulent organisms, such as *P. aeruginosa*.

Treatment usually involves aggressive topical and subconjunctival antibiotic therapy, prescribed on the basis of culture of corneal scrapings to determine the drug sensitivity of the infective organism. In severe cases, hospitalization is often necessary. The use of intravenous medication may be indicated if the integrity of the globe is threatened. Sequelae in the form of peripheral or central corneal opacities are to be expected if the stroma is involved, and subsequent surgical intervention may be necessary to restore useful vision.

Careful patient management can reduce the risk of corneal infection. It is important to emphasize to extended-wear patients that lenses must be removed and the practitioner contacted immediately if any unusual redness, discomfort, or blurred vision occurs, particularly in one eye only. Yamane and Kuwabara[243] recommended that extended-wear lens users perform a daily routine on awakening to check that their eyes "feel good, look good, and see good."

Rigorous patient instructions on lens disinfection and handling procedures are also necessary to reduce the risk of introducing pathogens into the eye. Written instructions on lens care and the required schedule of aftercare

visits should be provided to the patient. Signing of a written consent form may help to stress to the patient the importance of compliance to the prescribed lens-wearing and replacement schedules and the recommended lens care and aftercare regimens. Because few patients demonstrate complete compliance to lens care instructions,[244] it is recommended that the importance of correct lens care procedures be re-emphasized at aftercare visits (also see Compliance section, later in this chapter).

Finally, minimizing the chronic hypoxic stress experienced by the cornea during lens wear may help to maintain epithelial integrity and reduce the chances of bacterial attachment and invasion. This can be achieved by fitting lenses with high-Dk/t values, ensuring adequate lens movement, and instituting a regimen of frequent overnight lens removal. The significance of hypoxia as a risk factor for corneal infection becomes clearer with the wider use of novel high-Dk/t soft lenses, which are currently prescribed for up to 30 days of continuous wear. Early studies indicate equivalent levels of lens contamination with these new materials compared to hydrogels,[245] but the verdict with respect to corneal infection rates awaits large-scale, real world clinical experience. With current hydrogel lenses, however, it is believed that ocular health is best promoted by encouraging patients to avoid sleeping in lenses.

DISPOSABLE VERSUS CONVENTIONAL EXTENDED WEAR

The concept of regular lens replacement originated in Sweden and has been used in that country for many years. In the early 1980s, a similar approach, the Gold Card regular replacement scheme, was introduced in the United States by CooperVision (Fairport, NY) but did not achieve significant use. The Fresh Lens Pro-Care System from Bausch & Lomb, Inc. (Rochester, NY) was launched in the United States in 1986, with similar initial low acceptance. Typically, lenses worn for extended wear were replaced on a regular 3- or 6-month basis, and clinical reports suggested that this approach contributed significantly to increased success rates and low complication rates.[67,188,246-248]

For many years, the concept of disposable lenses that could be worn for a short period (1–2 weeks) and then discarded remained an unachievable goal because of the cost of such a system. Disposable lenses were first pioneered in Denmark as the Danalens. In the United States, manufacturing innovations by Vistakon (Jacksonville, FL) in the late 1980s allowed lenses (ACUVUE) to be produced cheaply enough to allow true disposability on a weekly, fortnightly, or monthly basis. Other companies soon followed suit, with the SeeQuence lens from Bausch & Lomb, Inc. (Rochester, NY) and NewVues from CIBA Vision (Duluth, GA), and an enormous range of disposable lens types is now available. Indeed, it is clear that disposable lenses now dominate the contact lens market in most countries.[10,11]

Disposable lenses were marketed initially as extended-wear lenses, to be worn for up to 2 weeks and then replaced with a fresh lens. After the U.S. Food and Drug Administration issued a recommendation in 1989 for a maximum 6-night extended-wear regimen, the recommended extended-wear period was reduced to 1 week before disposal. The attractions of the disposable lens modality for patients and practitioners included improved ocular health, freedom from complicated care and maintenance routines, and better patient compliance. Despite initial skepticism about cost and the potential for patient noncompliance (to save money by wearing lenses longer than recommended), early clinical studies indicated good compliance with the disposable regimen, and few complications were initially reported.[249-257] Later reports of serious infections with extended wear of disposable lenses[258-266] and improper care of these lenses with daily wear leading to severe complications[267] have shown that inappropriate use of this lens can have serious consequences.

Deposit-Related Complications

The rationale behind the regular replacement and disposable lens philosophies stemmed from the perceived role of lens deposits in many contact lens–related complications. Deposits on the lens surface are thought to provoke mechanical and immunologic complications, in particular GPC and CLPC. The pathogenesis of these palpebral conjunctival changes is believed to involve mechanical trauma to the tissue[163,164] and a delayed hypersensitivity response to antigens associated with front-surface lens deposits.[176] In addition, it has been suggested that deposits provide attachment sites for pathogens,[268-270] thereby implicating lens deposits as a contributing factor in contact lens–related corneal infections. In theory, by replacing the lens before deposits build up to a point at which they can trigger an adverse response, many contact lens complications should be avoided.

Most currently marketed disposable lenses fall into two U.S. Food and Drug Administration categories: low–water content nonionic lenses (group I; e.g., SeeQuence and Optima FW, Bausch & Lomb, Inc., Rochester, NY), and high–water content ionic lenses (group IV; e.g., ACUVUE and NewVues). It is well established that group IV lenses show a greater affinity for protein deposits than do group

I lens materials,[271] and Lin and coworkers demonstrated increased deposition on ACUVUE compared with See-Quence lenses.[272] Significantly, these researchers noted significant deposition after only 1 minute of lens wear, particularly for ACUVUE lenses, with increasing deposition up to 1 week of continuous wear. Lin et al. also commented on the significant individual variation in deposition rates in their subject group, a finding that has been confirmed by others[271,273] and is familiar to practitioners.

In addition to the variability in individual deposition rates, individual susceptibilities to challenge from lens deposits are also highly variable. This has been well known since the early work of Fowler and coworkers,[184] who found no difference in lens deposits from patients with and without palpebral conjunctival changes. Taken together, these observations suggest that some patients may develop upper eyelid changes in spite of regular replacement of lenses. This has been confirmed by a number of investigators. For example, Grant[187] reported a CLPC incidence of 5% with disposable extended-wear lenses (compared to 19% with conventional extended wear). Others have also reported the development of CLPC or GPC during extended wear of disposable lenses.[251,255,257]

The problem of lens deposition may be compounded if compliance with lens replacement schedules is poorly maintained.[255] Smith has reported that up to 69% of disposable lens patients may not comply with the lens replacement schedule.[274] It is not surprising, therefore, that although disposable lenses are associated with a significantly reduced incidence of CLPC and GPC, they do not eliminate this complication. In addition, the mechanical factor in the pathogenesis of CLPC should not be ignored. It may be that even a nondeposited lens can induce CLPC in some patients.

Lens Aging and Solution Sensitivities

A major potential advantage of the disposable lens regimen is avoidance of complications associated with aging of lens materials, lens deposits, and sensitivities to lens care solution preservatives that may be absorbed by the lens polymer over time. As a hydrogel lens ages, it may discolor, lose flexibility, and develop surface and edge defects. In addition, lens parameters may change, resulting in a tightening of the lens fit. These changes reduce vision and comfort and may predispose the wearer to complications associated with a tight lens fit, such as limbal compression,[275] conjunctival staining,[275] neovascularization,[276] and inflammatory responses to debris trapped behind the lens.[155] By replacing lenses before aging changes occur, these problems can be avoided. However, because of the relatively limited parameter range available in disposable lenses compared to conventional stock or custom-made lenses, problems associated with tight lens fitting have been reported occasionally in clinical studies of disposable lenses.[252,253,255]

Use of disposable lenses on a six-night extended-wear basis obviates the need for regular care and maintenance of the lens. This has been a major attraction of the disposable lens regimen, and the lenses have been marketed as *carefree*. This may in part explain the popularity of this lens modality among male contact lens wearers.[252] With a disposable extended-wear regimen, the lenses are not exposed to care solutions that may contain preservatives, and, thus, the problems associated with solution preservative sensitivities are avoided. Complications, such as superior limbic keratoconjunctivitis (which has been associated with thimerosal sensitivity)[277] and allergic or toxic keratitis, attributable to lens care products have not been reported with disposable lens extended wear.[249-257] The continuing development of new lens care solutions containing novel preservatives has also undoubtedly had a significant impact in reducing the incidence of solution-related adverse responses.

It is possible that the promotion of the disposable lens system as carefree may have its disadvantages. Inevitably, extended-wear patients must occasionally remove their lenses for cleaning or rinsing (e.g., in dusty environments, when swimming in chlorinated water, or because of foreign bodies). More important, extended-wear patients should be instructed to remove their lenses promptly if unusual unilateral redness, pain, or reduced vision occur. If contact lens solutions and cases are not provided to the patient, or if the patient incorrectly perceives that lens removal and cleaning are not appropriate in this regimen, a chance exists that minor problems may progress to more serious and vision-threatening sequelae. When disposable lenses are removed and reused, it is essential that they undergo careful mechanical surfactant cleaning and rigorous disinfection in the same way as any other hydrogel lens.

Hypoxia

Because available disposable lenses are manufactured from identical or similar polymers as those used for nondisposable hydrogel lenses, the oxygen transmissibility of these lenses differs little from conventional extended-wear lenses. This point has been clearly demonstrated by Weissman and colleagues,[278] who measured oxygen permeability of the ACUVUE material as 18, NewVues as 15, and SeeQuence as 9×10^{-11} $(cm^2 \times ml\ O_2)/(s \times ml \times mm\ Hg)$. This means that disposable hydrogel lenses in thicknesses comparable to conventional lenses have oxygen transmissi-

bilities in the range of $9-17 \times 10^{-9}$ $(cm \times ml\ O_2)/(s \times ml \times mm\ Hg)$.[279] This level of oxygen transmissibility gives rise to average overnight corneal edema levels of 10–12% (see Table 14-1), which is equivalent to those induced by conventional extended-wear hydrogel lenses.[38,187] Although disposable lenses are now often made thinner than conventional lenses because of the reduced emphasis on durability, the oxygen advantage obtained is modest; even the most transmissible of the current hydrogel disposable lenses achieves a Dk/t (in a –3.00 D lens) of only 27×10^{-9} $(cm \times ml\ O_2)/(s \times ml \times mm\ Hg)$, barely exceeding the Holden-Mertz criterion for daily wear.[35,44,280]

It must be stressed, therefore, that disposable hydrogel lenses worn for extended wear induce similar chronic hypoxic and hypercapnic changes in corneal structure and function as do conventional extended-wear lenses. Therefore, epithelial microcysts, reduced epithelial adhesion, endothelial polymegethism, and other subtle hypoxia-induced corneal tissue changes occur with the same frequency as with conventional extended-wear lenses.[187,249,251,254-257] Clearly, the low oxygen transmissibility of disposable hydrogel lenses militates against their use for extended wear at all. In fact, CCLRU studies have shown that only 6% of patients seem unaffected physiologically after 3 years of extended wear of even the highest-Dk/t disposable hydrogel lenses.[281]

Corneal Inflammation

Corneal inflammatory responses, such as infiltrative keratitis and the CLARE reaction, have been documented during extended wear of disposable lenses.[168,187,249,253-255,257] There have also been several reports of sterile corneal ulceration associated with infiltrates (CLPU),[163,167-171,187,249] which is thought to be inflammatory rather than infectious in etiology.[163]

Regular replacement of lenses has been shown to significantly reduce the incidence of the CLARE reaction.[188,247] Grant[187] reported a 3% incidence of CLARE reaction with disposable extended wear compared with an annual incidence of 15% during conventional extended wear. It is probable that regular disposal of lenses lessens the exposure of the cornea to factors that may provoke these inflammatory responses, such as bacterial toxins, preservatives absorbed by the lens polymer, and lens deposits. However, Grant and coworkers[163,187] have found that the annual incidence of CLPU is similar for disposable lenses (2.0%) and less frequently replaced conventional extended-wear hydrogel lenses (2.9%), which suggests that this complication may have a more complex etiology. As discussed earlier in the Contact Lens-Induced Peripheral Ulcers section, Willcox and colleagues have shown that these ulcers may be triggered by toxins secreted by gram-positive bacteria that colonize lenses during wear.[171,173–174]

Corneal Infection

Corneal infection is the most serious complication of hydrogel lens extended wear. It was hoped initially that the use of disposable lens regimens would reduce the frequency of corneal infection because the lenses would have little chance of becoming contaminated by exposure to contaminated lens cases or care solutions. Furthermore, because lenses are replaced before significant lens deposits accumulate, it has been suggested that there should be less bacterial attachment to lens surfaces. However, there have been an increasing number of reports of corneal infection during disposable lens extended wear, including severe infections with *P. aeruginosa*[168,169,258–264] and *Acanthamoeba*.[265,266] Evidence therefore suggests that the use of a disposable lens regimen does not reduce the risk of corneal infection during extended wear. Although case-control studies have presented some evidence that the risk might be enhanced compared with conventional extended wear,[201,202] reanalysis of these findings has confirmed no increased risk of infection with disposable lenses per se, with overnight lens wear emerging as the most important risk factor regardless of lens type.[12,13]

Several reasons can be advanced for the continuing problem of corneal infection during extended wear of disposable lenses. Poor patient compliance with wearing and disposal schedules[169,202,259,264] and inappropriate use of contaminated care solutions[202,261] have been implicated in a number of cases of corneal infection with disposable lenses. It may well be that marketing strategies that have promoted disposable lenses as carefree have tended to attract a group of patients who are less meticulous about lens hygiene and reporting of initial symptoms. Delay in seeking treatment is a major risk factor in the progression of corneal ulceration.[4,238] This stresses the importance of careful patient selection, instruction, and education for all forms of extended lens wear.

Although some studies have reported that bacteria preferentially attach to deposits on the lens surface,[268–270] other studies have questioned this finding. Duran et al.[282] showed that bacteria can attach avidly to unworn lenses, and Dart and Badenoch[283] found no difference in bacterial adherence between worn and unworn lenses. Williams and colleagues[284] did not demonstrate any facilitation of bacterial adherence in vitro by tear film constituents, such as lysozyme and lactoferrin. These findings suggest that replacement of lenses before significant deposits have accumulated may do little to reduce the chances of bacterial

adherence to the lens surfaces. Conversely, Taylor et al.[285] demonstrated that although deposition of albumin, which derives from serum and is present in high concentrations in closed-eye tear fluid, can reduce bacterial lens adherence compared to unworn lenses, bacterial adherence increases with increasing deposition of albumin. Increased concentrations of the sticky protein fibronectin in tear fluid in the closed eye[286] and in contact lens wearers[287] may also serve to enhance bacterial adherence to the lens, thus increasing the risk of infection.[288] Further work in this area is clearly needed to clarify the role of lens deposits in bacterial colonization of the lens and anterior ocular tissues.

Hypoxia has also been implicated as a major contributing factor in contact lens–related corneal infection. As discussed previously in the Effects of Hypoxia on Corneal Structure and Function section, chronic hypoxic stress reduces corneal sensitivity,[71,72] increases epithelial fragility,[70] and compromises epithelial adhesion.[74,75] More subtle effects on the epithelium, the primary barrier to invasion of pathogens, may also result from the continuous presence of the lens and the absence of blink-activated cleansing of the ocular surface. Because disposable extended-wear lenses induce similar levels of chronic hypoxia as conventional hydrogel extended-wear lenses and are present on the eye for similar periods, these risk factors are not significantly reduced with a disposable lens regimen. The virtual elimination of chronic hypoxia with the newly released high-Dk/t soft lenses helps to clarify the significance of hypoxia in the pathogenesis of corneal infections.

Finally, there were several reports of lens imperfections in early-generation disposable lenses, particularly the ACU-VUE lenses.[252,289–292] These imperfections, mainly at the lens edge, arose because of the manufacturing process, in which lenses were molded in a hydrated state, resulting in occasional excess material (flashing) at the lens edge. One study presented some evidence for slight compromise of ocular integrity associated with wear of imperfect disposable lenses,[292] and the authors presented the rather tenuous hypothesis that this compromise may be related to the development of severe ocular complications during extended wear. However, no evidence has been presented to support these claims.[293–295] Furthermore, technological advances in mass production of disposable lenses have virtually eliminated this quality control problem.

In summary, the use of disposable lenses for extended wear significantly reduces the incidence of (but does not eliminate) acute and chronic inflammatory ocular responses that are triggered by aging of lenses and lens deposits. However, complications attributable directly or indirectly to chronic hypoxic stress are not reduced in frequency because current disposable hydrogel lenses have oxygen transmission characteristics similar to conventional hydrogel extended-wear lenses. Furthermore, the continuing problems of corneal inflammation and infection with disposable lens extended wear should act as a reminder to practitioners that careful patient selection, rigorous instruction in lens care, and compliance with lens replacement and aftercare schedules, although important for optimizing success, are not sufficient to avoid the inevitable problems associated with hydrogel extended wear.

The use of disposable hydrogel lenses for daily wear is preferable to extended wear for maintaining long-term ocular health. The ultimate daily, hydrogel lens–wearing modality may well prove to be daily disposal, and improvements in manufacturing technology have allowed this goal to be reached. Early clinical reports of daily disposable lens wear support the view that this modality of lens wear has significant advantages over conventional and biweekly disposable regimens.[296] Further research is needed to quantify adverse response rates and levels of patient satisfaction and compliance with this lens regimen. It is clear that adverse responses still occur with these lenses, however, which are often but not always associated with poor compliance and misuse.

COMPLIANCE

Compliance with contact lens care and wearing instruction plays an important role in minimizing contact lens–related complications. This attains more significance during extended contact lens wear because of the higher incidence of complications in this modality compared to daily wear. However, the contact lens literature documents disturbingly high levels of noncompliance with lens care instructions, hygiene, wearing and replacement schedules, and aftercare attendance.

The medical literature in the area of compliance yields some important messages about levels of compliance with medical advice as well as factors that may influence compliance.[297] Noncompliance with medical advice is a well-recognized phenomenon, and it represents a major cause for treatment failure and increased health costs.[297] In an interesting summary of studies on medical compliance, Ley reported that noncompliance with medication regimens ranged between 38% and 61%, with similar high noncompliance levels to other forms of medical advice.[298] Compliance tends to be greater in the presence of symptomatic or acute disease, and noncompliance rates increase significantly for chronic disease and prophylactic treatments. A good example is the high rates of noncompliance reported in studies monitoring patient self-medication for glaucoma management.[299] Compliance with contact lens care instructions provides another important example.

It is clear that the level of compliance is strongly influenced by factors relating to the patient, the practitioner, and the nature of the treatment or regimen used.[300] The Health Belief Model[298,301-303] provides a useful template from which to appreciate patient factors relating to compliance. This psychosocial model, which addresses patients' attitudes or beliefs about their health status and proposed treatment, can be used to divide the relevant issues relating to compliance into beliefs about the following:

- *Susceptibility*: How likely am I to suffer consequences of noncompliance?
- *Severity*: How severe are the consequences if I do not comply?
- *Benefits*: Does this regimen work to prevent consequences?
- *Barriers*: Are there reasons why I should or should not use the regimen?

This model can be useful to explore a patient's reasons for noncompliance, and it can be used to devise and direct intervention and re-education strategies to encourage compliance.[297,301-303]

The relationship between the patient and practitioner strongly influences compliance because of the patient's perception of the practitioner's attitudes, interest, and confidence and the continuity of the relationship.[304] At a more fundamental level, the accuracy and quality of instructions given by the practitioner to the patient affect compliance. In developing countries, such as China, where practitioner training in contact lens management is minimal, the lack of awareness among lens fitters of the need for aftercare has led to extremely poor compliance and a high incidence of contact lens complications.[305,306] In more developed countries, a higher level of practitioner knowledge minimizes these problems, although instances of practitioner misunderstanding or misinformation have certainly occurred, leading to unintentional patient noncompliance.[307] An example is the early perception about disposable lenses that digital cleaning was not required before disinfection; the omission of this step was subsequently implicated in several cases of microbial keratitis.[267]

Claydon et al.[302] comment that the practitioner should attempt to provide information and instructions that are clear, simple, individualized to the patient's needs and lifestyle, and pitched at an appropriate level. Take-home written (or videotaped) instructions on lens care and handling and other aspects of the prescribed lens-wearing regimen, such as wearing and replacement schedules, aftercare appointments, and emergency advice, are also very useful in reinforcing patient instructions.[302] They act as a reminder for the patient who may have misunderstood or forgotten instructions. It is interesting to note that Ley[308] found that within minutes of completion of instruction, patients typically forget between one-third and one-half of medical advice given. Practice support staff also play a significant role in this regard because patients may ask them for advice in situations in which the patient does not want to admit confusion or in which problems arise that the patient regards as relatively trivial (such as lens discomfort or ocular redness).[309] Appropriate training of support staff is thus an important step in optimizing patient compliance.[304,309]

The nature of the treatment or product to be used also influences the level of compliance. In medical studies, the simplicity of the prescribed regimen[310] and the cost[311] have been shown to enhance compliance. Although these factors make intuitive sense, it is interesting to note that studies in the contact lens field have provided only equivocal support to confirm their significance,[307,312] which suggests that other factors may be of more importance.

Studies of compliance are fraught with difficulties and prone to error, thus making interpretation and comparison of findings difficult. For example, the definition of compliance varies across studies. Few studies differentiate between unintentional and intentional compliance, an important distinction, particularly when devising strategies to improve compliance. Unintentional noncompliance may arise because of ineffective or incorrect initial instruction by the practitioner, patient misunderstanding of instructions, or forgetfulness. In these situations, patients may not be aware that they are not complying with instructions, and intervention strategies are more likely to be successful.[304] On the other hand, many patients are aware of their noncompliance[313,314] but choose, for reasons of laziness, cost, or perceived minimal risk, to ignore instructions. The detection of these noncompliant patients is more difficult because they may avoid admitting their noncompliance to the practitioner or to investigators in research studies using interviews, questionnaires, or demonstration of lens care techniques to detect noncompliance.[302,304] For this reason, it is likely that most published studies of compliance give conservative estimates of the incidence of noncompliance.

In the 1990s, many studies have addressed the issue of compliance in contact lens care and wearing regimens, and all have revealed disturbingly high levels of noncompliance. In 1986, Collins and Carney[244] reported at least one aspect of noncompliant behavior in 74% of patients. They also found a significant correlation between noncompliance and the presence of epithelial staining and lens deposits, indicating that noncompliance with lens care instructions could affect the incidence of complications and patient success in lens wear. Since then, many

estimates for levels of noncompliance have been reported, ranging from 10%[315] to more than 90%.[312] Comparisons across studies are difficult, however, because of different criteria used to define compliance. Some studies record noncompliance if any part of the regimen is inadequate,[244] some accept occasional lapses in compliance (i.e., the patient frequently rather than always carries out required steps),[316] and others allow a leeway of two or three errors or omissions before noncompliance is recorded.[303] In some studies, an attempt is made to weigh the degree of compliance based on the clinical risk associated with the noncompliant behavior.[307,312,317] Using this approach, Turner and coworkers noted that compliance was greater for behaviors enhancing lens comfort than for behaviors that significantly affect safety.[312]

Despite differences between studies, several broad conclusions can be reached. The areas in which noncompliance to contact lens instructions is likely to have clinical consequences can be broadly defined as hygiene, lens care and use of solutions, wearing and replacement schedules, and the keeping of aftercare appointments.[302] The specific hygiene and lens care tasks that emerge from studies as most commonly associated with noncompliance among contact lens wearers are these:

- Omission of handwashing before handling lenses[244,307,312,318–320]
- Inadequate or irregular lens cleaning before disinfection[244,302,303,307,312,316,318,319]
- Inadequate or irregular lens case cleaning or replacement[244,307,312,319]
- Use of inappropriate solutions (including tap water[316,321] or saliva[307]) or old solutions[320]
- Not replacing used disinfection solution (instead, topping up)[244,307]
- Inappropriate frequency or technique for enzymatic cleaning[303,307,312]

Poor compliance with extended lens wearing schedules,[313,315,319] aftercare schedules,[302,303,313] and disposable lens replacement[274] has also been reported. Not disinfecting lenses before insertion is less frequent among the general contact lens–wearing population, but it has been reported in 72% of cases in one sample of patients with contact lens–induced microbial keratitis.[320] Chalmers et al. have also reported high levels of inappropriate self-management behavior associated with uncomfortable or damaged lenses, particularly among wearers of conventional rather than disposable lenses.[309]

Conclusions drawn from these studies are unclear about which factors encourage or discourage noncompliance. According to reports in the medical literature,[298] contact lens compliance does not appear to be related to patient gender, ethnicity, socioeconomic or educational level, occupation, or perceived risk of disease. Two studies have implicated age (older than 30 years[303,314] and older than 50 years[314]) as a factor in noncompliance, although other studies have found no effect of age.[244] Similar levels of noncompliance have been found for soft and rigid lens wearers,[307,314] although the areas of noncompliance differ.[307,321] Rigid lens wearers are more likely to use tap water to rinse their lenses before insertion[321] and to reuse disinfecting solution[307] but less likely to practice inappropriate lens case care compared to soft lens wearers.[307] It might be anticipated that more experienced lens wearers become less compliant over time owing to boredom and familiarity or the perception that time-saving shortcuts or omissions have no immediate effect on their lens-wearing comfort. However, there have been equivocal findings in this regard.[244,307,314]

Based on previous studies, it is expected that the complexity and cost of a lens care regimen may affect compliance, but findings are contradictory. Radford and coworkers found higher levels of compliance with the relatively simple chlorine-based disinfection systems than with hydrogen peroxide systems.[307] On the other hand, Turner and colleagues found similar levels of compliance with hydrogen peroxide and multipurpose chemical care systems.[312,317] Sheard and coworkers[316] found no difference in compliance levels between patients paying in full for their lens solutions and those paying a nominal low price.

Initial instruction or education on the need for lens care and the intensity or adequacy of this instruction might also be expected to affect the level of compliance. Claydon and coworkers,[302] however, found no differences in compliance levels between patients given basic lens care instructions and those given supplementary instructional materials, including posters, videotapes, and booklets. In contrast, Radford et al.[307] demonstrated the value of reinstruction, finding much improved compliance 3 months after reinstruction of noncompliant patients, but this is more likely to be effective for patients who were unaware of their noncompliance owing to misunderstanding, confusion, or forgetfulness. Patients who are intentionally noncompliant may be more resistant to changing their familiar habits unless the risks of their noncompliance are specifically pointed out.

In summary, because of the high levels of noncompliance found among contact lens wearers, practitioners should assume noncompliance, in at least some aspects of a contact lens regimen, in all contact lens patients. The practitioner is advised to review lens care, wear, replacement, and aftercare requirements at each aftercare appointment.[304] Care should be taken when presenting instructions to the new patient and to experienced patients who are refitted or prescribed a new lens care or wearing regimen. Instructions should be clear, simple, pitched at an appropriate level, and individualized to the patient's personality and lifestyle. The provision of written or videotaped supporting material is of some benefit. The patient-practitioner relationship is an important factor in enhancing compliance, and practice support staff also play a significant role. In the event of noncompliance, re-education can be successful. Application of the Health Belief Model (see previously in this section) can provide useful insights into the factors underlying intentional patient noncompliance.

It is clear that the prescription of simple, low-cost lens care regimens is likely to enhance compliance and thus promote safer and more successful lens wear. Indeed, to optimize compliance, it is highly desirable to make contact lenses as convenient and trouble-free as possible. The single-use (disposable) philosophy, whether it is applied on a daily, weekly, or monthly basis, may well meet this goal and should be supportable with appropriately designed and tested products that are safe, comfortable, and affordable.

SUMMARY

Despite almost 30 years of research, development, and clinical application, extended wear of hydrogel lenses continues to induce significant problems related to hypoxia, inflammation, and infection. Changes in the corneal epithelium, stroma, and endothelium induced by chronic hypoxia and acidosis can be seen in virtually all long-term hydrogel extended-wear patients, and acute or chronic inflammatory problems affect approximately 30% of wearers over a 12-month period when conventional (nondisposable) lenses are used. Although corneal infections are rare, they are of major concern because of their potential threat to ocular integrity.

Disposable extended wear is an attractive and convenient mode of lens wear for the prospective patient and has achieved widespread usage. It is unfortunate that the products currently available do not fulfill the needs of the eye. Although the incidence of inflammatory responses is halved with disposable lenses, hypoxic and hypercapnic changes occur at the same rate as with conventional hydrogel lens extended wear, and the problem of corneal infections remains.

Most prospective patients want safe, effective hydrogel extended or continuous lens wear. To realize this goal, it is clear that soft lenses with truly high Dk/t represent the next step in contact lens development. Large-scale real world clinical investigations of high-Dk/t soft lenses, based on novel polymer formulations, provide important information about the significance of hypoxia in extended-wear adverse responses. Minimization of chronic hypoxia, however, is unlikely to eliminate all complications associated with extended wear. A better understanding of factors that promote biocompatibility between contact lens surfaces and the ocular tissues is also essential to eliminate or reduce the risk of inflammation and infection during extended wear. It can be anticipated that continued efforts to conduct carefully planned and executed basic and clinical research, driving innovative technologic developments in the contact lens industry, will eventually provide the key to achieving the ultimate goal of safe and effective long-term extended or continuous contact lens wear.

Looking at the continuing evolution of refractive care, it is clear that to be responsive to the needs of an increasingly demanding ametropic public, contact lenses must be truly safe, effective, comfortable, and easy to care for. Contact lenses that are inserted once and then discarded on a daily, weekly, or monthly basis and that provide consistent, comfortable, and safe performance may well meet this goal. Unless such products are successfully developed, however, contact lenses will never truly challenge the comfort and convenience of spectacles or the permanence of refractive surgery.

REFERENCES

1. Holden BA: The Glenn A. Fry Award lecture 1988: the ocular response to contact lens wear. Optom Vis Sci 66:717, 1989
2. deCarle J: Developing hydrophilic lenses for continuous wearing. Aust J Optom 55:343, 1972
3. Ruben M: Acute eye disease secondary to contact lens wear. Lancet 1:138, 1976
4. Cooper RL, Constable LJ: Infective keratitis in soft contact lens wearers. Br J Ophthalmol 61:250, 1977
5. Zantos SG, Holden BA: Ocular changes associated with continuous wear of contact lenses. Aust J Optom 61:418, 1978
6. Weissman BA: Danger EXW. Optom Monthly 74:21, 1983
7. Barr JT: The Contact Lens Spectrum decade report: entering a new age of contact lenses. Contact Lens Spectrum Jan:20, 1996
8. Morgan PB, Efron N: Trends in UK contact lens prescribing 1998. Optom Vis Sci (suppl.)75:160, 1998
9. Pye DC, Badre P, Kazzi R: Current contact lens practice in Australia. Student project report, School of Optometry, University of New South Wales, Sydney, Australia, 1997
10. Schwartz CA: Contact lens update: The buzz is back. Optom Management 33:38, 1998
11. Tanner J: How do the demographics of your practice compare? Optician 213:30, 1997
12. Dart JKG, Stapleton F, Minassian D: Contact lenses and other risk factors in microbial keratitis. Lancet 338:651, 1991
13. Schein OD, Buehler PO, Stamler JF, et al: The impact of overnight wear on the risk of contact lens–associated ulcerative keratitis. Arch Ophthalmol 112:186, 1994
14. Smelser GK, Ozanics V: Importance of atmospheric oxygen for maintenance of the optical properties of the human cornea. Science 115:140, 1952
15. Hill RM, Fatt I: How dependent is the cornea on the atmosphere? J Am Optom Assoc 35:873, 1964
16. Riley MV: Glucose and oxygen utilization of the cornea. Exp Eye Res 8:193, 1969
17. Smelser GK, Ozanics V: Structural changes in corneas of guinea pigs after wearing contact lenses. Arch Ophthalmol 49:335, 1953
18. Freeman RD: Oxygen consumption by the component layers of the cornea. J Physiol 225:15, 1972
19. Zurawski CA, McCarey BE, Schmidt FH: Glucose consumption in cultured corneal cells. Curr Eye Res 8:349, 1989
20. Barr RE, Hennessey M, Murphy VG: Diffusion of oxygen at the endothelial surface of the rabbit cornea. J Physiol 270:1, 1977
21. Kwan M, Niinikoski J, Hunt TK: In vivo measurements of oxygen tension in the cornea, aqueous humor, and anterior lens of the open eye. Invest Ophthalmol 11:108, 1972
22. Efron N, Carney LG: Oxygen levels beneath the closed eyelid. Invest Ophthalmol Vis Sci 18:93, 1979
23. Langham M: Utilization of oxygen by the component layers of the living cornea. J Physiol 117:461, 1952
24. Holden BA, Sweeney DF: The oxygen tension and temperature of the superior palpebral conjunctiva. Acta Ophthalmol 63:100, 1985
25. Benjamin WJ, Rasmussen MA: The closed-lid tear pump: oxygenation? Int Eyecare 1:251, 1985
26. Smelser GK, Chen DK: Physiological changes in cornea induced by contact lenses. Arch Ophthalmol 53:676, 1955
27. Klyce SD: Stromal lactate accumulation can account for corneal oedema osmotically following epithelial hypoxia in the rabbit. J Physiol 321:49, 1981
28. Holden BA, Sweeney DF, Sanderson G: The minimum precorneal oxygen tension to avoid corneal edema. Invest Ophthalmol Vis Sci 25:476, 1984
29. Sarver MD: Striate corneal lines among patients wearing hydrophilic contact lenses. Am J Optom 48:762, 1971
30. Polse KA, Mandell RB: Etiology of corneal striae accompanying hydrogel lens wear. Invest Ophthalmol 15:553, 1976
31. Holden BA: High magnification examination and photography with the slit lamp. p. 335. In Brandreth RH (ed): Clinical Slit Lamp Biomicroscopy. Blaco, San Leandro, CA, 1977

32. La Hood D, Grant T: Striae and folds as indicators of corneal edema. Optom Vis Sci (suppl.)67:196, 1990

33. Hamano H, Hori M, Hamano T, et al: Effects of contact lens wear on mitosis of corneal epithelium and lactate content of aqueous humor of rabbit. Jpn J Ophthalmol 27:451, 1983

34. Williams LJ: Transient endothelial changes in the in vivo human cornea. PhD thesis. University of New South Wales, Sydney, Australia, 1986

35. Holden BA, Mertz GW: Critical oxygen levels to avoid corneal edema for daily and extended wear contact lenses. Invest Ophthalmol Vis Sci 25:1161, 1984

36. Mandell RB, Fatt I: Thinning of the human cornea on awakening. Nature 208:292, 1965

37. Mertz GW: Overnight swelling of the living human cornea. J Am Optom Assoc 51:211, 1980

38. La Hood D, Sweeney DF, Holden BA: Overnight corneal edema with hydrogel, rigid gas-permeable and silicone elastomer contact lenses. Int Contact Lens Clin 15:149, 1988

39. Andrasko GJ: Corneal deswelling response to hard and hydrogel extended wear lenses. Invest Ophthalmol Vis Sci 27:20, 1986

40. Holden BA, Sweeney DF, La Hood D, Kenyon E: Corneal deswelling following overnight wear of rigid and hydrogel contact lenses. Curr Eye Res 7:49, 1988

41. Cuklanz HD, Hill RM: Oxygen requirements of corneal contact lens systems. Am J Optom 46:228, 1969

42. Fatt I, Hill RM: Oxygen tension under a contact lens during blinking—a comparison of theory and experimental observations. Am J Optom 47:50, 1970

43. Polse KA: Tear flow under hydrogel contact lenses. Invest Ophthalmol Vis Sci 18:409, 1979

44. Holden BA, Mertz GW, McNally JJ: Corneal swelling response to contact lenses worn under extended wear conditions. Invest Ophthalmol Vis Sci 24:218, 1983

45. Holden BA, Sweeney DF, Seger RG: Epithelial erosions caused by thin high water contact lenses. Clin Exp Optom 69:103, 1986

46. Orsborn GN, Zantos SG: Corneal desiccation staining with thin high water content contact lenses. CLAO J 14:81, 1988

47. Alvord L, Court J, Davis T, et al: Oxygen permeability of a new type of high Dk soft contact lens material. Optom Vis Sci 75:30, 1998

48. MacDonald KE, Fonn D, Richter DB, Robboy M: Comparison of the physiological response to extended wear of an experimental high Dk soft lens versus a 38% HEMA lens. Invest Ophthalmol Vis Sci (suppl.)36:s310, 1995

49. Fonn D, du Toit R, Situ P, et al: Apparent sympathetic response of contralateral nonlens wearing eyes after overnight lens wear in the fellow eye. Invest Ophthalmol Vis Sci (suppl.)39:s336, 1998

50. Thoft RA, Friend J: Biochemical aspects of contact lens wear. Am J Ophthalmol 80:139, 1975

51. Masters BA: Effects of contact lenses on the oxygen concentration and epithelial mitochondrial redox state of rabbit cornea measured noninvasively with an optically sectioning redox fluorometer microscope. p. 281. In Cavanagh HD (ed): The Cornea: Transactions of the World Congress on the Cornea III. Raven, New York, 1988

52. Tsubota K, Laing RA: Metabolic changes in the corneal epithelium resulting from hard contact lens wear. Cornea 11:121, 1992

53. King JE, Augsburger A, Hill RM: Quantifying the distribution of lactic dehydrogenase in the corneal epithelium with oxygen deprivation. Am J Optom 48:1016, 1971

54. Ichijima H, Imayasu M, Ohashi J, Cavanagh HD: Tear lactate dehydrogenase levels—a new method to assess effects of contact lens wear in man. Cornea 11:114, 1992

55. Hill RM, Rengstorff RH, Petrali JP, Sim VM: Critical oxygen requirements of the corneal epithelium as indicated by succinic dehydrogenase reactivity. Am J Optom Physiol Opt 51:331, 1974

56. Burns RP: Meesman's corneal dystrophy. Trans Am Ophthalmol Soc 66:530, 1968

57. Bergmanson JPG, Chu LW-F: Corneal response to rigid contact lens wear. Br J Ophthalmol 66:667, 1982

58. Bergmanson JPG, Ruben CM, Chu LW-F: Epithelial morphological response to soft hydrogel contact lenses. Br J Ophthalmol 69:373, 1985

59. Hamano H, Hori M, Hirayama K, et al: Influence of soft and hard contact lenses on the cornea. Aust J Optom 58:326, 1975

60. Hamano H, Komatsu S, Hirayama K: Influence of oxygen deficiency on corneal potential. Contacto 13:14, 1969

61. Kwok S: Review: the effects of contact lens wear on the electrophysiology of the corneal epithelium. Aust J Optom 66:138, 1983

62. Humphreys JA, Larke JR, Parrish ST: Microepithelial cysts observed in extended contact-lens wearing subjects. Br J Ophthalmol 64:888, 1980

63. Zantos SG: Cystic formations in the corneal epithelium during extended wear of contact lenses. Int Contact Lens Clin 10:128, 1983

64. Holden BA, Sweeney DF: The significance of the microcyst response: a review. Optom Vis Sci 68:703, 1991

65. Bergmanson JPG: Histopathological analysis of the corneal epithelium after contact lens wear. J Am Optom Assoc 58:812, 1987

66. Madigan MC: Cat and monkey as models for extended hydrogel contact lens wear in humans. PhD thesis. University of New South Wales, Sydney, Australia, 1989

67. Holden BA, Sweeney DF, Vannas A, et al: Effects of long-term extended contact lens wear on the human cornea. Invest Ophthalmol Vis Sci 26:1489, 1985

68. Carney LG, Brennan NA: Time course of corneal oxygen uptake during contact lens wear. CLAO J 14:151, 1988

69. Lemp MA, Gold JB: The effects of extended-wear hydrophilic contact lenses on the human corneal epithelium. Am J Ophthalmol 101:274, 1986

70. O'Leary DJ, Millodot M: Abnormal epithelial fragility in diabetes and in contact lens wear. Acta Ophthalmol 59:827, 1981

71. Millodot M: Effect of soft lenses on corneal sensitivity. Acta Ophthalmol 52:603, 1974

72. Millodot M, O'Leary DJ: Effect of oxygen deprivation on corneal sensitivity. Acta Ophthalmol 58:434, 1980

73. Mindel JS, Szilagyi PIA, Zadunaisky JA, et al: The effects of blepharorrhaphy induced depression of corneal cholinergic activity. Exp Eye Res 29:463, 1979

74. Madigan MC, Holden BA, Kwok LS: Extended wear of contact lenses can compromise corneal epithelial adhesion. Curr Eye Res 6:1257, 1987

75. Madigan MC, Holden BA: Reduced epithelial adhesion after extended contact lens wear correlates with reduced hemidesmosome density in cat cornea. Invest Ophthalmol Vis Sci 33:314, 1992

76. Wallace W: The SLACH syndrome. Int Eyecare 1:220, 1986

77. Lindsay R, Lakkis C, Brennan NA: Focal loss of epithelium associated with hydrogel contact lens wear and trigeminal nerve defect. Int Contact Lens Clin 20:234, 1993

78. Mauger TF, Hill RM: Corneal epithelial healing under contact lenses: quantitative analysis in the rabbit. Acta Ophthalmol 70:361, 1992

79. Imayasu M, Petroll WM, Jester JV, et al: The relation between contact lens oxygen transmissibility and binding of *Pseudomonas aeruginosa* to the cornea after overnight wear. Ophthalmology 101:371, 1994

80. Kangas TA, Edelhauser HF, Twining SS, O'Brien WJ: Loss of stromal glycosaminoglycans during corneal edema. Invest Ophthalmol Vis Sci 31:1994, 1990

81. Holden BA, Sweeney DF, Efron N, et al: Contact lens wear can induce stromal thinning. Clin Exp Optom 71:109, 1988

82. Zantos SG, Holden BA: Transient endothelial changes soon after wearing soft contact lenses. Am J Optom Physiol Opt 54:856, 1977

83. Barr RE, Silver IA: Effects of corneal environment on oxygen tension in the anterior chamber of rabbits. Invest Ophthalmol 12:140, 1973

84. Stefansson E, Wolbarsht ML, Landers MB: The corneal contact lens and aqueous humor hypoxia in cats. Invest Ophthalmol Vis Sci 24:1052, 1983

85. Stefansson E, Foulks GN, Hamilton RC: The effect of corneal contact lenses on the oxygen tension in the anterior chamber of the rabbit eye. Invest Ophthalmol Vis Sci 28:1716, 1987

86. Holden BA, Zantos SG: Corneal endothelium: transient changes with atmospheric anoxia. p. 79. In The Cornea in Health and Disease (VIth Congress of the European Society of Ophthalmology), Royal Society of Medicine International Congress and Symposium Series No. 40. Academic Press and Royal Society of Medicine, London, 1981

87. Holden BA, Williams L, Zantos SG: The etiology of transient endothelial changes in the human cornea. Invest Ophthalmol Vis Sci 26:1354, 1985

88. Fatt I, Bieber MT, Pye SD: Steady state distribution of oxygen and carbon dioxide in the in vivo cornea of an eye covered by a gas-permeable contact lens. Am J Optom Physiol Opt 46:3, 1969

89. Holden BA, Ross R, Jenkins J: Hydrogel contact lenses impede carbon dioxide efflux from the human cornea. Curr Eye Res 6:1283, 1987

90. Bonanno JA, Polse KA: Measurement of the in vivo human corneal stromal pH: open and closed eye. Invest Ophthalmol Vis Sci 28:522, 1987

91. Bonanno JA, Polse KA: Corneal acidosis during contact lens wear: effects of hypoxia and CO_2. Invest Ophthalmol Vis Sci 28:1514, 1987

92. Bonanno JA, Polse KA: Effect of rigid contact lens oxygen transmissibility on stromal pH in the living human eye. Ophthalmology 94:1305, 1987

93. Rivera R, Gan C, Polse K, et al: Contact lenses affect corneal stromal pH. Optom Vis Sci 70:991, 1993

94. Giasson C, Bonanno JA: Corneal epithelial and aqueous humor acidification during in vivo contact lens wear in rabbits. Invest Ophthalmol Vis Sci 35:851, 1994

95. Giasson C, Bonanno JA: Acidification of rabbit corneal endothelium during contact lens wear in vitro. Curr Eye Res 14:311, 1995

96. Cohen SR, Polse KA, Brand RJ, Bonanno JA: Stromal acidosis affects corneal hydration control. Invest Ophthalmol Vis Sci 33:134, 1992

97. Cohen SR, Polse KA, Brand RJ, Bonanno JA: The association between pH level and corneal recovery from induced edema. Curr Eye Res 14:349, 1995

98. Gonnering R, Edelhauser HF, Van Horn DL, Durant W: The pH tolerance of rabbit and human corneal endothelium. Invest Ophthalmol Vis Sci 18:373, 1979

99. Jentsch T, Keller S, Wiederholt M: Ion transport mechanisms in cultured corneal endothelial cells. Curr Eye Res 4:361, 1985

100. Fischbarg J, Lim JJ: Role of cations, anions and carbonic anhydrase in fluid transport across rabbit corneal endothelium. J Physiol 241:647, 1974

101. Green K, Cheeks L, Hull DS: Effect of ambient pH on corneal endothelial sodium fluxes. Invest Ophthalmol Vis Sci 27:1274, 1986

102. Lyslo A, Kvernes S, Garlid K, Ratkje S: Ionic transport across corneal endothelium. Acta Ophthalmol 63:116, 1985

103. Bowman K, Elijah RD, Cheeks K, Green K: Intracellular potential and pH of rabbit corneal endothelial cells. Curr Eye Res 3:991, 1984

104. Khodadoust AA, Hirst LW: Diurnal variation in corneal endothelial morphology. Ophthalmology 91:1125, 1984

105. Schoessler JP, Woloschak MJ: Corneal endothelium in veteran PMMA contact lens wearers. Int Contact Lens Clin 8:19, 1981

106. Schoessler JP: Corneal endothelial polymegethism associated with extended wear. Int Contact Lens Clin 10:148, 1983

107. Hirst LW, Auer C, Cohn J, et al: Specular microscopy of hard contact lens wearers. Ophthalmology 91:1147, 1984

108. Stocker EG, Schoessler JP: Corneal endothelial polymegethism induced by PMMA contact lens wear. Invest Ophthalmol Vis Sci 26:857, 1985

109. MacRae SM, Matsuda M, Yee R: The effect of long-term hard contact lens wear on the corneal endothelium. CLAO J 11:322, 1985

110. MacRae SM, Matsuda M, Shellans S, Rich LF: The effects of hard and soft contact lenses on the corneal endothelium. Am J Ophthalmol 102:50, 1986

111. Carlson KH, Bourne WM, Brubaker RF: Effect of long-term contact lens wear on corneal endothelial cell morphology and function. Invest Ophthalmol Vis Sci 29:185, 1988

112. Lass JH, Dutt RM, Spurney RV, et al: Morphologic and fluorophotometric analysis of the corneal endothelium in long-term hard and soft contact lens wearers. CLAO J 14:105, 1988

113. Schoessler JP, Barr JT, Freson DR: Corneal endothelial observations of silicone elastomer contact lens wearers. Int Contact Lens Clin 11:337, 1984

114. Liberman G, Mandell RB: Corneal endothelial polymegethism in high-Dk contact lens wearers. Int Contact Lens Clin 15:282, 1988

115. Vannas A, Holden BA, Makitie J: The ultrastructure of contact lens induced changes. Acta Ophthalmol 62:320, 1984

116. Williams L, Holden BA: The bleb response of the endothelium decreases with extended wear of contact lenses. Clin Exp Optom 69:90, 1986

117. Bergmanson JPG: Histopathological analysis of corneal endothelial polymegethism. Cornea 11:133, 1992

118. Stevenson RWW, Kirkness CM: Corneal endothelial irregularity with long-term contact lens wear. Cornea 11:600, 1992

119. Holden BA, Vannas A, Nilsson KT, et al: Epithelial and endothelial effects from the extended wear of contact lenses. Curr Eye Res 4:739, 1985

120. Yamauchi K, Hirst LW, Enger C, et al: Specular microscopy of hard contact lens wearers II. Ophthalmology 96:1176, 1989

121. Sibug ME, Datiles MB, Kashima K, et al: Specular microscopy studies on the corneal endothelium after cessation of contact lens wear. Cornea 10:395, 1991

122. Rao GN, Shaw EL, Arthur EJ, Aquavella JV: Endothelial cell morphology and corneal deturgescence. Ann Ophthalmol 11:885, 1979

123. Rao GN, Aquavella JV, Goldberg SH, Berk SL: Pseudophakic bullous keratopathy: relationship to preoperative corneal endothelial status. Ophthalmology 91:1135, 1984

124. Bates AK, Cheng H: Bullous keratopathy: a study of endothelial cell morphology in patients undergoing cataract surgery. Br J Ophthalmol 72:409, 1988

125. Sweeney DF: Corneal exhaustion syndrome with long-term wear of contact lenses. Optom Vis Sci 69:601, 1992

126. Polse KA, Brand RJ, Cohen SR, Guillon M: Hypoxic effects on corneal morphology and function. Invest Ophthalmol Vis Sci 31:1542, 1990

127. McMahon TT, Polse KA, McNamara N, Viana MAG: Recovery from induced corneal edema and endothelial morphology after long-term PMMA contact lens wear. Optom Vis Sci 73:184, 1996

128. Dutt RM, Stocker EG, Wolff CH, et al: A morphological and fluorophotometric analysis of the corneal endothelium in long-term extended wear soft contact lens wearers. CLAO J 15:121, 1989

129. Aronson SB, Elliott JH: Introduction to inflammation. p. 3. In Aronson SB, Elliot JH: Ocular Inflammation. Mosby, St. Louis, 1972

130. Vannas A, Sweeney DF, Holden BA, et al: Tear plasmin activity with contact lens wear. Curr Eye Res 11:243, 1992

131. Willcox MDP, Morris CA, Thakur A, et al: Complement and complement regulatory proteins in human tears. Invest Ophthalmol Vis Sci 38:1, 1997

132. Sack RA, Underwood PA, Tan KO, et al: Vitronectin: possible contribution to the closed-eye external host defense mechanism. Ocular Immunol Inflam 1:327, 1993

133. Tan M, Thakur A, Morris C, Willcox MDP: Presence of inflammatory mediators in the tears of contact lens wearers and non-contact lens wearers. Aust NZ J Ophthalmol (suppl.)25:S27, 1997

134. Abelson MB, Soter NA, Simon MA, et al: Histamine in human tears. Am J Ophthalmol 83:417, 1977

135. Thakur A, Willcox MDP, Stapleton F: The proinflammatory cytokines and arachidonic acid metabolites in human overnight tears: homeostatic mechanisms. J Clin Immunol 18:61, 1998

136. Sack RA, Tan KO, Tan A: Diurnal tear cycle: evidence for a nocturnal inflammatory constitutive tear fluid. Invest Ophthalmol Vis Sci 33:626, 1992

137. Wilson C, O'Leary DJ, Holden BA: Cell content of tears following overnight wear of a contact lens. Curr Eye Res 8:329, 1989

138. Stapleton F, Willcox MDP, Morris CA, Sweeney DF: Tear changes in contact lens wearers following overnight eye closure. Curr Eye Res 17:183, 1998

139. Holden BA, Sweeney DF, Swarbrick HA, et al: The vascular response to long-term extended contact lens wear. Clin Exp Optom 69:112, 1986

140. McMonnies CW: Contact lens-induced corneal vascularization. Int Contact Lens Clin 10:12, 1983

141. Papas EB, Vajdic CM, Austen R, Holden BA: High-oxygen-transmissibility soft contact lenses do not induce limbal hyperaemia. Curr Eye Res 16:942, 1997

142. Dumbleton K, Richter D, Simpson T, Fonn D: A comparison of the vascular response to extended wear of conventional lower Dk and experimental high Dk hydrogel contact lenses. Optom Vis Sci (suppl.)75:170, 1998

143. Josephson JE, Caffery BE: Infiltrative keratitis in hydrogel lens wearers. Int Contact Lens Clin 6:223, 1979

144. Gordon A, Kracher GP: Corneal infiltrates and extended wear contact lenses. J Am Optom Assoc 56:198, 1985

145. Bates AK, Morris RJ, Stapleton F, et al: Sterile corneal infiltrates in contact lens wearers. Eye 3:803, 1989

146. Stapleton F, Dart J, Minassian D: Nonulcerative complications of contact lens wear: relative risks for different lens types. Arch Ophthalmol 110:1601, 1992

147. Thakur A, Willcox MDP: Chemotactic activity of tears

and bacteria isolated during adverse responses. Exp Eye Res 66:129, 1998

148. Sweeney DF, Holden BA, Sankaridurg PR, et al: Categorisation of corneal infiltrative responses observed during hydrogel lens wear. Invest Ophthalmol Vis Sci (suppl.)39:s337, 1998

149. Sweeney DF, Terry R, Papas E, et al: The prevalence of "infiltrates" in a non contact lens wearing population. Invest Ophthalmol Vis Sci (suppl.)37:s71, 1996

150. Zantos SC, Holden BA: Research techniques and materials for continuous wear of contact lenses. Aust J Optom 60:86, 1977

151. Zantos SG: Management of corneal infiltrates in extended-wear contact lens patients. Int Contact Lens Clin 11:604, 1984

152. Sweeney DF, Grant T, Chong MS, et al: Recurrence of acute inflammatory conditions with hydrogel extended wear. Invest Ophthalmol Vis Sci (suppl.)34:1008, 1993

153. Weissman BA: An introduction to extended-wear contact lenses. J Am Optom Assoc 53:183, 1982

154. Crook T: Corneal infiltrates with red eye related to duration of extended wear. J Am Optom Assoc 56:698, 1985

155. Mertz GW, Holden BA: Clinical implications of extended wear research. Can J Optom 43:203, 1981

156. Baleriola-Lucas C, Grant T, Newton-Howes J, et al: Enumeration and identification of bacteria on hydrogel lenses from asymptomatic patients and those experiencing adverse responses with extended wear. Invest Ophthalmol Vis Sci (suppl.)32:739, 1991

157. Baleriola-Lucas C, Holden BA, Gardner H, et al: Habitual bacterial contamination among users of daily and extended wear hydrogel contact lenses. Optom Vis Sci (suppl.)68:75, 1991

158. Holden BA, La Hood D, Grant T, et al: Gram-negative bacteria can induce contact lens related acute red eye (CLARE) responses. CLAO J 22:47, 1996

159. Sankaridurg PR, Willcox MDP, Sharma S, et al: *Haemophilus influenzae* adherent to contact lenses associated with production of acute ocular inflammation. J Clin Microbiol 34:2426, 1996

160. Fleiszig SMJ, Zaidi TS, Preston MJ, et al: Relationship between cytotoxicity and corneal epithelial cell invasion by clinical isolates of *Pseudomonas aeruginosa*. Infect Immunol 64:2288, 1996

161. Cowell BA, Willcox MDP, Hobden JA, et al: An ocular strain of *Pseudomonas aeruginosa* is inflammatory but not virulent in the scarified mouse model. Exp Eye Res 1999 (in press)

162. Cole N, Willcox MDP, Fleiszig SMJ, et al: Different strains of *Pseudomonas aeruginosa* isolated from ocular infections or inflammation display distinct corneal pathologies in an animal model. Curr Eye Res 17:730, 1998

163. Grant T, Chong MS, Vajdic C, et al: Contact lens induced peripheral ulcers during hydrogel contact lens wear. CLAO J 24:145, 1998

164. Stein RM, Clinch TE, Cohen EJ, et al: Infected vs sterile corneal infiltrates in contact lens wear. Am J Ophthalmol 105:632, 1988

165. Parker WT, Wong SK: Keratitis associated with disposable soft contact lenses. Am J Ophthalmol 107:195, 1989

166. Serdahl CL, Mannis MJ, Shapiro DR, et al: Infiltrative keratitis associated with disposable soft contact lenses. Arch Ophthalmol 107:322, 1989

167. McLaughlin R, Kelley CG, Mauger TF: Corneal ulceration associated with disposable EW lenses. Contact Lens Spectrum 4:57, 1989

168. Harris JK, Shovlin JP, Pascucci SE, et al: Keratitis associated with extended wear of disposable contact lenses. Contact Lens Spectrum 4:55, 1989

169. Dunn JP, Mondino BJ, Weissman BA, et al: Corneal ulcers associated with disposable hydrogel contact lenses. Am J Ophthalmol 108:113, 1989

170. Mertz PHV, Bouchard CS, Mathers WD, et al: Corneal infiltrates associated with disposable extended wear soft contact lenses: a report of nine cases. CLAO J 16:269, 1990

171. Willcox MDP, Sweeney DF, Sharma S, et al: Culture negative peripheral ulcers are associated with bacterial contamination of contact lenses. Invest Ophthalmol Vis Sci (suppl.)36:s152, 1995

172. Mondino BJ: Inflammatory diseases of the peripheral cornea. Ophthalmology 95:463, 1988

173. Sankaridurg PR, Sharma S, Willcox M, et al: Colonization of hydrogel lenses with *Streptococcus pneumoniae*: risk of development of corneal infiltrates. Cornea (in press), 1999

174. Holden BA, Reddy MK, Sankaridurg PR, et al: Contact lens induced peripheral ulcers with extended wear of disposable hydrogel lenses: histopathological observations on the nature and type of corneal infiltrate. Cornea (in press), 1999

175. Spring TF: Reactions to hydrophilic lenses. Med J Aust 1:449, 1974

176. Allansmith MR, Korb DR, Greiner JV, et al: Giant papillary conjunctivitis in contact lens wearers. Am J Ophthalmol 83:697, 1977

177. Herman JP: Clinical management of GPC. Contact Lens Spectrum 2:24, 1987

178. Schnider CM, Zabkiewicz K, Holden BA: Unusual complications associated with RGP extended wear. Int Contact Lens Clin 15:124, 1988

179. Abelson MB, Greiner JV, Chin TLN, Mooshian ML: Adaptive changes in the threshold sensitivity of the tarsus as measured with Cochet-Bonnet aesthesiometer. Invest Ophthalmol Vis Sci (suppl.)34:1006, 1993

180. Perryman F: The management of GPC with disposable lenses. Optician 196:21, 1988

181. Strulowitz L, Brudno J: The management of giant papillary conjunctivitis with disposables. Contact Lens Spectrum 4:45, 1989

182. Grant T, Chong MS, Holden BA: Management of GPC with daily disposable lenses. Am J Optom Physiol Opt (suppl.)65:89P, 1988

183. Holden BA, Swarbrick HA: Extended wear lenses. p. 566. In Phillips AJ, Stone J (eds): Contact Lenses. 3rd ed. Butterworths, London, 1989

184. Fowler SA, Greiner JV, Allansmith MR: Soft contact lenses from patients with giant papillary conjunctivitis. Am J Ophthalmol 88:1056, 1979

185. Sugar A, Meyer RF: Giant papillary conjunctivitis after keratoplasty. Am J Ophthalmol 91:239, 1981

186. Nirankari VS, Karesh JW, Richards RD: Complications of exposed monofilament sutures. Am J Ophthalmol 95:515, 1983

187. Grant T: Clinical aspects of planned replacement and disposable lenses. p. 8. In Kerr C (ed): The Contact Lens Year Book 1991. Medical and Scientific Publishing, Hythe, UK, 1991

188. Kotow M, Grant T, Holden BA: Avoiding ocular complications during hydrogel extended wear. Int Contact Lens Clin 14:95, 1987

189. Meisler DM, Krachmer JH, Goeken JA: Giant papillary conjunctivitis. Am J Ophthalmol 92:368, 1981

190. Kruger CJ, Ehlers WH, Luistro AE, Donshik PC: Treatment of giant papillary conjunctivitis with cromolyn sodium. CLAO J 18:46, 1992

191. Molinari J: Giant papillary conjunctivitis management: a review of management and a retrospective clinical study. Clin Eye Vis Care 3:68, 1991

192. Bartlett JD, Howes JF, Ghormley NR, et al: Safety and efficacy of loteprednol etabonate for treatment of papillae in contact lens–associated giant papillary conjunctivitis. Curr Eye Res 12:313, 1993

193. Asbell P, Howes J: A double-masked, placebo-controlled evaluation of the efficacy and safety of loteprednol etabonate in the treatment of giant papillary conjunctivitis. CLAO J 23:31, 1997

194. Wood TS, Stewart RH, Bowman RW, et al: Suprofen treatment of contact lens–associated giant papillary conjunctivitis. Ophthalmology 95:822, 1988

195. Dart JKG: Predisposing factors in microbial keratitis: the significance of contact lens wear. Br J Ophthalmol 72:926, 1988

196. Schein OD, Ormerod LD, Barraquer E, et al: Microbiology of contact lens-related keratitis. Cornea 8:281, 1989

197. Chalupa E, Swarbrick HA, Holden BA, Sjöstrand J: Severe corneal infections associated with contact lens wear. Ophthalmology 94:17, 1987

198. Schein OD, Glynn RJ, Poggio EC, et al: The relative risk of ulcerative keratitis among users of daily-wear and extended-wear soft contact lenses. N Engl J Med 321:773, 1989

199. Poggio EC, Glynn RJ, Schein OD, et al: The incidence of ulcerative keratitis among users of daily-wear and extended-wear soft contact lenses. N Engl J Med 321:779, 1989

200. MacRae S, Herman C, Stulting D, et al: Corneal ulcer and adverse reaction rates in premarket contact lens studies. Am J Ophthalmol 111:457, 1991

201. Buehler PO, Schein OD, Stamler JF, et al: The increased risk of ulcerative keratitis among disposable soft contact lens users. Arch Ophthalmol 110:1555, 1992

202. Matthews TD, Frazer DG, Minassian DC, et al: Risks of keratitis and patterns of use with disposable contact lenses. Arch Ophthalmol 110:1559, 1992

203. Adams CP, Cohen EJ, Laibson PR, et al: Corneal ulcers in patients with cosmetic extended-wear contact lenses. Am J Ophthalmol 96:705, 1993

204. Galentine PG, Cohen EJ, Laibson PR, et al: Corneal ulcers associated with contact lens wear. Arch Ophthalmol 102:891, 1984

205. Weissman BA, Mondino WC, Pettit TH, Hofbauer JD: Corneal ulcers associated with extended-wear soft contact lenses. Am J Ophthalmol 97:476, 1984

206. Koidou-Tsiligianni A, Alfonso E, Forster RK: Ulcerative keratitis associated with contact lens wear. Am J Ophthalmol 108:64, 1989

207. Fleiszig SMJ, Zaidi TS, Fletcher EL, et al: *Pseudomonas aeruginosa* invades corneal epithelial cells during experimental infection. Infect Immunol 62:3485, 1994

208. Fleiszig SMJ, Zaidi TS, Pier GB: *Pseudomonas aeruginosa* invasion of and multiplication within corneal epithelial cells in vitro. Infect Immunol 63:4072, 1995

209. Stern GA, Weitzenkorn D, Valenti J: Adherence of *Pseudomonas aeruginosa* to the mouse cornea. Arch Ophthalmol 100:1956, 1982

210. Stern CA, Lubniewski A, Allen C: The interaction between *Pseudomonas aeruginosa* and the corneal epithelium. Arch Ophthalmol 103:1221, 1985

211. Fleiszig SMH, Lee EJ, Wu C, et al: Cytotoxic strains of *Pseudomonas aeruginosa* can damage the intact corneal surface in vitro. CLAO J 24:41, 1998

212. Raber IM, Laibson PR, Kurz GH, Bernardino VB: *Pseudomonas* corneoscleral ulcers. Am J Ophthalmol 92:353, 1981

213. Fleiszig SMJ, Zaidi TS, Ramphal R, Pier GB: Modulation of *Pseudomonas aeruginosa* adherence to the corneal surface by mucus. Infect Immunol 62:1799, 1994

214. Faber E, Golding TR, Lowe R, Brennan NA: Effect of hydrogel lens wear on tear film stability. Optom Vis Sci 68:380, 1991

215. Moore MB, McCulley JP, Newton C, et al: *Acanthamoeba* keratitis: a growing problem in soft and hard contact lens wearers. Ophthalmology 94:1654, 1987

216. Auran JD, Starr MB, Jakobiec FA: *Acanthamoeba* keratitis: a review of the literature. Cornea 6:2, 1987

217. Moore MB, Ubelaker JE, Martin JH, et al: In vitro penetration of human corneal epithelium by *Acanthamoeba castellani*: a scanning and transmission electron microscopy study. Cornea 10:291, 1991

218. Simmons PA, Tomlinson A, Seal DV: The role of *Pseudomonas aeruginosa* biofilm in the attachment of *Acanthamoeba* to four types of hydrogel contact lens materials. Optom Vis Sci 75:860, 1998

219. Larkin DFP, Kilvington S, Easty DL: Contamination of contact lens storage cases by *Acanthamoeba* and bacteria. Br J Ophthalmol 74:133, 1990

220. Fleiszig SMJ, Efron N, Pier GB: Extended contact lens wear enhances *Pseudomonas aeruginosa* adherence to human corneal epithelium. Invest Ophthalmol Vis Sci 33:2908, 1992

221. Mondino BJ, Weissman BA, Farb MD, Pettit TH: Corneal

ulcers associated with daily-wear and extended-wear contact lenses. Am J Ophthalmol 102:58, 1986

222. Mowrey-McKee MF, Sampson HJ, Proskin HM: Microbial contamination of hydrophilic contact lenses. Part II: Quantification of microbes after patient handling and after aseptic removal from the eye. CLAO J 18:240, 1992

223. Ramachandran L, Sharma S, Sankaridurg PR, et al: Examination of the conjunctival microbiota after 8 hours of eye closure. CLAO J 21:195, 1995

224. Willcox MDP, Power KN, Stapleton F, et al: Potential sources of bacteria that are isolated from contact lenses during wear. Optom Vis Sci 74:1030, 1997

225. Cowell BA, Willcox MDP, Schneider RP: Growth of gram-negative bacteria in a simulated ocular environment. Aust NZ J Ophthalmol (suppl.)25:S23, 1997

226. Williams TJ, Willcox MDP, Schneider RP: Role of tear fluid in the growth of gram-negative bacteria on contact lenses. Aust NZ J Ophthalmol (suppl.)25:S30, 1997

227. Stapleton F, Dart JK, Matheson M, Woodward EG: Bacterial adherence and glycocalyx formation on unworn hydrogel lenses. J Br Contact Lens Assoc 16:113, 1993

228. Stapleton F, Dart J: *Pseudomonas* keratitis associated with biofilm formation on a disposable soft contact lens. Br J Ophthalmol 79:864, 1995

229. Rauschl RT, Rogers JJ: The effect of hydrophilic contact lens wear on the bacterial flora of the human conjunctiva. Int Contact Lens Clin 5:56, 1978

230. Tragakis MP, Brown SI, Pearce DB: Bacteriologic studies of contamination associated with soft contact lenses. Am J Ophthalmol 75:496, 1973

231. Callender MG, Tse LSY, Charles AM, Lutzi D: Bacterial flora of the eye and contact lens cases during hydrogel lens wear. Am J Optom Physiol Opt 63:177, 1986

232. Larkin DFP, Leeming JP: Quantitative alterations of the commensal eye bacteria in contact lens wear. Eye 5:70, 1991

233. Fleiszig SMJ, Efron N: Conjunctival flora in extended wear of rigid gas-permeable contact lenses. Optom Vis Sci 69:354, 1992

234. Stapleton F, Willcox MDP, Fleming CM, et al: Changes to the ocular biota with time in extended- and daily-wear disposable contact lens use. Infect Immunol 63:4501, 1995

235. Gopinathan U, Stapleton F, Sharma S, et al: Microbial contamination of hydrogel contact lenses. J Appl Microbiol 82:653, 1997

236. Carney FP, Morris CA, Willcox MDP: Effect of hydrogel lens wear on the major tear proteins during extended wear. Aust NZ J Ophthalmol (suppl.)25:S36, 1997

237. Cowell BA, Willcox MDP, Schneider RP: A relatively small change in sodium chloride concentration has a strong effect on adhesion of ocular bacteria to contact lenses. J Appl Microbiol 84:950, 1998

238. Lemp MA, Blackman HJ, Wilson LA, Leveille AS: Gram-negative corneal ulcers in elderly aphakic eyes with extended-wear lenses. Ophthalmology 91:60, 1984

239. Graham CM, Dart JKG, Wilson-Holt NW, Buckley RJ: Prospects for contact lens wear in aphakia. Eye 2:48, 1988

240. Eichenbaum JW, Feldstein M, Podos SM: Extended-wear aphakic soft contact lenses and corneal ulcers. Br J Ophthalmol 66:663, 1982

241. Spoor TC, Hartel WC, Wynn P, Spoor DK: Complications of continuous-wear soft contact lenses in a nonreferral population. Arch Ophthalmol 102:1312, 1984

242. Sjöstrand J, Linner E, Nygren B, et al: Severe corneal infection in a contact lens wearer. Lancet 1:149, 1981

243. Yamane SJ, Kuwabara DM: Ensuring compliance in patients wearing contact lenses on an extended-wear basis. Int Contact Lens Clin 14:108, 1987

244. Collins MJ, Carney LG: Compliance with care and maintenance procedures amongst contact lens wearers. Clin Exp Optom 69:174, 1986

245. Keay LJ, Harmis N, Corrigan K, et al: Comparison of bacterial populations on worn contact lenses following 6 nights extended wear of ACUVUE and 30 nights extended wear of investigational hydrogel lenses. Aust NZ J Ophthalmol (suppl.)27, 1999 (accepted abstract)

246. Nilsson SEG, Persson G: Low complication rate in extended wear of contact lenses: a prospective two-year study of nonmedical high water content lens wearers. Acta Ophthalmol 64:88, 1986

247. Kotow M, Holden BA, Grant T: The value of regular replacement of low water content contact lenses for extended wear. J Am Optom Assoc 58:461, 1987

248. Ames KS, Cameron MH: The efficacy of regular lens replacement in extended wear. Int Contact Lens Clin 16:104, 1989

249. Grant T, Holden BA: The clinical performance of disposable (58%) extended wear lenses. Trans Br Contact Lens Assoc 11:63, 1988

250. Davis RL: A clinical study of the Disposalens system. Contact Lens Spectrum 3:49, 1988

251. Donshik P, Weinstock FJ, Wechsler S, et al: Disposable hydrogel contact lenses for extended wear. CLAO J 14:191, 1988

252. Maskell RW: The ACUVUE experience—personal experience over 18 months. Contact Lens J 17:257, 1989

253. Nilsson SEG, Lindh H: Disposable contact lenses—a prospective study of clinical performance in flexible and extended wear. Contactologia 12:80, 1990

254. Port M: A European multicentre extended wear study of the NewVues disposable contact lens. Contact Lens J 19:86, 1991

255. Maguen E, Tsai JC, Martinez M: A retrospective study of disposable extended-wear lenses in 100 patients. Ophthalmology 98:1685, 1991

256. Marshall EC, Begley CG, Nguyen CHD: Frequency of complications among wearers of disposable and conventional soft contact lenses. Int Contact Lens Clin 19:55, 1992

257. Maguen E, Rosner I, Caroline P, et al: A retrospective study of disposable extended wear lenses in 100 patients: year 2. CLAO J 18:229, 1992

258. Glastonbury J, Crompton JL: *Pseudomonas aeruginosa* corneal infection associated with disposable contact lens use. Aust NZ J Ophthalmol 17:451, 1989

259. Kershner RM: Infectious corneal ulcer with overextended wearing of disposable contact lenses. JAMA 261:3549, 1989
260. Killingsworth DW, Stern GA: *Pseudomonas* keratitis associated with the use of disposable soft contact lenses. Arch Ophthalmol 107:795, 1989
261. Rabinowitz SM, Pflugfelder SC, Goldberg M: Disposable extended-wear contact lens–related keratitis. Arch Ophthalmol 107:1121, 1989
262. Kent HD, Sanders RJ, Arentsen JJ, et al: *Pseudomonas* corneal ulcer associated with disposable soft contact lenses. CLAO J 15:264, 1989
263. Capoferri C, Sirianni P, Menga M: *Pseudomonas* keratitis in disposable soft lens wear. Contactologia 13:61, 1991
264. Cohen EJ, Gonzalez C, Leavitt KC, et al: Corneal ulcers associated with contact lenses including experience with disposable lenses. CLAO J 17:173, 1991
265. Ficker L, Hunter P, Seal D, Wright P: *Acanthamoeba* keratitis occurring with disposable contact lens wear. Am J Ophthalmol 108:453, 1990
266. Heidemann DG, Verdier DD, Dunn SP, Stamler JF: *Acanthamoeba* keratitis associated with disposable contact lenses. Am J Ophthalmol 110:630, 1990
267. Efron N, Wohl A, Toma NG, et al: *Pseudomonas* corneal ulcers associated with daily wear of disposable hydrogel contact lenses. Int Contact Lens Clin 18:46, 1991
268. Fowler SA, Greiner JV, Allansmith MR: Attachment of bacteria to soft contact lenses. Arch Ophthalmol 97:659, 1979
269. Stern GA, Zam ZS: The pathogenesis of contact lens–associated *Pseudomonas aeruginosa* corneal ulceration. 1. The effect of contact lens coatings on adherence of *Pseudomonas aeruginosa* to soft contact lenses. Cornea 5:41, 1986
270. Butrus SI, Klotz SA, Misra RP: The adherence of *Pseudomonas aeruginosa* to soft contact lenses. Ophthalmology 94:1310, 1987
271. Minarik L, Rapp J: Protein deposits on individual hydrophilic contact lenses: effects of water and ionicity. CLAO J 15:185, 1989
272. Lin ST, Mandell RB, Leahy CD, Newell JO: Protein accumulation on disposable extended wear lenses. CLAO J 17:44, 1991
273. Tripathi PC, Tripathi RC: Analysis of glycoprotein deposits on disposable soft contact lenses. Invest Ophthalmol Vis Sci 33:121, 1992
274. Smith SK: Patient noncompliance with wearing and replacement schedules of disposable contact lenses. J Am Optom Assoc 67:160, 1996
275. Grant T, Terry R, Holden BA: Extended wear of hydrogel lenses: clinical problems and their management. p. 599. In Harris MG (ed): Problems in Optometry. Vol 2. No. 3. Lippincott, Philadelphia, 1990
276. McMonnies C: Risk factors in the etiology of contact lens induced corneal vascularization. Int Contact Lens Clin 11:286, 1984
277. Sendele DD, Kenyon KR, Mobilia EF, et al: Superior limbic keratoconjunctivitis in contact lens wearers. Ophthalmology 90:616, 1983
278. Weissman BA, Schwartz SD, Gottschalk-Katsev N, Lee DA: Oxygen permeability of disposable soft contact lenses. Am J Ophthalmol 110:269, 1990
279. Weissman BA, Schwartz SD, Lee DA: Oxygen transmissibility of disposable hydrogel contact lenses. CLAO J 17:62, 1991
280. Morgan PB, Efron N: The oxygen performance of contemporary hydrogel contact lenses. Contact Lens Ant Eye 21:3, 1998
281. Holden BA: Factors affecting the corneal response to contact lenses. p. 9. In Franz RP, Hanks AJ, Weisbarth RE (eds): Current Perspectives in Vision Care, CIBA Vision Monograph Series No. 1. CIBA Vision, Bulach/Zurich, Switzerland, 1992
282. Duran JA, Refojo MF, Gipson IK, Kenyon KR: *Pseudomonas* attachment to new hydrogel contact lenses. Arch Ophthalmol 105:106, 1987
283. Dart JK, Badenoch PR: Bacterial adherence to contact lenses. CLAO J 12:220, 1986
284. Williams TJ, Willcox MDP, Schneider RP: Interactions of bacteria with contact lenses: the effect of soluble protein and carbohydrate on bacterial adhesion to contact lenses. Optom Vis Sci 75:266, 1998
285. Taylor RL, Willcox MDP, Williams TJ, Verran J: Modulation of bacterial adhesion to hydrogel contact lenses by albumin. Optom Vis Sci 75:1, 1998
286. Fukuda M, Fullard RJ, Willcox MDP, et al: Fibronectin in the tear film. Invest Ophthalmol Vis Sci 37:459, 1996
287. Baleriola-Lucas C, Fukuda M, Willcox MDP, et al: Fibronectin concentration in tears of contact lens wearers. Exp Eye Res 64:37, 1997
288. Baleriola-Lucas C, Willcox MDP: The ability of ocular bacteria to bind to fibronectin. Clin Exp Optom 81:81, 1998
289. Seger RG, Mutti DO: Conjunctival staining and single-use CLs with unpolished edges. Contact Lens Spectrum 3:36, 1988
290. Wodis M, Hodur N, Jurkus J: Disposable lens safety: the reproducibility factor. Int Contact Lens Clin 17:96, 1990
291. Lowther GE: Evaluation of disposable lens edges. Contact Lens Spectrum 6:41, 1991
292. Efron N, Veys J: Defects in disposable contact lenses can compromise ocular integrity. Int Contact Lens Clin 19:8, 1992
293. Guillon M: Invited commentary: statistical significance vs. clinical significance. Int Contact Lens Clin 19:18, 1992
294. Holden BA: The Efron defect debate—a personal perspective. Int Contact Lens Clin 19:224, 1992
295. Levy B: Letter to the editor. Int Contact Lens Clin 19:228, 1992
296. Solomon OD, Freeman MI, Boshnick EL, et al: A 3-year prospective study of the clinical performance of daily disposable contact lenses compared with frequent replacement and conventional daily wear contact lenses. CLAO J 22:250, 1996
297. Trick LR: Patient compliance—don't count on it! J Am Optom Assoc 64:264, 1993

298. Ley P: Satisfaction, compliance and communication. Br J Clin Psychol 21:241, 1982

299. Kass MA, Meltzer DW, Gordon M, et al: Compliance with topical pilocarpine treatment. Am J Ophthalmol 101:515, 1986

300. Claydon BE, Efron N: Non-compliance in contact lens wear. Ophthalmol Physiol Opt 14:356, 1994

301. Rosenstock IM: Patients' compliance with health regimens. JAMA 234:402, 1975

302. Claydon BE, Efron N, Woods C: A prospective study of the effect of education on non-compliant behaviour in contact lens wear. Ophthalmol Physiol Opt 17:137, 1997

303. Sokol JL, Mier MG, Bloom S, Asbell PA: A study of patient compliance in a contact lens-wearing population. CLAO J 16:209, 1990

304. Claydon BE, Efron N, Woods C: Non-compliance in optometric practice. Ophthalmol Physiol Opt 18:187, 1998

305. Fan L, Jia Q, Jie C, Jun J: The compliance of Chinese contact lens wearers. Int Contact Lens Clin 22:188, 1995

306. Cho P, Conway R, Fung-Lian L: A report on contact lens practice in Tianjin, China. Int Contact Lens Clin 20:80, 1993

307. Radford CF, Woodward EG, Stapleton F: Contact lens hygiene compliance in a university population. J Br Contact Lens Assoc 16:105, 1993

308. Ley P: Memory for medical information. Br J Social Clin Psychol 18:245, 1979

309. Chalmers RL, Cutter GR, Roseman M: The self-management behaviors of soft contact lens wearers: the effect of lens modality. Int Contact Lens Clin 22:117, 1995

310. Cockburn J, Gibberd RW, Reid AL, et al: Determinants of non-compliance with short term antibiotic regimens. BMJ 295:814, 1987

311. Hughes JR, Wadland WC, Fenwick JW, et al: Effect of cost on the self-administration and efficacy of nicotine gum: a preliminary study. Preventive Med 20:486, 1991

312. Turner FD, Gower LA, Stein JM, et al: Compliance and contact lens care: a new assessment method. Optom Vis Sci 70:998, 1993

313. Koetting RA, Castellano CF, Wartman R: Patient compliance with EW instructions. Contact Lens Spectrum Nov:23, 1986

314. Chun MW, Weissman BA: Compliance in contact lens care. Am J Optom Physiol Opt 64:274, 1987

315. Lane I: Disposables increase patient compliance and referrals. Contact Lens Forum Dec:32, 1990

316. Sheard GM, Efron N, Claydon BE: Does solution cost affect compliance among contact lens wearers? J Br Contact Lens Assoc 18:59, 1995

317. Turner FD, Stein JM, Sager DP, et al: A new method to assess contact lens care compliance. CLAO J 19:108, 1993

318. Phillips LJ, Prevade SL: Replacement and care compliance in a planned replacement contact lens program. J Am Optom Assoc 64:201, 1993

319. Claydon BE, Efron N, Woods C: A prospective study of non-compliance in contact lens wear. J Br Contact Lens Assoc 19:133, 1996

320. Bowden FW, Cohen EJ, Arentsen JJ, Laibson PR: Patterns of lens care practices and lens product contamination in contact lens associated microbial keratitis. CLAO J 15:49, 1989

321. Davis LJ: Lens hygiene and care system contamination of asymptomatic rigid gas permeable lens wearers. Int Contact Lens Clin 22:217, 1995

15

Rigid Gas-Permeable Extended-Wear Lenses

CRISTINA M. SCHNIDER

GRAND ROUNDS CASE REPORT

Subjective:
A 36-year-old woman presented to pick up a replacement right eye (OD) contact lens. Patient has worn Fluoroperm 92 rigid gas-permeable (RGP) lenses for the past 5 months. She experienced discomfort OD for 2 days. She reported mostly daily-wear use but wore her lenses overnight 2 days ago with subsequent OD irritation on arising. The right eye remained irritable after she tried to reinsert the lens several hours later, so she wore only the left lens. Ocular history was positive for chronic blepharitis and meibomianitis as well as epidemic keratoconjunctivitis 6 months previously. Although fitted with extended-wear RGP lenses, she had been advised against full-time extended-wear use because of history of lid problems.

Objective:
- Entrance acuities: OD $^{20}/_{400}$ (uncorrected); OD best visual acuity $^{20}/_{20}$, left eye (OS) $^{20}/_{20}$ (with contact lenses)
- Biomicroscopy: OD a 1-mm peripheral oval corneal excavation at 8:30 o'clock was evident, surrounded by a 0.3-mm band of anterior stromal and subepithelial infiltrates; temporal conjunctiva showed 1+ injection; trace cells in anterior chamber; pupillary functions normal. OS light central superficial punctate keratitis and 1+ peripheral corneal desiccation; quiet conjunctiva and anterior chamber.

Assessment:
Peripheral corneal ulcer, presumed sterile because of location, small size, and lack of significant inflammatory response of cornea, conjunctiva, and anterior chamber.

Note: Corneal ulcers with RGP extended wear have been primarily associated with peripheral corneal desiccation (3 and 9 o'clock staining) and lens adherence.[1,2] Review of this patient's record did not reveal prior history of peripheral desiccation or lens adherence.

Plan:
Culture not taken owing to presumed sterile appearance and clinical findings. However, patient immediately treated with 1 drop 1% cyclopentolate, 1 drop 1% tropicamide, 1 drop 0.3% tobramycin (Tobrex), and 1 drop 1% prednisolone acetate (Pred Forte). Patient advised to continue use of Tobrex and Pred Forte q2h and to return the following morning.

The next day, corneal signs essentially the same; dosage changed to q4h for Tobrex and Pred Forte and gentamicin ointment added at bedtime for prophylaxis and lubrication through the night. Cycloplegia maintained with 1 drop 1% cyclopentolate. Patient instructed to return in 2 days.

At this visit, ulcer showed slight central staining with fluorescein, with underlying stromal haze. Tobrex discontinued. Continue with gentamicin at bedtime, Pred Forte three times a day, and return in 5 days for follow-up.

On this visit, the corneal excavation had filled in and epithelial layer showed light stipple staining over a trace of stromal haze. Gentamicin and Pred Forte were discontinued; preservative-free lubricating drops were begun three times a day and preservative-free ointment at bedtime.

Other:
Patient resumed wear with RGP lenses after ulcer resolved but continued to experience superficial punctate keratitis and itching OU. Examination revealed repeated daytime adherence of right contact lens, resulting in significant staining over area of prior ulcer. Patient dissatisfied with rigid lens wear, so no attempt to alter lens design was made. The patient was subsequently refitted with daily-wear hydrogel lenses with monthly planned replacement.

Nearly 30 million contact lens wearers exist in the United States. Although 8 million new wearers enter the market each year, an equal number stop wearing contact lenses. A major factor in the decision of many patients to discontinue use of contact lenses is the inconvenience associated with the care and maintenance of daily-wear lenses. In addition, the current popularity of spectacle frames as fashion accessories, combined with a surge in promotion of refractive surgery techniques, has led to re-evaluation of ways to increase the popularity of contact lenses for refractive correction. Although extended wear offers a much simplified care system, experience with traditional hydrogel extended wear has shown that the oxygen levels achieved are insufficient to maintain adequate corneal metabolism, as evidenced by changes in corneal thickness, epithelial microcysts, and endothelial polymegethism.[3] In addition, the negative publicity surrounding microbial keratitis associated with extended-wear soft lenses in the late 1980s significantly limited its use in the following years.[4,5] This trend occurred just as the first RGP materials were approved for extended wear.

Despite the negative publicity surrounding the risks of extended wear, interest in the modality remained quite high among patients wearing contact lenses. The appearance of novel rigid and soft lens materials in the 1990s that boasted oxygen transmissibility values in excess of 100 brought a renewed sense of optimism for prolonged wear of contact lenses. Rigid lens materials have continued to evolve with more stable, machinable formulations that have made prescribing highly permeable materials feasible for even daily-wear regimens and have made the possibility of continuous wear (30 days or more) a reality. The addition of silicone and sometimes fluorine to traditional hydrogel materials has significantly boosted the oxygen permeability (Dk) and transmissibility (Dk/t)

values for soft lenses as well. Approval of several rigid and soft lens materials for 30-day continuous wear in the early 2000s is expected. Oxygen-related complications are undoubtedly minimized as lenses with higher oxygen transmissibility become available. However, oxygen alone does not provide for problem-free extended wear.

COMPLICATIONS

Compared with extended wear of hydrogel lenses, even when oxygen transmissibility values are comparable, RGP lenses have fewer, more predictable, and therefore potentially avoidable complications. Problems are also usually less severe than those that occur with soft lenses. These benefits are largely the result of characteristics related to the materials themselves. Inappropriate patient selection, fitting, and patient management, however, can contribute to increased incidence of problems. Although complications associated with extended wear of RGP lenses are not significantly different from those of daily wear with the same lenses, they usually occur at an accelerated pace and require an enhanced follow-up regimen.

For the purposes of this discussion, complications associated with extended wear of RGP lenses are divided into those primarily associated with material properties of lenses and solutions and those caused by problems of fitting and lens design.

Material-Related Complications

Complications related to the properties of the polymers used to make the lenses, or the solutions used to care for them, tend to fall into one of three categories: hypoxia, lid complications, and ocular surface disorders.

TABLE 15-1. *Selected Extended-Wear Rigid Gas-Permeable and Disposable Soft Lens Materials*

Material	Composition	Dk[a]	L_{min} Used for calculation (–3.00 D lens)[b]	Dk/t_{min} (Calculated)[c]
Rigid Gas-Permeable Lenses				
Menicon Z[d]	Tisilfocon A (FS/A)	189	0.15	126
Menicon SF-P[d]	Melafocon A (FS/A)	159	0.18	88
Fluoropern 151[e]	Paflufocon D (FS/A)	151	0.18	84
Fluoroperm 92[e]	Paflufocon A (FS/A)	92	0.18	51
Boston Equalens[f]	Itafluorofocon A	64	0.15	43
Fluorocon[g]	Paflufocon B (FS/A)	60	0.12	50
Fluoroperm 60[e]	Paflufocon B (FS/A)	60	0.15	40
Paraperm EW[e]	Pasifocon C (S/A)	56	0.15	37
Hydrogel Lenses				
Focus NIGHT & DAY[h]	Lotrafilcon A	140	0.08	175
PureVision[i]	Balafilcon A	99	0.09	110
Focus 1-2 Week[h]	Vifilcon A 55%	16	0.06	27
Optima FW[i]	Polymacon 38.6%	8.4	0.035	24
ACUVUE[j]	Etafilcon A 58%	28	0.07	40

Dk = oxygen permeability; Dk/t = oxygen transmission; FS/A = fluorosilicone/acrylate; L_{avg} = average thickness; L_{min} = minimum thickness; S/A = silicone/acrylate.

[a]$\times 10^{-11}$ (cm²/sec) (ml O_2/ml × mm Hg); as stated by manufacturer (without edge correction).
[b]For minus lenses, L_{min} are generally less than L_{avg}+, resulting in an overestimation of Dk/t values.
[c]$\times 10^{-9}$ (cm/sec) (ml O_2/ml × mm Hg).
[d]Manufactured by Menicon USA, Clovis, CA.
[e]Manufactured by Paragon Vision Sciences, Mesa, AZ.
[f]Manufactured by Polymer Technology Corp., Rochester, NY.
[g]Manufactured by Wesley-Jessen, Des Plaines, IL.
[h]Manufactured by CIBA Vision, Duluth, GA.
[i]Manufactured by Bausch & Lomb, Inc., Rochester, NY.
[j]Manufactured by Vistakon, Jacksonville, FL.

Hypoxia

Holden and Mertz[6] performed the hallmark study in determining oxygen transmissibility values that are required to maintain good corneal health. They set various standards based on the equivalent oxygen percentage (EOP) required to maintain an edema-free state of the average cornea on different wearing schedules. Their results suggest an EOP requirement of 12% (standard atmospheric EOP is 21% at sea level) as a minimum for extended wear. This level enables the cornea to return to an edema-free state within a few hours of eye opening. This corresponds to a Dk/t of 34. However, if the non–lens-wearing state is taken as the goal, an EOP of 18% (corrected Dk/t of 87) is required to result in no lens-induced overnight corneal swelling. These results have been confirmed by Fatt,[7] who estimated that a material Dk of 126 for minus lenses (average thickness 0.17 mm) and a Dk of more than 200 for low-plus lenses (average thickness 0.27 mm) is required to provide a Dk/t of 75, which is short of the Holden and Mertz criteria for edema-free extended wear.

Table 15-1 lists the rigid lenses approved for extended-wear use by the U.S. Food and Drug Administration (FDA), along with some commonly used conventional soft extended-wear materials and two new silicone hydro-gels. In reviewing these numbers, it is obvious that presently available RGP materials are superior to traditional hydrogel lenses in providing the oxygen necessary for edema-free extended wear by virtue of Dk/t alone. Although Dk/t values are more comparable for the high-Dk silicone hydrogel materials, the added benefits of a smaller diameter and increased tear exchange owing to lens movement generally give the rigid lenses the advantage physiologically. RGP lenses typically result in a lower overnight swelling response for a given Dk/t and a faster deswelling response on eye opening.[8]

These Dk and EOP values are useful for comparing different materials, yet they are not sufficient to guarantee adequate on-eye lens performance on an individual basis. Even though the average nonlens overnight corneal swelling value is reported to be approximately 4%, the range is from approximately 2% to more than 10% for healthy individuals. It is likely that people on the high end of this range are less successful than average with extended wear and those on the low end may perform better than expected. Therefore, consideration of each patient as an individual, combined with skill and diligence during the aftercare process, is the only way of achieving success with this type of lens wear.

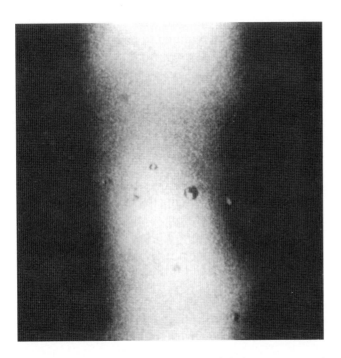

FIG. 15-1. *Slit-lamp photograph of epithelial microcysts and vacuoles. The small irregular lesions are microcysts, and the larger bubblelike objects are vacuoles (×30). (Courtesy of Cornea and Contact Lens Research Unit, Sydney, Australia.)*

Evidence of edema with contemporary rigid and soft lens materials is subtler than the frank central corneal clouding caused by polymethylmethacrylate (PMMA) lenses. The specific metabolic changes associated with these responses to hypoxia vary somewhat depending on the layer of the cornea affected. In the early 1970s, Schoessler and Lowther[9] evaluated slit-lamp findings associated with PMMA contact lens wear and suggested that epithelial edema is associated primarily with osmotic imbalances, whereas stromal edema relates to hypoxia. Since then, Klyce[10] has shown that hypoxia increases epithelial lactate production and that diffusion of the lactate into the stroma creates an osmotic imbalance, which leads to swelling. Bonnano and Polse[11] then demonstrated that tear film hypoxia is accompanied by a reduction in corneal stromal pH and, more specifically, that RGP contact lenses worn with the eyes closed reduce stromal pH, despite Dk values in the neighborhood of 100.[12]

This pH shift may well be a common mechanism for the many changes observed in the hypoxic cornea. Work by Madigan and colleagues[13] has shown that contact lens–induced chronic hypoxia in cats results in a severe reduction in epithelial adhesion. This finding may explain the etiology of soft lens–associated chronic hypoxia syndrome described by Wallace,[14] in which the corneal epithe-

lium is removed with a soft lens, creating a large epithelial erosion in long-term soft lens wearers. Mauger and Hill[15] found significant delays in epithelial healing rates for rabbits after corneal injury with contact lenses that produced oxygen levels less than approximately 9%.

Ren and coworkers provided even more compelling evidence to support the quest for ever-increasing Dk/t values in extended-wear contact lenses. They demonstrated an inverse correlation between lens oxygen transmissibility and the binding of *Pseudomonas aeruginosa* to exfoliated human epithelial cells.[16] Ren et al. also found that epithelial cell desquamation decreases and cell size increases with wear of all contact lenses, but these factors in the absence of hypoxia do not contribute to increased *P. aeruginosa* adherence.[17] These results suggest strongly that achieving oxygen transmissibility values in excess of 100 may offer a significant potential advance in safety for extended wear.

More studies like these are needed to truly understand the short- and long-term consequences of chronic hypoxia. In the meantime, if the non–lens-wearing cornea is taken as the standard and apply the dictum "above all, do no harm," one should strive to avoid the various clinical signs of hypoxic stress described in this chapter.

Epithelial Microcysts   Microcysts are tiny refractile lesions, irregular in shape, that can vary from 15 to 50 μm.[18] Under high magnification, they exhibit reversed illumination, which suggests that their refractive index is higher than that of the surrounding epithelial tissue. Histologic studies indicate that microcysts are pockets of dead and malformed cells that originate at the basement membrane and eventually migrate to the surface of the epithelium with the newly formed epithelial layers.[19] The exact cause of the cell disruption is not well understood, but because microcysts are rare in the absence of hypoxia, it is clear that they are an indication of chronic hypoxia or other metabolic disorder in the cornea.

Because these pockets of debris must move forward through the epithelial layers to be sloughed off with normal epithelial cells, they do not appear for some time after the creation of the hypoxic environment. Similarly, they may take some weeks to clear after elimination of the cause of hypoxia. Microcysts usually become noticeable after several weeks or months of extended wear, and they are most easily viewed in marginal retroillumination near the inferior pupil border. Although the relationship is not clear, they are often seen in the presence of vacuoles, which appear as larger, round, bubblelike objects showing unreversed illumination (Fig. 15-1). Microcysts do eventually move through the surface of the epithelium and can cause staining, as shown in Figure 15-2. Positive staining (bright fluorescent spots) represents areas where the cystic formations have broken through, whereas dark dots indicate negative staining or an elevation of the epithelium that does not hold the fluorescein and thus causes a relatively dark spot in the fluorescent film.

Because microcysts closely resemble tear film debris and endothelial pigment in size and appearance, it is important to use good biomicroscopy technique in observing them. Microcysts are refractile lesions and therefore are not visible in direct illumination, unlike tear debris and endothelial pigment, both of which are opaque. In addition, tear film debris moves with the blink, unlike microcysts or endothelial pigment. Endothelial pigment and microcysts are visible in retroillumination; however, only the pigment can be viewed directly in the parallelepiped and can be localized to the endothelial surface. Endothelial pigment displays a color similar to the iris pigment, whereas microcysts have no color and can be viewed only in retroillumination from the pupil or iris. The appearance of microcysts can be likened to that of salt on a jellyfish.

Several grading scales have been proposed for microcysts, some involving simply numbers of cysts and others incorporating staining as a criterion. However, because the eruption of microcysts is more a function of time than of severity, a system that involves the number of visible cysts is preferred for grading (Table 15-2). It should be remembered, however, that healthy corneas do not have more than a few microcysts,[20] and the presence of microcysts before lens wear should lead to a high suspicion of epithelial basement membrane dystrophy. Because of the higher-than-average chance of recurrent erosion with epithelial basement membrane dystrophy, it may be inadvisable to fit contact lenses at all, and extended wear should be avoided in all cases of suspected dystrophic conditions. Bear in mind, however, that microcysts may appear to increase temporarily for a few weeks or months when an extended-wear lens patient is given a different lens of significantly improved oxygen transmissibility. This occurs because the metabolic rate of the cornea is allowed to speed up with the increase in oxygen availability, and the malformed cells from the previous hypoxic period are pushed to the surface.

The literature has few reports of microcysts in RGP extended-wear patients, and when they occur, the microcystic response is graded as trace or mild. Rates range from 22–77% for low-Dk lenses, to 3–19% for moderate-Dk lenses, and 0–5% for high-Dk lenses.[21,22]

Striae and Folds   Striae and folds are indications of excessive corneal swelling resulting from edema, primarily in the stromal lamellae. The increase in stromal thickness is best measured by optical or ultrasonic pachometry, but striae and folds are indirect indications of levels of stro-

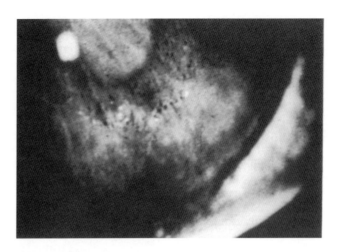

FIG. 15-2. *Fluorescein photograph showing positive and negative staining associated with an eruption of microcysts through the anterior epithelial layers. (Courtesy of Cornea and Contact Lens Research Unit, Sydney, Australia.)*

mal edema. Striae were first described in the early days of soft lens use[23-25] and were observed when the level of edema reached 5–6%.[26-28] They appear as fine, vertical grayish-white lines in the posterior stroma and are thought to represent a refractile effect caused by fluid separation of collagen fibrils.[29] They can be differentiated from corneal nerves, which they resemble, by use of an optic section. The corneal nerves run midway through the stroma and can be viewed on optic section as a pinpoint centered in the stroma, whereas the striae are not visible because they appear on the posterior surface.

When edema levels reach 10–12% with soft lenses, stromal folds may form. These appear as dark lines in the posterior stroma (Fig. 15-3) and represent actual buckling or creasing of the posterior corneal layers.[29] The observation of folds should warrant immediate cessation of overnight wear, followed by a change in lens or wearing schedule, or both. Striae that persist for more than a few hours after eye opening for an extended-wear patient indicate an inability of the cornea to deal with the level of edema that occurs during sleep, also warranting a change of lenses, wearing schedule, or both. Striae and folds, however, are much less likely to be observed in rigid lens wearers, despite correspondingly high levels of edema measured by optical pachometry.[26,30] Literature reports of striae in rigid lens wearers are exceedingly rare, although striae have been observed in daily- and extended-wear patients. Therefore, because most offices are not equipped with pachometers, patient symptoms may be the only indication that the level of edema is excessive.

Patients who experience high levels of edema on awakening often report hazy or foggy vision that does not clear

TABLE 15-2. *Clinical Grading Scales and Intervention Indications*

Grade	Clinical Implication and Intervention	Hyperemia/Redness	Papillae	Staining	Edema	Vascularization
0	Absence of sign. No intervention.	Rare in vascular tissues; may indicate anemia	Uniform satin appearance of conjunctiva	No staining of cornea or conjunctiva	Absence of microcysts, striae, folds, CCC	Vessels not dilated, no growth or buds
1	Minimal; normal in non–lens-wearing individual. No intervention.	Bulbar vessels of expected caliber; yellow appearance of tarsal plate	Uniform microscopic appearance	<25 discrete punctate dots or discrete patch; (>10%) of conjunctiva stains	<5% daytime edema; <25 microcysts, no striae, folds, or CCC	Vessels slightly dilatated, growth <0.25 mm beyond limbus
2	Mild; may be present before lens wear but not usual. Monitor.	Mild dilatation of vessels; pink appearance of tarsal plate	Nonuniform enlargement to 0.5 mm	>25 discrete dots, or mild coalescence; up to 25% of conjunctiva stains	5–10% daytime edema; >25 microcysts, striae that resolve during day; no folds or CCC	Vessels quiet and ≤1.5 mm beyond limbal arcade
3	Moderate; severity sufficient to contraindicate continued wear. Remove lens and modify material, fit, or wear schedule.	Marked dilatation of vessels; brick-red tarsal plate	Enlargement becoming uniform with some papillae >0.5 mm	Marked coalescence, dots not countable, penetration into deeper layers; up to 50% of conjunctiva stains	10–15% edema; uncountable microcysts; striae and folds present; CCC	Vessels engorged and ≤1.5 mm beyond limbus, or growth ≥2 mm beyond limbus but not in pupil area
4	Severe; potentially sight threatening. Discontinue lens wear and treat condition medically if indicated.	Severe congestion of vessels, blood-red appearance	Giant papillae >1 mm in diameter; tops stain with NaF	Loss of epithelium and penetration of fluorescein to stroma; >50% of conjunctiva stains	>15% edema; loss of transparency; reduced BVA	Vessels threaten visual axis

BVA = best visual acuity; CCC = central corneal clouding; NaF = sodium fluorescein.

within a few minutes of eye opening. Many patients report that the fogginess disappears when they shower or wash their face, which may, in fact, just be a coincidence of timing and not a result of the activity itself. Any patient wearing RGP extended-wear lenses who reports foggy vision persisting more than 15–20 minutes in the morning should be viewed with suspicion because this may indicate high levels of residual edema despite the absence of clinical signs.

Polymegethism   Hypoxia of the most posterior corneal layer is not as well understood as that of other layers. The hexagonally arranged cells are most definitely affected by hypoxia and show polymegethism (a change in cell size) and pleomorphism (a change in cell shape) as a result of hypoxia. These changes have been reported in response

to PMMA lens wear,[31] soft lens extended wear,[32] and lid ptosis,[33] and less rapid changes characterize the normal aging process as well.[34]

Little controversy exists about the morphology of the endothelial changes associated with chronic hypoxia. However, Bergmanson[35] presented a new theory on the mechanism of the apparent changes in size and shape based on evidence from electron microscopic studies of the endothelia of six humans, three of whom were contact lens wearers. Bergmanson proposed that a three-dimensional reorientation takes place, such that apparently small cells are oriented so that their larger face is not in the plane of regard and the volume of the cell remains the same. This is in contrast to thinking in a more two-dimensional perspective, in which the cells would have to gain and lose cell area to change size and shape. The observations of endothelial blebs, reported by Zantos, Holden, and Williams,[36,37] may be transient manifestations of this proposed morphologic change, and they are also produced in response to a change in corneal pH.[38] Regardless of the outcome of this new controversy, however, it is agreed that changes do occur in response to hypoxia. Clements[39] attributes these changes to corneal acidosis secondary to inhibited carbon dioxide efflux from the cornea and increased lactic acid production.

The functional significance of polymegethism and pleomorphism is far more nebulous than their morphology. Some authors maintain that long-term contact lens wear and the resultant endothelial changes do not cause functional abnormalities.[40] Other studies have shown functional losses in patients with higher amounts of polymegethism, as evidenced by localized corneal swelling over areas of enlarged endothelial cells[41] and an increase in postoperative corneal swelling.[42–44] Sweeney et al.[45] have also shown that corneal swelling in response to thick hydrogel contact lenses correlates with the subject's degree of polymegethism, and deswelling rates are inversely correlated to the degree of polymegethism. On the basis of evidence from these and other studies, Connor and Zagrod[46] have suggested that the shape changes may be a result of decreased endothelial adenosine triphosphate levels and disturbed calcium homeostasis resulting from corneal endothelial hypoxia.

Although little evidence exists that polymegethism can be reversed to any large degree, results for daily and extended wear have indicated that the increases in endothelial polymegethism have been minimal with high-Dk/t RGP lenses.[47,21] A more thorough discussion of complications relating to edema and the endothelial layer can be found in Chapters 2 and 3.

Lid Complications

Complications of the lids are rare with rigid lenses but can nevertheless occur, primarily in response to a soiled or improperly finished lens surface. In addition, the mechanical aspect of the interaction of the rigid lens and the lid can contribute to papillary hypertrophy and an apparent lid ptosis.[48,49] It should be obvious, however, that preexisting inflammatory reactions, blepharitis, meibomian gland dysfunction, and lid appositional problems constitute contraindications to extended wear and should be remedied before extended wear is attempted. These complications are discussed in detail in Chapters 6 and 9.

Contact Lens Papillary Conjunctivitis   The term *contact lens papillary conjunctivitis* has been coined to describe papillary hypertrophy of the superior tarsal plate specifically related to contact lens use. It is preferred to the term *giant papillary conjunctivitis* for describing mild-to-mod-

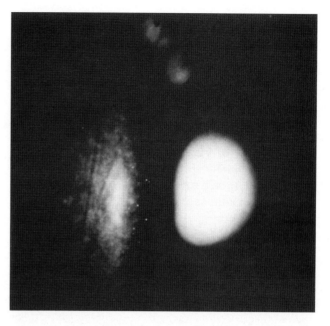

FIG. 15-3. *Endothelial folds, photographed in specular reflection, indicating corneal edema level more than 10%. (Photograph by Dr. C. Schnider; Courtesy of Cornea and Contact Lens Research Unit, Sydney, Australia.)*

erate papillary changes of the upper lid. Giant papillary conjunctivitis is a specific diagnostic entity consisting of an entire set of signs and symptoms, described by Allansmith et al. in 1977,[50] and is essentially the end stage of a progression of changes of the upper lid.

Papillary changes of the upper lid are unusual with rigid lens wear and present a slightly different appearance from those caused by soft lenses.[51,52] However, Schnider et al.[1] reported on a case in which a unilateral lens deposit problem caused increased hyperemia and papillary response in a patient wearing lenses on an extended-wear basis. A 2% incidence of lid inflammation was reported in another report on RGP extended-wear effects,[53] which was much lower than the 13% rate reported by the same center for soft lens extended-wear clinical studies.[54]

When lid changes do occur in patients using RGP extended-wear lenses, they are usually either a reinflammation of pre-existing papillary conjunctivitis or a secondary reaction to obvious deposits on the lens surface. The first sign is typically an increase in hyperemia of the upper tarsal plate, beginning in area 3 (the one-third of the lid closest to the lash margins, as described by Allansmith et al.[50]) and progressing toward the fold into areas 2 and 1. The papillary response usually follows the injection and, again, progresses from the lash margin to the fold. Figures 15-4 and 15-5 show a patient before beginning RGP extended wear and after 8 months

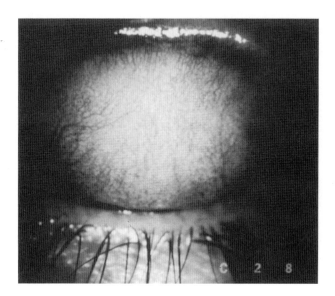

FIG. 15-4. *Prefitting appearance of upper tarsal conjunctival of a patient using extended-wear rigid gas-permeable lenses. (Photograph by Dr. C. Schnider; Courtesy of Cornea and Contact Lens Research Unit, Sydney, Australia.)*

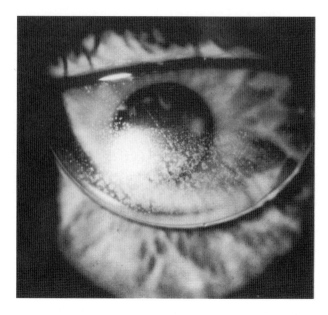

FIG. 15-6. *Lens with deposits worn by patient in Figures 15-4 and 15-5. (Photograph by Dr. K. Zabkiewicz; Courtesy of Cornea and Contact Lens Research Unit, Sydney, Australia.)*

of wearing a lens with obvious deposits (Fig. 15-6). This lens was inspected and was found to have a burned surface from overpolishing, resulting in a buildup of a mucoprotein deposit. Returning to a daily-wear schedule and replacing the lens with a well-manufactured lens resolved the deposit problem and the lid inflammation within 1 month, at which time the patient successfully returned to extended wear. Early changes such as these resolve

rapidly on replacement with a clean lens or with an enhanced cleaning routine designed to control the front surface deposits.

Woods and Efron studied the effect of quarterly replacement on a group of RGP extended-wear patients in comparison to a group with no scheduled replacements over a 12-month period.[55] They noted increases in mucous coating over time but found no difference in tarsal conjunctival response in the two groups of RGP extended-wear users during the study.

Further discussion of papillary conjunctivitis can be found in Chapter 7.

Ptosis Fonn and Holden[49] reported an apparent upper lid ptosis in many patients wearing RGP lenses. In an extended-wear study they conducted comparing rigid and soft lenses, five of 11 patients showed a narrowing of the aperture in the rigid lens–wearing eye at the end of 2 months. All cases resolved after cessation of lens wear, and the mechanism was believed to be edema or hypertrophy of the tissues of the upper lid in response to mechanical trauma from the rigid lens. Although it is a benign condition, it may present a cosmetic impediment to success with RGP lenses for some patients.

Fit-Related Complications

Even though RGP lenses can provide high levels of oxygen to the cornea during daily and extended wear, adherence to sound fitting principles is still necessary to ensure

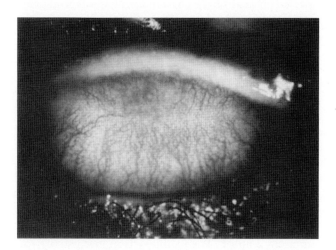

FIG. 15-5. *Appearance of lid of patient shown in Figure 15-4 after 8 months of wearing a lens (lens shown in Fig. 15-6). (Photograph by Dr. C. Schnider; Courtesy of Cornea and Contact Lens Research Unit, Sydney, Australia.)*

success. Difficulties related to the fitting characteristics of rigid lenses include ocular surface disorders such as staining, as well as inflammation and infection.

Staining

Because corneal staining represents a breakdown of the barrier function of the epithelium, it is obviously not a desirable state with extended wear. All potential extended-wear candidates should be thoroughly evaluated during a period of daily wear, and any staining classified as grade 2 or higher be considered a contraindication to extended wear. Similarly, when this level of staining is noted during the course of extended wear, an immediate change in the wearing schedule or lens design, or both, is indicated until the problem can be remedied.

As with daily wear, the primary staining problem with rigid lenses is that of peripheral corneal desiccation, or 3 and 9 o'clock staining. Toxic staining is rare because of the minimal use of solutions with an extended-wear regimen and, except in cases of lens adherence, the only other type of staining common to RGP extended wear is foreign-body tracking.

Peripheral Corneal Desiccation

The etiology and manifestation of peripheral corneal desiccation with RGP extended wear are similar to those with daily wear, except that the dry ocular environment during sleep can accelerate or exacerbate a mild condition. Extensive extended-wear studies from the Cornea and Contact Lens Research Unit[56] (CCLRU) in Australia found an incidence of significant peripheral corneal staining of 14.3% (Fig. 15-7). Schnider et al.[57] have demonstrated that individual patient characteristics are important in determining which patients are prone to significant staining, and these characteristics can be identified during the initial fitting and daily-wear follow-up period. This study showed that patients prone to staining exhibited higher baseline conjunctival hyperemia levels, had more tear film lipid and debris, faster lens drying times, higher blink interval to lens drying time ratios, and poorer lens centration and movement than did a matched group of non-stainers. These authors also found that the peripheral tear reservoir (or edge clearance) is the key lens design factor in minimizing staining in susceptible individuals.[58] As shown in Figures 15-8 and 15-9, significantly more severe staining was found when the edge clearance was either too shallow or too narrow. Figure 15-10 illustrates the difference between edge width and clearance.

Peripheral corneal desiccation that progresses after the onset of extended wear can sometimes be managed with lens design changes. The following steps are recommended in an attempt to reduce the levels of peripheral corneal desiccation in RGP extended-wear patients[59]:

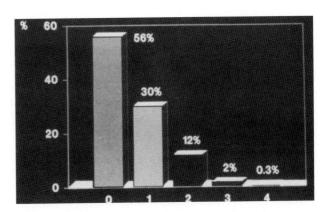

FIG. 15-7. *Distribution of peripheral corneal staining grades for patients in rigid gas-permeable extended-wear clinical studies at the Cornea and Contact Lens Research Unit in Sydney, Australia.*

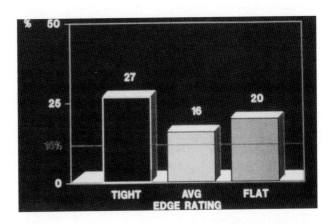

FIG. 15-8. *Percentage of rigid gas-permeable extended-wear patients displaying moderate-to-severe 3 and 9 o'clock staining for each edge clearance rating. (Cornea and Contact Lens Research Unit data, Sydney, Australia.)*

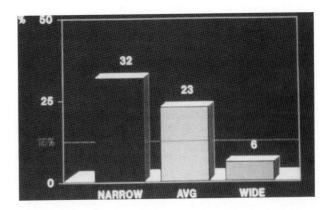

FIG. 15-9. *Percentage of rigid gas-permeable extended-wear patients displaying moderate-to-severe 3 and 9 o'clock staining for each edge width rating. (Cornea and Contact Lens Research Unit data, Sydney, Australia.)*

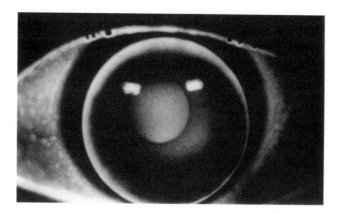

FIG. 15-10. *Examples of edge width and clearance. The right side of the lens displays insufficient edge width and depth, the inferior portion has a wide but shallow edge (dimmer appearance of fluorescein), and the left side has a wide edge with moderate or flat clearance. (Photograph by Dr. R. Terry; Courtesy of Cornea and Contact Lens Research Unit, Sydney, Australia.)*

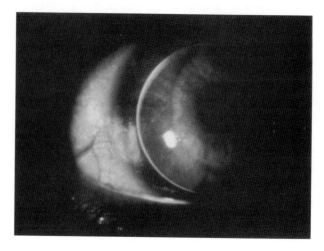

FIG. 15-11. *Corneal staining of nasal quadrant of left eye resulting from insufficient edge lift. (Photograph by Dr. C. Schnider.)*

- Blend the lens thoroughly. This ensures an adequate channel for passage of tears from center to edge behind the lens.
- Widen and, if necessary, flatten the peripheral curve system of the lens. This provides an adequate peripheral tear film reservoir to allow lens translation and corneal surface wetting over the flatter peripheral areas.
- Taper the anterior edge if edge thickness is excessive. This allows an uninterrupted flow of tears over the anterior surface of the lens.
- If edge lift is excessive, a new lens must be ordered.

If these changes are not sufficient to reduce the staining, extended wear should be terminated because of the risk of vascularization and ulceration. Lens adherence can cause a sudden and severe increase in the amount of peripheral staining observed, and it should be suspected when a sudden change is noted in an extended-wear patient.

Mechanical Staining

The most common form of mechanical staining is foreign-body tracking, which is largely an unavoidable consequence of RGP lens wear. Any deep or extensive foreign-body staining requires lens removal and a daily-wear schedule until the staining is resolved, after first ensuring that the foreign body itself has been removed. If the foreign body penetrated the epithelial layer, a prophylactic antibiotic may be indicated, depending on the extent of staining.

Other forms of mechanical staining include arcuate indentation lines, which can result from a decentered lens,

particularly if the transition zones are not well blended, and from lens adherence. Blending solves the transition zone problem, but if lens adherence is suspected, the lens design may have to be changed (see Adherence section).

Conjunctival Staining

Conjunctival staining with fluorescein is an indication of desiccation and is most often apparent in the quadrant opposite lens decentration or adjacent to an insufficient peripheral tear reservoir. It can be seen with or without corneal staining and, if allowed to persist, can result in rose bengal staining as the tissue becomes keratinized. Figures 15-11 and 15-12 show the nasal and temporal quadrants of a patient wearing an RGP lens with insufficient edge lift. The nasal side shows predominantly corneal staining, whereas the temporal side has mostly conjunctival staining. The use of a yellow barrier filter over the observation system (Wratten no. 12 [Kodak Corp., Rochester NY] or Tiffen no. 2 [Rochester, NY] photographic filters) is necessary to achieve the brightly fluorescent appearance shown in these photographs. Lissamine green has also been reported to be effective in the observation of conjunctival staining,[60] is much more comfortable than rose bengal,[61] and requires no special filters for viewing. It is available in liquid and strip forms. Lubrication with artificial tears, improved blinking habits, and punctal occlusion are also helpful in alleviating conjunctival staining caused by xerosis.

Arcuate bands of conjunctival staining can be a sign of xerosis as well, but often they also represent mechanical chafing of the conjunctiva in the case of a low-riding lens.

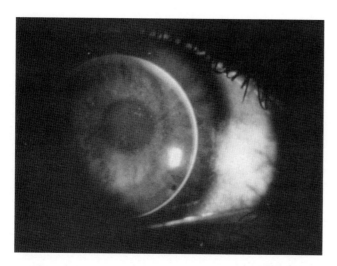

FIG. 15-12. *Conjunctival staining of temporal quadrant of left eye in same patient as in Figure 15-11. (Photograph by Dr. C. Schnider.)*

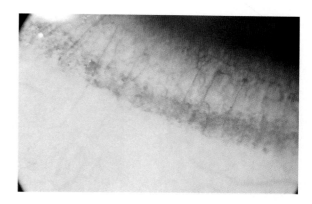

FIG. 15-13. *Rose bengal staining resulting from excessive lens movement and inferior positioning in a patient using rigid gas-permeable extended-wear lenses. (Photograph by Dr. M. Shiobara; Courtesy of Cornea and Contact Lens Research Unit, Sydney, Australia.)*

If the lens positions excessively high, the tear film breaks up at the bottom edge of the lens and results in inferior drying in a pattern parallel to the lens edge, forming a very regular arcuate band of staining on the inferior conjunctiva. If the lens rides low or drops quickly, the band is also quite regular but corresponds to the lowest position of the lens. In both cases, steps must be taken to improve lens centration and movement, or rose bengal staining can result (Fig. 15-13).

Adherence

Adherence of RGP lenses during sleep is by far the most significant complication of RGP extended wear. Swarbrick and Holden[62] estimate that although nearly 100% of patients exhibit lens adherence on awakening at some time, only approximately 22% have persistent problems with adherence. The figure of 32% adherence on eye opening with patched-eye studies reported by Kenyon et al.[63] is also in close agreement. If the adherence is allowed to persist for more than a few minutes, however, the consequences can be severe and include corneal distortion,[64] dellen formation, and ulceration.[1,65] In fact, lens adherence has been implicated in every case of peripheral corneal ulceration with RGP extended-wear lenses I have seen.

Lens adherence is characterized by an immobile lens on awakening, which may move spontaneously within a few blinks or may remain adherent until a lubricant is added or, in severe cases, until the lens is manipulated digitally. The latter circumstance is associated with the most severe signs and symptoms associated with lens adherence (Fig. 15-14). Symptoms of lens adherence are typically minimal owing

to the lack of movement but may include blurred vision, spectacle blur on lens removal, dryness or grittiness, and conjunctival injection that subsides during the day.[63] Signs include a nonmoving lens with trapped mucus and debris behind the lens, corneal indentation, central punctate staining, peripheral arcuate staining, and corneal distortion. Most of these signs disappear within 2 hours of the onset of lens movement, however, so patients should be examined as early as possible after awakening to detect them.

The most obvious indication of lens adherence is observation of the nonmoving lens, but this is rare in a conventional office setting. Other signs of a problem with lens adherence include a subtle arcuate pattern to the prelens tear film breakup, which often occurs over the site

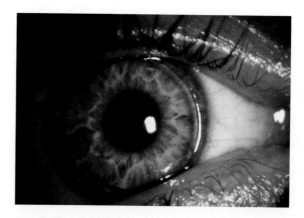

FIG. 15-14. *Imprint left after lens removal after an episode of severe adherence in a patient using rigid gas-permeable extended-wear lenses. (Photograph by Dr. C. Schnider; Courtesy of Cornea and Contact Lens Research Unit, Sydney, Australia.)*

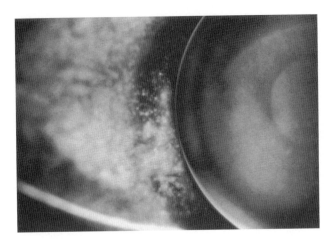

FIG. 15-15. *Peripheral staining in a patient with vascularized limbal keratitis. (Photograph by Dr. C. Schnider.)*

of the indentation long after the indentation itself is gone. Photokeratoscopy is most useful in identifying low-grade distortion because the small area of the keratometer is likely to miss the distorted section of the cornea. A well-demarcated area of apparent 3 and 9 o'clock staining can also indicate lens adherence. However, unlike traditional 3 and 9 o'clock staining, adherence staining tends to exactly follow the outline of the lens edge, creating a sharp arcuate interior border. Swarbrick and colleagues[62,66] also found that lenses adhere most often in a decentered position, usually nasally or superonasally, so the edge of the staining does not correspond to the resting position of the mobile lens. The best method of detecting lens adherence, however, is to have the patient actually observe the lens on eye opening. If the lens appears stuck, drops should be added and digital manipulation used if the lens still does not move. Repeated occurrences of lens adherence that require digital manipulation should signal the need to discontinue extended wear.

The phenomenon of lens adherence appears to be largely patient dependent,[66] but once the mechanism of adherence is understood, some design changes may help reduce the frequency and severity of occurrence.[67] Swarbrick's theory of mucous adhesion offers several avenues for managing problems with adherence. She proposes that a loss of aqueous tears causes an increase in viscosity of the post-lens tear film, creating an increase in the resistance to lens movement. The thin-film theory predicts that the adhesive forces are greater with larger lens diameters and smaller edge clearances, and this is borne out by her clinical data. In addition, work by Gilbard and associates[68] has demonstrated a decrease in tear osmolarity and tear volume on awakening, and they propose that these factors explain the problem of soft lens adherence during

sleep. Swarbrick's studies with fenestrated lenses have shown that negative pressure is not responsible for the adherence, nor is lens flexibility a major factor, so the advice of some authors to fit flatter and thicker lenses[4] is not supported. In fact, to achieve a sufficient quantity of aqueous component in the post-lens tear film to prevent the formation of a viscous film, the following steps are recommended to combat lens adherence:

- Reduce lens diameter (an overall diameter in the 8.8- to 9.2-mm range is suitable for most corneas, but some may require even smaller lens diameters).
- Fit with minimal apical clearance (0.25–0.50 D steeper than flat K) with moderate blending of the transition zones.
- Use lens designs with wide and moderately flat peripheral tear reservoirs.
- Avoid lens care solutions and medications that increase the mucous response or decrease aqueous volume. An increase in the frequency of daytime and overnight lens adherence has been observed in some patients using Boston Advance Conditioning Solution (Polymer Technology, Rochester, NY); this is usually resolved by changing to the original formulation of the Boston Conditioning Solution.

If these design changes do not reduce the problems with lens adherence, extended wear should be discontinued.

Inflammation

Inflammatory responses with rigid lenses are uncommon. They usually involve peripheral corneal desiccation, owing to the proximity of the limbal vasculature, and lens adherence, which causes stagnation of the tear film and is usually associated with limbal compression.

Vascularized Limbal Keratitis   Vascularized limbal keratitis (VLK) has been well described by Grohe and Lebow,[69] who suggest that it is most common in patients who began lens wear with PMMA lenses and switched to RGP extended-wear lenses. The majority of cases had common lens design parameters, including larger overall diameters (9.0–9.8 mm), low-edge lift designs, and poor lens movement. The condition results from chronic irritation in the 3 and 9 o'clock areas (Fig. 15-15) and causes hyperplasia of the peripheral corneal epithelium, followed by inflammation and infiltration of the affected area, peripheral corneal vascularization (Fig. 15-16), and eventual erosion. The patient can remain asymptomatic until the later stages of this condition.

Because peripheral corneal desiccation and lens adherence can contribute to these conditions, management is essentially the same. No patient who manifests significant peripheral corneal desiccation should be considered for extended wear, and patients observed to experience repeated lens adherence should be required to cease extended wear. However, even with these dicta, some patients still develop VLK sometime after commencement of an extended-wear schedule. Grohe and Lebow[69] reported that six of eight cases progressed to the later stages of the condition in less than 6 months. For this reason, it is imperative that these patients are followed on a routine basis, with not more than 3–4 months between visits.

The lens design changes to treat VLK are much the same as those for staining and adherence:

- Reduce wearing time to 6–8 hours daily.
- Increase edge lift (width and depth).
- Use lubricating drops or antioxidants, or both.
- Reduce lens diameter.
- Consider topical steroids and antibiotic therapy to manage cases with infiltrates and erosions.

Acute Red Eye   The only reported case of contact lens acute red eye (CLARE) with RGP extended-wear lenses was associated with lens adherence.[1] The mechanism of this condition, which consists of an infiltrative corneal response with severe conjunctival congestion, is thought to be the accumulation of debris beneath an immobile lens. It has been reported most often in association with soft lens extended wear, in which incidence rates are estimated at 15–20%.[70,71]

In the typical presentation of CLARE, the patient is awakened in the early hours of the morning with a hot, painful eye, accompanied by photophobia and excess lacrimation. Slit-lamp observation of the cornea usually reveals marginal corneal infiltrates and moderate-to-severe limbal and conjunctival congestion. The condition clears over a number of hours to days, depending on the severity of the case, although it can recur if the conditions that trigger the inflammatory response recur.

In the case of RGP extended wear, because lens adherence is the single most important factor associated with CLARE, procedures should be instituted to manage the adherence problem. Because CLARE is extremely rare with daily wear, cessation of extended wear usually solves the problem.

Infection

Infectious keratitis is one of the rarest complications of contact lens wear but one of the most widely publicized, particularly in the lay press. However, the incidence of infectious keratitis is quite small for rigid lens daily wear, being less than or equal to that quoted for soft lens daily wear.[4,5]

Ulcerative Keratitis

Although few statistical data exist for ulcerative keratitis rates with RGP extended wear, some peripheral

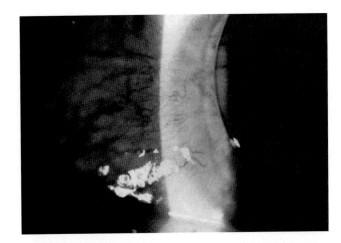

FIG. 15-16. *Vascularization of peripheral cornea of patient shown in Figure 15-15. (Photograph by Dr. C. Schnider.)*

corneal ulcers have been reported associated with this modality.[1,2,65,72] However, some debate exists about whether most of these reports represent infectious or inflammatory etiologies. Nevertheless, corneal ulceration, usually peripheral, does occur with RGP extended wear. All published reports to date, however, have been in association with high levels of peripheral corneal desiccation or lens adherence, or both. This implies that with proper patient selection and management, such complications can be avoided.

Figures 15-17 and 15-18 are typical representations of the peripheral corneal ulcers seen with RGP extended

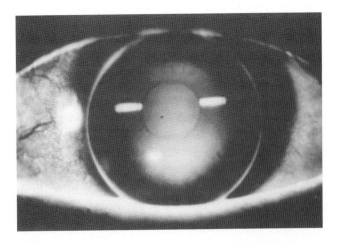

FIG. 15-17. *Peripheral corneal ulcer and lens fit with fluorescein. (Photograph by Dr. C. Schnider; Courtesy of Cornea and Contact Lens Research Unit, Sydney, Australia.)*

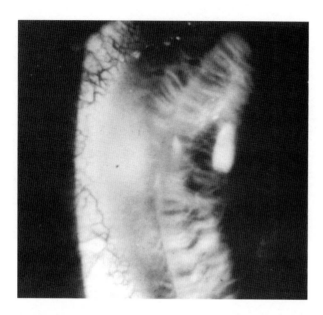

FIG. 15-18. *White-light photograph of patient shown in Figure 15-17, showing area of infiltration and limbal injection. (Photograph by Dr. C. Schnider; Courtesy of Cornea and Contact Lens Research Unit, Sydney, Australia.)*

wear. This patient experienced persistent high levels of 3 and 9 o'clock staining with his RGP lenses under daily- and extended-wear conditions. This ulcer, presumed sterile, resulted when he commenced wear of the low edge-lift design shown in Figure 15-17. The ulcer healed with a small scar after treatment with chloramphenicol by an ophthalmologist, and the patient returned to a daily-wear regimen with hydrogel lenses.

If peripheral corneal ulceration is observed in a rigid lens extended-wear patient, the practitioner should be highly suspicious of lens adherence, particularly if the patient has not shown a prior disposition to moderate-to-severe peripheral corneal staining. In addition, any epithelial loss with underlying stromal infiltration should be treated as potential infectious keratitis. Whenever possible, the area should be scraped and cultured and the lens case and solutions cultured to aid in establishing an optimal treatment plan. Initial treatment should include broad-spectrum antibiotics, such as a fluoroquinolone, and may include fortified topical antibiotics if the infectious organism can be identified.[73] Steroids are usually contraindicated as long as the epithelial layer is compromised.

When the cornea has healed completely, the decision to return the patient to extended wear depends on the presumed etiology of the ulceration. If staining or lens adherence is suspected or confirmed, the patient should not return to an extended-wear schedule unless the problems can be fully remedied.

MANAGEMENT OF RIGID GAS-PERMEABLE LENS EXTENDED-WEAR PATIENTS

Management of the extended-wear patient starts well before fitting begins, with careful consideration not only of which lens to fit but also of which patient to fit. Many of the problems discussed in this chapter can be avoided with adequate screening and patient education before extended wear begins.

Material Selection

Selection of a suitable lens material for a given patient involves understanding the inter-relationship of the many attributes of an RGP polymer. Because of the importance of oxygen in short-term and long-term success with extended wear, there should be little compromise in this area when materials are selected. Several studies have demonstrated the importance of oxygen in the success of extended wear. Armitage and Schoessler[74] and others[75] have presented evidence that extended-wear patients display lower mean overnight swelling responses than a matched group of non–lens wearers. This points to either adaptation or natural selection as an explanation. Although no good evidence exists for adaptation, Sweeney et al.[76] reported that voluntary dropouts and patients lost to follow-up from RGP and soft-lens extended-wear studies had a significantly higher rate of hypoxia-related findings, such as microcysts, than did successful patients.

With the earliest rigid lens materials for extended wear, compromises sometimes had to be accepted in other areas, such as flexibility and durability. Increasing oxygen transmission by increasing silicone content in silicone/acrylate (S/A) lenses results in a material with low flexural resistance and relatively high surface reactivity. The high silicone content creates manufacturing difficulties and a negative surface charge, which attracts, among other substances, positively charged lysozyme found in the precorneal tear film. The addition of fluorine to S/A materials to create fluorosilicone/acrylates (FS/A) yields a lower surface tension and, therefore, a lower tendency to bind the various proteins.[77] The clinical result of the addition of fluorine to RGP lenses is a lens that shows superior wetting characteristics and deposit resistance compared with S/A materials. However, flexibility can still be a problem with the higher-Dk FS/A materials, and the softer surfaces typical of FS/A can result in the lenses' greater susceptibility to damage during manufacturing and normal handling. The Menicon Z (Menicon USA, Clovis, CA) hyper-Dk material combines the traditional FS/A chemistry with styrene to achieve added stiffness while maintaining high permeability, thus enabling thin lens profiles without sacrificing flexure resistance.

Patient Selection

Patient Requirements

Perhaps the most important aspect of a successful RGP extended-wear experience is correct selection of potential patients.[78] Some studies[4] have shown a very strong link between patient factors (compliance with care regimen, personal hygiene, and habits such as smoking) and serious corneal complications resulting from extended wear. Some of the more important factors are vision correction, vocational needs, and patient expectations and experience.

Vision Correction

The increased rate of complications with this modality[79] should more than justify a careful assessment of the appropriateness of extended wear for vision need. The vision needs of those with high myopia, hyperopia, and aphakia are often particularly suited to extended wear in view of the optical distortions inherent in spectacle prescriptions. However, these prescriptions require thicker lenses and may be accompanied by poorer physiologic performance if anything but the hyper-Dk materials are used. These patients should be made aware of the limitations of their lenses as well as their relative advantages.

Vocational Needs

Contact lenses are often viewed in terms of social advantages, without consideration of their function in a work environment. Extended wear obviates the necessity for assessment of needs and potential hazards in the workplace. The use of air-conditioning systems, video display terminals, and forced-air heating or ventilation systems in the office environment can decrease the ambient humidity or alter the blink rate of contact lens wearers, leading to signs and symptoms of dryness and lens intolerance. Adequate instruction in maintaining normal blink habits, in-eye lubricants, or a humidifier, or all three, are often effective in reducing or eliminating these problems.

Patient Expectations and Experience

A clear understanding of the patient's perception of extended wear is necessary to provide an optimal extended-wear experience. Laziness, a prior history of noncompliance, or existing problems in daily wear are clear indications for patient education. All patients must be made aware of the responsibilities that accompany use of extended-wear lenses and should be encouraged to report any unusual occurrences promptly.

Practitioner Assessment

Selection of patients for extended wear requires careful inspection and consideration of all factors involved in the normal daily-wear assessment.

Ocular and General Health History   The same questions about ocular and general health required for daily-wear assessment apply to RGP extended wear and may be even more significant. Although allergies alone do not preclude extended wear, the use of certain antihistamines may cause unacceptable alterations in the tear film, leading to problems such as staining and binding. Diabetes[80] and any other conditions associated with poor wound healing, depressed sensitivity, or immunosuppression should rule out extended wear. Patients with ocular abnormalities, such as keratoconus, or a history of surgery, such as penetrating keratoplasty or radial keratotomy, are also not suited to extended wear.

Ocular Topography   Ocular topography includes assessment of the entire anterior bulbar surface, including the sclera and limbus, in addition to the cornea. Although unusual corneal topography can typically be managed with the appropriate lens design, limbal and scleral abnormalities, such as pingueculae and pterygia, may pose more difficult problems.[78] The presence of a pterygium usually contraindicates an extended-wear schedule owing to the proximity of vascular elements and the increased inflammatory potential. Patients with pingueculae may be successful in extended wear but should first be followed closely on daily wear before commencement of extended wear. Significant peripheral corneal or conjunctival staining, ocular redness, or engorgement of limbal vessels that cannot be managed with a change in diameter or edge configuration indicates a poor prognosis for extended wear.

Tear Layer Characteristics   Because of the less-frequent cleaning inherent in an extended-wear schedule, a good tear layer is essential. Observation of the oily layer with the use of specular reflection or a device for viewing the tear layer interference pattern[81,82] can be particularly useful. An excess of lipid or debris, evidenced by deeply colored fringes and dark globules in the marbled appearance of the oily layer of the tears, can be a sign of a heavy depositor of lipid. Although this is usually also evident with daily wear, the dry ocular environment during sleep and the decreased frequency of cleaning with extended wear can exacerbate the problem. Mucous- and aqueous-deficient tear films also generally represent poor extended-wear options.[83]

Lid Appearance   Careful documentation of lid redness and smoothness must be made before starting an extended-wear schedule. Lid problems can flare up quite suddenly with extended wear, particularly in patients with a prior

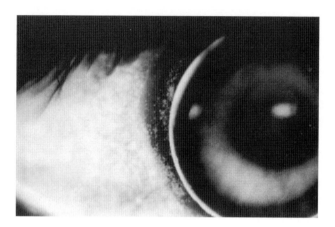

FIG. 15-19. *Fluorescein pattern of lens that is too large, showing a bull's eye–like appearance with apical alignment, midperipheral pooling, thin bearing, and an adequate peripheral edge clearance. This lens should be reduced in diameter to approximately the outer edge of the ring of pooling to provide unrestricted movement in all gazes. (Photograph by Dr. C. Schnider; Courtesy of Cornea and Contact Lens Research Unit, Sydney, Australia.)*

history of lid inflammation with rigid or soft lenses. Signs of chronic blepharitis, such as scaliness of the lids and lashes and hordeola, may indicate the potential for a secondary staphylococcal keratitis. These patients should be placed on an intensive lid hygiene regimen before beginning contact lens wear and should be monitored closely if placed on an extended-wear regimen.

Corneal Physiologic Status Assessment of corneal physiology must include limbus-to-limbus, epithelium-to-endothelium examination of the cornea with white light and sodium fluorescein. The presence of significant ghost vessels, neovascularization, or limbal engorgement with RGP daily wear may signal the potential for more rapid vascular involvement after future insult. Signs of possible high oxygen demand include epithelial microcysts, increased visibility of epithelial and stromal nerve fibers, decreased transparency of the stroma, and polymegethism of the endothelium. All these findings are frequently observed in cases of long-term chronic hypoxia and in corneal dystrophies. Hypoxic changes indicate the need for high oxygen-transmissibility levels in the lens material, and extended wear should be avoided completely with dystrophies.

Corneal staining should be minimal before commencement of extended wear. The presence of any significant corneal staining, whether large in extent or coalescent over a smaller area, should be viewed as a contraindication to extended wear. Heavy or localized conjunctival staining may indicate a marginal dry eye and, therefore, also a guarded prognosis for extended wear. The use of a yellow photographic filter over the objective or eyepieces of the slit lamp greatly enhances the appearance of fluorescein with cobalt blue light, and is invaluable in accurately assessing corneal and conjunctival staining and fluorescein patterns.

Fitting Guidelines

Aside from problems related primarily to hypoxia, most complications associated with RGP extended-wear lenses can be solved with intelligent fitting and lens design decisions. Although the requirements for successful RGP extended wear do not differ drastically from those of daily wear, the tolerances for error are smaller and the consequences can certainly be more serious.

Lens Design and Fitting

The selection of material is more limited in fitting for extended-wear applications, and choice of material can influence fitting characteristics and design decisions as well. Using the same material and design for diagnostic fitting and ordering should ensure that lens flexure, wetting, and concentration characteristics of the patient's lenses are similar to the diagnostic fit. With few exceptions, extended-wear materials are more flexible and more difficult to manufacture and may be manufactured with greater center-thickness values than are used for daily-wear lenses to compensate. This increases the mass of the lens and may necessitate a smaller or steeper lens design than is customary for daily wear to achieve good centration and movement characteristics.

To maximize success with extended wear, it is prudent to select the highest-Dk lens available with which a stable fit, vision, and good surface characteristics can be achieved. A minimum Dk of 60–90 may be suitable for the occasional overnight wearer, but Dk more than 100 is more likely to ensure success for the typical patient who wishes to wear lenses overnight for 6 consecutive days or more.

The choice of lens design is largely individual, but a few general rules apply. Lens diameter and base curve radius should be chosen to allow the lens to move freely across the cornea during the blink and normal gaze excursions. A lens that is too large displays a bull's eye–like appearance (Fig. 15-19), and its movement is obstructed during lateral gaze. Most contemporary designs feature lens diameters between 8.8 and 9.6 mm, although because of complications, it may be advisable to limit diameters for extended wear to 8.8–9.2 mm. Optic zone diameters can be determined by one of two methods: equal to the base curve radius[84] or a fixed amount smaller than the overall diameter.[85]

The final decision on lens fit and design should be based on the static and dynamic aspects of the fluorescein pattern evaluation. The lenses should be well centered, with minimal apical clearance and a wide and moderately flat peripheral tear reservoir, and should move smoothly and freely during the blink and gaze excursions. To minimize focal bearing areas and promote free exchange of tears and flushing of debris, lenses should be blended well at all peripheral curve junctions. It may be that aspheric designs help in this respect because of their ability to better approximate the corneal topography.[86,87] Many aspheric designs exist, however, and fitting characteristics can vary significantly between designs even when base curve and diameter are identical.[88] Because edge clearance on a given cornea is determined by the base curve and rate of flattening, it is not possible to manipulate edge clearance separately from base curve with aspheric designs. This means that the acceptability of an aspheric design for extended-wear usage must be determined on a case-by-case basis.

Follow-Up Care

Frequent and thorough follow-up care is essential to the success of all extended-wear patients. Timely intervention and sound patient management techniques can prevent many of the complications.

Wear Schedule

The FDA recommends no longer than 6 nights and 7 days of continuous wear. This requires removal of the lenses for 1 night per week, usually for a period of 8 hours or more. However, several studies provide evidence that first-generation RGP extended-wear materials may not be adequate for long-term extended wear. Specular microscopy of the epithelium of contact lens wearers showed alterations in cell size of contact lens wearers compared to healthy controls.[89] Scanning confocal microscopy of rabbit epithelium also shows alterations in the morphology of the superficial epithelial cells, even when the Dk/t is high enough to cause no residual corneal swelling after overnight wear.[90] These studies indicate that even when oxygen levels are sufficiently high to avoid hypoxic complications, there may still be alterations to the ocular surface that can limit the success of extended wear. For this reason, it is prudent to limit overnight lens wear to the minimal number of nights per week (never more than 6) to allow the ocular surface time to regenerate in the absence of a contact lens. It is anticipated, however, that one or more of the hyper-Dk RGP materials will be submitted to the FDA for 30-day

continuous-wear approval in the early 2000s. It remains to be seen whether such materials can indeed support long-term extended wear without compromise to the cornea.

Follow-Up Schedule

A necessary prerequisite for RGP extended wear should be successful RGP daily wear. Therefore, first-time wearers should be allowed to adapt to their lenses on a daily-wear basis before beginning an extended-wear schedule. Patients who wore PMMA or soft lens usually also benefit from daily-wear adaptation, although the process may be more rapid in these individuals. Daily-wear adaptation allows the patient time to gain confidence and proficiency in lens care and handling and an opportunity to identify any contraindication to extended wear. This usually takes from 1 to 4 weeks.

After the final daily-wear progress examination, the patient should be scheduled for an early morning visit after the first night of extended wear, at which time the practitioner should carefully check for signs or symptoms of excessive edema or lens adherence. If no indications of problems are present, the patient should be re-evaluated after 1 week, at 1–2 months, and then every 3–6 months of extended wear.[91] This ensures early detection of any adverse situation that might result in complications.

At every progress examination, the following procedures should be performed[59]:

- Case history. Ensure that the patient is performing the morning self-assessment for lens adherence and that no signs of excessive corneal swelling are present.
- Visual acuity with contact lenses.
- Over-refraction.
- Overkeratometry (to assess lens flexure on-eye).
- Biomicroscopy with lenses on (white light and fluorescein). Particular attention should be paid to lens surface wetting and deposits as well as lens movement. Note the presence of excessive mucus or back surface debris, which can be a sign of lens adherence. Any peripheral staining should be assessed for severity and location with respect to lens position to discern any possible relation to lens adherence.
- Biomicroscopy with lenses off (white light and fluorescein). Look carefully at the ocular surface characteristics, including the cornea, limbus, and bulbar and palpebral conjunctiva, to determine if signs of chronic irritation are present.
- Visual acuity through baseline (pre–extended-wear) refraction. This procedure divulges any corneal distortion or excessive corneal deformation caused by the

lenses. Visual acuities should usually be within one line of the prefitting best corrected acuity through the pre-fitting refraction.

- Postwear refraction. Rigid lenses typically cause slight corneal flattening and a sphericalization of toric corneas, resulting in less myopia with the rule cylinder, but best corrected visual acuity should not decrease after lens wear.

- Keratometry and photokeratoscopy (if available) to assess the curvature and regularity of the corneal surface. In the absence of a photokeratoscopy device, observe the keratometric mires when the patient fixates a peripheral location. If corneal distortion is present, this technique often reveals it.

- Lens inspection and verification. The lens should be free of deposits, scratches, and other surface defects and should be within manufacturing tolerances of the original parameters. Lenses not meeting these criteria should be replaced. Although modifications such as surface polishing are possible, the higher-Dk materials are more susceptible to damage, such as crazing,[92] so the risks more easily outweigh the benefits. Semiannual replacement of RGP extended-wear materials is recommended to maintain an optimal lens surface and to encourage patient and practitioner to upgrade into more advanced materials as they become available.[55]

Observations and Grading Scales

In addition to discussing the etiology of complications, it is helpful to establish a system for communicating the magnitude of the observation across time and observers. This is best accomplished by use of a standard grading system, supplemented by photographs or clinical descriptions whenever possible. In addition to descriptive information, the scale should also imply clinical relevance[93] and the need for intervention. Table 15-2 outlines the features of the grades used to describe the clinical findings discussed in this chapter as well as their implications for intervention and treatment.

Indications for Discontinuing Extended Wear

Using the grading scale outlined in the previous Observations and Grading Scales section, a grade of 2 is the fulcrum or decision point. On a daily-wear schedule, a finding of grade 2 severity merits closer supervision but not necessarily intervention. However, because of the magnifying effect of the extended-wear schedule, a grade 2 finding should warrant a change to daily wear until the problem can be managed. Any finding greater than grade 2 war-

rants immediate cessation of extended wear, and if the problem cannot be remedied with daily wear, cessation of all lens wear.

Extended wear should be considered a privilege rather than a right. The practitioner should remind the patient that the wearing schedule is part of the prescription and, as such, is under the control of the prescriber, not the user. Under no circumstances should a noncompliant patient or a patient with significant ocular complications be advised to continue with an extended-wear schedule.

REFERENCES

1. Schnider CM, Zabkiewicz K, Holden BA: Unusual complications associated with RGP extended wear. Int Contact Lens Clin 15:124, 1988

2. Levy B: Rigid gas-permeable lenses for extended wear—a 1-year clinical evaluation. Am J Optom Physiol Opt 62:889, 1985

3. Holden BA, Sweeney DF, Vannas A, et al: Effects of long term extended contact lens wear on the human cornea. Invest Ophthalmol Vis Sci 26:1489, 1985

4. Schein OD, Glynn RG, Poggio EC, et al: The relative risk of ulcerative keratitis among users of daily wear and extended wear soft contact lenses: a case control study. N Engl J Med 321:773, 1989

5. Poggio EC, Glynn RJ, Schein OD, et al: The incidence of ulcerative keratitis among users of daily wear and extended wear soft contact lenses. N Engl J Med 321:779, 1989

6. Holden BA, Mertz GW: Critical oxygen levels to avoid corneal edema for daily and extended wear contact lenses. Invest Ophthalmol Vis Sci 25:1161, 1986

7. Fatt I: The "super-permeable" rigid lens for extended wear. Contact Lens Spectrum 1:53, 1986

8. Holden BA, LaHood D, Sweeney D: Does Dk/L measurement accurately predict overnight edema response? Am J Optom Physiol Opt (suppl.)62:95P, 1985

9. Schoessler JP, Lowther GE: Slit lamp observations of corneal edema. Am J Optom Arch Am Acad Optom 49:666, 1971

10. Klyce SD: Stromal lactate accumulation can account for corneal oedema osmotically following epithelial hypoxia in the rabbit. J Physiol 321:49, 1981

11. Bonnano JA, Polse KA: Corneal acidosis during contact lens wear: effects of hypoxia and CO_2. Invest Ophthalmol Vis Sci 28:1514, 1987

12. Bonnano JA, Polse KA: Effect of rigid contact lens oxygen transmissibility on stromal pH in the living human eye. Ophthalmology 94:1305, 1987

13. Madigan MC, Holden BA, Kwok LS: Extended wear of contact lenses can compromise corneal epithelial adhesion. Curr Eye Res 6:1257, 1987

14. Wallace W: The SLACH syndrome. Int Eyecare 1:220, 1985

15. Mauger TF, Hill RM: Corneal epithelial healing under contact lenses. Quantitative analysis in the rabbit. Acta Ophthalmol 70:361, 1992

16. Ren DH, Petroll WM, Jester JV, et al: The relationship between contact lens oxygen permeability and binding of *Pseudomonas aeruginosa* to human corneal epithelial cells after overnight and extended wear. CLAO J 25:80, 1999

17. Ren DH, Petroll WM, Jester JV, et al: Short-term hypoxia downregulates epithelial cell desquamation in vivo, but does not increase *Pseudomonas aeruginosa* adherence to exfoliated human corneal cells. CLAO J 25:73, 1999

18. Zantos SG: Cystic formations in the corneal epithelium during extended wear of contact lenses. Int Contact Lens Clin 10:128, 1983

19. Henriquez AS, Kenyon KR, Hanninen L: Histopathology of corneal changes associated with an extended-wear contact lens: case report. Contact Lens J 18:209, 1990

20. Holden BA, Sweeney DF: The significance of the microcyst response: a review. Optom Vis Sci 68:703, 1991

21. Rivera RK, Polse KA: Corneal response to different oxygen levels during extended wear. CLAO J 17:96, 1991

22. Polse KA, Sarver MD, Kenyon E, et al: Gas permeable hard contact lens extended wear: ocular and visual responses to a 6 month period of wear. CLAO J 13:31, 1987

23. Sarver MD: Striate corneal lines among patients wearing hydrophilic contact lenses. Am J Optom Arch Am Acad Optom 48:762, 1971

24. Wechsler S: Striate corneal lines among patients wearing conventional contact lenses. Am J Optom Arch Am Acad Optom 49:177, 1972

25. Wechsler S: Striate corneal lines. Am J Optom Physiol Opt 51:852, 1974

26. Kerns RL: A study of striae observed in the cornea from contact lens wear. Am J Optom Physiol Opt 51:998, 1974

27. Polse KA, Sarver MD, Harris MG: Corneal edema and vertical striae accompanying the wearing of hydrogel lenses. Am J Optom Physiol Opt 52:185, 1975

28. Kame RT: Clinical management of hydrogel-induced edema. Am J Optom Physiol Opt 53:468, 1976

29. Efron N, Holden BA: A review of some common contact lens complications. Part I: The corneal epithelium and stroma. Optician 5057:21, 1986

30. LaHood D, Grant T, Holden BA: Characteristics of the overnight corneal edema contact lenses. Am J Optom Physiol Opt (suppl.)64:99P, 1987

31. Schoessler JP: The corneal endothelium following 20 years of PMMA contact lens wear. CLAO J 13:157, 1987

32. Schoessler JP: Corneal endothelial polymegethism associated with extended wear. Int Contact Lens Clin 10:148, 1983

33. Schoessler JP, Orsborn GN: A theory of corneal endothelial polymegethism and aging. Cur Eye Res 6:301, 1987

34. Laing RA, Sandstrom MM, Berrospi AR, Leibowitz HM: Changes in the corneal endothelium as a function of age. Exp Eye Res 22:587, 1976

35. Bergmanson JPG: Histopathological analysis of corneal endothelial polymegethism. Cornea 11:133, 1992

36. Zantos SG, Holden BA: Transient endothelial changes soon after wearing contact lenses. Am J Optom Physiol Opt 54:856, 1977

37. Williams L, Holden BA: The bleb response of the endothelium decreases with extended wear of contact lenses. Clin Exp Optom 69:90, 1986

38. Holden BA, Williams L, Zantos SG: The etiology of transient endothelial changes in the human cornea. Invest Ophthalmol Vis Sci 26:1354, 1985

39. Clements DL: Corneal acidosis, blebs and endothelial polymegethism. Contact Lens Forum 15:39, 1990

40. Carlson KH, Bourne WM, Brubaker RF: Effect of long term contact lens wear on corneal endothelial cell morphology and function. Invest Ophthalmol Vis Sci 29:185, 1988

41. Bron AJ, Brown NAP: Endothelium of the corneal graft. Trans Ophthalmol Soc UK 94:863, 1974

42. Bourne WM, Brubaker RF, O'Fallon WM: Use of air to decrease endothelial cell loss during intraocular lens implantation. Arch Ophthalmol 97:1473, 1979

43. Rao GN, Shaw EL, Arthur EJ, Aquavella JV: Endothelial cell morphology and corneal deturgescence. Ann Ophthalmol 11:885, 1979

44. Shaw EL, Rao GN, Arthur EJ, Aquavella JV: The functional reserve of corneal endothelium. Ophthalmology 85:640, 1978

45. Sweeney DF, Holden BA, Vannas A, et al: The clinical significance of corneal endothelial polymegethism. Invest Ophthalmol Vis Sci (suppl.)26:53, 1985

46. Connor CG, Zagrod ME: Contact lens induced corneal endothelial polymegethism: function, significance and possible mechanisms. Am J Optom Physiol Opt 63:539, 1986

47. Tanishima T, Nakakura S, Numaga J, et al: Corneal thickness changes and specular microscopic studies in gas permeable hard contact lens extended wear patients. J Jpn Contact Lens Soc 28:172, 1986

48. Fonn D, Holden BA: Extended wear of hard gas permeable contact lenses can induce ptosis. CLAO J 12:93, 1986

49. Fonn D, Holden BA: Rigid gas permeable vs. hydrogel contact lenses for extended wear. Am J Optom Physiol Opt 65:536, 1988

50. Allansmith M, Korb DR, Greiner JV, et al: Giant papillary conjunctivitis in contact lens wearers. Am J Ophthalmol 83:697, 1977

51. Korb DR, Allansmith MR, Greiner JB, et al: Prevalence of conjunctival changes in wearers of hard contact lenses. Am J Ophthalmol 90:336, 1980

52. Richmond PR: Giant papillary conjunctivitis: an overview. J Am Optom Assoc 50:343, 1979

53. Schnider CM, Holden BA, Terry R, et al: Effects of rigid gas permeable extended wear on the cornea. p. 287. In Cavanagh HD (ed): The Cornea: Transactions of the World Congress on the Cornea III. Raven, New York, 1988

54. Grant T, Kotow M, Holden BA: Hydrogel extended wear: current performance and future options. Contax May: 5,1987

55. Woods CA, Efron N: Regular replacement of extended wear rigid gas permeable contact lenses. CLAO J 22:172, 1996

56. Schnider CM, Terry RL, Holden BA: Clinical correlates of peripheral corneal desiccation. Invest Ophthalmol Vis Sci (suppl.)29:336, 1988

57. Schnider CM, Terry RL, Holden BA: Effect of patient and lens performance characteristics on peripheral corneal desiccation. J Am Optom Assoc 67:144, 1996

58. Schnider CM, Terry RL, Holden BA: Effect of lens design on peripheral corneal desiccation. J Amer Optom Assoc 68:163, 1997

59. Schnider CM, Bennett ES, Grohe RM: Rigid extended wear. p. 1. In Bennett ES, Weissman BA (eds): Clinical Contact Lens Practice. Lippincott, Philadelphia, 1991

60. Fowler WC, Kim J, Cox T, et al: Ocular staining characteristics of lissamine green and rose bengal in patients with keratoconjunctivitis sicca and primary Sjögren's syndrome. Invest Ophthalmol Vis Sci (suppl.)38:S151, 1997

61. Manning FJ, Wehrly SR, Foulks GN: Patient tolerance and ocular surface staining characteristics of lissamine green versus rose bengal. Ophthalmol 102:1953, 1995

62. Swarbrick HA, Holden BA: Rigid gas permeable lens binding: significance and contributing factors. Am J Optom Physiol Opt 64:815, 1987

63. Kenyon E, Polse KA, Mandell RB: Rigid contact lens adherence: incidence, severity and recovery. J Am Optom Assoc 59:168, 1988

64. Terry R, Schnider C, Holden BA: Complications associated with RGP extended wear: two case reports. Clin Exp Optom 72:19, 1989

65. Terry R, Holden BA, Schnider C: Peripheral corneal ulceration in rigid gas permeable extended wear: a case report. Int Contact Lens Clin 16:323, 1989

66. Swarbrick HA, Holden BA: Rigid gas permeable lens adherence: a patient dependent phenomenon. Optom Vis Sci 66:269, 1989

67. Swarbrick HA: A possible etiology for RGP lens binding (adherence). Int Contact Lens Clin 15:13, 1988

68. Gilbard JP, Cohen GR, Baum J: Decreased tear osmolarity and absence of the inferior marginal tear strip after sleep. Cornea 11:231, 1992

69. Grohe RM, Lebow KA: Vascularized limbal keratitis. Int Contact Lens Clin 16:197, 1989

70. Kotow M, Holden BA, Grant T: The value of regular replacement of low water content contact lenses for extended wear. J Am Optom Assoc 58:461, 1987

71. Holden BA, LaHood D, Grant T, et al: Gram-negative bacteria can induce contact lens acute red eye response (CLARE). CLAO J 22:47, 1996

72. Erlich M, Weissman BA, Mondino BJ: *Pseudomonas* corneal ulcer after use of extended wear rigid gas permeable contact lens. Cornea 8:225, 1989

73. Silbert JA: Complications of extended wear. Optom Clin 1:95, 1991

74. Armitage BS, Schoessler JP: Overnight corneal swelling response in adapted and unadapted extended wear patients. Am J Optom Physiol Opt 65:155, 1988

75. Ichikawa H, Kozai A, MacKeen DL, Cavanagh HD: Corneal swelling responses with extended wear in naive and adapted subjects with Menicon RGP contact lenses. CLAO J 15 :192, 1989

76. Sweeney DF, Holden BA, Grant T, Schnider C: Discontinuations from hydrogel and rigid gas permeable extended wear. Am J Optom Physiol Opt 64:83, 1987

77. Feldman G, Yamane SJ, Herskowitz R: Fluorinated materials and the Boston Equalens. Contact Lens Forum 12:57, 1987

78. Terry R, Schnider C, Holden B: Maximizing success with rigid gas permeable extended wear lenses. Int Contact Lens Clin 16:169, 1989

79. Chalupa E, Swarbrick HA, Holden BA, Sjostrand S: Severe corneal infections associated with contact lens wear. Ophthalmology 94:17, 1987

80. Azar DT, Spurr-Michaud SJ, Tisdale AS, et al: Altered epithelial basement membrane interactions in diabetic corneas. Arch Ophthalmol 109:537, 1992

81. Guillon JP, Guillon M: Tear film examination of the contact lens patient. Contax May:14, 1988

82. Opel H, Ris W: The tear film and its interference patterns. Contactologia 12E:181, 1990

83. Terry R, Schnider C, Holden BA: Rigid gas permeable lenses and patient management. CLAO J 15:305, 1989

84. Caroline PJ, Norman CW: A blueprint for RGP design. Contact Lens Spectrum 7:35, 1992

85. Bennett ES: Silicone/acrylate lens design. Int Contact Lens Clin 12:45, 1985

86. Seibel DB, Bennett ES, Henry VA, et al: Clinical evaluation of the Boston Equacurve. Contact Lens Forum 13:39, 1988

87. Barr JT. Aspheric update 1988: part 1. Contact Lens Spectrum 3:56, 1988

88. Caroline PJ, Garbus C, Garbus J, Norman CW: Comparison of aspheric RGP lens contours. Contact Lens Spectrum 7:43, 1992

89. Mathers WD, Sachdev MS, Pertoll M, Lemp MA: Morphologic effects of contact lens wear on the corneal surface. CLAO J 18:49, 1992

90. Ichijima H, Petroll WM, Jester JV, et al: Effects of increasing Dk with rigid contact lens extended wear on rabbit corneal epithelium using confocal microscopy. Cornea 11:282, 1992

91. Schnider CM: Rigid gas permeable extended wear. Contact Lens Spectrum 5:101, 1990

92. Schnider CM: An overview of RGP extended wear. Contax May:10, 1987

93. Lloyd M: Lies, statistics, and clinical significance. J Br Contact Lens Assoc 15:67, 1992

VI

Complications of Irregular Astigmatism

16

Contact Lens–Induced Distortion and Corneal Reshaping

EDWARD S. BENNETT AND VINITA ALLEE HENRY

GRAND ROUNDS CASE REPORT

Subjective:
A 39-year-old woman reports that her contact lenses are less comfortable than they used to be. She has worn Polycon II (Wesley-Jessen, Inc., Des Plaines, IL) rigid gas-permeable (RGP) lenses for the past 11 years, with a 15-year history of polymethylmethacrylate (PMMA) wear before this. Current lenses are 5 years old. She wears lenses all waking hours. She uses the Wet N' Soak Plus/Resolve care system from Allergan (Irvine, CA). The patient is interested in having a back-up spectacle prescription.

Objective:
- Visual acuity with contact lenses: right eye (OD) $20/25$ +1, left eye (OS) $20/25$
- Over-refraction: OD +0.25 –0.75 × 168 $20/20$, OS Pl –0.75 × 175 $20/20$
- Biomicroscopy: Both lenses position slightly inferiorly, with 3-mm lag with the blink. Fluorescein evaluation shows apical clearance in each eye (OU) with adequate edge lift. Numerous surface scratches are noted, in addition to a mucoproteinaceous film on the lenses.
- After lens removal, the following is noted OU:
  1. Grade 1+ central corneal clouding (CCC)
  2. Coalesced 3 and 9 o'clock staining
  3. Papillary hypertrophy
- Lens verification: base curve radius (BCR): OD 7.76 × 7.85 (warped), OS 7.87 × 7.97 (warped)
     Power: OD –5.50 D, OS –4.75 D
     Overall diameter (OAD)/optical zone diameter: 9.5/8.4 mm OU

Assessment:
Corneal warpage syndrome (CWS).

Plan:
1. Refit into a moderately higher–oxygen-permeability (Dk) RGP lens material (Dk 30–50); consider somewhat flatter BCR.
2. Patient should reduce current Polycon II wearing time to no more than 8–10 hours per day until new lenses are fabricated.

3. On receipt of new lenses, resume full-time wear.
4. Clean lens gently in palm of hand to reduce warpage.
5. Use a suitably strong cleaning regimen, such as abrasive cleaner supplemented by daily use of liquid enzyme.
6. Prescribe spectacles once the refraction has stabilized, typically 2–3 weeks after dispensing of new lenses.
7. Follow up at 1 month, 6 months, and then annually.

The application of any form of contact lens material or design can result in changes in corneal curvature and refractive error. These induced changes can either be deliberate (i.e., orthokeratology) or accidental.[1] With the exception of orthokeratology, in which RGP lenses are applied with the typical goal of reducing existing myopia, the goal of contact lens application is not to induce any change in the physiology and structure of the ocular tissue.[2]

The largest induced changes in corneal curvature and refractive error have resulted from PMMA lens wear. These changes are most likely the result of a combination of the mechanical pressure exerted by the contact lens and corneal edema induced by the absence of direct oxygen transmission through this lens material. Unpredictable changes in refractive error and corneal curvature can occur if PMMA lens wear is discontinued for more than 1 day. Conversely, prolonged wear of soft and RGP lenses has typically resulted in minimal to no change in refractive error and corneal curvature.

The hypoxic effects of prolonged wear of PMMA and even soft and first-generation RGP lens materials can ultimately result in a loss of tolerance for contact lens wear, or *corneal exhaustion syndrome*. Similarly, over time, the combined effects of mechanical pressure and edema can also result in corneal distortion. This is more likely to occur if, in fact, lens decentration is present. The combination of contact lens–induced corneal distortion and decreased postrefraction visual acuity has been termed corneal warpage syndrome (CWS).

The ability to refit patients into high–oxygen permeability lens materials often eliminates the aforementioned complications. However, careful monitoring of the patient's lens-to-cornea fitting relationship is important. This is also true with the monitoring of the patient's corneal topography. The use of computerized videokeratography (VKG) (see Chapter 24) can provide the practitioner with a much more comprehensive, reproducible, and accurate method of evaluating corneal curvature than that of keratometry. The presence of even subtle forms of corneal distortion can be diagnosed and monitored. The color map can be invaluable in differentiating subclinical ker-

atoconus from CWS, and multiple color maps can be used to show changes or differences in topography over time. This is especially beneficial with orthokeratology patients for evaluating the longitudinal effect of purposely inducing changes in corneal topography and comparing the differences between visits.

The purpose of this chapter is to describe the etiology and management of contact lens–induced changes, accidental and deliberate. How to minimize undesirable changes, notably corneal distortion, is emphasized.

CONTACT LENS–INDUCED CORNEAL CURVATURE AND REFRACTIVE CHANGES

Complications of Polymethylmethacrylate and Low-Dk Rigid Gas-Permeable Lenses

Numerous induced changes to refraction, corneal curvature, and ocular physiology have been reported from long-term wear of PMMA and first generation low-Dk RGP materials.

Hypoxia
PMMA contact lenses have an oxygen permeability (Dk) value of 0; thus, the tear pump is the primary source of oxygen to the cornea. Oxygen deprivation caused by PMMA wear results in symptoms such as prolonged blur with spectacles (greater than 30 minutes) on removal of contact lenses (i.e., spectacle blur), discomfort, haloes around lights, cloudy or hazy vision, and reduced wearing time. Despite published reports to the contrary,[3,4] even patients who appear to be symptom free reveal subtle to pronounced clinical signs resulting from long-term oxygen deprivation.[5,6] During open-eye lens wear, PMMA and thick hydrogel contact lenses induce corneal edema levels of approximately 6–8%.[7,8] Hypoxia-related complications, including CCC, edematous corneal formations, and endothelial polymegethism can be induced by PMMA lens wear. CCC has been reported in 98% of PMMA wearers.[9] It may result in the subjective complaint of specta-

cle blur on contact lens removal. The edema caused by PMMA lenses may lead to corneal curvature changes and corneal distortion and is often accompanied by an increase in myopia, astigmatism, or both.[10]

Corneal Exhaustion Syndrome

Characterized by loss of tolerance to contact lens wear, ocular discomfort, reduced vision, and photophobia, corneal exhaustion syndrome is often reported in long-term wearers of PMMA lenses but can also occur after long-term wear of first-generation RGP or soft lenses.[6,11–13] Posterior corneal changes include distortion of the endothelial mosaic and moderate-to-severe endothelial polymegethism. According to Sweeney,[12] long-term hypoxia and acidosis accompanying long-term PMMA and thick hydrogel lens wear may be responsible for this syndrome, which results in inadequate regulation of corneal hydration and subsequent intolerance to contact lens wear owing to endothelial dysfunction. Because patients tend to vary in their corneal edema response to contact lens wear,[14] it makes sense that the high responders are most prone to this condition.

Pence[13] identified this complication, which he termed *corneal fatigue syndrome*, in long-term wearers of first-generation RGP lens materials. He refit patients wearing PMMA lenses into low-Dk (i.e., typically 10–15) RGP lens materials after they presented with symptoms of corneal fatigue syndrome. Four to 6 years later, these patients reappeared with the identical symptoms. He successfully managed these patients by refitting them into medium- to high-Dk RGP lens materials. According to Holden and Mertz,[15] a contact lens material requires an oxygen transmission (Dk/t) value of 24 for edema-free daily wear. For the myopic patient, this can be approximated or exceeded by an RGP material with a minimum Dk of 30; for the hyperope, approximately twice the oxygen permeability or a minimum Dk of 60 is necessary.

Corneal Curvature and Refractive Changes

Much is owed to the extensive clinical research on this subject performed by Rengstorff. Several studies have found that during adaptation to PMMA lenses, the corneal curvature usually steepens initially,[16–26] then flattens toward the baseline value, and by 1 year, is slightly flatter than the baseline keratometry values.[24,25–27] In comparison, the corneal curvature of non–contact-lens wearers is stable.[28,29] Although a relationship does appear to be present between refractive and corneal curvature changes (i.e., flat-fitting relationships induce plus power; steep-fitting relationships induce minus power), the corneal curvature change is only approximately one-half of the refractive change.[30,31]

After one or more years of wearing PMMA contact lenses, keratometry and refractive changes become greater, demonstrating a more prominent diurnal variation. During the first 8 hours of lens wear, the corneal curvature becomes steeper and myopia increases, followed by a flattening of the cornea and a decrease in myopia from 8–16 hours of contact lens wear.[32–34] Conversely, measurements on non–lens wearers showed stable corneal curvature[28] values and refractive error findings.[35]

Corneal asphericity, or the rate of change of the corneal radius from center to periphery, has been found to be reduced by PMMA contact lens wear.[23,36–40] Carney[23,36] found that during adaptation, flat-, steep-, and alignment-fitting PMMA lenses all reduced the asphericity of the cornea. After adaptation, the steep-fitting lenses continued to reduce corneal asphericity; however, the flat-fitting lenses actually increased asphericity. When the edema reaction was compensated by introducing 100% oxygen to the cornea, flat and steep lenses reduced corneal asphericity; therefore, the corneal swelling caused by uneven oxygen distribution under the lens was eliminated.

Corneal rigidity was found to change with the length of time contact lenses were worn. Corneal rigidity was high for individuals who had worn contact lenses 3.5 years or less and low for individuals who had worn contact lenses for an average of 5.5 years.[41]

Rengstorff described a pattern of refractive and corneal curvature changes after PMMA wear was discontinued.[42–49] It was found that for individuals who had worn PMMA lenses for at least 1 year, progressive corneal flattening occurred followed by corneal steepening through 48 days after discontinuation of lens wear.[44] Most flattening occurred within the first week of discontinuation of lens wear, with greater flattening occurring in the horizontal meridian, resulting in an increase in with-the-rule astigmatism. This astigmatic change then tends to decrease over time and revert toward baseline.[49,50] Variation in corneal curvature is typically quite small after 21 days.

The refractive change typically accompanied the corneal curvature change. With discontinuation of PMMA lens wear, an average of 1.0–1.5 D reduction in myopia resulted in the first 3 days (Fig. 16-1).[47,51] This was followed by an increase in myopia approaching baseline until stability was reached at approximately 21 days. Bennett and Tomlinson[50] found that, in the absence of corneal distortion after discontinuation of lens wear, the refractive error stabilized, on the average, in approximately 2 weeks.

Refractive and corneal curvature changes after PMMA lens removal, however, can be quite variable, with several diopters of change reported in many cases.[44,47,52,53] In one case, a patient who had lost a PMMA lens increased 10 D in myopia, accompanied by keratometric mire dis-

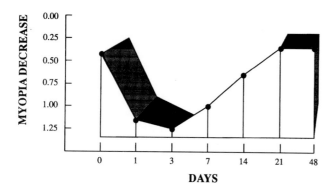

FIG. 16-1. *Reduction in myopia in the first 3 days after discontinuation of polymethylmethacrylate lens wear. (Modified from RH Rengstorff: Variations in myopia measurements: an aftereffect observed with habitual wearers of contact lenses. Am J Optom 44:149, 1967; and MM Hom: Thoughts on contact lens refractive changes. Contact Lens Forum 11:16, 1986.)*

tortion within 1 week after lens loss.[52] Similarly, the amount of astigmatic change can be large, unpredictable, and permanent.[53] It has been theorized that the amount of refractive change and corneal distortion experienced by these patients is caused by sudden exposure to high oxygen levels resulting from abrupt cessation of PMMA lens wear.[54] The amount of distortion is related to the number of years of PMMA lens wear, with the greatest change occurring the first few days after lens removal.

Corneal Distortion
Long-term wear of PMMA lenses has been commonly associated with corneal distortion.[16,39,48,52-67] It has been found that, on lens removal, 38% of patients have mild corneal distortion and 23% have moderate corneal distortion.[42] In a retrospective study, 50 patients acquired 1 D or more of irregular astigmatism as a result of long-term contact lens wear.[60] This change in astigmatism correlated with the duration of PMMA lens wear. Corneal distortion observed after long-term PMMA contact lens wear has been associated with corneal hypoxia and irregular astigmatism. The term *CWS* refers to distorted keratometry mires with or without irregular astigmatism and decreased visual acuity on postwear refraction. If the syndrome is not diagnosed early, these PMMA wearers can exhibit keratoconuslike changes and inconsistent, unpredictable refractive changes.

CWS is most likely caused by a sequence of events resulting from a combination of corneal hypoxia, resulting in typically central corneal steepening and irregular astigmatism and the mechanical effects of a rigid lens on the cornea. Eventually a change in the lens-to-cornea fitting

relationship can occur, resulting in decentration. Studies by Wilson et al.[61-64] have concluded that once decentration has occurred, significant changes in corneal topography typically result. The topographic abnormalities that result correlate with the decentered resting position of the contact lens on the cornea. For example, superiorly decentered lenses produced superior flattening with a steeper contour inferiorly simulating the topography of early keratoconus (*pseudokeratoconus*). In one study, 21 eyes of 12 predominantly PMMA lens–wearing patients (i.e., 13 PMMA, three RGP, five soft) with contact lens–induced warpage were followed with topography.[61] The corneal topography of these patients was characterized by central irregular astigmatism, loss of radial symmetry, and frequent reversal of the normal topographic pattern of progressive corneal flattening from center to periphery. Sixteen of the 21 eyes returned to a normal topography after discontinuation of contact lens wear, although it took as long as 5 months with rigid-lens wearers. Detection of corneal warpage that persisted for months was attributable to the increased sensitivity of computer-assisted topographic analysis relative to keratometry and other previous techniques.

Corneal distortion is a particularly significant complication owing to its gradual onset, which may mask the true nature of the problem for some time. Although most cases are reversible, recovery times have significant individual variation. In some cases, the cornea may need as long as 2–8 months to return to regularity; in other cases, the corneal distortion can be permanent.[48,53,61,64-67]

Management

Evaluation and Patient Education
A comprehensive evaluation of the eye is necessary, including a comprehensive case history.[68-71] Important issues to cover during the case history include the following:

- Length of PMMA lens wear
- Number of hours lenses are worn daily
- Symptoms the patient may be experiencing
- History of corneal abrasion

Tests with lenses on the eye should include visual acuity, over-refraction, and biomicroscopy (evaluating surface quality and fluorescein pattern). Biomicroscopy, keratometry, and post–lens wear refraction should be performed after lens removal. The current lens parameters should also be verified. This is not absolutely necessary, but it can be extremely beneficial when lens design changes are deemed indicated. When performing the examination, symptoms and signs of long-term PMMA-related changes, such as CCC, edematous corneal formations, corneal abrasion, irregular astigmatism, keratometric mire distortion, retinoscopic scissors reflex, and reduced vision with best subjective refraction, should be noted. All examination findings should be documented before refitting into another lens material.

If the PMMA (or low-Dk RGP) lens wearer is having symptoms resulting from hypoxia and long-term wear, he or she is easier to convince that a change is necessary. Those who have not yet noticed symptoms require a more comprehensive educational process about why refitting into another contact lens material is important. This can be initiated by explaining the oxygen needs of the cornea and emphasizing that PMMA lenses provide little to no oxygen, unlike RGP lenses, which provide oxygen directly through the lens material. This provides the wearer with long-term physiologic benefits of good health and long-term wear. Pamphlets, posters, photograph albums, and videotapes that emphasize the benefits of RGP wear and the complications associated with corneal edema reinforce verbal education. The Contact Lens Manufacturers Association videotape entitled "RGP Problem-Solving: Part II" addresses refitting and demonstrates hypoxia-induced complications. Most likely, the patient has experienced spectacle blur, which can be used as evidence to confirm the presence of edema. After refitting, he or she experiences an added benefit in being able to wear spectacles with acceptable vision after contact lens removal. A philosophy of "if it's not broken, don't fix it" has often been used by patients and practitioners to justify maintaining a patient in PMMA lenses.[72]

The patient needs to know that some disadvantages may be associated with rehabilitating the cornea with RGP contact lenses. Although it is more oxygen permeable than PMMA, the RGP lens is a softer, less-durable material. A typical life span for an RGP contact lens is 1–4 years, as opposed to 5–10 years and longer for a PMMA lens. The RGP lens is more easily scratched and warped, but proper handling techniques can minimize the incidence of these problems. After refitting, some patients may notice more dryness with the RGP lens; however, the newer RGP fluoro-silicone/acrylate lens materials have improved wettability compared to their predecessors. Finally, as the cornea becomes healthier, a few patients may become more aware of the RGP lenses than they were of their previous PMMA lenses. This should be seen as a sign of a healthier cornea, no longer desensitized from corneal hypoxia. Whatever disadvantages there might be, they are far outweighed by the benefits of RGP lenses over PMMA lenses for providing long-term comfort and eye health.

Refitting Procedure

Three primary techniques, or some combination of these three, can be used for refitting a PMMA lens wearer to another material: "cold turkey" lens discontinuation, de-adaptation, and immediate refitting.

A method commonly used in the past was to cease all contact lens wear ("cold turkey") in an effort to allow the cornea to rehabilitate. Sudden discontinuation of PMMA or low-Dk RGP lens wear has been found to result in large fluctuations in keratometry and refractive readings.[44,47] Some patients may return to normal values, but others may develop irreversible decrements in corneal curvature and visual acuity.[54,73] According to Rengstorff,[69] practitioners who routinely advise immediate discontinuation of lens wear may be responsible for inducing permanent and undesirable corneal and refractive changes. In addition, the patient is inconvenienced during the period of no contact lens wear, and the refractive changes often result in variable vision through a spectacle correction. In addition, these patients must readapt to rigid lens wear after being refit.

A second method is to de-adapt the patient from lens wear until corneal curvature and refractive stabilization has occurred and the patient can be refit.[74,75] Typically, lens wear is decreased 1–2 hours per day. The idea behind this method is to provide a more gradual exposure to new oxygen levels. The cornea is able to rehabilitate, and refraction and corneal curvature changes are monitored until they stabilize.[76] Gradually decreasing the wearing time has been found to reduce the incidence of visual acuity loss and corneal distortion during rehabilitation.[77-79] The disadvantage of this method is that the patient must decrease contact lens wear. Wearing spectacles may not be desirable to the patient or the spectacle prescription may not provide acceptable visual acuity. Like the "cold-turkey" method, de-adaptation may also result in a cornea that must adapt once again to new RGP lenses when refit. Although refitting PMMA patients to hydrogel lenses is rarely the desired method, if the patient is going to change to hydrogel lenses, this method of de-adaptation is recommended. Once the cornea has stabilized, the patient may be refit with hydrogel lenses.

Refitting the patient immediately into RGP lens wear is the most desirable method of rehabilitating the cornea of a previous PMMA or very low-Dk RGP lens wearer. This method results in little to no loss in lens wearing time. The stabilizing force of the RGP lens acts on the cornea while the cornea is exposed to a healthier, more oxygen-rich environment. The cornea is rehabilitating while oxygen is transmitted through the higher-Dk RGP lens material. Bennett and Tomlinson[50] found that immediate refitting of a PMMA wearer into RGP lenses did not inhibit

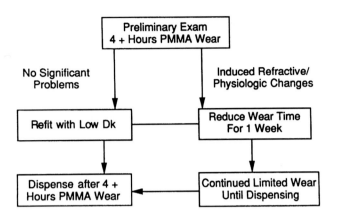

FIG. 16-2. *Flow chart for refitting polymethylmethacrylate (PMMA) and very-low-oxygen permeability (Dk) rigid gas-permeable lens wearers into higher-Dk rigid gas-permeable lenses. (Reprinted with permission from ES Bennett: Treatment options for PMMA-induced problems. p. 275. In ES Bennett, RM Grohe [eds]: Rigid Gas-Permeable Contact Lenses. Professional Press, New York, 1986.)*

corneal rehabilitation and that vision was better and more stable than in a group of wearers who had completely ceased contact lens wear. Astigmatic changes were significant in the spectacle-wearing group but not in the immediate-refit group. Novo et al.[58] found that immediate refitting of long-term PMMA lens wearers into RGP materials of similar fit allowed a slightly more regular and symmetric corneal shape, resulting in an improvement in spectacle visual acuity. The general corneal topographic patterns of contact lens–induced warpage did not change, however. Another study showed that when PMMA wearers were immediately refit into Boston II lenses (Polymer Technology, Rochester, NY), no significant deviation occurred in the horizontal or vertical meridians with keratometry, which was similar to a group of new RGP wearers.[80]

When immediately refitting the myopic patient, a low-to medium-Dk (i.e., 30–50) fluoro-silicone/acrylate RGP lens material should provide sufficient oxygen while exhibiting durability, good surface wettability properties, and stability to the cornea without excessive changes in oxygen levels. As the patient becomes more accustomed to handling RGP lenses and the cornea has stabilized, the practitioner may want to fit the patient into a higher-Dk RGP lens. In addition to the aforementioned possible compromises if a PMMA or first-generation RGP lens wearer is refit into a high-Dk material, a significant problem is *warpage.* Former PMMA wearers have been found to be much more prone to warpage of their RGP lenses than are first-time contact lens wearers.[81] The stability and scratch resistance of PMMA lenses can induce some poor

care habits, which can be detrimental to long-term successful RGP wear. This would be especially true if these patients are fit into high-Dk polymers because of their greater tendency for warpage.[82] To minimize problems associated with the softer RGP lens materials, the patient should clean the lens in the palm of the hand with the little finger immediately on removal at night to remove fresh lens deposits. In addition, the lenses must be stored in fresh disinfecting solution. Patients should never drag the lens across a hard surface; instead, the fingertip should be wetted with solution and the lens lifted straight up. At each follow-up visit, former PMMA/low-Dk RGP wearers refit into a higher-Dk polymer should have care instructions reinforced to ensure compliance.

It is advantageous to know the parameters of the PMMA lenses the patient has been wearing; however, it may or may not be desirable to duplicate these parameters for the new RGP lens, especially if the current fitting relationship is undesirable. RGP lens materials often benefit from a different design than traditional PMMA designs, including a larger overall diameter, a flatter BCR, a lower edge clearance, and in many cases, a greater center thickness owing to the increased flexibility of the lens material.[83]

In cases of the cornea exhibiting corneal warpage as a result of PMMA wear, a combination of de-adapting and immediate refitting may be used.[84] Typically, the wearing time is gradually reduced to 8–10 hours a day for a week and then the cornea is re-evaluated. When the cornea appears improved and more stable, the patient is refit with RGP lenses. The patient continues the desired wearing time (i.e., 8–10 hours) until RGP lenses are dispensed (Fig. 16-2).

Occasionally, the patient who is refit immediately into RGP lenses requires some lens changes as the cornea rehabilitates, especially in cases of CWS. A corneal rehabilitation fee should be charged in such cases. In addition, ordering the lenses on a warranty basis from the laboratory aids in providing appropriate lens changes to the patient as needed. However, warranties do expire after a specified time, so the patient should be educated about the potential costs involved if reordering lenses is necessary. Another alternative is to provide the patient with a low-Dk RGP "loaner" lens to wear while the cornea stabilizes, thereby eliminating any lens reordering.

Rigid Gas-Permeable Lens–Induced Complications

Daily Wear

The use of daily-wear RGP lenses has typically resulted in little to no change in refractive error or corneal curvature.[80,85–92] As with PMMA lenses, when corneal curvature does change, it is typically equal to approximately one-half of the refractive change.[80,89,90] In addition, a sphericalization effect can result, just as with PMMA. This effect appears to be greater with aspheric versus spheric RGP lens designs. In a study in which a biaspheric lens was compared to a spheric design, the aspheric design resulted in a greater reduction in keratometric astigmatism.[93] It was concluded that the aspheric design might have more closely aligned with the corneal surface, creating a greater mechanical molding effect.

The molding effect of an RGP lens against the eye can induce corneal curvature and refractive changes, even in lieu of corneal hypoxia.[94] These changes can result from a decentered lens position resulting in loss of an alignment fitting relationship.[61,62,95,96] Corneal flattening results in a region of lens bearing which is accompanied by adjacent corneal steepening. Eventually, these regions of corneal bearing can result in corneal warpage.

Extended Wear
Although some studies found little change in refractive error or corneal curvature in RGP extended wear,[97–99] most studies have found a trend toward corneal flattening during the first few months of lens wear, followed by steepening toward the baseline.[81,100–102] The vertical meridian typically flattens more than the horizontal, resulting in as much as 1 D of change in the first few months of wear.[102] A sphericalization effect then occurs with mild-to-moderate, with-the-rule astigmatic patients. This effect appears to be slightly greater in extended wear than in daily wear,[90,103] and the changes appear to be the result of corneal molding. The combination of lid forces during sleep with uneven pressure distribution of the lens against the eye can induce changes in corneal shape.[81,104,105] When corneal topography and refractive error were evaluated on subjects who were fit 1 D *flatter than K, on-K,* and *steeper than K* in rigid extended wear, the trend was toward keratometric flattening in all groups.[105] Cases of inferior steepening were induced by the flat-fitting lenses, which resulted in the most irregular changes.

Lens-to-cornea adherence can occur during extended wear. Because the lens typically adheres during sleep, it can remain immobile on awakening in as many as 50% of RGP extended-wear users.[98,100,106] Numerous theories have been proposed for the etiology of lens adherence. One theory is that a large tear volume between the back surface of the lens (i.e., an apical clearance fitting relationship) and the front of the eye produces adherence via the negative centration force exerted by the high pressure.[107] However, Swarbrick[106] has found adherence to occur primarily via changes in the tear film. Specifically, thinning of the post-lens tear film during sleep leaves a very thin, highly

viscous layer of mucus-rich tears between the lens and the cornea. The lens may remain adherent until the mucus film is diluted and thinned by the gradual penetration of aqueous tears after awakening. Adherence has been known to occur more often in large-diameter and low–edge clearance lens designs,[106,108] although in many cases it is independent of the lens design of the material.[109] Adherence has been associated with acute red-eye reactions[110] and corneal ulceration.[99] (See Chapter 15 for more detailed information on extended wear of RGP lenses.)

Management
The most important management plan is regular monitoring of the RGP lens-wearing patients' corneal topography, refractive error, and ocular health. To rule out hypoxia as a possible cause of corneal curvature and refractive error changes, the RGP lens material should meet the *Holden-Mertz criteria* for an edema-free state of the cornea (i.e., Dk/t of 24 for daily wear and 34 for extended wear, with no residual corneal swelling).[15] To approximate or meet these criteria, a lens material with a minimum Dk/t of 30 should be selected for myopic daily wear. A material with a minimum Dk/t of 60 should be selected for hyperopic daily wear and myopic flexible wear and one with a minimum Dk/t of 100 used for hyperopic extended wear using the oxygen transmission guidelines (incorporating thickness) provided in Table 16-1.[111–114]

In addition to hypoxia, the lens-to-cornea fitting relationship should be monitored to rule out the corneal shape changes resulting from a decentered lens. Good oxygen transmission is important but only when supplemented by an acceptable lens-to-cornea fitting relationship. A lens design factor for optimizing comfort is achieved with a well-centered or slightly superior positioned lens-to-cornea fitting relationship.[115,116] Lenticularizing the edge (or other similar manufacturing procedure) to thin the high–minus power lens edge or increase the edge thickness in low-minus and all plus lenses is very important.[117,118] Typically, a *plus-edge lenticular* is recommended for powers exceeding –5.00 D. Similarly, as the center of gravity of all plus-power lenses is more anterior, it is important to have sufficient edge thickness for proper interaction with the upper lid. Therefore, a *minus lenticular* is beneficial for minus lens powers less than –1.50 D and all plus-power lenses. Second, a thin lens design is very important. As the center thickness increases, the potential for inferior decentration (and resulting symptoms and clinical signs of dryness) increases.[119–121] The introduction of lens materials in ultrathin designs (i.e., 0.10–0.13 mm for –3.00 D power) has assisted in achieving an optimum lens-to-cornea fitting relationship. Management of rigid lens decentration is summarized in Table 16-2.

TABLE 16-1. *Rigid Gas-Permeable Lens Material Selection*

Dk	Recommendation
Low-to-medium (12–25)	Daily wear only
High (26–50)	Flexible wear (i.e., 1–3 nights)
Super (51–80)	Extended wear in myopic patients
	Flexible wear in hyperopic patients
Hyper (>80)	Extended wear

Dk = oxygen permeability.

If a patient has been experiencing rigid lens adherence, consideration should be given to increasing center thickness, increasing edge clearance (i.e., widening the peripheral curve width or flattening the peripheral curve radius, or both), or changing the BCR, depending on the fluorescein pattern. Maintaining good surface wettability properties via an aggressive cleaning program is recommended, including regular enzyme use (even liquid enzyme used nightly if necessary) and careful cleaning in the palm of the hand on removal. If this regimen is not successful, the cause could be the patient. Therefore, the patient should decrease to daily wear (if an extended-wear patient) and possibly to a hydrogel lens if he or she is currently wearing lenses on a daily-wear basis.

Refitting an RGP wearer who is experiencing problems is occasionally necessary. Calossi et al.[95] showed that corneal warpage induced by a poor lens-to-cornea fitting relationship with RGP lenses was eliminated after refitting into a high–water content soft lens. When this is the case, it is important to gradually de-adapt the patient from RGP lens wear until corneal curvature and refraction have stabilized.[122] Because these patients have often been satisfied with their vision through RGP lenses, it is important to provide a correction as close to their refractive error as possible.

Hydrogel Lens–Induced Complications

Daily Wear

As a result of the flexible nature of a soft lens, less likelihood exists of significant refractive error and corneal curvature change when less opportunity exists for large localized areas of molding to develop.[1] Similarly, although epithelial edema may be present, the corneal curvature does not tend to change significantly because the edema is typically uniform across the cornea.[24,123–125] Compared to PMMA patients, therefore, soft lens wearers rarely experience spectacle blur.

Several early studies using relatively thick hydrogel lenses resulted in little change in corneal curvature.[24,126–128] When changes did occur with these lenses, typically they consisted of slight corneal flattening accompanied by a small (<0.50 D) decrease in myopia during the adaptation period. This would often be accompanied by a return to baseline or perhaps even a slight residual steepening and myopia increase.[24,39,129–131]

A study in which myopic patients were fit with a thin (0.06-mm) hydrogel lens for a 3-month period also found very little central steepening of the cornea. However, significant midperipheral steepening (0.5–0.62 D) was found 4 mm away from the center.[132] It has been theorized, however, that this change has little effect on visual performance because the slight steepening along all the meridians in the midperiphery of the cornea is accompanied by an increase in the spheric aberration of the eye. This effect was based on the soft lens exhibiting flexure to maintain alignment with the corneal contour.[133] In addition, because all the subjects were myopic, the region of greatest steepening accompanied the region of greatest lens thickness, the edge of the front optical zone.

Corneal distortion has also been found with hydrogel lenses. Wilson et al.[61] found that it took an average of 5.2 weeks for the topography of five soft lens–wearing patients with corneal distortion to return to normal. In addition, significant corneal wrinkling accompanied by distortion has been reported with ultrathin lenses with excessively thick peripheries, which cause a ripple effect in the center of the lens.[127,134] This rippling is transferred to the cornea, perhaps as a result of dehydration and mechanical pressure.[125] It can significantly reduce vision but is

TABLE 16-2. *Management of Rigid Gas-Permeable Lens Decentration*

Symptoms	Possible Causes	Management

Vision varies with blink
Lens awareness
	Decentered apex
	Unusual corneal topography
	Tight or loose lid tension
	Thick lens design
		For inferior decentration:
		  Minus lenticular.
		  Lid attachment design.
		  Flatten base curve.
		  Reduce center thickness.
		For superior decentration:
		  Plus lenticular.
		  Increase center thickness.
		  Steepen base curve.
		For lateral decentration:
		  Increase overall diameter or steepen base curve.
		  Use aspheric design.

fully correctable after discontinuation of lens wear. This wrinkling is visible with retinoscopy, keratometry, and with fluorescein application.[135]

Annular tinted contact lenses have been reported to cause irregular astigmatism and reduce visual acuity.[136–140] Bucci et al.[140] reported on the VKG findings of five patients who were wearing annular tinted contact lenses and presented with bilateral blurred vision and a loss of best corrected visual acuity. The study concluded with 10 characteristic symptoms and clinical signs of this *annular tinted contact lens syndrome* (Table 16-3). It was found that a distinct ring-shaped pattern of irregular astigmatism was present, characterized by concentric areas of relative steepening, flattening, and steepening with a diameter of approximately 4 mm. It was theorized that forces acting at the junctional zone between the clear pupillary area and the tinted region are inducing structural abnormalities of the corneal surface. Refitting into another nonannular tinted lens design typically eliminated the topographic irregularity.

Extended Wear
Although Rengstorff and Nilsson[141] found little change in refraction and corneal curvature after discontinuation of hydrogel extended wear, several reports of a slow increase in myopia, or *myopic creep*, have been reported.[39,142,143] It appears to result from long-term, low-level, chronic epithelial edema with subtle changes in corneal contour, and it can be permanent if not diagnosed early and properly managed.

Hydrogel lens adherence to the cornea can also occur, although the magnitude of changes in refraction and corneal curvature are not as great as with RGP lenses.[1] Adherence is often the result of lens dehydration, which can result in a steeper fitting relationship and edema via reduced oxygen transmission.[144,145]

Management
Management of hydrogel-induced complications depends on the cause of the problem. If corneal distortion is present, refitting into RGP lenses is an option to be considered. Iacona[146,147] refit 50 patients manifesting some degree of corneal distortion into new RGP lenses. In this group, 25 had been wearing soft lenses and 25 had worn RGP lenses. After 1 week of RGP lens wear, corneal topographic mires, which were distorted with hydrogel lens wear, had cleared up completely. In addition, RGP lenses have been found to provide the most optimal visual acuity and least residual aberrations.[148] If the patient has hydrogel-induced complications, such as corneal distortion and reduced vision, there should not be any hesitancy in recommending RGP lenses. In one retrospective

TABLE 16-3. *Characteristic Clinical Signs and Symptoms of Annular Tinted Contact Lens Syndrome*

Concentric areas of steepening and flattening correspond to the diameter of the clear pupil via topographic analysis.
Visual acuity is typically reduced to 20/25- to 20/40 level.
A circular shadow is observed with retinoscopy.
Symptoms do not begin until after months to years of lens wear.
Rapid recovery of best corrected vision occurs with almost any mode of correction other than annular tinted lenses.
No discomfort or excessive lens awareness is present.
A higher incidence is present with more heavily pigmented annular lenses.
In more severe cases, slit-lamp evaluation may reveal a circular depression at the surface of the cornea with fluorescein pooling.
A rapid onset of symptoms occurs if the same pair of annular lenses are retained and used at a later date.
It is difficult to photograph this entity with the biomicroscope.

Source: Modified from FA Bucci, RE Evans, KJ Moody, et al: The annular tinted contact lens syndrome: corneal topographic analysis of ring-shaped irregular astigmatism caused by annular tinted contact lenses. CLAO J 23:161, 1997.

study consisting of 200 consecutive patients refit into another material, 46% were refit from rigid into hydrogel lenses.[149] These patients should be provided with a realistic explanation of the adaptation process to RGP lenses, using terms such as *lid sensation* and *lens awareness* rather than *discomfort*.[150] The use of a topical anesthetic has been recommended at the fitting visit to help ease the patient into adaptation.[151]

When a patient has low-level hypoxia resulting in myopic creep but is otherwise satisfied with soft lens wear, changing to an ultrathin or higher–water content lens design to increase oxygen transmission should be considered. In addition, the patient's wearing time may need to be reduced to minimize change. When adherence is present, altering the lens fit (i.e., flattening the BCR or decreasing the lens diameter) and decreasing the water content of the lens should provide an improvement in lens lag. Young[152] has found that soft lenses with flatter base curves do not necessarily show increased lens movement with the blink. Ensuring that the lens exhibits movement when performing the push-up test has been found to be an important indicator of a good fitting relationship.

Frequent replacement of lenses—assuming a good fitting relationship—can be beneficial in maintaining a regular corneal topographic pattern.[153] When the topographic maps of patients who had worn the same soft lenses for more than 12 months were compared to those of newly worn replacement lenses (with identical parameters), irregular topographic patterns were observed only in color-coded maps of worn lenses, not in maps of replacement lenses.

TABLE 16-4. *Nomenclature for Keratoconus and Corneal Warpage Syndrome*

Corneal warpage syndrome: Contact lens–induced corneal distortion that is often remediated after discontinuation of contact lens wear. This syndrome has none of the biomicroscopic signs characteristic of keratoconus (i.e., corneal thinning, Fleischer's ring, or Vogt's striae).
Clinical keratoconus: Actual or true keratoconus in which one or more of the classic biomicroscopic signs are present.
Subclinical keratoconus: Typically used for cases in which keratoconus is diagnosed subsequently.
Pseudokeratoconus: A keratoconuslike condition in which typically the topographic pattern and possibly the retinoscopic findings are similar to keratoconus. This can be caused by a superiorly decentered rigid gas-permeable lens, a decentered corneal apex, inadvertent external pressure on the globe, or misalignment of the videokeratoscope.

CORNEAL WARPAGE VERSUS KERATOCONUS

Definitions

One of the most confusing factors pertaining to differentiating CWS from keratoconus is the terminology used to label these conditions or variants thereof. CWS is a contact lens–induced condition in which irregular astigmatism, corneal distortion, edema, and refractive changes are present.[154] Unlike keratoconus, progressive corneal steepening does not occur, and in most cases, this condition improves with proper management. Although CWS, like keratoconus, presents with irregular astigmatism, the hallmark biomicroscopic clinical signs, such as corneal scarring, corneal thinning, Vogt's striae, and Fleischer's ring, are absent.

Waring[155] has differentiated these conditions into clinical keratoconus, subclinical keratoconus, and pseudokeratoconus. Clinical keratoconus is the actual or true keratoconus in which one or more of the classic biomicroscopic signs are present. *Subclinical keratoconus* is a term typically used for cases in which keratoconus had been diagnosed subsequently. *Pseudokeratoconus* is a keratoconuslike condition in which typically the topographic pattern and possibly the retinoscopic findings are similar to keratoconus. This can be caused by a superiorly decentered RGP lens, a decentered corneal apex, inadvertent external pressure on the globe, or misalignment of the videokeratoscope (Table 16-4).

Differential Diagnosis

Keratoconus and corneal warpage often can be differentiated by way of a combination of case history and com-

prehensive clinical examination including videokeratoscopy. Patients with CWS, typically have a long-term *history* of contact lens wear. This condition occurs as a combination of corneal hypoxia and the mechanical effects induced by the contact lens. It has been most often reported with PMMA lens wear, although soft and RGP lenses can induce CWS, with the latter via a poor lens-to-cornea fitting relationship.

Although much is still unknown about the etiology, keratoconus is associated with a history of atopic disease in as many as 50% of those manifesting this condition.[156-159] Similarly, eye rubbing via mechanical pressure has been implicated as a cause, often in association with atopic etiology.[160] A small correlation with heredity has been found: Typically, fewer than 10% of patients with keratoconus have a blood relative with this condition.[161-163] Although contact lens wear has been described as a possible etiologic factor, this is still controversial.

With a comprehensive clinical examination, these conditions can often be differentiated. Although corneal distortion and often a scissorslike retinoscopy reflex are present in both conditions, patients with CWS typically manifest signs of corneal hypoxia but rarely exhibit corneal steepening beyond 50 D.[154] In addition, the degree of mire irregularity or misalignment is typically less with CWS than with keratoconus. Keratoconus can often be differentiated with a comprehensive biomicroscopic examination. Clinical signs, such as Fleischer's ring, Vogt's striae, and in moderate-to-severe cases, corneal scarring, are present in keratoconus and not typically associated with CWS, which is limited to changes in corneal contour.[164] In addition, corneal thinning is typically present in keratoconus, often in the inferotemporal region, diagnosed via slit-lamp optic section or from pachometry.[165-167] The affected corneal region is limited in keratoconus, often of variable size, encompassing some of the central and inferior regions. *Photodiagnosis* using direct ophthalmoscopic observation at a 2-ft distance from a dilated pupil can be beneficial in determining the conical area.[168] Keratoconus, unlike CWS, typically progresses over a 5–10-year period, often resulting in a protruding conical region.

With CWS, discontinuation of contact lens wear or refitting into lens material with greater oxygen permeability results in a healthy, regular cornea exhibiting a well-centered lens-to-cornea fitting relationship.

Role of Videokeratography

VKG plays an important role in differentiating CWS from keratoconus: It is an excellent screening method for detecting subclinical keratoconus.[166] In fact, several VKG systems have applications for the screening and diagnosis of keratoconus.[167,168–179] This is particularly important because the presence of keratoconus is a contraindication for refractive surgery, and up to 5–7% of refractive surgery candidates have subclinical keratoconus.[173,174]

With the cone apex aligned with the optical system of a VKG, Mandell[175,176] determined that a true apex power reading can be obtained and therefore compared to the normal range in the detection of keratoconus. He concluded that if the cone apex power is 48–49 D, the patient should be considered a keratoconus suspect. For powers of 49–50 D, a high likelihood of keratoconus exists, and for powers more than 50 D, the diagnosis is almost certain. The modified Rabinowitz-McDonnell (R-M) method[167,177,178] uses the following guidelines:

- If the central corneal power is more than 47.2 D or if the difference between the inferior and superior paracentral corneal regions (i.e., I–S value) is more than 1.4 D, the cornea is considered suspect for keratoconus.
- If the central corneal power is more than 48.7 D or the I–S value is more than 1.4 D, the cornea is classified as keratoconic.

Cochet and Dezard[170] found that the R-M method was not totally diagnostic of keratoconus, particularly with regard to the criterion of central corneal power. They found that individuals with clinical keratoconus had an average difference between the central corneal radius and the radius at the apex of the cone equal to 0.55 mm compared to an average of 0.11 mm for those with pseudokeratoconus. In addition, corneal eccentricity was found to be an important factor, with an average eccentricity value of 0.94 in clinical keratoconus versus a more normal value of 0.56 in pseudokeratoconic individuals. Perhaps the most sophisticated and accurate method using VKG to detect keratoconus was developed by Maeda et al.[179,180] Their Expert System Classifier (ESC) incorporates eight topographic indices representing specific topographic features often associated with keratoconus, including asymmetry, fine and gross irregularities, and generalized or localized areas of steepness. They compared this system to simulated keratometry (Sim K) and the modified R-M test in ability to screen for and diagnose keratoconus. The ESC was significantly more sensitive as a measure than simulated keratometry readings (i.e., 98% versus 84%) but similar to the modified (R-M) test (96%). However, the ESC was significantly more specific in its detection of keratoconus than was either of the other two methods (i.e., 99% versus 86% for Sim K and 85% for modified R-M). The authors concluded that

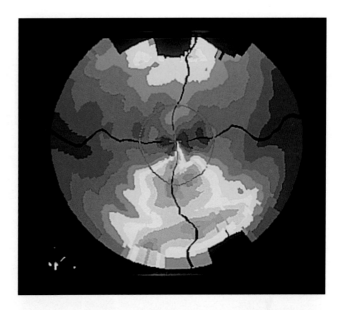

FIG. 16-3. *Enlarged view of corneal topography map, indicating a suspicious red zone in the inferior section of the cornea. Although a normal cornea may plot a red zone, it can also be a beneficial early clue of subclinical keratoconus or possibly corneal warpage. (Courtesy of Dr. Robert Grohe.)*

for screening candidates for refractive surgery, in which high sensitivity is required, either the ESC method or modified R-M method is suitable; for diagnosing keratoconus, in which high specificity is more beneficial, the ESC method is most appropriate.

Using VKG to differentiate keratoconus from CWS (as opposed to normals) appears to be much more difficult. Both demonstrate irregular astigmatic patterns (Figs. 16-3 and 16-4). Similarly, the presence of a superiorly decentered lens-to-cornea fitting relationship can induce a pseudokeratoconic topography pattern. The ESC system was applied to 106 VKGs of 53 patients presenting for an opinion on refractive surgery.[181] The ESC system was quite sensitive and specific in keratoconus detection, but it identified three patients as keratoconic who were rigid contact lens wearers and, in fact, were probably pseudokeratoconic. They concluded that keratoconuslike topography patterns in rigid contact lens wearers may be difficult to distinguish from patterns in true keratoconus, even when sophisticated quantitative algorithms are applied to the analysis.

However, the use of serial VKGs can be beneficial in differentiating these conditions.[166,182] In cases of corneal warpage, after contact lens removal, the cornea typically becomes less irregular, whereas the keratoconic cornea either remains unchanged or becomes progressively steeper in the affected region. This can be supplemented by the use of pachometry to evaluate corneal thickness, which

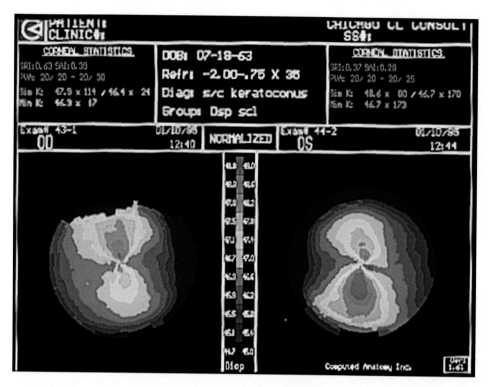

FIG. 16-4. *Bilateral corneal topography maps of a patient exhibiting symptoms (i.e., ghosting, slight loss of best corrected visual acuity) of subclinical keratoconus. Note that each map has red zone areas that are comparatively asymmetric in pattern and power, as is common with irregular astigmatism found in corneal warpage or subclinical keratoconus. (Courtesy of Dr. Robert Grohe.)*

should remain relatively unchanged in CWS while demonstrating a much thinner profile in keratoconus.[167] A method to differentiate clinical keratoconus from CWS uses quantitative measures based on VKG data.[183] A *corneal irregularity coefficient* (CIC) and a *corneal power coefficient* (CPC) were derived from multiple measures of mean corneal power and its variance for VKGs of normal, warped, clinical keratoconus, and keratoconus-suspect corneas. CIC was plotted against CPC, creating a distribution of points, grouping together all maps. Normal, steep, abnormal, and warped zones were defined by CIC and CPC cutoff values chosen to distinguish normal from keratoconus corneas graphically. A differential diagnosis of CWS and keratoconus is given in Table 16-5.

It is also important to differentiate other potentially misleading VKG results, including those resulting from pressure on the globe or from artifact. When pressure is exerted on the globe by an instrument or by a probe used to open the lids, the globe can be distorted, producing an area of steepness that could be mistaken for a keratoconic pattern.[166] In addition, in cases in which the cone apex is not aligned with the optical system of the VKG, error can result.[175,184–186] Mandell et al.[184] found that when the VKG optic axis alignment does not coincide with the corneal apex, an optical distortion produces a color map that is similar to a map expected for a cornea with true corneal asymmetry. An asymmetric or angled bow-tie appearance of a VKG color map suggests a decentered apex rather than asymmetric corneal toricity. This can be reduced or eliminated by realigning the VKG with the corneal apex. It is also important to rule out keratoconuslike VKGs produced by early pellucid marginal degeneration, inflammatory corneal thinning, and previous ocular surgery.[177,187] The use of serial VKGs assists in diagnosing the exact condition.

INTENTIONAL CONTACT LENS–INDUCED CORNEAL CURVATURE AND REFRACTIVE CHANGES: ORTHOKERATOLOGY

Overview

Orthokeratology is generally defined as a reshaping of the corneal contour with a series of RGP contact lenses with progressively flatter base curve radii to reduce, modify, or eliminate myopia and astigmatism. The theory proposed is that as the curvature of the eye changes, the patient's myopia is reduced and visual acuity improves. As additional lens changes are made, the patient's natural vision is theorized to continue to improve. At the end of the therapy, RGP lenses are worn on a part-time *retainer* basis to maintain the improved vision. The procedure is also used to slow down or halt the progression of myopia in young people. Because much individual variation on myopia reduction exists, the usefulness of orthokeratology for most patients depends on the magnitude of change and whether any prolonged therapeutic effect exists.

History

The idea of using rigid contact lenses to deliberately reduce refractive error was first reported in 1962.[188] Interest was initiated by the unintentional reduction in myopia found in some wearers of conventional hard contact lenses. It gained popularity in the 1960s and 1970s, but by the 1980s, the technique of orthokeratology had lost favor, largely because of the unpredictability reported in several controlled studies in the late 1970s and early 1980s.[189–197] With the introduction of *reverse-geometry* lens designs, RGP materials with greater oxygen permeability, and the use of VKG to evaluate corneal topography, interest in orthokeratology is renewed.

Mechanism of Action

Many theories exist to explain the mechanism of orthokeratology, with the most widely accepted being corneal sphericalization.[193,198–201] The non–contact lens–wearing cornea is generally characterized as aspheric, with the central cornea having the steepest curvature and becoming progressively flatter toward the periphery. RGP contact lens wear is postulated to cause central corneal flattening accompanied by paracentral steepening, which results in a *corneal shape factor* that approaches zero (i.e., spheric). This process is accelerated by the use of reverse-geometry lens designs, which have a steeper secondary curve to allow less resistance to the adjacent steepening of the midperipheral cornea. In other words, when a rigid contact lens applies pressure to the cornea in one area, the cornea yields to that force and pushes out in another area where less force exists. Therefore, flattening of the apex of the central cornea is accompanied by midperipheral steepening, and this is the basis for changes occurring in orthokeratology.

Efficacy

Orthokeratology appears to be quite successful in patients with less than 2 D of myopia. Early studies reported only a 1 D decrease in myopia.[189,196,197,202] Research with newer designs reported approximately twice as much myopia reduction.[198,203–205] Contex Laboratories conducted a study of 138 eyes, of which 110 eyes completed a minimum of 3 months of contact lens wear.[204] The spheric myopia value decreased an average of 1.69 D, with a range of 0.25–4.25 D. A total of 43 (39%) eyes achieved 20/20 or bet-

TABLE 16-5. *Corneal Warpage Syndrome versus Keratoconus: Differential Diagnosis*

	Corneal Warpage Syndrome	Keratoconus
Case history	Long-term rigid lens wear: often polymethyl methacrylate or low-Dk rigid gas-permeable lenses	Not limited to rigid lens wear Often atopic history
Slit-lamp evaluation	Corneal hypoxia and possibly lens decentration	Corneal thinning in affected region Fleischer's ring Vogt's striae Scarring (in later stages)
Corneal topography	Rarely steeper than 50 D	Often steeper than 50 D at apex of cone
	Mire irregularity often mild, improves with discontinuation of contact lens wear or refitting into higher-Dk material	Continues to progress with increasing mire irregularity and steepening of affected region
	Videokeratography shows irregularity; not limited in location; if inferior steep region, must rule out superior decentration	Location of steepest is often inferior
	CIC versus CPC is in the "warped" zone	CIC versus CPC is in the "keratoconus" zone

CIC = corneal irregularity coefficient; CPC = corneal power coefficient; Dk = oxygen permeability.

ter unaided visual acuity, and 78 (71%) achieved 20/40 or better visual acuity (Table 16-6).

Predicting Amount of Change

Predicting the amount of myopia reduction in a given orthokeratology candidate has been difficult. Mountford[198] has indicated that as the corneal eccentricity tends to decrease and approach zero (i.e., a sphere) owing to the sphericalization effect of orthokeratology, the amount of myopia reduction can be predicted from the amount of baseline corneal eccentricity. This relationship is described as

$$y = 0.21x$$

in which y is corneal eccentricity and x is the refractive change in diopters. Because the average corneal eccentricity is approximately 0.5, according to this formula, the potential reduction in refractive error to obtain a spheric

TABLE 16-6. *Percentage of Eyes That Achieved Full or Partial Temporary Reduction of Myopia*

Initial Myopia (D)	Full Temporary Reduction (%)	Up to 0.50 D under Full Reduction (%)	Final Visual Acuity 20/20 or Better (%)	Final Visual Acuity 20/40 or Better (%)
≤ –1.00	52	84	78	100
–1.25 to –2.00	36	55	74	96
–2.25 to –3.00	18	35	48	72
–3.25 to –4.00	4	13	16	64

Source: Data from Contex Laboratories, Sherman Oaks, CA, and the U.S. Food and Drug Administration, 1997.

cornea is approximately 2.50 D. For high corneal eccentricity, such as 0.6, the potential reduction is 3.00 D, and for low eccentricity, such as 0.4, it is 2.00 D.[206] However, this theory is controversial because total corneal sphericalization is not a common finding.[207] Newer lens designs have been reported to reduce myopia by as much as 4 D or more.[208–210]

Candidate Selection

Individuals with low myopia who are motivated to explore nonsurgical means of reducing nearsightedness are good candidates for orthokeratology. The advantages of this process over refractive surgery include the fact that it is noninvasive and, because it is reversible, the potential for irreversible sequelae with refractive surgery is avoided. An occupational or recreational need or requirement motivates many individuals.[211,212] For example, airline employees, military personnel, police officers, and firefighters are among the individuals who may use orthokeratology as a means of meeting an unaided visual acuity requirement. Prospective candidates must be given a realistic overview of the expectations in terms of how much myopia may be reduced, the cost, the time frame, and the patient's availability for visits. Although the cost and the number of visits are often reduced as a result of the more rapid changes occurring with reverse-geometry lens designs, patients must be advised that as many as 10–12 visits may be necessary for monitoring any design changes over a 6-month period or longer. The patient's goals also should be considered. Whereas 20/20 unaided visual acuity is often desirable, it may not be the required end point of therapy for a highly myopic individual who desires an improvement in unaided vision. Young, progressive myopic patients are good candidates, although as the axial length of young people continues to grow, promises of emmetropia are not realistic. Highly astigmatic individuals are not good candidates, nor are hyperopes. For the hyperope, lenses with progressively steeper base curves are necessary, and their impact on corneal change is less than with myopic individuals. Similarly, patients with low

hyperopic refractive errors are often asymptomatic without correction owing to the use of the accommodative system for compensation. Finally, individuals who are current rigid lens wearers most likely have already experienced some sphericalization of the cornea; therefore, orthokeratology may have little further impact.

Retainer Lens Wear

When no further refractive change has been elicited or the corneal topography shows a uniform, spheric corneal contour, the orthokeratology patient enters a retainer lens–wear regimen. Usually, the patient gradually reduces wearing time until he or she first experiences a decrease in unaided visual acuity.[211] The lower the amount of presenting myopia, the less time necessary for retainer wear. Overnight retainer lens wear has been promoted.[213–215] This has the benefits of eliminating the effects of dust and wind occurring with daily wear, the patient experiences little to no discomfort, and the speed of refractive change can be enhanced via the closed-lid effect at night. This technique has also been recommended for the initial phase of orthokeratology as well. A high-Dk lens material is required, but overnight orthokeratology has not yet received approval from the U.S. Food and Drug Administration.

Complications

Complications of orthokeratology include

- Decreased quality or variability of vision
- Increased with-the-rule corneal astigmatism
- Peripheral corneal distortion
- Visual problems at near
- Corneal staining
- Adherence
- Regression toward prefit level
- Ethical considerations

Decreased Quality and Variability of Vision

As a result of corneal changes, particularly after lens removal, patients may report variable or decreased vision, or both.[192,197] Because the amount of refractive change reduction is rather unpredictable, some patients may not obtain satisfactory unaided visual acuity.[189,191,202] The need for a retainer lens after completion of the orthokeratology process and the individual variation in the number of hours of lens wear necessary to maintain the refractive end point can contribute to these symptoms.

Increased with-the-Rule Astigmatism
Several reports of an increase in with-the-rule corneal astigmatism have been documented.[192,196,197] Often, this is the result of a lens that exhibits superior decentration, inducing changes in corneal topography.

Peripheral Corneal Distortion
In some cases, because of the effect of a flat-fitting lens on the cornea, peripheral corneal distortion can occur.[192,205,212] Often, this can result from an excessively aggressive approach (i.e., BCR is too flat).

Visual Problems at Near
Visual problems at near distances can occur as orthokeratology proceeds. This may be a result of a hyperactivity of the accommodative system.[1]

Corneal Staining
Over time, corneal staining can become a problem, especially if the lens is fitting too flat, resulting in a mechanical abrasion of the central epithelium, or if a tight-fitting lens results in adherence.[212,216] There have been a few reports of permanent corneal damage resulting from orthokeratology.[217,218]

Adherence
The introduction of centrally positioned but tighter-fitting reverse-geometry lens designs typically results in approximately 1 mm of lens movement with the blink but can potentially result in adherence.[219] With adherence, corneal edema, distortion, and staining can result.

Regression toward Prefit Level
Once retainer lens wear has been initiated, and even more so if contact lens wear is discontinued altogether, the refractive error tends to regress toward baseline values.[189,197]

Ethical Considerations
It is important for patients and practitioners to exercise appropriate ethical behavior when fitting lenses for myopia reduction. An example of unethical activity is to prescribe orthokeratology lenses for a patient

to meet an unaided vision requirement and then to discontinue lens wear afterward, thereby circumventing the vision requirement process.[220] Patients must be monitored and maintain retainer lens wear once the first phase of orthokeratology is complete. In addition, practitioners must be cautious in their promotion of orthokeratology to the public. In 1997 and 1998, the Federal Trade Commission investigated two practitioners for alleged false guarantees about the effectiveness of orthokeratology.[221] This is especially true because the first orthokeratology lens design was newly approved by the U.S. Food and Drug Administration (in May 1998, the OK series of lenses from Contex, Sherman Oaks, CA, was approved).

Management
Appropriate management of orthokeratology patients to minimize induced complications is a threefold process involving: high-Dk lens material, reverse-geometry lens design, and careful monitoring, including use of VKG.

High-Dk Lens Material
To ensure the absence of corneal edema, the selection of a high-Dk (i.e., more than 50) lens material is recommended. This is especially important if overnight orthokeratology is being used (indeed, if retainer lenses are to be used for overnight wear, the Dk should approach 100).

Reverse-Geometry Lens Design
With a rigid lens fitted flatter than K, the cornea tends to shift into the steeper secondary curve region. The principle behind reverse-geometry lenses is to use a steeper secondary curve to accommodate the change in corneal topography, thus enhancing lens centration. These lenses have demonstrated faster topographic changes than conventional lens designs and, therefore, the term *accelerated orthokeratology* has been applied.[222] In fact, clinically significant changes in myopia reduction have occurred in as little as 30 minutes of lens wear. The initial phase is often completed within 3 months, compared to 6–12 months for traditional orthokeratology. These lens designs often use a large overall diameter with a small optical zone. The reverse curve is typically anywhere from 2 to 7 D steeper than the base curve, with an average value of 3 D. The base curve is fitted 1.5–2.0 D flatter than K in an effort to achieve a 4–5-mm band of central bearing, a 2–3-mm band of midperipheral tear pooling, and approximately 1 mm of lens movement with the blink.[199] The most commonly used lens design is the OK series from Contex Laboratories. This series

TABLE 16-7. *The OK* Lens Design and Lens Selection Guidelines*

Lens	OZD (mm)	Reverse Curve	Rate of Corneal Change	Recommendations
OK-1	6.00	1 D steep	Minimal	Retainer
OK-2	6.00	2 D steep	Moderate-to-fast	Retainer; night therapy
OK-3	6.00	3 D steep	Fast	Often lens of first choice
OK-4	6.00	4 D steep	Fast	Useful for centration
OK-5	6.00	5 D steep	Fast	High shape factor
OK-61	6.50	1 D steep	Moderate-to-fast	For larger pupils; low myopia
OK-62	6.50	2 D steep	Moderate	Useful for centration
OK-63	6.50	3 D steep	Fast	Useful for centration
OK-64	6.50	4 D steep	Fast	Useful for centration
OK-65	6.50	5 D steep	Fast	Useful for centration
OK-71	7.00	1 D steep	Slow	Retainer or large pupils
OK-72	7.00	2 D steep	Slow	Retainer; night therapy
OK-73	7.00	3 D steep	Slow	Retainer; night therapy

OZD = optical zone diameter.
*Manufactured by Contex, Sherman Oaks, CA.
Source: Modified from J Mountford: Orthokeratology. p. 653. In AJ Phillips, L Speedwell (eds): Contact Lenses. Butterworth–Heinemann, Oxford, 1997.

of lenses and their recommended applications are provided in Table 16-7.[216]

It is important to evaluate the lens-to-cornea fitting relationship as soon as 1 hour after dispensing to determine if the fitting relationship has changed and to ensure that sufficient movement is still present. If the central fluorescein pattern has changed to an alignment or apical clearance pattern, a 0.50-D flatter lens should be dispensed. For this reason, it is advisable to order two pairs of lenses in which to begin. The patient should be evaluated 1–2 days later and then every 2–3 weeks. When no further unaided visual improvement can be realized and the central cornea has reached an end point, retainer lens wear can begin. The retainer lens can either be the last orthokeratology lens or a lens with a slightly flatter BCR or a larger optical zone diameter, or both. Lens-wearing time can be gradually decreased (i.e., 1 hour/day) until an effect on refractive error and unaided visual acuity is observed. The alternative is to have the patient wear the lenses overnight for retainer purposes. The number of nights of wear can be gradually reduced until an effect is observed.

Careful Monitoring, Including Videokeratography

It is important to carefully monitor every orthokeratology patient, to ensure compliance with lens wear and to ensure that corneal integrity is still optimal. The use of VKG is quite valuable in monitoring these patients. Often, these instruments can provide corneal eccentricity values, which can assist in predicting the amount of change as well as how much change is occurring from visit to visit. The color map itself can rule out poor candidates (i.e., corneal distortion and subclinical keratoconus) and provide beneficial information on the corneal topography in general. In addition, the use of difference maps can show how much change has occurred from visit to visit (Fig. 16-5).

Another potential management option that adds to the permanence of orthokeratology, *corneaplasty*, is under investigation. Corneal intrastromal injection of an enzyme combined with orthokeratology lenses could enable longer maintenance of the modified corneal contour after orthokeratology, thereby minimizing the need for retainer lens wear. One study has reported a dramatic improvement in unaided visual acuity in as short a period as a few weeks.[223]

FIG. 16-5. *Double difference map in orthokeratology. (Courtesy of EyeSys Technologies, Inc.)*

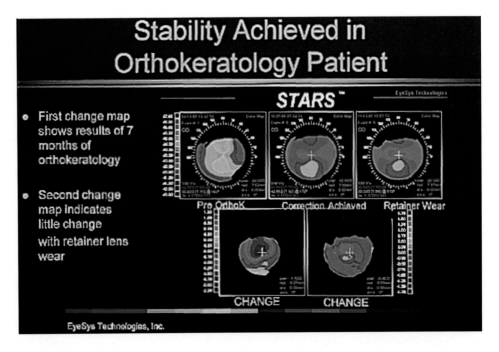

REFERENCES

1. Bennett ES: Contact lens-induced changes in corneal topography and refractive error. p. 69. In Tomlinson A (eds): Complications of Contact Lens Wear. Mosby–YearBook, St. Louis, 1992

2. Lowther GE: Induced refractive changes. p. 1035. In Ruben M, Guillon M (eds): Contact Lens Practice. Chapman & Hall, London, 1994

3. Sorkin A: The merits of PMMA. Contact Lens Spectrum 6:55, 1991

4. Sorkin A: Lifeblood of the cornea or contact cement. Contact Lens Spectrum 8:53, 1993

5. Bennett ES: Refitting PMMA and hydrogel lens wearers into RGP's. p. 201. In Harris MG (ed): Problem-Solving in Optometry. Lippincott, Philadelphia, 1990

6. Holden BA: Suffocating the cornea with PMMA. Contact Lens Spectrum 4:69, 1989

7. Fonn D, Holden BA, Roth P, et al: Comparative physiologic performance of polymethylmethacrylate and gas-permeable contact lenses. Arch Ophthalmol 102:760, 1984

8. Sarver MD, Baggett DA, Harris MG, Louie K: Corneal edema with hydrogel lenses and eye closure: effect of oxygen transmissibility. Am J Optom Physiol Opt 58:386, 1981

9. Finnemore VM, Korb JE: Corneal edema with polymethylmethacrylate versus gas permeable rigid polymer contact lenses of identical design. J Am Optom Assoc 51:271, 1980

10. Pratt-Johnson JA, Warner DM: Contact lenses and corneal curvature changes. Am J Ophthalmol 60:852, 1965

11. Holden BA, Sweeney DF: Corneal exhaustion syndrome (CES) in long-term contact lens wearers: a consequence of contact lens–induced polymegethism? Am J Optom Physiol Opt 65:95P, 1988

12. Sweeney DF: Corneal exhaustion syndrome with long-term wear of contact lenses. Optom Vis Sci 69:601, 1992

13. Pence NA: Corneal fatigue syndrome: the sequel. Contact Lens Spectrum 3:64, 1988

14. Hill RM: Corneas: in search of the right stuff. Int Contact Lens Clin 18:114, 1991

15. Holden BA, Mertz GW: Critical oxygen levels to avoid corneal edema for daily and extended wear contact lenses. Invest Ophthalmol Vis Sci 25:1161, 1984

16. Miller D: Contact lens-induced corneal curvature and thickness changes. Arch Ophthalmol 80:420, 1968

17. Hazlett RD: Central circular clouding. J Am Optom Assoc 40:268, 1969

18. Manchester PT: Hydration of the cornea. Trans Am Ophthalmol Soc 68:425, 1970

19. Masnick K: A preliminary investigation into the effects of corneal lenses on central corneal thickness and curvature. Aust J Optom 54:87, 1971

20. Farris RL, Kubota Z, Mishima S: Epithelial decompensation with corneal contact lens wear. Arch Ophthalmol 85:651, 1971

21. Westerhout D: A clinical survey of oedema, its signs, symptoms and incidence. Contact Lens 3:3, 1971

22. Berman MR: Central corneal curvature and wearing time during contact lens adaptation. Optom Weekly 63:27, 1972

23. Carney LG: The basis for corneal shape change during contact lens wear. Am J Optom Physiol Opt 52:445, 1975

24. Hill JF: A comparison of refractive and keratometric changes during adaptation to flexible and non-flexible contact lenses. J Am Optom Assoc 46:290, 1975

25. Saks SJ: Fluctuation in refractive state in adapting and long-term contact lens wearers. J Am Optom Assoc 37:229, 1966

26. Schapero M: Tissue changes associated with contact lenses. Am J Optom Arch Am Acad Optom 43:477, 1966

27. Rengstorff RH: Studies of corneal curvature changes after wearing contact lenses. J Am Optom Assoc 40:298, 1969

28. Rengstorff RH: Diurnal constancy of corneal curvature. Am J Optom 49:1002, 1972

29. Grosvenor TP: Contemporary Contact Lens Practice. p. 79. Professional Press, Chicago, 1972

30. Williams B: Orthokeratology update. Contacto 20:34, 1976

31. Kroll JR: Preliminary report on refractive changes in orthokeratology patients using automated refractors. Ophthalm Optician 18:39, 1978

32. Rengstorff RH: Diurnal variations in corneal curvature after wearing of contact lenses. Am J Optom 48:239, 1971

33. Rengstorff RH: Diurnal variations in myopia measurements after wearing contact lenses. Am J Optom 47:812, 1970.

34. Rengstorff RH: Circadian rhythm: corneal curvature and refractive changes after wearing contact lenses. J Am Optom Assoc 49:443, 1978

35. Rengstorff RH: Refractive changes after wearing contact lenses. p. 527. In Stone J, Phillips AJ (eds): Contact Lenses. 2nd ed. Butterworth, Stoneham, MA, 1984

36. Carney LG: Corneal topography changes during contact lens wear. Cont Lens J 3:5, 1974

37. Binder PS, May CH, Grant SC: An evaluation of orthokeratology. Am Acad Ophthalmol 87:729, 1980

38. Freeman R: Predicting stable changes in orthokeratology. Contact Lens Forum 3:321, 1978

39. Hovding G: Variation of central corneal curvature during the first year of contact lens wear. Acta Ophthalmol 61:117, 1983

40. Kerns RL: Research in orthokeratology—part VIII: results, conclusions and discussion of techniques. J Am Optom Assoc 49:308, 1978

41. Ong J, Bowling R: Effect of contact lens on cornea and lid on a 10-year wearer. Am J Optom 49:932, 1972

42. Rengstorff RH: The Fort Dix Report—a longitudinal study of the effects of contact lens wear. Am J Optom 42:153, 1965

43. Rengstorff RH: An investigation of overnight changes in corneal curvature. J Am Optom Assoc 39:262, 1968

44. Rengstorff RH: Variations in corneal curvature measurements: an after-effect observed with habitual wearers of contact lenses. Am J Optom Arch Am Acad Optom 46:45, 1969

45. Rengstorff RH: Changes in corneal curvature associated with contact lens wear. J Am Optom Assoc 50:375, 1979

46. Rengstorff RH: Relationship between myopia and corneal curvature changes after wearing contact lenses. Am J Optom Arch Am Acad Optom 46:357, 1969

47. Rengstorff RH: Variations in myopia measurements: an after-effect observed with habitual wearers of contact lenses. Am J Optom 44:149, 1967

48. Rengstorff RH: Corneal curvature and astigmatic changes subsequent to contact lens wear. J Am Optom Assoc 36:996, 1965

49. Rengstorff RH: Astigmatism after contact lens wear. Am J Optom Physiol Opt 54:787, 1977

50. Bennett ES, Tomlinson A: A controlled comparison of two techniques of refitting long-term PMMA contact lens wearers. Am J Optom Physiol Opt 60:139, 1983

51. Hom MM: Thoughts on contact lens refractive changes. Contact Lens Forum 11:16, 1986

52. Bennett ES, Gilbreath MK: Handling PMMA-induced corneal distortion: a case study. Optom Monthly 74:529, 1983

53. Hartstein J: Corneal warping due to contact lenses: a report of 12 cases. Am J Ophthalmol 60:1103, 1965

54. Rengstorff RH: Prevention and treatment of corneal damage after wearing contact lenses. J Am Optom Assoc 46:277, 1975

55. Rengstorff RH: The relationship between contact lens base curve and corneal curvature changes. J Am Optom Assoc 43:291, 1973

56. Koetting RA, Castellano CF, Keating MJ: PMMA lenses worn for twenty years. J Am Optom Assoc 57:459, 1986

57. Mobilia EF, Kenyon KR: Contact lens-induced corneal warpage. Int Ophthalmol Clin 26:43, 1986

58. Novo AG: Corneal topographic changes after refitting polymethylmethacrylate contact lens wearers into rigid gas permeable materials. CLAO J 21:47, 1995

59. Hill JF, Rengstorff RH: Relationship between steeply fitted contact lens base curve and corneal curvature changes. Am J Optom Physiol Opt 51:340, 1974

60. Levenson DS: Changes in corneal curvature with long-term PMMA contact lens wear. CLAO J 9:121, 1983

61. Wilson SE, Lin DTC, Klyce SD, et al: Topographic changes in contact lens–induced corneal warpage. Ophthalmol 16:177, 1990

62. Wilson SE, Lin DTC, Klyce SD, et al: Rigid contact lens decentration: a risk factor for corneal warpage. CLAO J 16:177, 1990

63. Wilson SE, Klyce SD: Advances in the analysis of corneal topography. Surv Ophthalmol 35:269, 1991

64. Ruiz-Montenegro J, Mafra CH, Wilson SE, et al: Corneal topographic alterations in normal contact lens wearers. Ophthalmol 100:128, 1993

65. Rubin ML: The tale of the warped cornea: a real-life melodrama. Arch Ophthalmol 80:430, 1968

66. Levenson DS, Berry CV: Finding on follow-up of corneal warpage patients. CLAO J 9:121, 1983

67. Colossi A, Casalboni F, Zanella SG: Same PMMA contact lenses worn for over 30 years: a case report. Int Contact Lens Clin 21:196, 1994

68. Bennett ES: Treatment options for PMMA-induced problems. p. 275. In Bennett ES, Grohe RM (eds): Rigid Gas-Permeable Contact Lenses. Fairchild Publications, New York, 1986

69. Rengstorff RH: Contact lens–induced corneal distortion. p. 351. In Silbert JA (ed): Anterior Segment Complications

of Contact Lens Wear. Churchill Livingstone, New York, 1994

70. Rengstorff RH: Corneal rehabilitation. p. 1. In Bennett ES, Weissman BA (eds): Clinical Contact Lens Practice. Lippincott, Philadelphia, 1992

71. Elliott LJ, Grohe RM, Bennett ES: Problem-solving. p. 1. In Bennett ES, Weissman BA (eds): Clinical Contact Lens Practice. Lippincott, Philadelphia, 1992

72. Diamond PA, Spinell MR: Should you fix it if it's not broken? Contact Lens Spectrum 7:49, 1992

73. Rengstorff RH: A study of visual acuity loss after contact lens wear. Am J Optom 43:431, 1966

74. Arner RS: Prescribing new contact lenses or spectacles for the existing contact lens wearer. J Am Optom Assoc 41:253, 1970

75. Arner RS: Corneal deadaptation: the case against abrupt cessation of contact lens wear. J Am Optom Assoc 48:339, 1977

76. Bennett ES: Rigid gas permeable lens problem-solving. p. 143. In Bennett ES, Henry VA (eds): Clinical Manual of Contact Lenses. Lippincott, Philadelphia, 1994

77. Rengstorff RH: Corneal curvature: patterns of change after wearing contact lenses. J Am Optom Assoc 42:264, 1971

78. Rengstorff RH: Refitting long-term wearers of hard contact lenses. Rev Optom 116:75, 1979

79. Rengstorff RH: Strategies for refitting PMMA lens wearers. Rev Optom 118:49, 1981

80. DeRubeis MJ, Shily BG: The effects of wearing the Boston II gas permeable contact lens on central corneal curvature. Am J Optom 62:497, 1985

81. Henry VA, Bennett ES, Forrest JF: Clinical investigation of the Paraperm EW rigid gas permeable contact lens. Am J Optom Physiol Opt 64:313, 1987

82. Ghormley NR: Rigid EW lenses: complications. Int Contact Lens Clin 14:219, 1987

83. Bennett ES: Silicone/acrylate lens design. Int Contact Lens Clin 12:45, 1985

84. Bennett ES: Immediate refitting of gas permeable lenses. J Am Optom Assoc 54:239, 1983

85. Iacona GD: Corneal contour changes with contact lenses: part I. Contact Lens Spectrum 4:54, 1989

86. Bennett ES, Bennett DS, Liesemeyer BH: A clinical investigation of the "Paraperm O_2 Plus" rigid gas-permeable contact lens. Int Eyecare 1:489, 1985

87. Hurd KK, Bennett ES: A clinical investigation of the Boston IV silicone/acrylate rigid contact lens for daily wear. Int Eyecare 2:564, 1986

88. Lowther GE, Paramore JE: Clinical comparison of silicon resin lenses to PMMA, C.A.B. and Polycon lenses. Int Contact Lens Clin 9:106, 1982

89. Sevigny J: The Boston lens clinical performance. Int Contact Lens Clin 10:73, 1983

90. Sevigny J: Clinical comparison of the Boston IV contact lens under extended wear versus the Boston II under daily wear. Int Eyecare 2:260, 1986

91. Pole JJ, Lowther GE: Clinical comparison of low, moderate and high rigid gas permeable lenses. Contact Lens Forum 12:47, 1987

92. Lydon D, Guillon M: Effect of center thickness on the performance of rigid gas permeable lenses. Am J Optom Physiol Opt 61:23, 1984

93. Schwallie JD, Barr JT, Carney LG: The effects of spherical and aspheric rigid gas permeable contact lenses: corneal curvature and topography changes. Int Contact Lens Clin 22:67, 1995

94. Fonn D: Progress evaluation procedures. p. 1. In Bennett ES, Weissman BA (eds): Clinical Contact Lens Practice. Lippincott, Philadelphia, 1991

95. Calossi A, Verzella F, Zanell SG: Corneal warpage resolution after refitting an RGP contact lens wearer into hydrophilic high water content material. CLAO J 22:242, 1996

96. Maeda N, Klyce SD, Hamano H: Alteration of corneal asphericity in rigid gas permeable contact lens induced warpage. CLAO J 20:27, 1994

97. Odby A, Rengstorff RH: The Boston lens: clinical study in Sweden. Int Contact Lens Clin 12:104, 1985

98. Polse KA, Rivera RK, Bonanno J: Ocular effects of hard gas permeable lens extended wear. Am J Optom Physiol Opt 65:358, 1988

99. Levy B: Rigid gas-permeable lenses for extended wear—a 1-year clinical evaluation. Am J Optom Physiol Opt 62:889, 1985

100. Polse KA, Sarver MD, Kenyon E, et al: Gas-permeable hard contact lens extended wear: ocular and visual responses to a 6-month period of wear. CLAO J 13:31, 1987

101. Schnider CM, Bennett ES, Grohe RM: Rigid extended wear. p. 1. In Bennett ES, Weissman BA (eds): Clinical Contact Lens Practice. Lippincott, Philadelphia, 1991

102. Thompson E, Henry VA, Bennett ES, Moser L: A clinical investigation of the Fluoroperm rigid gas-permeable contact lens. Contact Lens J 17:79, 1989

103. Zantos SG, Zantos PO: Extended wear feasibility of gas permeable hard lenses for myopes. Int Eyecare 1:66, 1985

104. Holden BA, Swarbrick HA: Extended wear: physiologic considerations. p. 1. In Bennett ES, Weissman BA (eds): Clinical Contact Lens Practice. Lippincott, Philadelphia, 1991

105. Badowski L: Refractive error and corneal topographical changes with daily and extended wear of rigid gas permeable contact lenses. Master's thesis. Ohio State University College of Optometry, Columbus, OH, 1991

106. Swarbrick HA, Holden BA: Rigid gas permeable lens binding: significance and contributing factors. Am J Optom Physiol Opt 64:815, 1987

107. Bennett ES, Grohe RM: How to solve 'stuck lens' syndrome. Rev Optom 124:51, 1987

108. Grohe RM, Lebow KA: Vascularized limbal keratitis. Int Contact Lens Clin 16:197, 1989

109. Swarbrick HA, Holden BA: Rigid gas-permeable lens adherence: A patient-dependent phenonemon. Optom Vis Sci 66:269, 1989

110. Schnider CM, Zabkiewicz K, Holden BA: Unusual complications associated with RGP extended wear. Int Contact Lens Clin 15:124, 1988

111. Johnson J, Bennett ES: Material selection. p. 1. In Bennett ES, Weissman BA (eds): Clinical Contact Lens Practice. 2nd ed. Lippincott, Philadelphia, 1998

112. Benjamin WJ: EOP and Dk/L: the quest for hyper transmissibility. J Am Optom Assoc 64:196, 1993

113. Bennett ES, Grohe RG. RGP extended wear revisited. Optom Today 6:67, 1998

114. Bennett ES: RGPs: when oxygen is a priority. Contact Lens Spectrum 13:18, 1998

115. Sorbara L, Fonn D, Holden BA, Wong R: Centrally fitted versus upper lid-attached rigid gas permeable lenses. Part I. Design parameters affecting vertical decentration. Int Contact Lens Clin 23:99, 1996

116. Sorbara L, Fonn D, Holden BA, Wong R: Centrally fitted versus upper lid–attached rigid gas permeable lenses. Part II. A comparison of the clinical performance. Int Contact Lens Clin 23:121, 1996

117. Bennett ES: Lens design, fitting, and evaluation. p. 41. In Bennett ES, Henry VA (eds): Clinical Manual of Contact Lenses. Lippincott, Philadelphia, 1994

118. Bennett ES: RGP fitting: how to increase comfort. Practical Optom 8:148, 1997

119. Bennett ES: RGP Grand rounds: management of RGP lens decentration. Presented at RGP Lens Practice: Today and Tomorrow, St. Louis, MO, July 1990

120. Andrasko G: Center thickness: an important RGP parameter. Contact Lens Forum 14:40, 1989

121. Hill RM, Brezinski SD: The center thickness factor. Contact Lens Spectrum 2:52, 1987

122. Henry VA, Campbell RC, Connelly S, Koch T: How to refit contact lens patients. Contact Lens Forum 16:19, 1991

123. Hill JF: Variation in refractive error and corneal curvature after wearing ultra-thin hydrophilic contact lenses. Int Contact Lens Clin 3:23, 1976

124. Mandell RB: Symptomatology and aftercare. p. 598. In Mandell RB: Contact Lens Practice. 4th ed. Thomas, Springfield, IL, 1988

125. Brennan N, Efron N: Problems with soft lenses. p. 221. In Harris MG: Problems in Optometry. Lippincott, Philadelphia, 1990

126. Bailey NJ, Carney LG: Corneal changes from hydrophilic contact lenses. Am J Optom Arch Am Acad Optom 50:299, 1973

127. Baldone JA: Corneal curvature changes secondary to the wearing of hydrophilic gel contact lenses. Contact Lens Intraocular Lens Med J 1:175, 1975

128. Masnick KB: Corneal curvature changes using hydrophilic lenses. Aust J Optom 54:240, 1971

129. Harris MG, Sarver MD, Polse KA: Corneal curvature and refractive error changes associated with wearing hydrogel contact lenses. Am J Optom Physiol Opt 52:313, 1975

130. Grosvenor T: Changes in corneal curvature and subjective refraction in soft contact lens wearers. Am J Optom Physiol Opt 52:405, 1975

131. Barnett WA, Rengstorff RH: Adaptation to hydrogel contact lenses: variations in myopia and corneal curvature measurements. J Am Optom Assoc 48:363, 1977

132. Collins MJ, Bruce AS: Soft contact lenses and corneal topography. Int Contact Lens Clin 20:187, 1993

133. Bibby MM: A model for lens flexure—validation and predictions. Int Contact Lens Clin 7:124, 1978

134. Lowe R, Brennan NA: Corneal wrinkling caused by a thin medium water contact lens. Int Contact Lens Clin 14:403, 1987

135. Hom MM: Soft lens design, fitting, and physiologic response. p. 179. In Hom MM: Manual of Contact Lens Prescribing and Fitting. Butterworth–Heinemann, Boston, 1997

136. Lobby P: Tinted lenses responsible for corneal distortion. Rev Optom 124:114, 1987

137. Clements D, Augsburger A, Barr JT, et al: Corneal imprinting associated with wearing a tinted hydrogel lens. Contact Lens Spectrum 3:65, 1988

138. Shovlin JP, Meshel LG, Weissman BA, et al: Tinted contact lenses: cosmetic and prosthetic application. p. 1. In Bennett ES, Weissman BA (eds): Clinical Contact Lens Practice. Lippincott, Philadelphia, 1991

139. Schanzer MC, Mehta RS, Arnold TP, et al: Irregular astigmatism induced by annular tinted contact lenses. CLAO J 15:207, 1989

140. Bucci FA, Evans RE, Moody KJ, et al: The annular tinted contact lens syndrome: corneal topographic analysis of ring-shaped irregular astigmatism caused by annular tinted contact lenses. CLAO J 23:161, 1997

141. Rengstorff RH, Nilsson KT: Long-term effects of extended wear lenses: changes in refraction, corneal curvature and visual acuity. Am J Optom Physiol Opt 62:66, 1985

142. Miller JP, Coon LJ, Meier RF: Extended wear of Hydrocurve II 55 soft contact lenses. J Am Optom Assoc 51:225, 1980

143. Kame R, Herskowitz R: The corneal consequences of hypoxia. p. 21. In Bennett ES, Grohe RM (eds): Rigid Gas-Permeable Contact Lenses. Professional Press, New York, 1986

144. Kohler JE, Flanagan GW: Clinical dehydration of extended-wear lenses. Int Contact Lens Clin 12:152, 1985

145. Andrasko G: The amount and time course of soft contact lens dehydration. J Am Optom Assoc 53:207, 1982

146. Iacona GD: Corneal contour changes with contact lenses: part I. Contact Lens Spectrum 4:54, 1989

147. Iacona GD: Corneal contour changes with contact lenses: part II. Contact Lens Spectrum 4:34, 1989

148. Griffiths M, Zahner K, Collins M, Carney L: Masking of irregular corneal topography with contact lenses. CLAO J 24:76, 1998

149. Connelly S: Why do patients want to be refit? Contact Lens Spectrum 7:39, 1992

150. Bennett ES, Stulc S, Bassi CJ, et al: Effect of patient personality profile and verbal presentation on successful rigid contact lens adaptation, satisfaction, and compliance. Optom Vis Sci 75:500,1998

151. Bennett ES, Smythe J, Henry VA, et al: The effect of topical anesthetic use on initial patient satisfaction and overall success with rigid gas permeable contact lenses. Optom Vis Sci 75:800, 1998

152. Young G: Soft lens fitting reassessed. Contact Lens Spectrum 7:56, 1992
153. Hamano H, Hamano T, Hamano T, et al: Comparison between old and new soft contact lenses' surface shape during wear. J Jpn Contact Lens Soc 34:53, 1992
154. Shovlin JP, DePaolis MD, Kame RT: Contact lens–induced corneal warpage syndrome. Contact Lens Forum 11:32, 1986
155. Waring GE III: Nomenclature for keratoconus suspects. Refract Corneal Surg 9:220, 1993
156. Gasset AR, et al: HLA antigen and keratoconus. Ann Ophthalmol 9:767, 1977
157. Taylor B, et al: Transient IgA deficiency and pathogenesis of infantile atopy. Lancet 7821:111, 1973
158. Rahi A, et al: Keratoconus and coexisting atopic disease. Br J Ophthalmol 61:761, 1977
159. Rahi A, Davies P, Ruben M, et al: Keratoconus and coexisting atopic disease. Br J Ophthalmol 61:761, 1977
160. Ridley F: Contact lenses in treatment of keratoconus. Br J Ophthalmol 40:295, 1956
161. Reinke AR: Keratoconus: a review of research and current fitting techniques. Part I. Int Contact Lens Clin 2:66, 1975
162. Hallerman W, Wilson EJ: Genetische Betrachtungen uber den keratokonus. Klin Monatsbl Augenheilkd 170:906, 1977
163. Hammerstein W: Zur genetik des keratoconus. Graefes Arch Klin Exp Ophthalmol 190:293, 1974
164. Davis LJ: Keratoconus: current understanding of diagnosis and management. Clin Eye Vis Care 9:13, 1997
165. Colin J, Sale Y, Malet F, Cochener B: Inferior steepening is associated with thinning of the inferotemporal cornea. J Refract Surg 12:697, 1996
166. Klyce SD: Role of corneal topography in keratorefractive surgery. p. 2039. In Krachmer JH, Mannis MJ, Holland EJ (eds): Cornea. Vol. III: Surgery of the Cornea and Conjunctiva. Mosby, St. Louis, 1997
167. Probst LE: Case 13: Lasik with forme fruste keratoconus. p. 504. In Machat JL, Slade SG, Probst LE (eds): The Art of Lasik. 2nd ed. SLACK, Inc., Thorofare, NJ, 1999
168. Bennett ES: Keratoconus. p. 297. In Bennett ES, Grohe RM (eds): Rigid Gas-Permeable Contact Lenses. Professional Press, New York, 1986
169. Caroline PJ, Andre MP: Help for screening abnormal corneal topographies. Contact Lens Spectrum 13:56, 1998
170. Cochet P, Dezard X: Pseudokeratoconus and its relevance to contact lens wear. Contactologia 16E:153, 1994
171. Klyce SD: Corneal topography in refractive keratectomy. p. 19. In Thompson FB, McDonnell PJ (eds): Color Atlas/Text of Excimer Laser Surgery: The Cornea. Igaku-Shoin, New York, 1993
172. Wilson SE, Klyce SD, Husseini ZM: Standardized color-coded maps for corneal topography. Ophthalmol 100:1723, 1993
173. Wilson SD, Klyce SD: Screening for cornea topographic abnormalities before refractive surgery. Ophthalmol 101:147, 1994
174. Nesburn AB, Bahri S, Berlin M, et al: Computer-assisted corneal topography (CACT) to detect mild keratoconus in candidates for photorefractive keratectomy. Invest Ophthalmol Vis Sci (suppl.) 33:995, 1995
175. Mandell RB: Contemporary management of keratoconus. Int Contact Lens Clin 24:43, 1997
176. Mandell RB, Barsky BA, Klein SA: Taking a new angle on keratoconus. Contact Lens Spectrum 9:44, 1994
177. Rabinowitz YS, McDonnell PJ: Computer-assisted corneal topography in keratoconus. Refract Corneal Surg 5:400, 1989
178. Rabinowitz YS: Keratoconus. Surv Ophthalmol 42:297, 1998
179. Maeda N, Klyce SD, Smolek MK: Comparison of methods for detecting keratoconus using videokeratography. Arch Ophthalmol 113:870, 1995
180. Maeda N, Klyce SD, Smolek MK, Thompson HW: Automated keratoconus screening with corneal topography analysis. Invest Ophthalmol Vis Sci 35:2749, 1994
181. Kalin NS, Maeda N, Klyce SD, et al: Automated topographic screening for keratoconus in refractive surgery candidates. CLAO J 22:164, 1996
182. Bennett ES, Gans L: Corneal topography in pre- and post-surgical contact lens fitting. p. 1. In Harris MG (ed): Contact Lenses in Pre- and Post-surgical Contact Lens Fitting. Mosby, St. Louis, 1998
183. Smolek MK, Klyce SD, Maeda N: Keratoconus and contact lens–induced corneal warpage analysis using the keratomorphic diagram. Invest Ophthalmol Vis Sci 35:4192, 1994
184. Mandell RB, Chiang CS, Yee L: Asymmetric corneal toricity and pseudokeratoconus in videokeratography. J Am Optom Assoc 67:540, 1996
185. Hubbe RE, Foulks GN: The effect of poor fixation on computer-assisted topographic corneal analysis. Pseudokeratoconus. Ophthalmol 101:1745, 1994
186. Keller PR, van Saarloos PP: Perspectives on corneal topography: a review of videokeratoscopy. Clin Exp Optom 80:18, 1997
187. Rabinowitz YS: Videokeratographic indices to aid in screening for keratoconus. J Refract Surg 11:371, 1995
188. Wesley GN: Orthofocus techniques. Contacto 6:200, 1962
189. Polse KA, Brand RJ, Schwalbe JS, et al: The Berkeley orthokeratology study, Part II: efficacy and duration. Am J Optom Physiol Opt 60:187, 1983
190. Polse KA, Brand RJ, Vastine DW, Schwalbe JS: Corneal change accompanying orthokeratology. Arch Ophthalmol 101:1873, 1983
191. Kerns RL: Research in orthokeratology, Part III: Results and observations. J Am Optom Assoc 47:1505, 1976
192. Kerns RL: Research in orthokeratology, Part IV: Results and observations. J Am Optom Assoc 48:227, 1977
193. Kerns RL: Research in orthokeratology, Part V: Results and observations—recovery aspects. J Am Optom Assoc 48:345, 1977
194. Kerns RL: Research in orthokeratology, Part VI: Statistical and clinical analyses. J Am Optom Assoc 47:1134, 1976
195. Kerns RL: Research in orthokeratology, Part VII: Examination and techniques, procedures and control. J Am Optom Assoc 48:1541, 1977

196. Kerns RL: Research in orthokeratology, Part VIII: Results, conclusions and discussion of techniques. J Am Optom Assoc 49:308, 1978
197. Binder PS, May CH, Grant SC: An evaluation of orthokeratology. Ophthalmol 87:729, 1980
198. Mountford J: An analysis of the changes in corneal shape and refractive error induced by accelerated orthokeratology. Int Cont Lens Clin 24:128, 1997
199. Marsden HJ, Kame RT: Orthokeratology: advanced fitting techniques. In Bennett ES, Weissman BA (eds): Clinical Contact Lens Practice. Lippincott, Philadelphia, 1997
200. May CH, Grant SC: Orthokeratology today: part II. Contact Lens Forum 2:25, 1977
201. Freeman RA: Orthokeratology and the corneascope computer. Optom Weekly 67:90, 1976
202. Coon LJ: Orthokeratology Part II: Evaluating the Tabb method. J Am Optom Assoc 55:409, 1984
203. Joe JJ, Marsden HJ, Edrington TB: The relationship between corneal eccentricity and improvement in visual acuity with orthokeratology. J Am Optom Assoc 67:87, 1996
204. Contex Laboratories, Sherman Oaks, CA and Food and Drug Administration data, 1997
205. Swarbrick HA, Wong G, O'Leary DJ: Corneal response to orthokeratology. Optom Vis Sci 75:791, 1998
206. Bennett ES: Taking the mystery out of orthokeratology. Cont Lens Spectrum 12:18, 1997
207. Marsden HJ, Joe JJ, Edrington TB: Changes in corneal eccentricity with orthokeratology. Optom Vis Sci 71(12s):94, 1994
208. Hom MM. Advanced orthokeratology. Int Cont Lens Clin 24:187, 1997
209. Day JH, Reim T, Bard R, et al: Advanced orthokeratology using custom lens designs. Contact Lens Spectrum 12:34, 1997
210. Tabb RL, Day JH: Advanced methods lead to improved results with orthokeratology. Primary Care Optom News 2:19, 1997
211. Marsden HJ: Orthokeratology. p. 176. In Schwartz CA: Specialty Contact Lenses: A Fitter's Guide. Saunders, Philadelphia, 1996
212. Lebow KA: Orthokeratology. In Bennett ES, Weissman BA (eds): Clinical Contact Lens Practice. Lippincott, Philadelphia, 1991
213. Winkler T, Kame RT: Night therapy. p. 69. In Winkler T, Kame RT: Orthokeratology Handbook. Butterworth–Heinemann, Boston, 1994
214. Grant S: Orthokeratology: night therapy and night retention. Contact Lens Spectrum 7:28, 1992
215. Hunter WA: Reconsider orthokeratology. Contact Lens Spectrum 8:47, 1993
216. Mountford J: Orthokeratology. p. 653. In Phillips AJ, Speedwell L: Contact Lenses. Butterworth–Heinemann, Oxford, 1997
217. Levy B: Permanent corneal damage in a patient undergoing orthokeratology. Am J Optom Physiol Opt 59:697, 1982
218. Waring GO: Orthokeratology. Surv Ophthalmol 24:291, 1980
219. Winkler T, Kame RT: Basic techniques of accelerated orthokeratology. p. 21. In Winkler T, Kame RT: Orthokeratology Handbook. Butterworth–Heinemann, Boston, 1994
220. Winkler T, Kame RT: Patient care and practice management. p. 91. In Winkler T, Kame RT: Orthokeratology Handbook. Butterworth–Heinemann, Boston, 1994
221. Federal Trade Commission: Vision correction procedures. Available at: www.ftc.gov/bcp/conline/pubs/health/vision.htm. November 1997
222. Wlodyga RJ, Bryla C: Corneal molding: the easy way. Contact Lens Spectrum 4:58, 1989
223. Karageozian H, Baker P, Kenney M, et al: Intrastromal application of ACS-005 enzyme for reshaping of human corneas. Invest Ophthalmol Vis Sci 37:S68, 1996

17

Keratoconus

KARLA ZADNIK AND TIMOTHY B. EDRINGTON

GRAND ROUNDS CASE REPORT

Subjective:
A 20-year-old woman presents with a history of decreasing vision in her left eye (OS) for the past 6 years. Prescription glasses have not improved the vision in her left eye, and no prior contact lens evaluation has been undertaken. Ocular and medical history are unremarkable except for hay fever. Familial history is also unremarkable.

Objective:
- Unaided distance acuity: right eye (OD) $20/20-$, OS $20/200$
- Keratometry: OD 44.75/46.50 @ 18 (1+ distortion), OS 46.00/59.50 @ 160 (3+ distortion)
- Best manifest refraction: OD $+0.25 -0.25 \times 005$ ($20/20-$), OS $+8.50 -4.00 \times 045$ ($20/200$)
- Potential acuity: with diagnostic rigid gas-permeable (RGP) lens OS $20/25$
- Biomicroscopy: OD cornea clear; no signs of keratoconus; OS full Fleischer's ring. No other corneal signs of keratoconus.

Assessment:
Keratoconus OS, nipple type. Incipient (subclinical) keratoconus OD.

Plan:
1. Perform corneal topography.
2. Fit with RGP contact lens OS.
3. Monitor for clinical signs of keratoconus OD at follow-up examinations.

Discussion:
Despite keratoconus being a bilateral disease, asymmetric clinical presentation is the norm. RGP lens wear for OS is indicated for visual acuity, which should improve from $20/200$ to $20/25$ and allow clear, binocular vision. It is highly probable that OD will develop signs of keratoconus. Contact lens treatment will be initiated for OD as signs and acuity changes warrant. Atopic history is a common finding.

TABLE 17-1. *Characteristics of Corneal Degenerations and Dystrophies*

Degenerations	Dystrophies	? Keratoconus
Unilateral	Bilateral	Bilateral
Asymmetric	Symmetric	Asymmetric
Peripheral	Axial	Axial
No inheritance	Heritable	Unknown
Late onset	Early onset	Early onset
Secondary disease	Primary disease	Unknown
Inflammatory	Noninflammatory	Noninflammatory

Keratoconus is a progressive, noninflammatory ectasia resulting in protrusion, thinning, and distortion of the central cornea. It is typically bilateral and asymmetric.[1,2] The onset of keratoconus is usually at puberty or later,[3] with the initial development of central corneal thinning[4] and irregular corneal astigmatism. Scarring is not present at this stage of keratoconus, and most patients can achieve good visual acuity with spectacles or contact lenses.

Many facts and much speculation about keratoconus are found in the ophthalmic literature. Although it is a rare disease by epidemiologic criteria, it is a common diagnosis among patients in specialty contact lens or tertiary cornea practices. Keratoconus patients represent challenging cases for contact lens practitioners, and it is a common diagnosis for which penetrating keratoplasty is performed. Therefore, optometrists and ophthalmologists alike, especially cornea and external disease specialists, manage keratoconus patients on a regular basis.

The role of contact lenses in keratoconus is an example of the speculation surrounding the disease and its natural history. Suspicion exists that rigid contact lenses actually cause keratoconus in some cases.[5] Some investigators believe that rigid contact lenses may cause or hasten the apical corneal scarring present in keratoconus.[6] Because rigid contact lenses are the mainstay of keratoconus management, such relations are difficult to identify and characterize.

The availability of corneal tissue with keratoconus from corneal transplant patients has made the biochemical and cellular changes seen in this disease a fertile area of research. However, the story of what has gone awry in keratoconus and what layer of the cornea is "to blame" for the disease is far from clear.

Intriguing associations with various ocular and systemic diseases stimulate discussions of etiology and cause and effect. Association with such diverse conditions as Down syndrome (trisomy 21), connective tissue diseases, retinitis pigmentosa, atopic disorders, and other corneal diseases has been reported in the past but may not be a true, meaningful association.[7] Do these represent coincidences in small numbers of keratoconus patients or a genetic or environmental association between one or more of these diseases and keratoconus?

The etiology of keratoconus remains a mystery, a nature-versus-nurture debate. Advancements in corneal topography measurement have rekindled interest in genetic theories.[8] Eye rubbing is indicted consistently, either as an independent causative factor or through the atopic or itching connection. The very classification of keratoconus as either a corneal degeneration or a corneal dystrophy depends on resolving the genetics-versus-environment debate. Table 17-1 shows the characteristics that define a condition as degenerative or dystrophic. Its third column indicates which category keratoconus falls into for each characteristic. It is clear that keratoconus falls somewhere between corneal degenerations and corneal dystrophies; however, it would be defined as a dystrophy if its inheritance pattern were demonstrated conclusively.

INCIDENCE AND PREVALENCE OF KERATOCONUS

Estimates of the incidence and prevalence of keratoconus in any population sample depend heavily on the diagnostic criteria used. The application of stringent criteria decreases estimates of the impact of the disease in a sample, and using lax diagnostic criteria results in estimates of higher prevalence and incidence.

Investigators studied the epidemiology of keratoconus in Olmsted County, Minnesota.[9] All cases of keratoconus newly diagnosed by ophthalmologists at the Mayo Clinic and other county medical facilities from 1935 to 1982 were included in the sample studied. The diagnosis of keratoconus was "based on the examiner's description of characteristic irregular light reflexes observed during ophthalmoscopy or retinoscopy or irregular mires detected at keratometry." They found an average annual incidence of keratoconus of 2 in 100,000 and a prevalence rate of 54.5 in 100,000. The incidence rate did not change significantly over the 48 years sampled. Duke-Elder and Leigh[10] estimate the prevalence of keratoconus at 4 per 100,000 population. Using a conservative annual incidence rate of 2 per 100,000 population,[7] 4,500 new cases of keratoconus appear in the United States each year. A high prevalence rate of 370 in 100,000 was based only on keratoscopic analysis of approximately 13,000 volunteers at the 1957 Indiana State Fair.[11] The reasons for these wide variations lie in the method of diagnosis and the population sampled.

No racial or gender predilection exists for keratoconus. Early reports[12,13] suggest a higher incidence of keratoconus among females, but data indicate no significant difference between the genders.[9]

Keratoconus is typically a bilateral disease. It is, however, markedly asymmetric in its presentation, with one eye usually diagnosed before the other—sometimes separated by years—and with one eye more advanced than the other throughout the course of the disease (Fig. 17-1). Estimates of the number of truly unilateral cases are difficult to make. If one selects a point in time to determine whether both eyes are involved, the cases that proceed to second eye involvement are not counted. As in the case of diagnostic criteria, the description of keratoconus in an eye directly influences the number of unilateral versus bilateral cases.[1] If inferior steepening on corneal topography is diagnostic of keratoconus in the fellow eye,[8,14,15] far fewer unilateral cases are observed than if biomicroscopic signs of the disease are required.

Keratoconus, after its classically described onset at puberty, progresses with age, over a period estimated at 10–20 years, to variable endpoints.[3] Some patients progress to the point of significant corneal thinning, with visual needs still well managed with contact lenses, whereas others develop significant corneal scarring, resulting in impaired vision and the need for corneal surgery. Other patients progress rapidly in the early stages of the disease to require relatively early penetrating keratoplasty or epikeratoplasty because of inadequate visual acuity even with rigid contact lenses or corneas so steep that tolerable contact lens wear cannot be achieved.

Although rigorous studies of the natural history of the disease have not been conducted, some observations about the clinical course of keratoconus are warranted. Typically, the younger the age of onset, the worse is the disease. Some researchers associate onset of the disease after rigid contact lens wear with less severe keratoconus.[5]

A specific mechanism for the development of keratoconus and its relation to heredity and environment has not been forthcoming but has been the impetus for endless speculation. Various etiologies have been proposed, but adequate scientific evidence does not exist for any of them. Some evidence exists that keratoconus might be a hereditary disease,[8,9,16-19] endocrine in nature,[20] or a degenerative, acquired disorder associated with ectodermal defects.[21] Other theories include collagen abnormalities in the form of abnormal collagen cross-linking,[22] increased levels of collagenase activity,[23-26] decreased corneal tensile strength,[27] increased corneal distensibility,[28] increased corneal fragility,[29] or stromal apoptosis in response to epithelial insult.[30] Keratoconus has been associated with atopic disease,[7,31-36] connective tissue disorders,[37] Down syndrome,[38] and previous rigid contact lens wear,[5,32,39-42] but results have

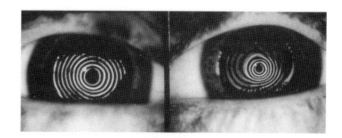

FIG. 17-1. *Corneascope photographs from a keratoconus patient's right and left eyes, showing marked asymmetry of the disease.*

not confirmed the association with rare systemic diseases as previously reported.[7]

A retrospective study of hundreds of patients examined the association between rigid contact lens wear and the onset of keratoconus.[5] The authors' conclusion was that rigid contact lens wear preceded diagnosis in less severe cases of keratoconus. The association of contact lens wear and keratoconus is suggested even after elimination of patients who are known to have corneal warpage from contact lens wear.[43] Macsai and coworkers [5] appear to have sorted their sample of keratoconus patients into two groups based on the relative timing of disease diagnosis and rigid lens wear. Difficulties with this study include the definition of keratoconus, uncertainty about the advent of contact lens wear, and whether the division is based solely on disease severity rather than on contact lens history.

Keratoconus has been linked to eye rubbing,[7,44-46] with estimates of the prevalence of significant eye rubbing among keratoconus patients ranging from 66% to 73%. This argument is strengthened by the apparent increased prevalence of atopic disease associated with keratoconus,[7,31,32,34,35] which presumably results in increased symptoms of ocular itching, partly alleviated by eye rubbing. However, other workers have not demonstrated a significant association between atopy and keratoconus.[33,36] Eye rubbing can also be postulated as the cause of keratoconus seen in patients with Down syndrome and infantile tapetoretinal degeneration (Leber's congenital amaurosis). Both groups exhibit an incidence of keratoconus far greater than that seen in the general population, and both engage in frequent, vigorous eye rubbing.

PATHOGENESIS

Debate rages over whether keratoconic corneas are inherently more deformable than normal corneas.[47,48] Contact lens practitioners who have encountered keratoconus patients whose corneas mold to the back surface of any applied rigid lens in a matter of hours certainly believe so. In a carefully controlled study of 55 patients with keratoconus and appropriate controls, Foster and Yamamoto[48] disproved the generalization that keratoconus is characterized by abnormally low ocular rigidity.

Keratoconic corneas are structurally and biochemically different from normal corneas. The distribution of stromal fibers is uneven. The results of a number of investigations indicate that intercellular substance is increased and total collagen is decreased, accompanied by an increase of structural glycoprotein component.[26,49,50] However, others argue that correction for age negates these observations.[51] In 1963, Teng[21] demonstrated early changes in keratoconus in the basal epithelium, indicating that enzymes may be released from fragile basal epithelial cells to cause fragmentation, fibrillation, and liquefaction of the anterior stroma, with invasion of fibroblasts and resultant scarring. Fibrin and fibrinogen are decreased in the epithelial basement membrane in keratoconus.[52] In scarred areas of keratoconic corneas, collagen type III predominates.[23,37] Some studies have found high amounts of lysinonorleucine in keratoconic corneas, indicating abnormal collagen cross-linking,[22] whereas others have not corroborated this finding.[26] Increased collagenase activity in excised keratoconic corneas has also been observed.[24] There has been speculation as to the role of programmed cell death, or apoptosis, in the corneal stroma in keratoconus.[30]

Corneas from keratoconus patients contain less protein per milligram of dry weight than those of healthy subjects. Reduced protein content may indicate the presence of increased nonproteinaceous materials. A high amount of polyanions, including glycosaminoglycans, is observed.[53] Higher levels of nucleoside monophosphates and choline phosphate and lower levels of adenosine diphosphate are present in postmortem keratoconic corneas.[54] Plasma membranes of keratoconus patients' stromal cells may contain elevated amounts of glyco-conjugates, which may influence cell differentiation and migration by mediating differences between wounded (or migrating) and nonwounded corneal epithelial cells. Although no certainty exists that these variations are associated with the pathogenesis of keratoconus, these variations are of great interest.[55]

OCULAR AND SYSTEMIC DISEASE CORRELATES

Keratoconus has been described in association with a large variety of ocular and systemic diseases. These include some of the connective tissue disorders, primarily Ehlers-Danlos syndrome and osteogenesis imperfecta, but also oculodentodigital syndrome, Rieger's syndrome, Marfan's syndrome, and focal dermal hypoplasia,[37] as well as Down syndrome,[38] infantile tapetoretinal degeneration (Leber's congenital amaurosis),[56] and atopic disease.[31-36,57] However, of the more than 1,200 patients enrolled in the Collaborative Longitudinal Evaluation of Keratoconus (CLEK) Study, none report having any of the systemic diseases traditionally associated with keratoconus, with the exception of atopy.[7]

Ocular diseases associated with keratoconus include retinitis pigmentosa,[8] posterior polymorphous corneal dystrophy,[58-60] floppy eyelid syndrome[61] (perhaps indicative of an association with obesity), and retrolental fibroplasia.[62]

Heredity

Quotable values for a positive family history in keratoconus patients are in the range of 6–13%.[7,9,18] A study of the corneal topography of 28 family members of five keratoconus patients demonstrated an increased prevalence of abnormal corneal topography, including high astigmatism, inferior corneal steepening, and asymmetric central corneal curvature.[8] These findings point to an autosomal dominant inheritance pattern with variable penetrance of the gene.

Atopy

Most clinicians associate atopic disease with keratoconus, in the sense that they expect keratoconus patients to more frequently exhibit the signs and symptoms of hay fever, allergy, asthma, or eczema than the general population. How marked the difference is depends on the sample studied. In a tertiary referral sample of keratoconus patients, the prevalence of atopy was 24%.[63] In another clinical population of 57 keratoconus patients, the prevalence of atopy was 42%.[64] In the CLEK Study, 53% of the patients self-report having hay fever, 15% self-report having asthma, and 8% self-report having atopic dermatitis.[7]

Specific aspects of atopy in keratoconus have been investigated. In one study of 53 keratoconus patients with vernal conjunctivitis, researchers found an increased incidence of hydrops, frequent eye rubbing, and overall decreased contact lens success.[65] In another study of 67 keratoconus patients, atopic status was not associated with gender or age of keratoconus onset. Atopy was less common in unilateral cases of keratoconus, and the involved eye in uni-

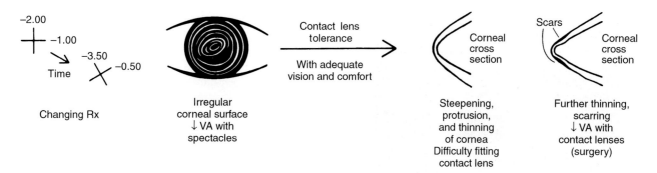

FIG. 17-2. *Progression of keratoconus. (Rx = eyeglasses prescription; VA = visual acuity; ↓ = decreased.) (Courtesy of Joseph T. Barr, OD, MS.)*

lateral cases was more frequently on the same side as the dominant hand.[57]

Biomicroscopic Signs

Keratoconus is a progressive disease with associated thinning of the apical cornea, steepening and distortion of the cornea, scarring, and treatment-related sequelae, such as abrasions from contact lens wear and surgical complications (Fig. 17-2). Although various geometries of keratoconus have been described,[66,67] it is not usually possible to identify these types in the early stages of the disease. The exception to this is keratoglobus.[1]

Biomicroscopy reveals several characteristic features, which increase as the keratoconus progresses.[1] These include an inferiorly displaced, thinned protrusion of the cornea (Fig. 17-3), visually evident corneal thinning over the apex, Vogt's striae[68] at the level of Descemet's membrane (Fig.

17-4), superficial scars at the level of Bowman's membrane, anterior clear spaces (interruptions of Bowman's membrane),[69] and Fleischer's ring (of iron) at the base of the cone, either full or partial (Fig. 17-5). Vogt's striae and Fleischer's ring are considered pathognomonic of keratoconus and tend to be associated with more severe disease.[70]

Central anterior corneal epithelial staining formations resulting from trauma are typical in keratoconus.[71] Central corneal sensitivity is reduced in keratoconus, especially in contact lens–wearing patients. This reduction of sensitivity correlates with disease severity in the contact lens–wearing subgroup.[29,72]

Clinical Symptoms

The typical patient with undiagnosed or early keratoconus complains of deteriorating vision, usually in one eye first, at distance and near. Near visual acuity may improve if

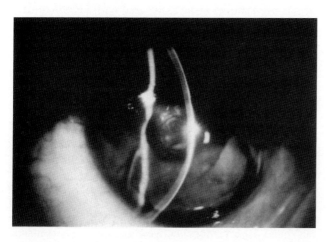

FIG. 17-3. *An inferiorly displaced cone with corneal thinning in keratoconus.*

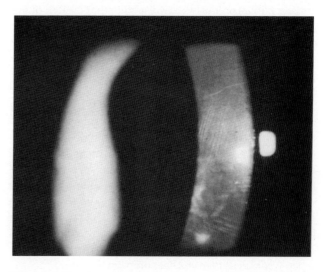

FIG. 17-4. *Vogt's striae in the posterior stroma in keratoconus.*

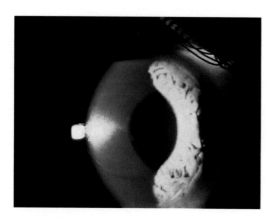

FIG. 17-5. *Fleischer's ring of iron at the base of the thinned area (cone) in keratoconus.*

the patient is allowed to squint or to hold the printed material closer. Keratoconus patients often report monocular diplopia, multiple images, or ghosting of images. Typically, they describe distortion of vision rather than the kind of blur typical of an uncorrected myope. Keratoconus patients often report a history of frequent spectacle changes without much improvement in vision. Even in the absence of contact lens wear, patients with early keratoconus complain of ocular irritation, sensitivity to glare, and photophobia.

VISION

Visual symptoms in early keratoconus are as described in the previous Clinical Symptoms section. As the disease progresses, patients report visual disability that is often out of proportion to Snellen visual acuity, as measured in the darkened examination room. Although they also report variable vision, visual acuity in keratoconus is highly repeatable across occasions.[73] Vision typically improves over the uncorrected or spectacle-corrected level with a pinhole or stenopaic slit but usually does not improve with a change in subjective refraction. When meaningful subjective refraction results can be obtained, they reveal moderate, irregular, compound myopic, or mixed astigmatism. The degree and the orientation of refractive astigmatism often change from visit to visit, and corneal toricity seldom correlates with refractive astigmatism, but subjective refraction in keratoconus is reasonably repeatable.[74] Speculation exists as to whether visual acuity is correlated with the type of rigid contact lens fitted (i.e., whether patients see better when wearing flat lenses that compress the cone).[1,6,75]

Because the corneal curvature changes in keratoconus, with rare exceptions, result in myopia and astigmatism,

patients require some type of visual correction from the earliest stages of the disease. Most practitioners prescribe spectacles very early. Limitations on the use of spectacle correction in keratoconus include high amounts of corneal toricity and resultant refractive astigmatism, the correction of which may not be tolerable in spectacle form. Other limitations are changing refractive error, either diurnally or from week to week, for which spectacles cannot be prescribed and inadequacy of visual acuity with spectacles because of uncorrected irregular astigmatism. Even given these problems, however, spectacles are the first form of optical management of the disease.

The corneal distortion inherent in keratoconus manifests as significant visual dysfunction in the form of contrast sensitivity abnormalities in the middle and high spatial frequencies. Even with contact lens correction and good visual acuity, vision, as measured by contrast sensitivity, is not normal.[76–79] Contrast sensitivity is restored to near normal after penetrating keratoplasty,[78] especially when postoperative contact lens correction is used.[80]

OTHER CONSIDERATIONS IN KERATOCONUS

The keratoconus patient is afflicted by a chronic, slowly progressive disease that requires contact lens wear for best visual correction because spectacles often do not correct vision to a useful level. As visual acuity declines, even at $20/40$, vision is no longer adequate for many occupations that require vast amounts of reading.

Anxiety is a common finding in keratoconus patients,[45,81–83] presumably owing to the unknown rate of disease progression and the resulting loss of visual acuity. Type A behavior has been shown to be associated with keratoconus.[84] Karseras and Ruben[45] had 75 patients with keratoconus and 231 healthy controls complete a personality inventory and found no increased incidence of such psychoneuroses as anxiety, phobias, depression, obsession, and hysteria. Besançon and associates[81] interviewed 34 keratoconus patients at the time of admission for corneal surgery and found no specific constellation of psychotic symptoms, but these authors claimed a greater prevalence of neurologic and psychosomatic traits (without comparison to controls). However, results differ when keratoconus patients are compared with patients with nonkeratoconic chronic eye disease. Mannis and coworkers[82] found significant differences in responses on a standardized personality inventory (the Millon Clinical Multiaxial Inventory) between eye disease patients (52 with keratoconus, 25 with chronic eye disease other than keratoconus) and healthy age-matched controls. They were unable to demonstrate those same differences between the keratoconus patients and the patients with chronic eye disease; in fact, the abnormalities documented between the two groups were remarkably similar.[82] In contrast, Swartz et al.[83] used the Minnesota Multiphasic Personality Inventory to compare 28 keratoconus patients with 16 herpetic keratitis patients. They found that significantly more of the keratoconus patients exhibited abnormal responses.

Patients with keratoconus must be seen frequently for eye examinations, contact lens fitting, and follow-up examinations for changes in corneal curvature and topography as the disease progresses. The time required for such doctors' office visits and the unmeasurable effects of mild-to-moderate acuity reduction translate into decreased productivity in the workplace. One report showed that four of 18 U.S. Air Force aviators with keratoconus were grounded either because of the need for surgery or because of contact lens intolerance.[85]

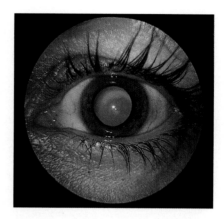

FIG. 17-6. *The so-called oil or honey droplet reflex observed with direct ophthalmoscopy in keratoconus. (Courtesy of Dr. Dennis Burger.)*

CORNEAL TOPOGRAPHY

Diagnosis of early keratoconus depends primarily on assessment of the corneal topography.[1] An irregular, scissoring motion can be detected by viewing the retinoscopic or ophthalmoscopic reflex (Fig. 17-6).[61] Inferior corneal steepening[72,86] and irregular mires are observed with the keratometer. Central corneal curvature at initial presentation (as measured by keratometry) is widely variable.[9] Devices that document corneal topography, such as a handheld Placido disk or a corneascope, show inferior corneal steepening as well as irregular astigmatism (see Fig. 17-1).[87] Some clinicians emphasize the value of documented increases in keratometric curvature of the cornea over time in diagnosing early keratoconus.[1] Lack of agreement between corneal toricity and refractive astigmatism is also a sign of early keratoconus, especially when accompanied by documented irregular astigmatism.

Sophisticated corneal modeling systems have been used to characterize the topography of the disease and to diagnose early keratoconus.[8,14,15,88,89] The advent of these computerized systems for the measurement of corneal topography has resulted in increased information about corneal shape in keratoconus.[88,90] Topographic patterns include the classic inferior steepening (Fig. 17-7) but extend to include some corneas with steepening above the horizontal midline and others with flattening in the superior nasal quadrant.[82] Investigators have touted corneal modeling as a tool for identifying subclinical keratoconus.[8,14,15] However, it remains to be seen if these "early" cases are keratoconus that never progresses beyond this early stage, representing some "form fruste" or aborted form or variable expression of the keratoconus gene,[88] or if these

patients go on to develop classic keratoconus. Longitudinal studies of these patients are required to make this differentiation.

The reliability and validity of these devices for normal corneas have only been sporadically investigated,[91–93] and studies have yet to explore the reliability and validity of videokeratography findings for keratoconic corneas. For example, the following questions remain unanswered about topographic measurement with a corneal modeling device in keratoconus:

- Is the position of the corneal apex consistent between measurements?
- Are the absolute values for corneal curvature consistent in the steep corneal areas and the normal corneal areas?

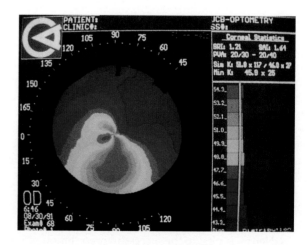

FIG. 17-7. *Corneal modeling in keratoconus.*

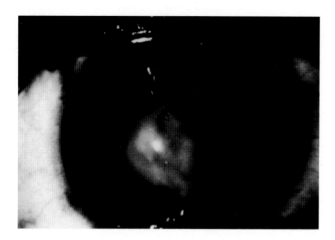

FIG. 17-8. *Corneal hydrops in keratoconus.*

- Is the overall pattern of corneal steepening, regardless of absolute values, consistent between measurements?
- How dramatic a change in apex position, absolute curvature values, and topographic pattern is necessary to document disease progression?

In addition to the technological development of videokeratographic instruments, a robust, repeatable assessment of corneal curvature in keratoconus has been developed for the CLEK Study. It involves the evaluation of fluorescein patterns with standard trial lenses to determine the flattest trial lens that just clears the corneal apex, the "first definite apical clearance lens."[94]

See Chapter 24 for a more detailed discussion of corneal topography.

CONE TYPES

Some attention has been paid to categorizing the type of conus present. The two most frequently described appearances are the round or nipple-shaped cone and the oval or sagging cone.[66,67] Some debate exists about whether the visual axis is more involved in either type, but the consensus is that more of the inferior cornea is ectatic in the oval or sagging cone.[67] The keratoconus must be moderate to advanced to make such a distinction on a given patient. The identification of the cone type may aid in contact lens fitting because nipple cones are easier to fit. Oval cones are more prone to hydrops, scarring, and difficulty in contact lens fitting.[66] In any event, application of trial lenses is vital to the successful prescription of rigid contact lenses in keratoconus.

HYDROPS

Rarely, corneal hydrops from an acute rupture of Descemet's membrane can also occur (Fig. 17-8).[95] Presenting symptoms include acute onset of blurred vision, pain on contact lens insertion, and the patient's observation of a "white spot on the eye." Contact lens wear must be discontinued temporarily and patients are treated with topical hypertonic agents. The post-hydrops cornea is often flatter in curvature, and contact lenses may be easier to fit and wear after an episode of hydrops. If the resulting scar is dense enough, surgery is indicated.

Hydrops occurs more frequently in keratoconus patients who tend to traumatize their corneas in an uncontrolled fashion (e.g., Down syndrome and Leber's amaurosis patients)[1] but can occur in any keratoconus patient with advanced disease and thin corneas. Spontaneous full-thickness perforation, however, is rare.[1]

DIFFERENTIAL DIAGNOSIS

Keratoconus must be differentiated from many other similar ectatic disorders. Some of the major disorders are corneal warpage resulting from rigid contact lens wear, postoperative or post-traumatic irregular corneal astigmatism, pellucid marginal degeneration, keratoglobus, posterior keratoconus, keratotorus, and Terrien's marginal degeneration (Table 17-2).

FACTORS LEADING TO CORNEAL SCARRING

It is possible that some keratoconus patients are destined to scar rapidly, regardless of contact lens treatment. For example, two groups of keratoconus patients have been identified on the basis of stromal collagen content. Group I has collagen similar to healthy controls, and group II has reduced collagen content.[46] To date, this differentiation cannot be performed in vivo. Even so, it appears that a biochemically altered, hypoesthetic, and fragile cornea, when further traumatized by a contact lens, may succumb to sterile, mechanical epithelial erosion, with resultant release of collagenase or similar destructive substances. With a reduced capacity for healing, the cornea may scar.

Scarring in keratoconus can reduce visual function beyond the possibility of optical correction. Methods have been developed to measure corneal scarring in a repeatable fashion.[96] Investigators have demonstrated that corneal scarring is associated with the diffusive, visually disabling blur of keratoconus.[97,98]

TABLE 17-2. *Differential Diagnosis of Disorders with an Irregular Corneal Surface*

	Keratoconus	Corneal Warpage	Postoperative/ Post-Traumatic Irregular Astigmatism	Pellucid Marginal Degeneration	Keratoglobus	Posterior Keratoconus	Terrien's Marginal Degeneration
Inflammation	—	—	—	—	—	—	Present
Irregular astigmatism	Present	Present	Present	Present (marked against-the-rule)	Present	Present	Present (marked against-the-rule)
Corneal thinning	Central	—	—	Inferior	Generalized/inferior	—	—
Corneal protrusion	Present	—	—	Present	Present	—	—
Stress lines	Present	—	—	—	—	Present	—
Iron ring	Present	—	—	Present	Present	—	—
Scarring	Present	—	Present	—	Present	Present	—
Progression	Present	—	Present	Present	Present	Present	—

SUMMARY

Keratoconus is a noninflammatory ectasia of the central cornea that leads to corneal thinning and protrusion. It is usually bilateral, asymmetric, and progressive. A multitude of etiologies and associations with ocular and systemic diseases have been proposed, including genetic factors, connective tissue disorders, atopic disease, and rigid contact lens wear. Several topographic presentations are manifested, the most prevalent being an inferiorly displaced nipple-type cone. Because keratoconus is progressive, with onset at puberty or later, the diagnosis of mild presentations is often tentative. Corneal distortion, as revealed by keratometry mires or the ophthalmoscopic/retinoscopic reflex accompanied by a Fleischer's ring or Vogt's striae, has served as the primary clinical diagnostic feature of keratoconus. With the increased use of sophisticated corneal topography mapping instruments, it may become possible to diagnose and manage keratoconus earlier when it presents in more subtle forms.

REFERENCES

1. Krachmer JH, Feder RS, Belin MW: Keratoconus and related noninflammatory corneal thinning disorders. Surv Ophthalmol 28:293, 1994
2. Rabinowitz YS: Keratoconus. Surv Ophthalmol 42:297, 1998
3. Amsler M: Le keratocone fruste au javal. Ophthalmology 96:77, 1938
4. Mandell RB, Polse KA: Keratoconus: spatial variation of corneal thickness as a diagnostic tool. Arch Ophthalmol 82:182, 1969
5. Macsai MS, Varley GA, Krachmer JH: Development of keratoconus after contact lens wear. Arch Ophthalmol 108:435, 1990
6. Korb DR, Finnemore VM, Herman JP: Apical changes and scarring in keratoconus as related to contact lens fitting techniques. J Am Optom Assoc 53:199, 1982
7. Zadnik K, Edrington TB, Everett DF, et al. and the CLEK study group: Baseline findings in the Collaborative Longitudinal Evaluation of Keratoconus (CLEK) study. Invest Ophthalmol Vis Sci 39:2537, 1998
8. Rabinowitz YS, Garbus J, McDonnell PJ: Computer-assisted corneal topography in family members of patients with keratoconus. Arch Ophthalmol 108:365, 1990
9. Kennedy RH, Bourne WM, Dyer JA: A 48-year clinical and epidemiologic study of keratoconus. Am J Ophthalmol 101:267, 1986
10. Duke-Elder S, Leigh AG: Keratoconus. Henry Kimpton, London, 1965
11. Hofstetter HW: A keratoscopic survey of 13,395 eyes. Am J Optom Arch Am Acad Optom 36:3, 1959
12. Thomas PF: The keratoconus patient. Aust J Optom 13:50, 1969
13. Hall KGC: A comprehensive study of keratoconus. Br J Physiol Opt 20:215, 1963
14. Maguire LJ, Bourne WM: Corneal topography of early keratoconus. Am J Ophthalmol 108:107, 1989
15. Maguire LJ, Lowry JC: Identifying progression of subclinical keratoconus by serial topography analysis. Am J Ophthalmol 112:41, 1991
16. Redmond KB: The role of heredity in keratoconus. Trans Ophthalmol Soc Austr 27:52, 1968
17. Falls HF, Allen AW: Dominantly inherited keratoconus. Report of a family. J Genet Hum 17:317, 1969
18. Hammerstein W: Zur genetik des keratoconus. Graefes Arch Klin Exp Ophthalmol 190:293, 1974

19. Forstot SL, Goldtein JH, Damiano RE, Dukes DK: Familial keratoconus. Ophthalmology 105:92, 1988
20. Leigh AG: The problems of keratoconus. Trans Ophthalmol Soc UK 80:373, 1960
21. Teng CC: Electron microscope study of the pathology of keratoconus: part I. Am J Ophthalmol 55:18, 1963
22. Cannon DJ, Foster CS: Collagen crosslinking in keratoconus. Invest Ophthalmol Vis Sci 17:63, 1978
23. Newsome DA, Foidart JM, Hassell JR, et al: Detection of specific collagen types in normal and keratoconus corneas. Invest Ophthalmol Vis Sci 20:1981
24. Rehany U, Lahav M, Shoshan S: Collagenolytic activity in keratoconus. Ann Ophthalmol 14:751, 1982
25. Kao WWY, Vergues JP, Ebert J, et al: Increased collagenase and gelatinase activities in keratoconus. Biochem Biophys Res Commun 107:929, 1982
26. Critchfield JW, Calandra AJ, Nesburn AB, Kenney MC: Keratoconus: I. Biochemical studies. Exp Eye Res 46:953, 1988
27. Andreassen TT, Simonsen AH, Oxlund H: Biomechanical properties of keratoconus and normal corneas. Exp Eye Res 31:435, 1980
28. Edmund C: Assessment of an elastic model in the pathogenesis of keratoconus. Acta Ophthalmol 65:545, 1987
29. Millodot M, Owens H: Sensitivity and fragility in keratoconus. Acta Ophthalmol 61:908, 1983
30. Wilson SE, Kim W-J: Keratocyte apoptosis: implications on corneal wound healing, tissue organization, and disease. Invest Ophthalmol Vis Sci 39:220, 1998
31. Copeman PW: Eczema and keratoconus. Br Med J 2:977, 1965
32. Gasset AR, Hinson WA, Frias JL: Keratoconus and atopic diseases. Ann Ophthalmol 10:991, 1978
33. Lowell FS, Carroll JM: A study of the occurrence of atopic traits in patients with keratoconus. J Allerg Clin Immunol 46:32, 1970
34. Khan MD, Kundi N, Saud N, et al: Incidence of keratoconus in spring catarrh. Br J Ophthalmol 72:41, 1988
35. Rahi A, Davies P, Ruben M, et al: Keratoconus and coexisting atopic disease. Br J Ophthalmol 61:761, 1977
36. Wachtmeister L, Ingemansson S, Moller E: Atopy and HLA antigens in patents with keratoconus. Acta Ophthalmol 60:113, 1982
37. Maumenee IH: The cornea in connective tissue disease. Ophthalmology 85:1014, 1978
38. Pierse D, Eustace P: Acute keratoconus in mongols. Br J Ophthalmol 55:50, 1971
39. Hartstein J: Corneal warping. Am J Ophthalmol 60:1103, 1965
40. Hartstein J: Keratoconus that developed in patients wearing corneal contact lenses. Arch Ophthalmol 80:728, 1968
41. Hartstein J: Keratoconus and contact lenses. JAMA 208:539, 1969
42. Nauheim JS, Perry HD: A clinicopathologic study of contact-lens-related keratoconus. Am J Ophthalmol 100:543, 1981

43. Wilson SE, Lin DTC, Klyce SD, et al: Topographic changes in contact lens–induced corneal warpage. Ophthalmology 97:734, 1990
44. Ridley F: Eye-rubbing and contact lenses. Br J Ophthalmol 45:631, 1961
45. Karseras AG, Ruben M: Aetiology of keratoconus. Br J Ophthalmol 60:522, 1976
46. Gritz DC, McDonnell PJ: Keratoconus and ocular massage. Am J Ophthalmol 106:757, 1988
47. Hartstein J, Becker B: Research into the pathogenesis of keratoconus. A new syndrome. Low ocular rigidity, contact lenses, and keratoconus. Arch Ophthalmol 84:728, 1970
48. Foster CS, Yamamoto GK: Ocular rigidity in keratoconus. Am J Ophthalmol 86:802, 1978
49. Yue BYJT, Sugar J, Benveniste K: Heterogeneity in keratoconus. Possible biochemical basis. Proc Soc Exp Biol Med 175:336, 1984
50. Robert L, Schillinger G, Moczar M, et al: Biochemical study of keratocone. Arch Ophthalmol Fr 30:590, 1970
51. Zimmermann DR, Fischer RW, Winterhalter KH, et al: Comparative studies of collagens in normal and keratoconus corneas. Exp Eye Res 46:431, 1988
52. Millin JA, Golub BM, Foster CS: Human basement membrane components of keratoconus and normal corneas. Invest Ophthalmol Vis Sci 27:604, 1986
53. Yue BYJT, Sugar J, Schrode K: Histochemical studies in keratoconus. Curr Eye Res 7:81, 1988
54. Greiner JV, Lass JH, Reinhart WJ, et al: Phosphatic metabolites in keratoconus. Exp Eye Res 49:799, 1989
55. Yue BYJT, Panjwani N, Sugar J, Baum J: Glycoconjugate abnormalities in cultured keratoconus stromal cells. Arch Ophthalmol 106:1709, 1988
56. Karel I: Keratoconus in congenital diffuse tapetoretinal degeneration. Ophthalmologica 155:8, 1968
57. Harrison RJ, Klouda PT, Easty DL, et al: Association between keratoconus and atopy. Br J Ophthalmol 73:816, 1989
58. Weissman BA, Ehrlich M, Levenson JE, Pettit TH: Four cases of keratoconus and posterior polymorphous corneal dystrophy. Optom Vis Sci 66:243, 1989
59. Gasset AR, Zimmerman TJ: Posterior polymorphous dystrophy associated with keratoconus. Am J Ophthalmol 78:535, 1974
60. Bechara SJ, Grossniklaus HE, Waring GO, Wells JA: Keratoconus associated with posterior polymorphous dystrophy. Am J Ophthalmol 112:678, 1991
61. Donnenfeld ED, Perry HD, Gibralter RP, et al: Keratoconus associated with floppy eyelid syndrome. Ophthalmology 98:1674, 1991
62. Lorfel RS, Sugar JS: Keratoconus associated with retrolental fibroplasia. Ann Ophthalmol 8:449, 1976
63. Lass JH, Lemback RG, Park SB, et al: Clinical management of keratoconus: a multicenter analysis. Ophthalmology 97:433, 1990
64. Swann PG, Waldron HE: Keratoconus: the clinical spectrum. J Am Optom Assoc 57:204, 1986

65. Cameron JA, Al-Rajhi AA, Badr HA: Corneal ectasia in vernal keratoconjunctivitis. Ophthalmology 96:1615, 1989

66. Perry HD, Buxton JN, Fine BS: Round and oval cones in keratoconus. Ophthalmology 87:905, 1980

67. Caroline PJ, McGuire JR: Preliminary report on a new contact lens design for keratoconus. Contact Intraocular Lens Med J 4:69, 1978

68. Vogt A: Reflexlinien durch faltung spiegelnder grenzflachen im bereiche von corneo, linsenkapsel und netzhaut. Albrecht von Graefes Arch Ophthalmol 99:296, 1919

69. Shapiro MB, Rodrigues MM, Mandel MR, Krachmer JH: Anterior clear spaces in keratoconus. Ophthalmology 93:1316, 1986

70. Zadnik K, Gordon MO, Barr JT, Edrington TB, et al. and the CLEK study group: Biomicroscopic signs and disease severity in keratoconus. Cornea 15:139, 1996

71. Dangel ME, Kracher GP, Stark WJ: Anterior corneal mosaic in eyes wearing hard contact lenses. Arch Ophthalmol 102:888, 1984

72. Zabala M, Archila EA: Corneal sensitivity and topogometry in keratoconus. CLAO J 14:210, 1988

73. Gordon MO, Schechtman KB, Davis LJ, et al. and the CLEK study group: Repeatability of visual acuity in keratoconus. Impact on sample size. Optom Vis Sci 75:249, 1998

74. Davis LJ, Schechtman KB, Begley CG, et al. and the CLEK study group: Repeatability of refraction and corrected visual acuity in keratoconus. Optom Vis Sci. 75:887, 1998

75. Zadnik K, Mutti DO: Contact lens fitting relation and visual acuity in keratoconus. Am J Optom Physiol Opt 64:698, 1987

76. Carney LG: Contact lens correction of visual loss in keratoconus. Acta Ophthalmol 60:795, 1982

77. Carney LG: Visual loss in keratoconus. Arch Ophthalmol 100:282, 1982

78. Mannis MJ, Zadnik K, Johnson CA: The effect of penetrating keratoplasty on contrast sensitivity in keratoconus. Arch Ophthalmol 102:1513, 1986

79. Zadnik K, Mannis MJ, Johnson CA, Rich D: Rapid contrast sensitivity assessment in keratoconus. Am J Optom Physiol Opt 65:693, 1987

80. Wicker D, Sanislo S, Green DG: Effect of contact lens correction on sine wave contrast sensitivity in keratoconus patients after penetrating keratoplasty. Optom Vis Sci 69:342, 1992

81. Besançon G, Baikoff G, Deneux A, et al: Note preliminaire sur l'etat psychologique et mental des porteurs de keratocone. Bull Soc Ophthalmol Fr 80:4, 1980

82. Mannis MJ, Morrison TL, Zadnik K, et al: Personality trends in keratoconus: an analysis. Arch Ophthalmol 105:798, 1987

83. Swartz MS, Cohen EJ, Scott DG, et al: Personality and keratoconus. CLAO J 16:62, 1990

84. Thalasselis A, Taie HF, Etchepareborda J, Selim A: Keratoconus, magnesium deficiency, type A behavior, and allergy. Am J Optom Physiol Opt 65:449, 1988

85. Carlson DW, Green RP: The career impact of keratoconus on Air Force aviators. Am J Ophthalmol 112:557, 1991

86. Edmund C: Corneal apex in keratoconic patients. Am J Optom Physiol Opt 64:905, 1987

87. Poster MG, Gelfer DM, Greenwald I, Posner JM: An optical classification of keratoconus: a preliminary report. Am J Optom Arch Am Acad Optom 45:216, 1968

88. McMahon TT, Robin JB, Scarpulla KM, Putz JL: The spectrum of topography found in keratoconus. CLAO J 17:198, 1991

89. Rabinowitz YS, McDonnell PJ: Computer-assisted corneal topography in keratoconus. Refract Corn Surg 5:400, 1989

90. Wilson SE, Lin DT, Klyce SD: Corneal topography of keratoconus. Cornea 10:2, 1991

91. Heath GG, Gerstman DR, Wheeler WH, et al: Reliability and validity of videokeratoscopic measurements. Optom Vis Sci 68:946, 1991

92. Hannush SB, Crawford SL, Waring GO, et al: Accuracy and precision of keratometry, photokeratoscopy, and corneal modeling on calibrated steel balls. Arch Ophthalmol 107:1235, 1989

93. Hannush SB, Crawford SL, Waring GO, et al: Reproducibility of normal corneal power measurements with a keratometer, photokeratoscope, and video imaging system. Arch Ophthalmol 108:539, 1990

94. Edrington TB, Szczotka LB, Begley CG, et al. and the CLEK study group: Repeatability and agreement of two corneal curvature assessments in keratoconus: keratometry and the first definite apical clearance lens (FDACL). Cornea 17:267, 1998

95. Fanta H: Acute Keratoconus. In Bellows JG (ed): Contemporary Ophthalmology. Williams & Wilkins, Baltimore, 1972

96. Barr JT, Gordon MO, Zadnik K, et al. and the CLEK study group: Photodocumentation of corneal scarring. J Refr Surg 12:492, 1996

97. Yackels T: Factors influencing vision in keratoconus. Master's thesis. Ohio State University, 1991

98. Burger D, Bullimore MA, McMahon TT: Determining the nature of visual loss in keratoconus. Optom Vis Sci (suppl.) 67:96, 1990

18

Effects of Contact Lenses in Keratoconus

DENNIS BURGER AND JOSEPH T. BARR

GRAND ROUNDS CASE REPORT

Subjective:
Patient has a 10-year history of keratoconus with contact lens wear. Reports that the contact lenses have become increasingly uncomfortable and that the left lens pops out of the eye. History of seasonal allergies and asthma. Vision has also decreased in both eyes with the left having a more noticeable decline. Wants to improve his contact lens comfort and fit.

Objective:
- Visual acuity with contact lenses: right eye (OD) $^{20}/_{40}$, left eye (OS) $^{20}/_{50}$
- Over-refraction: OD –1.00 = –0.25× 15, $^{20}/_{20-}$; OS –0.25 = –1.25× 140, $^{20}/_{30+}$
- Slit lamp with contacts on: Both contact lenses are flat. The right lens has 3 mm of bearing and centers well with an adequate peripheral system. The left lens has 6 mm of bearing, is not stable, and rests primarily on the apex. On lens removal, OD shows Vogt's striae with minimal corneal haze. OS shows a Fleischer's ring, Vogt's striae, and dense corneal scarring with staining at the corneal apex.
- Keratometry: OD 49.25/51.75 @ 110 (grade 1+ distorted), OS 51.50/56.25 @ 55 (grade 2+ distorted)
- Present contact lenses:

	Base Curve (mm)	Back Vert Power (D)	Diameter (mm)	Optical Zone Diameter (OZD) (mm)
OD	7.50	–3.25	9.0	7.8
OS	7.35	–4.75	9.0	7.8

The left lens showed some warpage.

Assessment:
The patient is fit with flat lenses. The patient's left lens is excessively flat, resting on the apex only, causing staining and possibly scarring. The decreased visual acuity is the result of the power being off in OD. The decreased vision in OS is related to power and corneal scarring.

Plan:
Refit the patient with new contact lenses that are steeper, correcting the power as indicated. The lenses ordered were made of Fluoroperm 30, with a medium blend OD (0.1 mm wide) and a heavy blend OS (0.2 mm wide). Specifications are as follows:

	Base Curve (mm)	Back Vert Power (D)	Diameter (mm)	Optical Zone Diameter (OZD) (mm)	Secondary Curve/Width	Peripheral Curve/Width	Center Thickness
OD	7.18	–6.25	8.8	7.0	8.5/0.4	10.5/0.4	0.15
OS	6.03	–15.00	8.8	6.4	8.0/0.6	10.0/0.4	0.15

Follow-up:

At dispensing when the lenses were inserted, a bubble was present under the left lens. The bubble disappeared after 20 minutes. The right lens looked steep initially, but after 20 minutes the lens fit looked minimally steep. The peripheral systems were adequate, allowing good contact lens movement. Bearing was achieved in the secondary area, and the lens was well centered and stable. At the first follow-up visit, central alignment was minimal apical clearance OD, with alignment to light touch OS. No staining was present. The lenses centered and moved well. Visual acuity with the contact lenses was OD 20/20, OS 20/30+. The patient reported good comfort with all-day wearing time. Both lenses were stable and the left lens no longer popped out.

Contact lenses have been the standard of care for improving vision in keratoconus patients ever since Fick[1] and Panas[2] used them for that purpose. Some reports[3-5] suggest that contact lenses cause keratoconus, but if they did, keratoconus would be more prevalent. Also improbable is that contact lenses inhibit progression of the disease except to temporarily flatten the cornea.

When keratoconus is first diagnosed, a patient should be informed of the following:

- Contact lenses eventually become necessary.
- The cornea may change and become scarred even if contact lenses are not worn.
- The prognosis is unpredictable and disease progression is variable.
- Annual or more frequent eye examinations are mandatory.
- The disease does not cause blindness but may complicate life, although patients usually retain the ability to drive and to read.
- Approximately 20% of patients ultimately need surgery.[6]

FITTING PROCEDURE

Specific procedures to facilitate fitting or refitting the keratoconus patient are described in this section, including management of complications associated with keratoconic lens wear.

Corneal Topography

Corneal topography is a useful aid in the diagnosis of keratoconus, especially when no other signs are present.

However, many of the algorithms underestimate the degree of the cone. Fluorescein pattern simulation software helps the practitioner to select an initial diagnostic lens. The practitioner cannot fully rely on this method to fit patients, however, because lenses may position differently on the eye or the topography of the cornea may not be properly represented.

Keratometry

Although keratometric readings may be of limited use in fitting keratoconus patients, such readings may help practitioners to select trial lenses and estimate disease progression. The keratometric range should be extended as necessary. To extend the range of the keratometer, an ancillary lens is placed on the front of the keratometer (Fig. 18-1). Using a +1.25 D lens extends the range to 60 D. To record a reading, 8 D is added to the drum reading (e.g., if the drum reads 45 D, the addition of 8 D yields an actual reading of 53 D). A +2.25 D lens extends the range to 68 D by adding 16 D to the reading.

Refraction

Careful refraction is mandatory. Patients with keratoconus often have unpredictably good best corrected visual acuity. High amounts of cylinder, frequently at an increasingly oblique axis, are commonly found. Retinoscopic and keratometric findings are an excellent starting point for determining subjective refraction. Careful refinement of cylinder axis and avoidance of so-called over-minusing are necessary. Accurate refraction provides a baseline best visual acuity without contact lenses, which serves as a reference point for expected contact lens–corrected acuity. Subjective refraction results are often prescribed, espe-

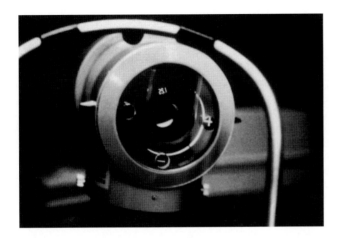

FIG. 18-1. *Ancillary lens mounted on keratometer.*

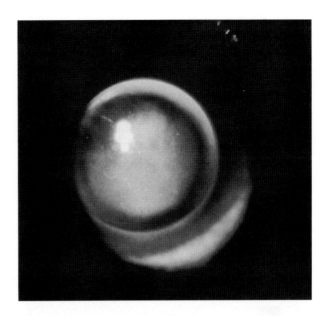

FIG. 18-2. *Apical clearance lens design.*

cially until contact lenses become necessary (i.e., when spectacles no longer suffice), in spectacles used as the backup mode of correction for patients who wear contact lenses or in spectacles used as the primary mode of correction for contact lens–intolerant patients.

Trial Lens Fitting

Trial diagnostic contact lens fitting is vital in fitting keratoconus patients. No formula exists for predicting proper lens fit. The initial trial lens should have a base curve that either splits the two keratometric readings or is steeper than the average corneal curvature. Initially, apical bearing can assist in determining the patient's best contact lens–corrected visual acuity. This information is especially important if the final objective is an apical clearance fit. If the patient has never worn contact lenses, instilling a topical corneal anesthetic may be helpful in obtaining an accurate visual acuity measurement without excessive tearing. During trial lens fitting, striae may become more apparent and thus help to confirm the diagnosis.[7]

Fluorescein Pattern Analysis

Apical Clearance

The ideal keratoconic fluorescein pattern depends on the lens design chosen. A minimum apical clearance design is preferred whenever possible. The apical clearance philosophy works well for cones that have central apexes or for apexes that are displaced only slightly inferior to the visual axis.[8] This method is best for small cones but is impractical for larger cones. When properly fitted, the lens vaults the central cornea, providing clearance over the apex (Fig. 18-2). Korb et al.[9] suggested that apical

bearing may increase the rate of abrasion or corneal scarring and proposed that the apical clearance design is relatively less traumatic. Apical clearance lenses are small in diameter (8.00–8.50 mm) and have small optical zones (5.8 mm) (Table 18-1). The fluorescein pattern should show central clearance, intermediate bearing, and peripheral clearance. Lens movement must be adequate to permit proper tear exchange. Possible disadvantages of the apical clearance design are slightly reduced visual acuity as well as increased fitting time to achieve the appropriate lens fitting relationship.[10] One approach is to describe the first definite apical clearance lens.[11] This is the flattest lens from a standardized trial set (Table 18-2) that first vaults the corneal apex. This base curve correlates well with the steepest K reading.

For analysis of fit, the fluorescein pattern should be divided into two areas: the central portion (Fig. 18-3), including the entire area under the optic zone, and the peripheral zone (Fig. 18-4). The two areas should be analyzed separately. The location and amount of bearing should be observed. Analysis of fluorescein patterns in these two regions may lead to the following observations:

- If central bearing is present, the base curve radius should be steepened (Fig. 18-5).
- If pooling in the periphery is absent, the peripheral systems should be made flatter (Fig. 18-6).
- When lens movement is insufficient and excessive bearing is present in the area of the secondary curves, the secondary curve is too tight, preventing lens movement.

TABLE 18-1. *Specifications for 8-mm Diameter, 5.8-mm Optical Zone Diameter Diagnostic Set*

Curve (mm)	Power (D)	CT (mm)	Secondary Radius (mm)[a]	R3 Width/Radius (mm)	R4 Width/Radius (mm)
6.00	–12.00	0.13	8.3	0.5/9.5	0.2/10.5
6.10	–12.00	0.13	8.4	0.5/9.6	0.2/10.6
6.20	–11.00	0.13	8.5	0.5/9.7	0.2/10.7
6.30	–11.00	0.13	8.6	0.5/9.8	0.2/10.8
6.40	–10.00	0.13	8.7	0.5/9.9	0.2/10.9
6.50	–10.00	0.13	8.8	0.5/10.0	0.2/11.0
6.60	–9.00	0.13	8.9	0.5/10.1	0.2/11.1
6.70	–9.00	0.13	9.0	0.5/10.2	0.2/11.2
6.80	–8.00	0.14	9.1	0.5/10.3	0.2/11.3
6.90	–8.00	0.14	9.2	0.5/10.4	0.2/11.4
7.00	–7.00	0.14[b]	9.3	0.5/10.5	0.2/11.5
7.10	–7.00	0.14[b]	9.4	0.5/10.6	0.2/11.6
7.20	–6.00	0.14[b]	9.5	0.5/10.7	0.2/11.7
7.30	–6.00	0.14[b]	9.6	0.5/10.8	0.2/11.8
7.40	–5.00	0.14[b]	9.7	0.5/10.9	0.2/11.9
7.50	–4.00	0.14[b]	9.8	0.5/11.0	0.2/12.0

CT = center thickness.

[a]Lenses blended to 5.6-mm zone with radius 1.0 mm flatter than base curve.

[b]Lenticular construction increases edge thickness and thus prevents creating center thickness >0.14 mm.

Source: Reprinted with permission from DR Korb, VM Finnemore, JP Herman: Apical changes and scarring in keratoconus as related to contact lens fitting techniques. J Am Optom Assoc 53:199, 1982.

- Absence of fluorescein in the secondary or peripheral area may result from lens seal-off.
- Location, size, and persistence of any air bubbles under the lens should be carefully noted. The presence of a central air bubble may indicate that the lens is too steep (Fig. 18-7); presence of paracentral air bubbles, on the other hand, may indicate that the optical zone is too large (Fig. 18-8).

Figures 18-9 through 18-16 show a series of trial lenses that increase in base curve and have a relatively constant diameter. Note the decreased central bearing, decreased peripheral edge lift, and increased intermediate touch as the base curve increases. Trial lenses must settle for at least 10 minutes. When apical clearance is initially obtained, the tear film thins and the paracentral

TABLE 18-2. *Collaborative Longitudinal Evaluation of Keratoconus Study Diagnostic Contact Lens Set**

Base Curve (mm)	Power (D)	Diameter (mm)	Optical Zone Diameter (mm)
7.35	–4.00	8.6	6.5
7.20	–5.00	8.6	6.5
7.05	–6.00	8.6	6.5
6.90	–7.00	8.6	6.5
6.75	–6.00	8.6	6.5
6.60	–7.00	8.6	6.5
6.50	–7.00	8.6	6.5
6.35	–7.00	8.6	6.5
6.25	–7.00	8.6	6.5
6.15	–8.00	8.6	6.5
6.00	–7.00	8.6	6.5
5.90	–7.00	8.6	6.5
5.80	–7.00	8.6	6.5
5.70	–9.00	8.6	6.5
5.60	–8.00	8.6	6.5

*Material is polymethylmethacrylate; secondary curve/width is 8.3/0.85 mm; peripheral curve/width is 11.0/0.2 mm; thickness is 0.13 mm.

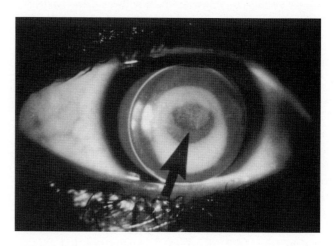

FIG. 18-3. *Central zone of contact lens (arrow).*

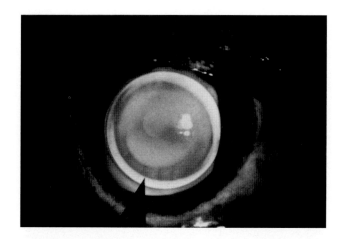

FIG. 18-4. *Peripheral zone of contact lens* (arrow).

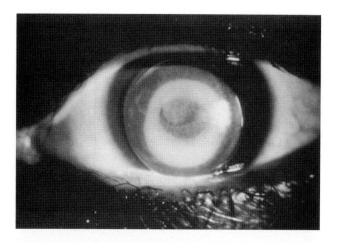

FIG. 18-6. *Tight peripheral curve.*

corneal epithelium may be compressed; in time, the lens may touch the corneal apex.

Three-Point Touch

An alternative to the apical clearance fit is the *three-point touch* design. This design is the most popular, most commonly used, and longest-advocated technique for fitting keratoconus patients.[12,13] *Three-point touch* refers to a rigid lens with a fitting relationship showing central bearing as well as two other areas of bearing at the corneal midperiphery, which are usually in the horizontal meridian.[14] The three-point touch design works well for a cone that either is centrally located or is not displaced too far inferiorly.[8] Lens diameter is usually 7.8–8.5 mm. The area of central bearing is approximately 2–3 mm in diameter

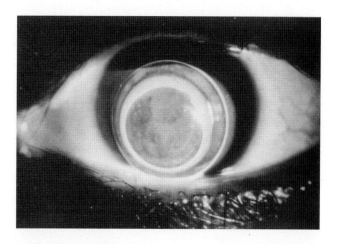

FIG. 18-7. *Central air bubble.*

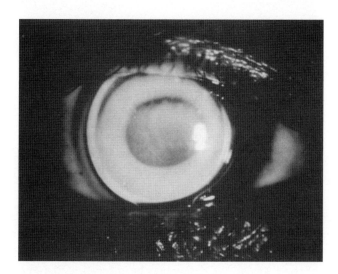

FIG. 18-5. *Excessive central bearing.*

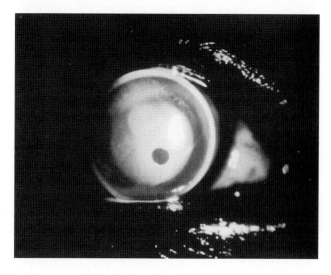

FIG. 18-8. *Paracentral air bubble.*

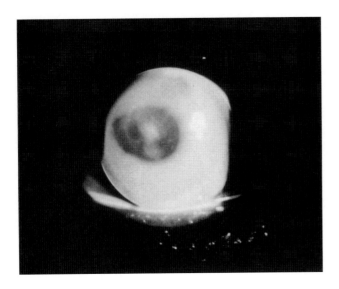

FIG. 18-9. *Base curve 48.00 D (7.03 mm), diameter 8.4 mm, optical zone diameter 7.0 mm.*

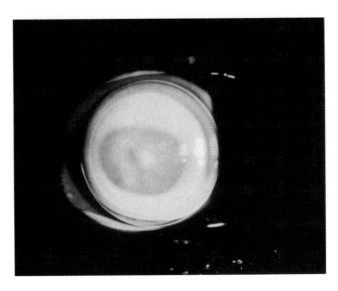

FIG. 18-11. *Base curve 51.50 D (6.55 mm), diameter 8.4 mm, optical zone diameter 7.0 mm.*

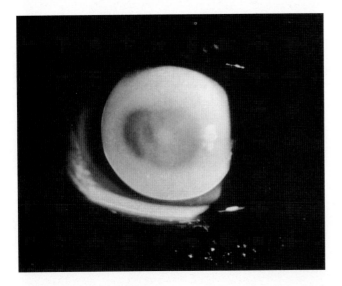

FIG. 18-10. *Base curve 49.50 D (6.82 mm), diameter 8.4 mm, optical zone diameter 7.0 mm.*

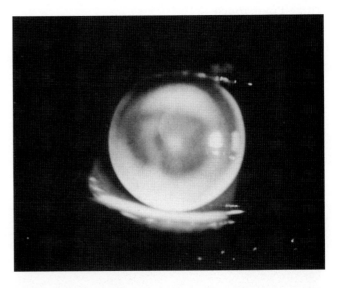

FIG. 18-12. *Base curve 53.00 D (6.37 mm), diameter 8.4 mm, optical zone diameter 7.0 mm.*

(Figs. 18-17, 18-18).[12,13,15] Distribution of lens weight among the three areas of bearing decreases lens rocking and provides a more even distribution of the lens surface and mass. Apical bearing should not exceed 2–3 mm; increased bearing may cause punctate staining or corneal erosion. Peripheral seal-off, which restricts lens movement, must be carefully avoided. Steep peripheral curves may prevent fluid interchange and lens movement. The three-point touch technique (with small lenses) cannot be used in fitting large-diameter cones or cones that are greatly displaced inferiorly (so-called sagging or oval cones) because poor lens centration usually occurs.

Corneal apex position can be evaluated on the basis of rigid trial lens fluorescein pattern or corneal mapping. As keratoconus develops, the corneal apex is usually displaced inferiorly.[16–18] Depending on steepness, size, or location of the cone, a small lens design may be impractical. If a small lens is placed on an inferiorly displaced apex, the lens tends

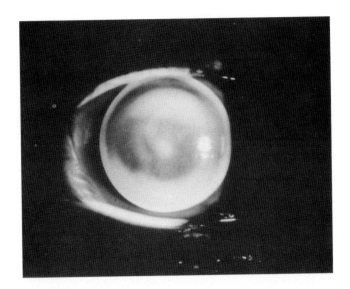

FIG. 18-13. *Base curve 54.00 D (6.24 mm), diameter 8.0 mm, optical zone diameter 6.6 mm.*

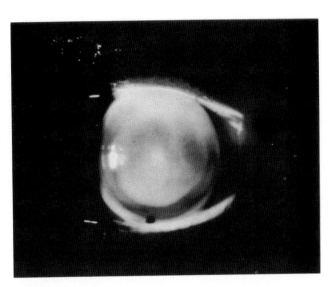

FIG. 18-15. *Base curve 57.00 D (5.92 mm), diameter 8.0 mm, optical zone diameter 6.6 mm.*

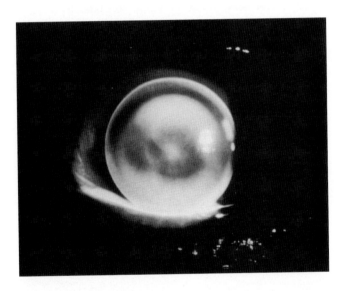

FIG. 18-14. *Base curve 55.00 D (6.14 mm), diameter 8.0 mm, optical zone diameter 6.6 mm.*

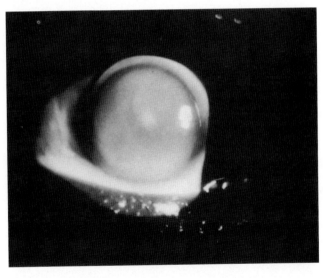

FIG. 18-16. *Base curve 59.50 D (5.67 mm), diameter 8.0 mm, optical zone diameter 6.6 mm.*

to position low and often orients in such a way that normal blinking may dislocate it. In such cases, a larger-diameter lens is preferable. The fitting objective is to position the lens so that its upper edge is always under the upper lid, thus preventing lens dislocation during blinking (Fig. 18-19). This lens is usually fitted flat, with a lens diameter of 9–10 mm. The lens peripheral curve system must also be flat enough to allow for lens movement, typically 1–2 mm flatter than standard lens designs. Large lenses are often too steep in the peripheral area and may bind to the cornea. Observing and interpreting the fluorescein pattern facilitate necessary modifications. Conversely, a very flat lens without secondary bearing often rocks and is uncomfortable (Fig. 18-20). The disadvantage of large flat lenses is that the area of bearing is often larger than with the three-point touch fit; the eye may therefore be more prone to erosion or scarring.[9]

A common clinical belief is that apical-bearing (flat-fitting) lenses, including three-point touch designs, provide bet-

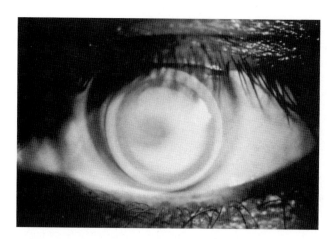

FIG. 18-17. *Acceptable three-point touch fit.*

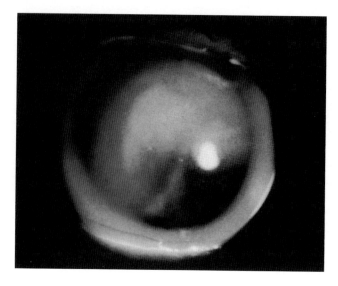

FIG. 18-19. *Lid attachment fit.*

ter long-term comfort (if central corneal epithelial erosion is absent) and better vision. This perceived advantage of flat-fitting lenses, however, is not supported by careful study.[10] Standard rigid gas-permeable (RGP) lens designs are often used for flat fitting in keratoconus, yet such indiscriminate fitting is not recommended. Apical clearance lenses may yield poorer vision and limited wearing time unless tear flow with adequate edge lift is maintained.

Aspheric lenses also have been advocated for fitting keratoconus patients. Spheric lenses have a constant radius of curvature in the optical zone area and different curvatures ground or polished into the lens periphery. Aspheric lenses, however, gradually flatten from the central area to the periphery. The *eccentricity*, or *e-value*, determines the rate of flattening and is independent of the base curve. The e-value of an average cornea is up to approximately

0.65.[14] Decreasing the lens e-value decreases the rate of flattening, whereas increasing the e-value increases the rate of flattening. When an aspheric lens is fitted, good centration is desirable. Because they have higher e-values, aspheric lenses are usually fitted with a steeper base curve than that of the three-point touch design. The fluorescein pattern should show central alignment or slight central bearing.[14] The peripheral system should show edge clearance, and lens movement should be apparent. The advantage of this lens is reduction of excessive para-apical or peripheral corneal bearing. Aspheric lenses that center over the visual axis are desirable because, when

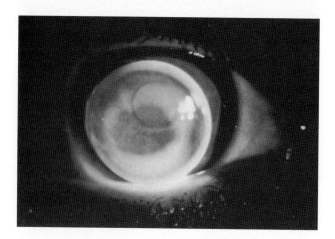

FIG. 18-18. *Unacceptable three-point touch fit.*

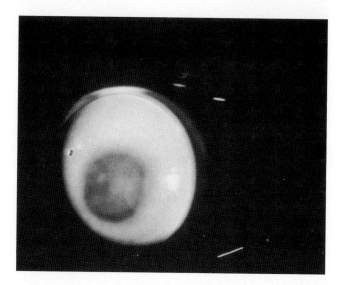

FIG. 18-20. *Excessively flat lens.*

TABLE 18-3. *Burger Keratoconus Trial Lens Set*[a,b]

Base Curve (D)	Base Curve (mm)	Power (D)	Optical Zone Diameter (mm)	Secondary Curve Diameter (mm)	Width (mm)	Blend (mm)	Peripheral Curve Width (mm)	Center Thickness (mm)
61.00	5.53	–18.00	8.4	6.0	7.5/0.6	8.5	9.5/0.4	0.15
60.00	5.63	–17.00	8.4	6.0	7.5/0.6	8.5	9.5/0.4	0.15
59.00	5.72	–16.00	8.4	6.0	8.0/0.6	9.0	10.0/0.4	0.15
58.00	5.82	–15.00	8.4	6.0	8.0/0.6	9.0	10.0/0.4	0.15
57.00	5.92	–14.00	8.8	6.4	8.0/0.6	9.0	10.0/0.4	0.15
56.00	6.03	–13.00	8.8	6.4	8.0/0.6	9.0	10.0/0.4	0.15
55.00	6.14	–12.00	8.8	6.4	8.0/0.6	9.0	10.0/0.4	0.15
54.00	6.24	–11.00	8.8	6.4	8.5/0.6	9.5	10.5/0.4	0.15
53.00	6.37	–10.00	8.8	6.4	8.5/0.6	9.5	10.5/0.4	0.15
52.00	6.49	–9.00	8.8	6.4	8.5/0.6	9.5	10.5/0.4	0.15
51.00	6.62	–8.00	8.8	6.4	8.5/0.6	9.5	10.5/0.4	0.15
50.00	6.75	–7.00	8.8	6.4	8.5/0.6	9.5	10.5/0.4	0.15
49.00	6.89	–6.00	8.8	6.4	8.5/0.6	9.5	10.5/0.4	0.15
48.00	7.03	–5.00	8.8	6.4	8.5/0.6	9.5	10.5/0.4	0.15
47.00	7.18	–4.00	8.8	6.4	8.5/0.6	9.5	10.5/0.4	0.15

[a]Material is Oxyflow F30.
[b]Allow 0.2 mm for heavy blend.

they decenter, visual acuity may be reduced (because of induced astigmatism). In theory, this approach is ideal; in practice, it may be less than ideal. Finding the correct e-value for the cornea and reproducing the lens are also difficult.

Other reports have described the use of small lenses (7.0–8.0 mm in diameter),[19] thin lens designs,[20] Polycon (Wesley-Jessen, Chicago, IL) lenses,[21-23] and aspheric silicone lenses.[24] Some clinicians believe that lower–oxygen permeability (Dk) RGP lenses are more desirable for keratoconus patients because such lenses are relatively stable (less warpage occurs), they are easily manufactured, and their use minimizes corneal epithelial injury (which is more likely when hydrophobic, higher-Dk materials are used). Regardless of the material, the desired outcome is to maximize vision and wearing time while minimizing corneal insult.

FITTING RECOMMENDATIONS

Early Keratoconus

When spectacles are no longer adequate for correcting vision, patients are fitted with contact lenses. A standard lens design (such as Polycon) may suffice in the earliest stages of keratoconus but not in the more advanced stages. Diagnostic fitting must be done carefully, using a trial lens set of known parameters (Tables 18-2 and 18-3) and striving to achieve apical clearance or minimal apical touch.

After allowing a suitable time for diagnostic lens setting, peripheral clearance and adequate edge lift must be present. The optical zone and secondary curve junction must be heavily blended. The secondary curve in all keratoconus lenses should be only approximately 1 mm flatter than the base curve to minimize the junction between the base curve and secondary curve and thereby allow this junction to be easily and optimally blended. Because the secondary curve may be steep (e.g., for a lens with a 6.45-mm base curve, the secondary curve should be 7.5 mm), multiple flatter peripheral curves are needed (such as 9.0-mm and 12.5-mm curves, of equal width and well blended). A good guideline is to keep the optical zone of the lens roughly equal to the base curve, estimated to the nearest 0.1 mm.

Because keratoconus lenses may have very high edge-lift values (nearly 0.25 mm compared with 0.1 mm for standard lenses), lenticular designs are needed when thin lenses are desired. Modification of lens peripheral curves, blending, and edging are necessary practitioner skills.

Advanced Keratoconus

In fitting advanced keratoconus patients with contact lenses, keeping the posterior surface of the lens clean is extremely important. Because apical clearance is minimal or impossible to achieve, deposits may erode the epithelium. For oval, sagging cones, use a larger lens with apical touch; for central, nipple cones, strive for minimal apical touch.

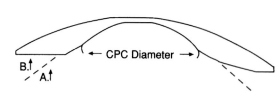

The second curve used on each lens A. (43.00 or 45.00) is to facilitate the placement in that area of the parabolic peripheral and intermediate curves, which creates a "ski-like" configuration B. to fit over the flat peripheral area of the cornea. The diameter of the CPC is critical as it is used to calculate the sagittal depth of the lens.

		Sagittal Depth (mm)	CPC (D)	Power (D)	Lens Diameter (mm)	Thickness (mm)	CPC Diameter (oz mm)
Moderate Cone	Try first						
	A	0.68	48.00/43.00	- 4.5	7.5	0.10	6.0
	B	0.73	52.00/45.00	- 8.50	7.5	0.10	6.0
	C	0.80	56.00/45.00	- 12.50	7.5	0.10	6.0
	D	0.87	60.00/45.00	- 16.50	7.5	0.10	6.0
Advanced Cone	Try first						
	E	1.00	52.00/45.00	- 8.50	8.5	0.10	7.0
	F	1.12	56.00/45.00	- 12.50	8.5	0.10	7.0
	G	1.22	60.00/45.00	- 16.50	8.5	0.10	7.0
Severe Cone	Try first						
	H	1.37	52.00/45.00	- 8.50	9.5	0.10	8.0
	I	1.52	56.00/45.00	-12.50	9.5	0.10	8.0
	J	1.67	60.00/45.00	-16.50	9.5	0.10	8.0

Note: The sagittal value (vaulting effect) of lens H (a 52.00D) is much greater than lens D (a 60.00D) because of the much larger diameter (9.5 mm) of the H lens.

FIG. 18-21. *Soper keratoconic system. (CPC = central posterior curve.) (Reprinted with permission from D Burger, K Zadnik: Contact lenses in ocular disease: keratoconus. p. 643. In MG Harris [ed]: Problems in Optometry. Vol. 2. Lippincott, Philadelphia, 1990.)*

KERATOCONUS LENS SYSTEMS

Many lens systems exist for fitting keratoconus patients. Often, these systems provide a cookbook approach in suggesting, for example, that lens diameter be increased as the cone progresses. However, small apical clearance or minimal apical touch lenses in advanced keratoconus are typically preferred unless the apex is quite decentered or oval.

Soper Lens System

The fitting objective of the Soper lens system, popularized by Soper and Jarrett,[25] is based on sagittal depth. The principle on which this system was developed is that spe-

cific base curves and secondary curves with increased diameter result in increased sagittal depth and thus a steeper-fitting lens.[8] The lenses included in the fitting set are categorized as mild (7.5-mm diameter, 6.0-mm optical zone diameter [OZD]), moderate (8.5-mm diameter, 7.0-mm OZD), and advanced (9.5-mm diameter, 8.0-mm OZD). The initial trial lens is selected on the basis of degree of advancement of the cone (Fig. 18-21 and Table 18-4).[8,26] The more advanced the cone, the larger the diameter of the recommended lens; the smaller and more centrally located the apex, the smaller the diameter of the lens. The smallest-diameter lens is best for nipple cones, whereas the advanced, largest-diameter lens is recommended for larger, oval (sagging) cones. Soper (personal communication, 1992) states that his lens, when properly manufactured, is not a

TABLE 18-4. *Cellulose Acetate Butyrate Soper Cone Trial Lens Set**

Lens	CPC (D)	CPC (mm)	Power (D)	Sagittal Depth (mm)	Lens Diameter (mm)	Thickness (mm)	CPC Diameter (mm)
1	47.75/43.00	7.07/7.85	−7.87	0.68	7.85	0.15	6.0
2	52.50/45.00	6.43/7.50	−8.37	0.74	7.90	0.15	6.0
3	56.75/45.00	5.96/7.50	−12.62	0.82	7.80	0.15	6.0
4	59.50/45.00	5.67/7.50	−15.50	0.86	7.85	0.17	6.1
5	52.25/45.00	6.46/7.50	−8.50	1.05	8.80	0.16	7.2
6	56.75/45.00	5.95/7.50	−8.75	1.17	8.80	0.18	7.2
7	59.75/45.00	5.64/7.50	−15.75	1.22	8.80	0.17	7.0
8	52.25/45.00	6.46/7.50	−8.25	1.37	9.90	0.15	8.0
9	56.75/45.00	5.95/7.50	−12.50	1.59	9.90	0.17	8.2
10	59.50/45.00	5.68/7.50	−16.00	1.72	9.90	0.16	8.2

CPC = central posterior curvature (bicurve lens).
*All lenses have 26 D (0.2 mm wide) diamond-tool generated and polished curves and are blended with 37 D (0.2 mm wide) and 40 D (0.1 mm wide) velveteen tools.
Source: Reprinted with permission from IM Raber: Use of CAB Soper Cone contact lenses in keratoconus. CLAO J 9:237, 1983.

bicurve lens but incorporates the following curvatures: a 26-D curve (0.2 mm wide), initially generated using a diamond tool; a 37-D curve (0.2 mm wide), generated using a velveteen tool; and a 40-D curve (0.1 mm wide), generated using a velveteen tool. When carefully manufactured (according to Soper), these curves are all blended together. Many laboratories, however, inappropriately manufacture this lens as a bicurve lens with a peripheral system, which may be too steep. The secondary curve, 7.5 mm (45 D), remains the same regardless of whether the base curve is 52 D or 62 D. When central alignment is achieved, clearance in the periphery is often inadequate, resulting in inadequate lens movement and tear exchange and the need to modify (flatten) the lens periphery.

McGuire Lens System

The McGuire keratoconic system is a modification of the Soper lens design.[27] In the McGuire system, fitting sets are categorized as nipple (8.1-mm diameter, 5.5-mm OZD), oval (8.6-mm diameter, 6-mm OZD), and globus (9.1-mm diameter, 6.5-mm OZD) (Table 18-5).[28] The McGuire system has four peripheral curves; the three inner curves are 0.3 mm wide and the peripheral curve is 0.4 mm wide. From most central to most peripheral, the curves are 3 D (0.5 mm), 9 D (1.5 mm), 17 D (3 mm), and 27 D (5 mm) flatter than the base curve. This lens system allows adequate edge clearance and movement.

Ni-Cone Lens System

The Ni-Cone lens system (Lancaster Contact Lens Co., Lancaster, PA) is promoted as having three base curves and one constant peripheral curve of 12.25 mm.

Ni-Cone fitting sets are designated by numbers 1–3. The no. 1 cone set is for patients with K readings 40–52 D, the no. 2 set is for patients with K readings of 53–65 D, and the no. 3 set is for patients with K readings more than 65 D. The preferred lens alignment is a *feather touch*.[29] The *second base curve* is a 0.3-mm transition zone between the central base curve and the *third base curve*, which rests on the normal peripheral cornea. The manufacturer indicates that "lathe cut, optically polished peripheral base curves prevent optical distortion that ground curvatures create in a lens."[29] In reality, these additional base curves are peripheral curves added to improve lens performance. The lens diameter and all other parameters vary, depending on lens steepness. A disadvantage of this system is that the p-values the manufacturer uses for the peripheral curvatures are unknown (owing to their patented design). Not knowing the curvatures of the lens in the peripheral areas limits the practitioner's ability to modify the lens and necessitates relying on the laboratory for fitting design changes.

Rose K Design

The Rose K design is a unique keratoconus lens design. The system (26-lens set) allows the practitioner to choose lens options based on a systematic fitting approach. The design starts with a standard 8.7-mm diameter that incorporates a decreasing optic zone as the base curve steepens, coupled with an intrinsic, computer-designed peripheral curve system. The lens is provided through Lens Dynamics, Inc. (Denver, CO) and is manufactured on a DAC lathe. Like the Ni-Cone lens, the Rose K lens has an unknown peripheral curve system, but the Rose K system provides the practitioner some latitude in design-

TABLE 18-5. *McGuire Lens Fitting Sets*

Base Curve (D)	Power (D)	Diameter (mm)	Optical Zone (mm)	Peripheral Curves (Radius [D]/Width [mm])			
Oval-cone fitting set							
50.00	−8.00	8.6	6.0	47.00/0.3	41.00/0.3	33.00/0.3	23.00/0.4
51.00	−8.00	8.6	6.0	48.00/0.3	42.00/0.3	34.00/0.3	24.00/0.4
52.00	−10.00	8.6	6.0	49.00/0.3	43.00/0.3	35.00/0.3	25.00/0.4
53.00	−10.00	8.6	6.0	50.00/0.3	44.00/0.3	36.00/0.3	26.00/0.4
54.00	−12.00	8.6	6.0	51.00/0.3	45.00/0.3	37.00/0.3	27.00/0.4
55.00	−12.00	8.6	6.0	52.00/0.3	46.00/0.3	38.00/0.3	28.00/0.4
56.00	−14.00	8.6	6.0	53.00/0.3	47.00/0.3	39.00/0.3	29.00/0.4
57.00	−14.00	8.6	6.0	54.00/0.3	48.00/0.3	40.00/0.3	30.00/0.4
58.00	−16.00	8.6	6.0	55.00/0.3	49.00/0.3	41.00/0.3	31.00/0.4
59.00	−18.00	8.6	6.0	56.00/0.3	50.00/0.3	42.00/0.3	32.00/0.4
60.00	−18.00	8.6	6.0	57.00/0.3	51.00/0.3	43.00/0.3	33.00/0.4
61.00	−18.00	8.6	6.0	58.00/0.3	52.00/0.3	44.00/0.3	34.00/0.4
Nipple-cone fitting set							
50.00	−8.00	8.1	5.5	47.00/0.3	41.00/0.3	33.00/0.3	23.00/0.4
52.00	−10.00	8.1	5.5	49.00/0.3	43.00/0.3	35.00/0.3	25.00/0.4
54.00	−12.00	8.1	5.5	51.00/0.3	45.00/0.3	37.00/0.3	27.00/0.4
56.00	−14.00	8.1	5.5	53.00/0.3	47.00/0.3	39.00/0.3	29.00/0.4
58.00	−16.00	8.1	5.5	55.00/0.3	49.00/0.3	41.00/0.3	31.00/0.4
60.00	−18.00	8.1	5.5	57.00/0.3	51.00/0.3	43.00/0.3	33.00/0.4
"Globus" cone fitting set							
50.00	−8.00	9.1	6.5	47.00/0.3	41.00/0.3	33.00/0.3	23.00/0.4
52.00	−10.00	9.1	6.5	49.00/0.3	43.00/0.3	35.00/0.3	25.00/0.4
54.00	−12.00	9.1	6.5	51.00/0.3	45.00/0.3	37.00/0.3	27.00/0.4
56.00	−14.00	9.1	6.5	53.00/0.3	47.00/0.3	39.00/0.3	29.00/0.4
58.00	−16.00	9.1	6.5	55.00/0.3	49.00/0.3	41.00/0.3	31.00/0.4
60.00	−18.00	9.1	6.5	57.00/0.3	51.00/0.3	43.00/0.3	33.00/0.4

Source: Adapted from PJ Caroline, JR McGuire, DJ Doughman: Preliminary report on a new contact lens design for keratoconus. Contact Intraocul Lens Med J 4:69, 1978.

ing the peripheral lens system with the many options available. Flatter peripheral curves, as well as steeper peripheral curves, are available if the standard lens lift is inadequate. Additional lens diameters are available when needed (8.3 mm, 9.0 mm). Peripheral curves as well as base curves can be configured in a toric design if necessary. Front surface cylinder using truncation for stability is an additional option.

SOFT LENS AND COMBINATION LENS ALTERNATIVES

Use of soft lenses as well as combination lens alternatives has been advocated in fitting keratoconus patients.

SoftPerm Lens

The SoftPerm lens (Wesley-Jessen, Chicago, IL) is a hybrid lens, with an RGP center surrounded by a soft hydrophilic skirt (Fig. 18-22). This lens may be indicated for patients with displaced corneal apexes or for rigid lens–intolerant patients. Advantages of the lens are its one-piece design, better centration on displaced apexes, and improved comfort compared to RGP lenses. The Soft-

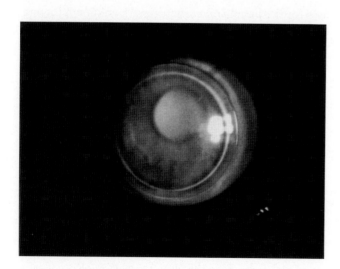

FIG. 18-22. *SoftPerm lens.*

FIG. 18-23. *Flexlens Piggyback Lens design (Paragon Vision Sciences, Mesa, AZ). (Reprinted with permission from PJ Caroline, DJ Doughman: A new piggyback lens design for correction of irregular astigmatism: a preliminary report. Contact Lens J 13:39, 1979.)*

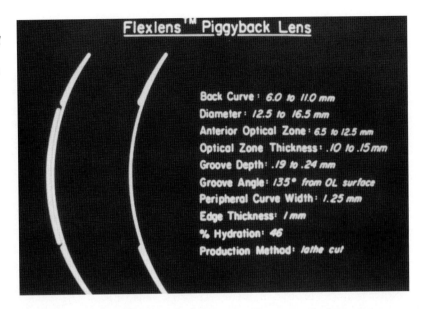

Perm lens does have limitations, however. In early keratoconus, most patients can be successfully fitted with rigid lenses. SoftPerm lenses may fit such patients too tightly, providing inadequate lens movement. For patients with advanced keratoconus, in which a larger-diameter lens is useful, the range of steep base curves is limited (its steepest base curve is 6.5 mm). In addition, the lens material has a low Dk value (rigid lens, 14 Dk; soft portion, 5.5 Dk). The major problems associated with this lens are difficult handling (problems occurring with lens removal), lack of lens movement, corneal edema, and neovascularization.

Piggyback Lens Designs

A piggyback lens system consists of a rigid lens fitted on top of a soft lens.[30] Indications for this technique are rigid lens intolerance or mechanical problems, such as recurrent corneal erosion. The combination of rigid and soft lenses results in visual acuity equal to that achieved using a rigid lens alone.[31] Another advantage of this system is that because the soft lens decreases the corneal curvature difference between the central and peripheral cornea, the base curve of the rigid lens used in combination with the soft lens is often flatter than the base curve of a rigid lens alone. Only highly oxygen-transmitting materials should be used for both components.

The most important factor in successfully fitting patients with this system is that the soft lens should move adequately. If the lens binds, the patient typically encounters physiologic problems. The RGP lens should have minimal center and edge thickness to promote centration

and comfort, as well as a rounded edge to prevent tearing the soft lens. Keratometry over the soft lens aids in the selection of the initial rigid lens. To evaluate the fit of the rigid lens, the presence and location of oxygen bubbles under the rigid lens should be noted. Central bubbles indicate a steep lens, whereas bubbles near the lens edge indicate a flat fit. Patients should use soft lens solutions with a piggyback system. Many rigid lens solutions contain preservatives, which may be toxic to the cornea in high concentrations, and soft lenses may absorb these solutions.

Piggyback systems are often used in difficult keratoconic cases but not as the preferred lens system because caring for three or four lenses on a long-term basis is often difficult. An example of an indication for use of a piggyback lens system is noninfectious mechanical epithelial erosion. Because the patient has keratoconus, discontinuing contact lens wear would severely handicap the patient visually. One option is to use a disposable lens (lowest minus power) as a bandage while allowing the patient to wear a high-Dk RGP lens over the soft lens. Wearing time should be minimal in these instances.

A unique type of piggyback system is the Flexlens Piggyback Lens (Paragon Vision Sciences, Mesa, AZ) (Figs. 18-23, 18-24).[32] This thick soft lens, available in 45% or 55% water-content materials and diameters ranging from 12.5 mm to 16.00 mm, has a counter-sunk groove that accepts an RGP lens. The rigid lens is designed so that thickness of the lens plus the tear reservoir is equal to the groove depth. If the rigid lens is too thick, it protrudes from the groove and may be blinked out; if the lens is too thin, the entire system may dislocate if the lid catches the groove during blinking. To permit tear

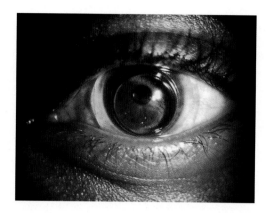

FIG. 18-24. *Piggyback contact lens system.*

exchange, the rigid lens should be made 0.1–0.2 mm smaller than the groove diameter. The rigid lens fit is evaluated by observing the location of any oxygen bubbles. The main objective of this system is to ensure centration of the rigid lens in advanced keratoconus while providing a comfortable lens system. The disadvantages of counter-sunk piggyback lenses include the inconvenience of a two-lens system, corneal edema, neovascularization, and ripping of the soft lens at the groove junction. In addition to applications for advanced keratoconus, this lens system can also be used for postkeratoplasty or trauma conditions.

Hydrogel Lenses

Keratoconus patients who are rigid lens intolerant or patients with early disease are occasionally fitted with conventional soft lenses.[33,34] The main advantage is greater comfort. Use of a soft lens may partly correct irregular astigmatism, thus permitting spectacle overcorrection.

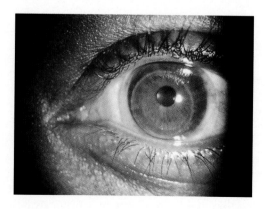

FIG. 18-25. *Soft keratoconus lens.*

Power to reduce anisometropia also can be placed in the soft lens. Compared with rigid lenses, the disadvantages of soft lenses are reduced visual acuity and the need for spectacle overcorrection for best visual acuity.

Specialized soft lenses are also available for keratoconus. Because these lenses are extremely thick (0.3–0.5 mm), they sometimes correct keratoconus as effectively as rigid lenses. This lens design is most often indicated for patients in whom a rigid lens cannot be fitted because of severe apical displacement, an extremely steep cone, or a particularly large-diameter cone. In such cases, the large diameter of the hydrogel lens (14–15 mm) allows it to bear on the sclera and the corneal apex (Fig. 18-25), enabling centration of the lens, which may not be possible with smaller rigid lenses. One available custom soft lens for incipient keratoconus is the Flexlens Harrison Keratoconus Lens (Paragon Vision Sciences, Mesa, AZ), which is available in 45% and 55% water-content materials. It can be made in any spheric power, in a base curve range from 6.0 to 9.9 mm. Diameters range from 10.0 to 16.0 mm, and the lens has a center thickness of 0.25 mm at –3.00 D.

For moderate or more advanced keratoconus, the Flexlens Tricurve Keratoconus Lens (Paragon Vision Sciences, Mesa, AZ) is available. This is thicker than the Harrison Lens, with a standard and recommended center thickness of 0.40 mm. The center thickness can be customized. For example, a center thickness of 0.30 mm may be selected to maximize oxygen transmissibility to the cornea, whereas a thicker lens (up to 0.60 mm) could be considered to improve visual performance. This lens is available in a base curve range from 6.0 mm to 10.0 mm, in diameters from 10.0 mm to 16.0 mm, and in powers from +30.00 D to –30.00 D. When high-molecular-weight fluorescein is instilled in the eye wearing this lens, the fluorescein pattern under the lens may appear similar to that of a rigid lens (Fig. 18-26). Lens movement is vital for a successful fit, and patients should be monitored for the potential development of corneal edema and vascularization.

Another soft cone lens is the Fre-Flex Cone Lens (Optech, Inc., Englewood, CO). This lens design is based on sagittal depth. The base curve (8.4 mm) and diameter (14 mm) of the lens are held constant. The OZD is varied to produce different fitting relationships. The larger the OZD, the steeper fitting the lens becomes. These lenses, which are made of 55% water-content material, are ordered as Cone A (5.9-mm OZD), Cone B (6.9-mm OZD), or Cone C (7.9-mm OZD). The Cone A lens, although the flattest, is often successful even for steep cones and should be tried before the steeper B and C lenses. As with the Flexlens, the Fre-Flex lens must be monitored for the potential development of corneal edema and vascularization.

PROBLEM SOLVING

The practitioner is often called on to solve a number of problems related to fitting contact lenses to a keratoconus patient. These problems may include lack of lens movement, reduced visual acuity, poor lens centration, rapidly changing lens-fitting relationships, and corneal staining. Successful fitting often depends on solving these problems.

Lack of Contact Lens Movement

Lack of lens movement (also termed *lens binding*) may be caused by peripheral curve seal-off, secondary curve seal-off, or a sharp junction at the optic zone border.

Peripheral curve seal-off occurs when the peripheral curve is too steep, which causes the lens to bind at the edge and thus prevent lens movement and tear interchange (see Fig. 18-6). Keratoconus is a disease of the central cornea and usually does not affect the peripheral cornea.[16,17] The peripheral curvature radii of the lens should be chosen accordingly. For example, a normal cornea with a central curvature of 43.00–43.50 D requires a peripheral contact lens curvature of approximately 10.5 mm. If the practitioner orders peripheral curves based on the same relationship of peripheral curve to base curve as is used with conventional (nonkeratoconic) lenses, the peripheral curve system is excessively steep. As a result, these lenses do not have adequate edge lift and bind to the cornea. This problem can be corrected by specifying flatter peripheral curves when the lens is ordered.

The second most common reason for lack of lens movement is excessive tightness of the secondary curve. Adequate edge lift is evident in the fluorescein pattern from pooling (which indicates a tear reservoir), accompanied by a large, dark intermediate (or secondary) bearing area (Fig. 18-27). In such cases, the tight intermediate area restricts lens movement. This tightness results when the secondary curve is too steep or too wide and thus prevents fluid interchange and lens movement. This deficiency is corrected either by using a flatter curvature or by decreasing the intermediate curve width (i.e., increasing peripheral curve width).

The third reason for lack of lens movement is a sharp junction between the secondary curve and base curve at the optic zone border, leading to lens seal-off, which may cause discomfort and epithelial erosion. This problem is remedied by blending this area heavily so that the lens has a rounded junction, enabling increased lens movement.

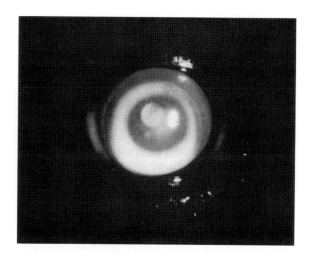

FIG. 18-26. *Fluorescein pattern of soft cone lens.*

Reduced Visual Acuity

Another problem in keratoconus patients is reduced visual acuity, which may result from incorrect power, corneal scarring, lens flexure, lens deposits, residual astigmatism, too steep a lens, or poor centration.

A common reason for reduced visual acuity (in addition to scarring) is overminusing. In fitting keratoconus patients, many practitioners tend to prescribe too much minus power. Overminusing is more likely to occur when a patient is tearing profusely and has not adapted to the lenses.

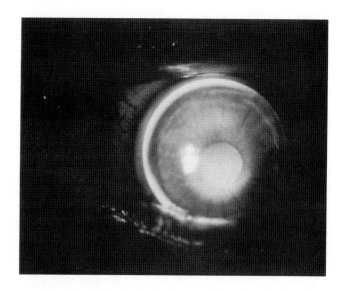

FIG. 18-27. *Excessive secondary bearing.*

One way to prevent overminusing is to use a topical anesthetic to prevent reflex tearing. Another approach is to compare the total effective power of each trial lens system to achieve consistency.

Example:

	Base Curve (D)	Back Vertex Power (D)	Over-refraction (D)	Net Power (D)
Trial lens 1	50.00	–10.00	–2.00	–12.00
Trial lens 2	53.00	–11.00	–4.00	–15.00

In this example, steepening the base curve by 3.00 D creates a fluid lens of +3.00 D. To compensate, an equal amount of minus power (–3.00 D) must be added. Therefore, a lens with parameters of 50.00/–12.00 is in theory equal to a lens with parameters of 53.00/–15.00. Although this guideline may not hold as precisely for keratoconus patients as for patients with normal corneas, it is a useful guide to prevent overminusing. In addition, over-refraction at follow-up visits is essential to check the power of the system as the patient adapts.

Another cause of reduced visual acuity is corneal scarring. Corneal scarring in the visual axis reduces visual acuity.[35] The denser the scarring, the greater the reduction in visual acuity. Korb et al.[9] believe that the incidence of corneal scarring can be minimized by fitting lenses with apical clearance.

Lens flexure also may reduce visual acuity. Keratoconus lenses are very steep and of high power; if they are made too thin, the lenses may flex. Lens flexure, which manifests as residual astigmatism,[36] can be measured by performing keratometry over the contact lens (i.e., over-K). If flexure is absent, the keratometric reading is spheric; if flexure is present, the keratometric reading is not spheric. Using a thicker lens and a moderate-Dk lens polymer instead of a high-Dk lens can help to prevent lens flexure. The higher the Dk, the softer the lens material is likely to be and the more the lens flexes.

Deposits on lens surfaces, or anything that reduces lens clarity, also may reduce visual acuity. Lenses should be cleaned daily with a surfactant and weekly with an enzymatic cleaner. The lens surface should be free of scratches because deposits may collect in such irregular areas. Polishing the lens surface or replacing the lens when indicated minimizes these problems.

Another cause of reduced visual acuity is residual astigmatism. Like lens flexure, such astigmatism occurs while the lens is in place. However, unlike lens flexure, over-Ks read spheric. Residual astigmatism, in this case, is caused either by the crystalline lens or, more likely, the corneal surfaces. Keratoconus is a disease of the entire cornea, not just the front surface.[37] A contact lens corrects the front surface corneal irregularity but not an irregular back surface or distorted corneal stroma. Therefore, some patients, especially in advanced keratoconus, have residual astigmatism.

To correct residual astigmatism, the practitioner has two prescription alternatives: overglasses containing the residual correction or a toric contact lens. The toric lens design may be either a front cylinder, prism-ballast lens or a cylindrical power effect bitoric lens. Although both lenses can be prescribed for keratoconus, they are prescribed only rarely because obtaining properly designed lenses is difficult. Therefore, overglasses appear to be the best choice when residual astigmatism is present.

A lens that is too steep also may reduce visual acuity. Steep lenses that have tight peripheral systems may produce less than optimal correction. In some cases, when an apical clearance fit is obtained, vision is apparently degraded.[10,37] Therefore, some patients need a lens that bears to some extent on the corneal apex for best vision.

The last reason for reduced visual acuity is poor centration. As keratoconus develops, the corneal apex decenters inferiorly, often causing the contact lens to ride low. As a result, the patient may use the peripheral area of the lens instead of the optical zone area. To correct this problem, the practitioner must change the fitting approach, increasing the lens diameter or using a larger, flatter-fitting lens to achieve a lid attachment fit.

Poor Lens Centration

Poor lens centration is caused by either a decentered corneal apex or an extremely flat-fitting lens. The steeper the cornea becomes, the more decentered (usually inferior) the apex becomes and the more difficult it is to fit a contact lens to the eye. In these cases, the lens often rides low. In addition, if a small lens is fitted to a decentered apex, the lens may become decentered when the patient blinks. In such cases, a larger, flatter lens can be used to create a lid attachment fit.

Excessively flat-fitting lenses may also cause poor lens centration. A lens may be so flat that it rocks on the corneal apex and never establishes a proper contact lens fitting relationship (see Fig. 18-20). When the patient blinks, the lens may decenter inferiorly, temporally, nasally, or superiorly and may eject. In such cases, the contact lens fit must be steepened appropriately by conducting a complete diagnostic trial lens fitting.

Rapidly Changing Fitting Relationships

Another problem in fitting keratoconus patients is rapidly changing fitting relationships between the contact lens

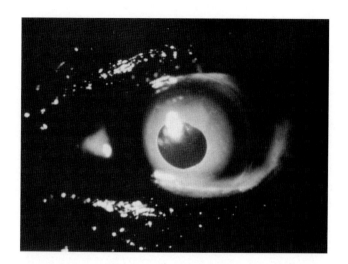

FIG. 18-28. *Initial lens evaluation of 6.25-mm base curve after removal of a lens with a 7.35-mm base curve.*

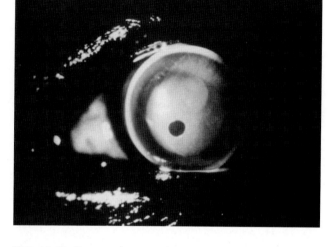

FIG. 18-29. *Lens evaluation of patient shown in Figure 18-28 after 20 minutes.*

and the cornea. Keratoconus patients often have rapid corneal steepening (or cone advancement), necessitating frequent contact lens changes (which may be needed as often as every 3–4 months). The rapid advancement stage in keratoconus usually does not exceed 5 years, after which changes occur much less frequently.[38]

Changing fitting relationships may often be observed when the practitioner does not allow the diagnostic keratoconic lens to settle adequately during fitting. For example, the practitioner places a diagnostic lens on the eye; if the lens appears to be too flat, the practitioner may remove it and place a steeper lens on the eye. Evaluating the lens immediately, the practitioner may determine it to be aligned and order it on the basis of this observation. After the patient wears the lens for some time, the lens pattern often appears too flat at the first progress visit. Diagnostic lenses should be allowed to settle for at least 10–20 minutes. Keratoconic corneas are very pliable, especially if the previous lens was flat. In a patient who is refitted after wearing a flat lens, the cornea may change dramatically (steepening as much as 4–6 D) in 15–20 minutes. If the lens has not settled long enough at the fitting, a fit that was apparently appropriate at the diagnostic lens fitting and that looked good on dispensing looks too flat at the first progress visit. The error is compounded if the practitioner then simply places another lens on the eye, evaluates it quickly, and, if the fit looks appropriate, reorders the lens, not allowing for corneal recovery time or time for the lens to settle.

Adequate lens settling time allows the cornea to unmold from a flat lens. Figures 18-28, 18-29, and 18-30 show steepening of the cornea during a 40-minute period after

removal of a flat lens. Diagnostic fitting may require 1–2 hours to allow ample time for effects of previous contact lenses to be neutralized. Practitioners may find that subsequent lenses appear substantially steeper when diagnostic lenses are given ample time to settle.

Corneal Staining

Another primary cause for concern is corneal staining, which may be either central or peripheral. Peripheral staining may occur because of tight peripheral curves, poor blending, dryness, or partial blinking.

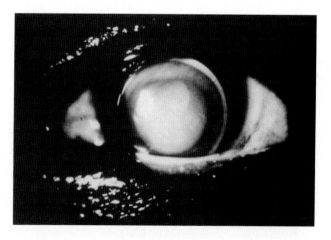

FIG. 18-30. *Lens evaluation of patient shown in Figure 18-28 after 40 minutes.*

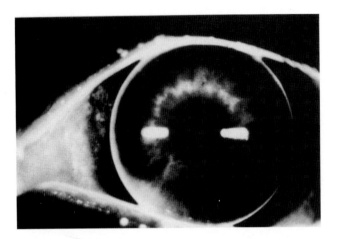

FIG. 18-31. *Three and 9 o'clock staining. (Courtesy of Dr. Cristina Schnider.)*

Tight peripheral curves result in staining at the edges of the lens and a lens indentation mark. This problem is corrected by using flatter, well-blended peripheral and secondary curves. Staining of the peripheral cornea (3 and 9 o'clock) also may be present, as a result of either dryness or partial blinking (Fig. 18-31). Edge improvements, lubricants, and blinking exercises should be prescribed as necessary.

Central corneal staining may be caused by lack of normal epithelial cells or lenses that are excessively flat or have many deposits on the posterior surface. The earliest histopathologic sign in keratoconus appears in the basal layer of the epithelium.[39] The cells of this layer are destroyed, and because the cornea heals itself from the posterior forward, epithelial cell dropout results. The corneal epithelium is regenerated from the periphery by mitosis, resulting in the *swirl staining* characteristic of keratoconus (Fig. 18-32).[40-42] This staining pattern may occur even when lenses are not being worn. Excessively flat lenses may abrade the cornea. Staining may appear as enhanced swirl staining or may advance to corneal erosion (Fig. 18-33). The base curves of the lenses must be steepened to eliminate central bearing, which reduces mechanical trauma. In prescribing steeper lenses to decrease central staining, proper secondary and peripheral curve designs must be incorporated to reduce trauma to the central cornea and prevent peripheral lens seal-off and resultant peripheral staining. Some surgeons remove the stained, raised epithelial lesion that may occur in advanced keratoconus (the so-called proud nebula) by superficial keratectomy.[43] After bandage lens therapy and total epithelial healing, rigid contact lens wear may resume sooner with this treatment than without it.

Lens Discomfort

Another problem encountered in fitting keratoconus patients is contact lens discomfort. Many keratoconus patients find contact lenses uncomfortable. The possible causes of discomfort (assuming edges are properly manufactured) include flat lenses, steep lenses, excessive edge lift, and general lens intolerance. Flat lenses that rock on the corneal apex are uncomfortable and may also cause corneal erosion. A lens that is fitted too steep or that has peripheral curve seal-off may feel fine initially but, after a period of wear, causes discomfort because of improper tear circulation and peripheral epithelial erosion.

Discomfort may also result from a very flat lens periphery. When excessive edge lift results in edge standoff, the lens is uncomfortable and is likely to decenter. A

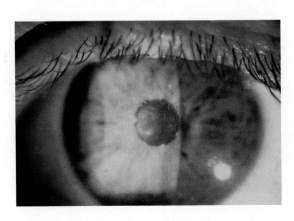

FIG. 18-32. *Swirl staining. (Courtesy of Dr. Lisa Badowski.)*

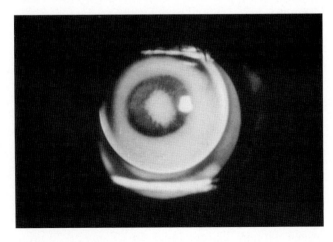

FIG. 18-33. *Corneal erosion.*

lens that has an adequate peripheral curve, neither too tight nor too flat, is more comfortable.

If a lens fitting relationship looks good but the patient is still uncomfortable, the patient may be contact lens intolerant. In such cases, a piggyback system may provide the patient with adequate comfort and wearing time. This may be the only viable option for correcting vision in advanced keratoconus (short of penetrating keratoplasty) when spectacles are inadequate.

Well-blended secondary and peripheral curve systems are important in successfully fitting keratoconus patients. Lenses that are poorly blended are uncomfortable and may bind to the cornea. The practitioner must design the lens to incorporate the blended area. A medium blend occupies 0.1 mm and a heavy blend 0.2 mm. A traditional lens (e.g., diameter 8.0 mm, OZD 6.0 mm, secondary curve 8.5/0.6 mm, and peripheral curve 10.5/0.4 mm) is therefore only lightly blended. Either the peripheral system or the OZD must be reduced to compensate for heavier blends. This reduction may explain the variability between duplicated keratoconic lenses. If the laboratory compensates, the OZD may be reduced one time and the peripheral system may be reduced the next time.

Specifying all lens parameters increases the accuracy of lens reproduction. To control the design, the manufacturer must be told exactly where a particular part of the lens must be changed. Careful measurement is essential: If a lens with a specific base curve–to–OZD fitting relationship is ordered and the manufacturer supplies a lens with a different base curve–to–OZD fitting relationship, the resultant fit is either too steep or too flat.

MODIFICATIONS

In fitting keratoconus patients, the ability to make lens modifications is vital. Returning the contact lens to the manufacturer for modifications is often impractical. A patient who needs a lens with parameters of 50.00/−16.00 D cannot see without the lens. Figures 18-34, 18-35, and 18-36 show how a lens with a tight peripheral system leaves an imprint on the cornea and how the lens appears after modification.

Many modification units are available, but the most efficient ones have multiple spindles for grinding and polishing (Fig. 18-37).[8] An extensive selection of tools, especially for creating steep curvatures, is necessary. Diamond-impregnated brass tools are recommended for making major modifications. Tools should range from 7.5 to 12.00 mm (45.00–27.00 D) in 0.5-mm steps. To polish out the rough cut, polishing laps with radii of 6.60–12.00 mm (51.00–27.00 D) are recommended. The

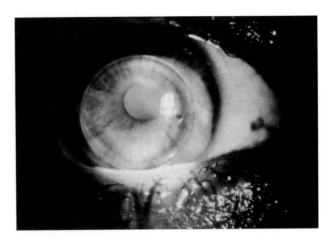

FIG. 18-34. *Tight contact lens.*

differences in laps should be 0.15 mm at the steep end (6.60–7.50 mm), 0.5–1.0 mm at the flat end (9.0–12.0 mm), and 0.2–0.5 mm in the normal corneal curvature range (7.8–9.0 mm). These ranges of diamond tools and polishing laps should suffice for modifying most secondary and peripheral curves. A polishing lap steeper than the diamond tool is often needed to remove tool marks completely. Waterproof adhesive tape, velveteen, and RGP polish are needed for polishing curves and blending. Using liberal amounts of polish, minimizing dwell times (short application, done within seconds), and limiting the amount of pressure on the lap during polishing are essential to prevent distortion and lens damage.

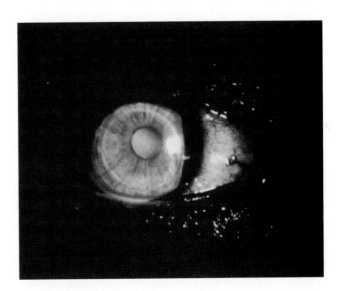

FIG. 18-35. *Imprint of the tight lens shown in Fig. 18-34 on the patient's cornea.*

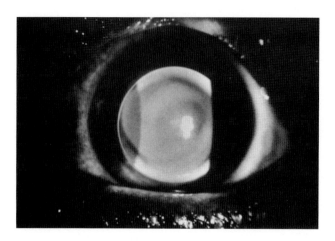

FIG. 18-36. *Contact lens of Fig. 18-34 modified to loosen the peripheral system.*

SURGICAL REFERRAL CRITERIA

In 15–20% of keratoconus patients, a corneal transplant (usually penetrating keratoplasty) is eventually required.[6] When should the patient be referred for a transplant? The generally accepted referral criteria are these:

- *Contact lens intolerance*: The patient cannot wear the lens, even if the fit looks adequate.
- *Inability to fit the patient for a contact lens*: The patient can tolerate the lens, but fitting a lens that performs adequately is impossible.

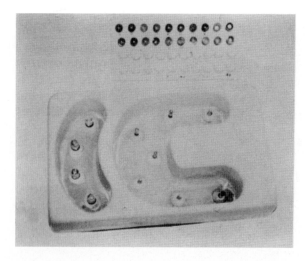

FIG. 18-37. *Modification unit. (Reprinted with permission from D Burger, K Zadnik: Contact lenses in ocular disease: keratoconus. p. 643. In MG Harris [ed]: Problems in Optometry. Vol. 2. Lippincott, Philadelphia, 1990.)*

- *Reduced vision*: The patient wants contact lenses and wears them successfully, but reduced vision (generally secondary to scarring) inhibits or prevents performance of necessary visual tasks. Depending on the visual needs of the patient, referral criteria based on visual acuity may vary. For some patients, visual acuity may be $20/60$; for other patients, it may be $20/100$.
- *Large cone with progressive thinning in the periphery*: Because the donor button is sutured to the peripheral cornea during surgery, the larger the cone, the more difficult the surgery.
- *Danger of perforation*: In extremely rare cases, the cornea becomes so thin that it is in danger of becoming perforated.

All patients should be informed of the long healing process that follows a corneal transplant. Visual rehabilitation normally takes approximately 9–10 months. Contact lenses may be needed after penetrating keratoplasty.

SURGICAL ALTERNATIVES

Various types of surgery are available for keratoconus patients.

Penetrating Keratoplasty

Penetrating keratoplasty is the most common surgical procedure for keratoconus.[44] The central area of the keratoconic cornea is removed, and a full-thickness donor corneal button is sutured in its place (Fig. 18-38). Depending on the criteria for success, this procedure is 90–95% successful.[6,45-48] Contact lenses are often required after surgery for best visual correction.

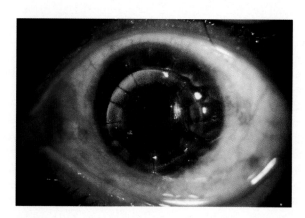

FIG. 18-38. *Penetrating keratoplasty.*

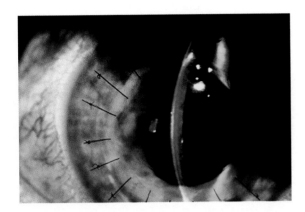

FIG. 18-39. *Epikeratoplasty. (Courtesy of Dr. Karla Zadnik.)*

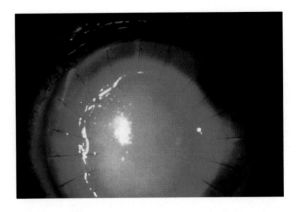

FIG. 18-40. *Fluorescein under epikeratoplasty. (Courtesy of Dr. Karla Zadnik.)*

Lamellar Keratoplasty

Lamellar keratoplasty is a partial, not a full-thickness, corneal transplant. The keratoconic cornea is removed to the depth of Descemet's membrane and the donor button is sutured in place. This technique is technically difficult, and visual acuity is inferior to that achieved with penetrating keratoplasty.[48] As a result, lamellar keratoplasty is usually done only in patients with large cones or for keratoglobus.[48] The advantages of this technique are shorter recovery time and less chance for corneal graft rejection.[49] The disadvantages are vascularization and haziness of the graft.

Thermokeratoplasty

In thermokeratoplasty, a hot ring is placed along the base of the cone. The cornea is heated and traumatized. As a result, the cornea develops a scar, which reduces corneal curvature and enables fitting of a flatter lens.[50] This procedure is rarely performed in the United States.[51]

Epikeratoplasty

Epikeratoplasty is appropriate primarily for contact lens–intolerant patients.[44,52] Prospective epikeratoplasty patients must be able to attain vision of at least $^{20}/_{40}$ with a contact lens and must have minimal or no scarring.[44,52,53] In this procedure, the central host epithelium is débrided and the donor cornea is sutured over the keratoconic cornea. The donor button is regular in shape and thus creates the uniform surface necessary for good visual correction (Figs. 18-39 and 18-40). Advantages of this procedure are that it is not penetrating, the mechanical integrity of the globe is retained, and the normal host endothelium is retained, precluding risk of epithelial rejection.[44,49] Contact lenses are occasionally required for best visual correction.[52]

Phototherapeutic Keratectomy

Phototherapeutic keratectomy is a surgical alternative for the patient with keratoconus who has superficial corneal scarring. For these patients, central scarring causes a decrease of visual acuity. The excimer laser is used to reduce the scarring and to improve vision. This procedure is also used for patients with a proud nebula with recurrent erosions. In this case, the reduction of the pronounced corneal apex allows the continued wearing of a rigid contact lens. Some corneal surgeons prefer to remove these lesions with a blade.

CONCLUSION

Before fitting contact lenses for keratoconus, educating patients about prognosis, dependence on contact lenses, and the need for ongoing care is critical. Patients with early-stage keratoconus may be fitted with standard lens designs, but, as in more advanced cases, excessive apical or peripheral cornea contact lens bearing must be prevented, otherwise, epithelial erosion is hastened. If the clinician has no diagnostic lens sets, a laboratory can fabricate a set or the practitioner can borrow a keratoconus fitting set from an RGP lens laboratory. Careful, methodical lens fitting with an appropriate array of diagnostic keratoconic trial lenses, allowing for adequate settling time, careful over-refraction, and precise lens verification is critical. RGP lenses for keratoconus patients must be well blended and manufactured with close adherence to ordered specifications and tolerances. The patient must thoroughly clean and disinfect the lenses daily, with close adherence to recommended wearing schedules.

When epithelial erosion occurs, the following steps should be taken: Allow the cornea to heal before resuming RGP lens wear (if necessary, use a disposable, bandage piggyback approach); redesign the fit to reduce contact between the lens and the abraded area; and re-evaluate the patient at least every 6 months.

To fit and manage patients with moderate-to-advanced keratoconus, the practitioner must be able to easily modify RGP contact lenses. Insurance companies often do not automatically reimburse the keratoconus patient for contact lens services. The provider must convince the insurer that the lenses are medically necessary for the patient and are not prescribed simply for cosmetic purposes.

Acknowledgment

The medical editing department of Kaiser Foundation Hospitals, Inc., provided editorial assistance.

REFERENCES

1. Fick AE: Eine Contactbrille. Arch Augenheilk 18:279, 1888. (English translation by May C: A contact lens.) Arch Ophthalmol 17:215, 1888
2. Panas P: Traitement optique du kératocône. Ann d'Oculistique 99:293, 1888
3. Hartstein J: Keratoconus that developed in patients wearing corneal contact lenses: report of four cases. Arch Ophthalmol 80:345, 1968
4. Steahly LP: Keratoconus following contact lens wear. Ann Ophthalmol 10:1177, 1978
5. Gasset AR, Houde WL, Garcia-Bengochea M: Hard contact lens wear as an environmental risk in keratoconus. Am J Ophthalmol 85:339, 1978
6. Smiddy WE, Hamburg TR, Kracher GP, Stark WJ: Keratoconus: contact lens or keratoplasty? Ophthalmology 95:487, 1988
7. Davis L, Barr J, VanOtteren D: Transient rigid lens–induced striae in keratoconus. Optom Vis Sci 70:216, 1993
8. Burger D, Zadnik K: Contact lenses in ocular disease: Keratoconus. p. 643. In Harris MG (ed): Problems in Optometry. Vol. 2. Lippincott, Philadelphia, 1990
9. Korb DR, Finnemore VM, Herman JP: Apical changes and scarring in keratoconus as related to contact lens fitting techniques. J Am Optom Assoc 53:199, 1982
10. Zadnik K, Mutti DO: Contact lens fitting relation and visual acuity in keratoconus. Am J Optom Physiol Opt 64:698, 1987
11. Edrington TB, Barr JT, Zadnik K, et al: Standardized rigid contact lens fitting protocol for keratoconus. Optom Vis Sci 73:6369, 1996
12. Chiquiar-Arias V, Liberatore JC: A new technique of fitting contact lenses on keratoconus. Contacto 3:393, 1959
13. Moss HI: The contour principle in corneal contact lens prescribing for keratoconus. J Am Optom Assoc 30:570, 1959
14. Bennett ES: Keratoconus. p. 297. In Bennett ES, Grohe RM (eds): Rigid Gas-Permeable Contact Lenses. Professional Press Books, New York, 1986

15. Mandell RB: Keratoconus. p. 824. In Mandell RB (ed): Contact Lens Practice. 4th ed. Thomas, Springfield, IL 1988
16. Wilson SE, Lin DTC, Klyce SD: Corneal topography of keratoconus. Cornea 10:2, 1991
17. Maguire LJ, Bourne WM: Corneal topography of early keratoconus. Am J Ophthalmol 108:107, 1989
18. McMahon TT, Robin JB, Scarpulla KM, Putz JL: The spectrum of topography found in keratoconus. CLAO J 17:198, 1991
19. Gould HL: Management of keratoconus with corneal and scleral lenses. Am J Ophthalmol 70:624, 1970
20. Gasset AR, Lobo L: Dura-T semiflexible lenses for keratoconus. Ann Ophthalmol 7:1353, 1975
21. Mobilia EF, Foster CS: A one-year trial of Polycon lenses in the correction of keratoconus. Contact Intraocul Lens Med J 5:37, 1979
22. Cohen EJ, Parlato CJ: Fitting Polycon lenses in keratoconus. Int Ophthalmol Clin 26:111, 1986
23. Maguen E, Espinosa G, Rosner IR, Nesburn AB: Long-term wear of Polycon contact lenses in keratoconus. CLAO J 9:57, 1983
24. Lembach RG, Keates RH: Aspheric silicone lenses for keratoconus. CLAO J 10:323, 1984
25. Soper JW, Jarrett A: Results of a systematic approach to fitting keratoconus and corneal transplants. Contact Lens Med Bull 5:50, 1972
26. Raber IM: Use of CAB Soper Cone contact lenses in keratoconus. CLAO J 9:237, 1983
27. Caroline PJ, McGuire JR, Doughman DJ: Preliminary report on a new contact lens design for keratoconus. Contact Intraocul Lens Med J 4:69, 1978
28. Caroline PJ, Doughman DJ, McGuire JR: A new contact lens design for keratoconus: a continuing report. Contact Lens J 12:17, 1978
29. Siviglia N: The Ni-Cone Keratoconus lens [pamphlet]. Lancaster Contact Lens, Lancaster, PA, 1987
30. Soper JW: Fitting keratoconus with piggy-back and Saturn II lenses. Contact Lens Forum 11:25, 1986
31. Woo GC, Callender MG, Egan DJ: Vision through corrected keratoconic eyes with two contact lens systems. Int Contact Lens Clin 11:748, 1984
32. Caroline PJ, Doughman DJ: A new piggyback lens design for correction of irregular astigmatism: a preliminary report. Contact Lens J 13:39, 1979
33. Hartstein J: The correction of keratoconus with hydrophilic contact lenses. Contact Lens Med Bull 7:36, 1974
34. Koliopoulos J, Tragakis M: Visual correction of keratoconus with soft contact lenses. Ann Ophthalmol 13:835, 1981
35. Burger D, Bullimore MA, McMahon TT: Determining the nature of visual loss in keratoconus. Presented at the American Academy of Optometry Annual Meeting, Nashville, TN, December 6–10, 1990
36. Herman JP: Flexure. p. 137. In Bennett ES, Grohe RM (eds): Rigid Gas-Permeable Contact Lenses. Professional Press Books, New York, 1986

37. Krachmer JH, Feder RS, Belin MW: Keratoconus and related noninflammatory corneal thinning disorders. Surv Ophthalmol 28:293, 1984

38. Duke-Elder S, Leigh AG: Corneal diseases. p. 950. In Duke-Elder S, Leigh AG (eds): System of Ophthalmology. Vol. 8, Part 2. Diseases of the Outer Eye. Mosby, St. Louis, 1965

39. Teng CC: Electron microscope study of the pathology of keratoconus: part I. Am J Ophthalmol 55:18, 1963

40. Mackman GS, Polack FM, Sydrys L: Hurricane keratitis in penetrating keratoplasty. Cornea 2:31, 1983

41. Kawabara T, Perkins DG, Cogan DG: Sliding of the epithelium in experimental corneal wounds. Invest Ophthalmol 15:4, 1976

42. Bron AJ: Vortex patterns of corneal epithelium. Trans Ophthalmol Soc UK 93:455, 1973

43. Moodaley L, Buckley RJ, Woodward EG: Surgery to improve contact lens wear in keratoconus. CLAO J 17:129, 1991

44. Dietze TR, Durrie DS: Indications and treatment of keratoconus using epikeratophakia. Ophthalmology 95:236, 1988

45. Boruchoff SA, Jensen AD, Dohlman CH: Comparison of suturing techniques in keratoplasty for keratoconus. Ann Ophthalmol 7:433, 1975

46. Troutman RC, Gaster RN: Surgical advances and results of keratoconus. Am J Ophthalmol 90:131, 1980

47. Paton RT, Swartz G: Keratoplasty for keratoconus. Arch Ophthalmol 61:370, 1959

48. Richard JM, Paton D, Gasset AR: A comparison of penetrating keratoplasty and lamellar keratoplasty in the surgical management of keratoconus. Am J Ophthalmol 86:807, 1978

49. Steinert RF, Wagoner MD: Long-term comparison of epikeratoplasty and penetrating keratoplasty for keratoconus. Arch Ophthalmol 106:493, 1988

50. Gasset AR: Keratoconus. Contact Lens Forum 2:38, 1977

51. Itoi M, Nakaji Y, Nakae T: Keratoconus: the Japanese experience. CLAO J 9:254, 1983

52. Lembach RG, Lass JH, Stocker EG, Keates RH: The use of contact lenses after keratoconic epikeratoplasty. Arch Ophthalmol 107:364, 1989

53. McDonald MB, Safir A, Waring GO III, et al: A preliminary comparative study of epikeratophakia or penetrating keratoplasty for keratoconus. Am J Ophthalmol 103:467, 1987

VII

Postsurgical Complications of Contact Lens Wear

19

Complications after Corneal Refractive Surgery

David T. Gubman

GRAND ROUNDS CASE REPORT

Subjective:
A 34-year-old male tool machinist complained of blurry near vision along with shadows and haloes at distance and near since his radial keratotomy (RK) corneal refractive procedure 2 years prior. He was a previous soft toric contact lens wearer with reported spheric equivalent refraction of –2.00 D.

Objective:
- Keratometry values showed grade 1+ mire distortion with the following values: right eye (OD) –1.25 × 145 axis meridian (AM) 41.25; left eye (OS) –0.75 × 130 AM 42.50
- Corneal topography revealed irregular astigmatism OD and distortion with inferior steepening OS.
- Uncorrected distance visual acuity was $^{20}/_{30}$ OD, $^{20}/_{30-}$ OS, and $^{20}/_{25-}$ each eye (OU).
- Manifest refraction showed hyperopic astigmatism as follows: OD +1.25 –1.00 × 035, $^{20}/_{20}$; OS +1.75 –1.50 × 010, $^{20}/_{20}$.
- Corneal evaluation revealed four radial incisions and four arcuate incisions (Fig. 19-1).

Assessment:
Overcorrected radial and astigmatic keratotomy with symptomatic irregular astigmatism.

Plan:
Rigid gas-permeable (RGP) contact lens fitting for corneal and visual rehabilitation. Reverse-geometry design lenses were not required because the standard design, with a 9.0 diameter and 8.0 optical zone and hyperbolic peripheral curves, proved adequate.

Follow-up:
Despite initial reluctance to adopt rigid contact lens wear, this patient achieved stable visual acuity of $^{20}/_{20}$ in each eye along with the crisp quality of vision he was unable to achieve either uncorrected or with glasses.

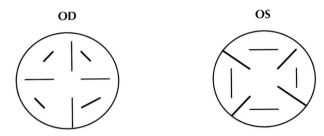

FIG. 19-1. *In Grand Rounds Case Report, corneal evaluation revealed four radial incisions and four astigmatic incisions.*

Early promise of the exquisite precision of the excimer laser in the treatment of refractive errors led some to worry that this technology would make glasses and contact lenses obsolete. Similar concerns were heard related to the potential displacement of glasses by soft contact lenses around their introduction in the early 1970s. Time and increasing knowledge and experience with both of these methods have proved these concerns unfounded. Rather, the late 1990s saw the emergence of refractive surgery procedures into the mainstream of the ophthalmic community and the public.

Although the first excimer laser application on the human eye occurred in 1987,[1,2] refractive surgical procedures have a much earlier history. RK originated in Japan in the 1930s. Dr. Sato is credited with its development after his observation of a keratoconus patient who sustained an incident of corneal hydrops with significant corneal flattening as a result. He set out to create more standardized radial incisions applied to the correction of myopia in nonkeratoconic patients.[3] The function and details of the posterior endothelial layer of the cornea were unknown at this time. Dr. Sato's incisions were placed on the anterior and posterior corneal surface and often led to subsequent corneal edema and opacification 10–20 years after the procedure.[4] The Russian ophthalmologist Fyodorov modernized RK in the early 1970s, restricting the procedure to the anterior corneal surface and refining the incision technique.[5] American ophthalmic surgeons traveled to learn his technique and bring the procedure to the United States in the late 1970s and early 1980s.[6] In this country, RK enjoyed increasing popularity until the mid-1980s. Long-term data on the stability of outcomes after RK indicated 43% of patients experienced a 1 D or greater shift toward hyperopia at 10 years.[7,8] Ultimately, questions about the technique's stability and effectiveness for moderate and higher levels of myopia and the potential for the experimental excimer laser as an alternative began to limit RK.[9] Studies of the efficacy, safety, and stability of photorefractive keratectomy (PRK) from other countries as well as from the U.S. Food and Drug Administration clinical trials for myopia

up to 7 D began to capture the attention of ophthalmic practitioners, with increasing recommendations for patients to wait for PRK approval.[10]

Along a parallel developmental timeline, procedures to correct high myopia, known as *keratomileusis*, were being pioneered by Barraquer in 1949. He first worked on human eyes in 1964.[11] Myopic keratomileusis was originally performed by using a microkeratome to create a partial-thickness central corneal lenticule, which was removed, frozen, lathed with a cryolathe like a contact lens, and then returned to the corneal surface and sutured in place. Development of this technique saw the elimination of freezing of the tissue and the creation of the in situ version by Ruiz,[12] who performed the refractive cut on the stromal bed. Keratomileusis was later combined with the excimer laser: A hinged corneal flap created using a keratome was followed by laser sculpting of the exposed stromal bed and sutureless replacement of the corneal flap.[13] This, known as *LASer In-situ Keratomileusis* (LASIK), is now the refractive procedure of choice for most refractive errors.

INDICATIONS AND CONTRAINDICATIONS TO CORNEAL REFRACTIVE SURGERY

Refractive Error Analysis

The heart of the field of refractive surgery is the patient's refractive error. Uncorrected visual acuity and best corrected visual acuity should be documented OD, OS, and OU. The nature and magnitude of the baseline refraction determine the refractive treatments and procedures available to the patient. Objective retinoscopy followed by subjective refractive refinement to best corrected acuity defines the starting point for refractive error analysis. Cycloplegia is recommended with 1% cyclopentolate (2 drops, 5 minutes apart) because of its rapid onset (20–45 minutes), relatively short duration of action (8–24 hours), and most important, its efficacy resulting in minimal residual accommodation.[14] One drop of 2.5% phenylephrine is also used for maximal dilation and retinal evaluation. Objective and subjective retinoscopy should then be repeated and the results compared with the dry or noncycloplegic data to rule out any accommodative component or pseudomyopia. These baseline data should be recorded and the refraction repeated on at least one additional occasion to demonstrate refractive stability. Unstable refractive findings may result from undiagnosed or borderline diabetes, corneal distortion from contact lens wear, or accommodative infacility or hysteresis. Pro-

TABLE 19-1. *Contraindications to Corneal Refractive Surgery*

Ocular relative contraindications
  Unstable refractive error
  Keratoconjunctivitis sicca
  Blepharitis
  Recurrent or active ocular disease
  Irregular astigmatism by topography
  Exposure keratitis or lagophthalmos
  Herpes simplex keratitis (active/inactive)
  Previous ocular surgery
Ocular absolute contraindications
  Cataract
  Glaucoma
  Keratoconus
  Amblyopia (monocular function)

TABLE 19-2. *Relative and Absolute Contraindications to Corneal Refractive Surgery*

Systemic relative contraindications
  Diabetes mellitus
  Atopy (severe allergy, eczema, asthma)
Systemic absolute contraindications
  Pregnant and lactating women
  Rheumatoid arthritis
  Systemic lupus erythematosus
  Collagen vascular disease

gressive refractive changes, as evidenced by consistent changes in refractive prescription, have led to a minimum age requirement of 18 years of age to eliminate the younger age bracket with the highest incidence of physiologic refractive progression.[15] Refractive fluctuation has the potential to cause serious over- or undercorrection and must therefore be detected, diagnosed, and treated before any permanent refractive procedure.

Ocular and Systemic History

As with any procedure, the history should document the patient's chief complaint and symptoms, especially previous experience and intolerance to optical aids. Previous ocular trauma and family ocular history, including relatives with cataracts and glaucoma and the age of onset, should be reviewed and compared with relative versus absolute contraindications (Table 19-1). Systemic history and current medications are reviewed and compared with relative versus absolute contraindications (Table 19-2).

Contact Lens History

The length of time glasses and contact lenses have been worn as well as any complications of these treatments should be recorded. Daily or extended wearing times, vision, comfort, and care systems in all lens types worn comprise the patient's contact lens experience and compliance. Patients currently in lens wear must discontinue all contact lens wear for 1–2 weeks for hydrogel wearers and 2–4 weeks for hard lens wearers. Polymethylmethacrylate (PMMA) wearers, especially those displaying even the mildest signs of microcystic edema, will benefit from a temporary refit into RGP material before any refractive procedure. This minimizes the chances of corneal distortion on discontinuation of PMMA lens wear.[16] Ulti-

mately, corneal stability and therefore refractive stability at the patient's true baseline is the preprocedure goal. Guidelines for the number of days or weeks to discontinue lens wear, whether RGP or hydrogel, are based on achieving demonstrable corneal stability and are therefore at the practitioner's discretion, based on evaluation of the lens impact on a particular patient's cornea.

Corneal Curvature

Keratometry values with demonstrable stability and repeatability, especially in light of any contact lens wear, are critical before any corneal procedure. Mire quality should be recorded and any distortion of the mire reflection described. A simple observation of the mires between blinks is a valuable and noninvasive method of evaluating ocular surface tear breakup time. A further comparison of corneal toricity and overall astigmatic refractive error allows for an accurate interpretation of residual astigmatism, an important factor for a given patient's prognosis. A diagnostic spheric rigid contact lens trial evaluation confirms the visual significance of any residual astigmatism. Corneal topography is an essential tool because of the increased number of data points analyzed and the additional information revealed about the peripheral corneal surface. Furthermore, corneal topography has proved to be the most sensitive clinical instrument in detecting early keratoconus or other peripheral degenerations.[17–21]

Binocular Vision

Binocular function often has a significant impact on refractive error and stability. Evaluation for high phoria, intermittent strabismus, and accommodative dysfunction must also be completed before refractive surgery to ensure an optimal outcome. A patient with undiagnosed accommodative infacility may habitually wear stronger refractive correction than indicated by the true refractive error. Similarly, a patient with convergence insufficiency may be using accommodative convergence to maintain fusion. A sudden change in refractive status has the potential to create diplopia owing to the previously undetected binocular dysfunction.[22] Furthermore, binocular inefficiency in the vergence or accommodative systems can easily be the underlying etiology for visual and refractive fluctuation. Once again, these conditions must therefore be detected, diagnosed, and treated before any permanent refractive procedure. Because refractive surgery does not treat presbyopia, ocular dominance should be determined and a monovision result considered.

Ocular Health Assessment

Anterior segment evaluation should rule out pre-existing disease, such as blepharitis, keratoconus, corneal dystrophy, and any notable lens changes or early cataracts. Corneal scarring or vascularization from contact lens wear should also be described.

Pupil size, especially in dim illumination, should be measured and compared with the known treatment zone sizes for refractive surgery procedures. Large pupil size is a significant risk factor for visual disturbances, such as glare and haloes, particularly at night.

Intraocular pressure is measured and used as a baseline guide to rule out risk factors for glaucoma and because the patient may require temporary topical steroid administration after a refractive procedure.

Complete dilated funduscopic evaluation is required, especially in the population of myopes who are at increased risk for retinal disease. Prophylactic treatment may be indicated for peripheral retinal lesions or atrophic holes.

Patient Expectations

Despite a healthy and stable ocular evaluation, not every ametropic patient is a qualified candidate for a keratorefractive procedure. Direct marketing efforts to patients through print, radio, and television media by individual doctors and laser vision companies has served to increase the awareness about refractive procedures and contributed to unrealistic patient expectations. Because keratorefractive procedures do not cure presbyopia, patients cannot reasonably expect to avoid all optical aids for the rest of their lives. Several studies of RK and PRK indicate that 10–35% of patients use some form of optical aid, either glasses or contact lenses, on at least a part-time basis 1 year after a refractive procedure.[9,23,24] The benefits of keratorefractive procedures depend on their success in transforming the lifestyles of patients who have been 100% dependent on prosthetic optical aids for all their

visual tasks to one in which they become relatively (or absolutely) independent of glasses and contact lenses. Factors such as patient occupation and avocation and their respective visual demands as well as the variables involved in postprocedure healing responses dictate the degree of freedom from glasses and contact lenses any particular patient may achieve. Patient personality and psychology also play a role in the level of visual clarity demanded and expected. Some patients are content with $^{20}/_{30}$ visual acuity, whereas others are bothered by even the mildest blur, despite $^{20}/_{20}$ or $^{20}/_{15}$ acuity. Therefore, an optimal clinical outcome after a refractive procedure may be experienced as a failure by a patient who has unrealistic expectations.

Prevalence and Effectiveness of Corneal Refractive Procedures

The efficacy, safety, and stability of keratorefractive procedures have improved to provide patients with a reasonable clinical alternative to glasses and contact lenses for the treatment of refractive error. Incisional procedures did not represent new technology and were not subject to the U.S. Food and Drug Administration approval process. The Prospective Evaluation of Radial Keratotomy study represents one of the best controlled analyses of RK with prospective analysis and standardized follow-up. This study used a standardized eight-incision procedure.[25] Modifications in technique led Waring and Casebeer to publish results with accuracy of outcomes within ±1.00 D improving to 89% and uncorrected visual acuity of $^{20}/_{40}$ or better at 93%.[23] Casebeer's technique allowed for an initial procedure with a minimal number of incisions, with additional incisions added only when necessary. In comparison, clinical results of PRK indicated that 78% achieved ±1.00 D and 93% achieved $^{20}/_{40}$ or better after a single procedure.[24] LASIK and its predecessor, automated lamellar keratomileusis, were originally used for the treatment of higher levels of myopia. LASIK has become the treatment of choice for even lower levels of myopia. When evaluated by correspondingly similar refractive errors, LASIK results are comparable to PRK and drop off somewhat with the more challenging cases of higher myopia. Farah et al. analyzed data from peer-reviewed clinical results of LASIK studies and summarized abstracts of clinical results presented at the major ophthalmic meetings in 1996 and 1997 (Table 19-3).[26]

Hyperopic excimer laser treatment has shown similar results. Jackson reported on 65 eyes between +1.00 and +4.00 D; 80% achieved ±0.50 D and 98% were within ±1.00 D of the intended correction at 1 year after

TABLE 19-3. *Published Clinical Results of Corneal Refractive Surgical Procedures*

Procedure	RK	RK	PRK	LASIK			LASIK
Study	Waring et al. (PERK)[25]	Waring and Casebeer[23]	Thompson et al.[24]	Farah et al.[26] (journal)			Farah et al.[26] (abstracts)
Year	1982–1998	1992–1993	1997	1987–1997			1996–1997
No. of eyes	435	615	612	1,028			11,397
Mean follow-up	1 yr	1 yr	2 yrs	6–12 mos			10 days–12 mos
Preoperative error	–2 to –8 D	–1 to –8.25 D	–1 to –6 D	–1 to –6 D	–6 to –12 D	> –12 D	–1 to –31 D
Loss ≥ 2 lines	3%	1%	7%	n/a	n/a	n/a	0.9%
± 1.00 D	60%	89%	78%	93%	74%	42%	83%
UCVA ≥ 20/40	78%	93%	93%	93%	67%	41%	83%
UCVA ≥ 20/20	47%	54%	67%	n/a	n/a	n/a	57%

LASIK = laser in situ keratomileusis; n/a = data not available; PERK = Prospective Evaluation of Radial Keratotomy study; PRK = photorefractive keratectomy; RK = radial keratotomy; UCVA = uncorrected visual acuity.

PRK with the VISX STAR laser. Correspondingly, 72% of eyes had uncorrected visual acuity of 20/25 or better.[27]

COMPLICATIONS OF CORNEAL REFRACTIVE PROCEDURES

Complications of refractive procedures may occur during surgery and during the healing process. Both types of complication can adversely affect the physiologic outcome as well as the refractive result and therefore influence the necessity for glasses or contact lenses after the procedure.

Radial Keratotomy

RK has evolved from incisions numbering as high as 32 to correct higher levels of myopia to a limited technique restricted to four incisions for 3 D or less. The advent of the excimer laser has meant a significant decrease in the performance of incisional procedures. Nevertheless, a substantial number of patients have keratotomized corneas, and some of them will experience complications.

Corneal perforation and clear zone decentration are intraprocedural problems. Because the greatest flattening effect occurs with the deepest incisions, incisional techniques are designed to penetrate 95% or more of the corneal thickness. Perforation or microperforation, in which only a few drops of aqueous humor are lost, is relatively common, with an estimated incidence of 2–10% of cases that are usually self-sealing.[28] Macroperforations allow more aqueous loss, and shallowing of the anterior chamber may result; its incidence is estimated at less than 0.5%.[28,29] Macroperforation represents an increased risk of infection and endophthalmitis.

Clear zone decentration results when the radial incisions are placed such that the untouched central clear zone is not centered over the pupil. Light scatter from the incision scars then causes visual disturbances, such as glare, haloes, and the starburst phenomenon. Centrifugal incisions that begin at the periphery and end at the clear zone edge carry a risk of incisional errors that compromise the visual axis. Surgeon error or patient movement at this critical point may cause this rare but serious complication.

Fluctuation of Vision

Visual fluctuations in the first few months after incision placement in RK is relatively common, with an incidence between 2% and 60%[30] of cases and as much as 1.5 D of refractive shift.[31] This early refractive fluctuation has been linked to variability in individual incision healing and stability. However, significant visual fluctuation of 1–3 D has been shown in 10–30% of patients 1–4 years after the procedure.[25,32,33]

Infection

Corneal infection is a possibility early in the postprocedure period, as the epithelium heals, and several months to several years later. Even the late-occurring infections have been shown to originate within the keratotomy scars.[34–37]

Irregular astigmatism, vascularization of the incision scars, and decreased globe integrity are additional complications of RK. Although the potential for globe rupture along the incision sites is insignificant under normal conditions, it has been documented in laboratory conditions and reported clinically resulting from extreme trauma associated with motor vehicle accidents.[38,39]

Photorefractive Keratectomy Complications and Management

Central Islands

Central islands have been defined as a topographic abnormality consisting of a centrally elevated or steeper corneal zone 1–3 D high relative to the surrounding paracentral cornea and having a diameter of 1–3 mm. Generally detected 1 month postoperatively, central islands can be associated with symptoms of glare, image ghosting, monocular diplopia, and decreased visual acuity, corrected and uncorrected. The incidence of topographic islands has been estimated at 80% 1 week after treatment but drops to 15% by 3 months and less than 5% at 6 months.[40] Flat or non–gaussian beam energy profiles, single-zone treatment programs, and treatment zone sizes of 6 mm and greater along with higher degrees of myopia (>6 D) are factors in central island development. Central island formation is characteristic of broad-beam excimer laser delivery systems, as evidenced by the high initial incidence. Scanning lasers that use a small, spot beam that rapidly jumps around the intended treatment zone do not produce central islands. The etiology of this phenomenon has been linked to fluid dynamics within the central region of the cornea during broad-beam treatment. Laser pulse–induced acoustic shock waves may drive fluid toward the corneal center.[40] Lin has described a naturally occurring increase in stromal hydration of the central anterior cornea relative to the periphery.[41] Fluid accumulation serves to effectively block the excimer beam and therefore diminish its ablative effect on the corneal tissue. Time and monitoring are the appropriate treatments for the vast majority of central islands detected after PRK. For those cases with persistent islands, a phototherapeutic keratectomy (PTK)–like ablation may be indicated to reduce or eliminate the island to the level of the surrounding original ablation.

Ablation Decentration

Centration of corneal refractive procedures depends on choosing the appropriate reference point around which to center the procedure and then succeeding in applying the treatment to the intended location. There has been less than universal consensus about the most advantageous method of centration. Some have advocated the visual axis as the center point.[42] Several reasons, including the Stiles-Crawford Effect, suggest that the pupil is the optimal central point for clinically optimal centration results.[43,44] Decentration of 1.0 mm or greater has been shown to produce clinically significant symptoms, including glare, haloes, and starburst effects, especially at night or in other dim illumination conditions.[45] Laser retreatment is often problematic but may be attempted by one of two methods. An increase in the treatment zone diameter around the originally decentered treatment may allow incorporation of the pupil within the larger zone. Second, but more difficult, is a PTK-type attempt to create centration by ablating previously untreated tissue adjacent to the first procedure. It is difficult to achieve the desired refractive and optical result using ablation over this uneven

surface. Whether centration problems result from incorrect procedure planning or errant patient fixation during the procedure, topographically linked ablations and eye tracking devices used during laser treatment are technological advances that are likely to minimize centration problems. Prevention is the preferable and eminently achievable solution to ablation decentration.

Infection

The risk of infection with PRK is higher than with other corneal refractive procedures because of the large epithelial defect created to ablate the superficial stroma. Incidence of corneal infection after PRK has been estimated at 0.1%, compared to 0.02% for LASIK.[46] Treatment consists of removal of the bandage hydrogel lens and frequent topical antibiotics with careful monitoring.

Topical Therapeutic Complications

Immediate postprocedure therapy usually consists of topical antibiotics, nonsteroidal anti-inflammatory agents, and a bandage hydrogel lens. Toxicity, infiltrative responses, lens-induced edema, chemosis, and injection are possibilities. Subsequent topical steroid treatment to modulate the corneal healing reaction carries well-documented risks for ptosis, intraocular pressure elevation, herpes simplex virus reactivation,[47] and posterior capsular cataract formation.[48]

Haze

Abnormal corneal haze must be clinically distinguished from normal haze formation characteristic of the typical PRK healing profile. Normal haze formation is detected at 1 month in a diffuse pattern and trace amount progressing to a peak at 3 months, with ultimate and complete resolution between 6 and 12 months.[49] Alternatively, persistent, confluent, and reticular haze that is not self-limiting and is associated with significant myopic regression is an abnormal reaction attributable to an individual patient's healing response. Several studies have estimated the incidence of abnormal corneal haze as 3%.[10,50] Seiler et al. described increasing risk for abnormal haze formation with increasing levels of attempted myopic correction. They observed abnormal haze formation in 0% of those treated for –3.00 D or less, in 1.1% of those with 3–6 D, in 17.5% of those with 6–9 D, and in 16.7% of those more than 9.00 D.[51] Later work by Machat indicated smaller incidences of 0.5% for those with less than –3.00 D, 1.0% with 4–6 D, 2–3% with 7–9 D, and 4–5% with 10–15 D.[40] This increasing risk of corneal haze at higher levels of myopia spurred the development of LASIK for higher levels of correction. Treatment initially consists of increased prescription of topical steroids and nonsteroidal agents to minimize the haze response. Secondarily, epithelial or haze débridement with or without additional laser ablation is performed, followed by early and aggressive topical steroid and nonsteroidal treatment.

Laser In Situ Keratomileusis Complications and Management

Procedural Complications

LASIK is a refractive procedure that combines the precision of the excimer laser to remove corneal tissue with the microkeratome's accessibility to the inner stroma and Bowman's membrane. The advantage of LASIK over PRK for high myopia is the preservation of the corneal epithelium and Bowman's layer. This preservation of corneal tissue reduces the effect of corneal haze associated with surface PRK.

LASIK involves ablation of the stroma of the cornea via creation of a corneal flap with a microkeratome. The corneal flap is usually one-third of corneal thickness, at approximately 130–160 μm thick. This flap has a nasal hinge to ensure proper realignment of the flap. The excimer laser used for ablation is a 193-nm argon-fluoride laser. Corneal flap reposition is sutureless.[52]

Compared to PRK, LASIK is a more invasive procedure because of the partial-thickness corneal flap and, therefore, it carries a greater intraoperative risk of complications. Problematic performance with the suction ring or the microkeratome leads to flap complications. An incomplete, irregular, or thin flap may result, either because of poor gear advancement or jammed gears resulting from incomplete exposure or incomplete or poor suction. A free cap is created when the microkeratome does not stop at the intended hinge position. A free cap increases the incidence of irregular astigmatism and epithelial ingrowth after the procedure. A simple free cap procedure may be continued with the corneal cap temporarily stored in an antidesiccation chamber with the epithelial side in balanced solution. The stromal side is not hydrated in storage to reduce edema of the cap stroma.[46] The flap is then replaced on the cornea after ablation is completed.

Eyes with narrow palpebral fissures, deep-set globes, or keratometric values less than 41.00 D[53] create conditions with greater risk of keratome complications. Such patients are better suited for an alternative procedure, such as PRK. Critical complications of intraocular penetration during flap formation may become an ocular reconstructive emergency. Although rare in the reported literature, this complication is linked to incomplete microkeratome assembly and may result in expulsion of globe contents because of elevated intraocular pressure.[54] Once the flap is successfully created, laser ablation decentration and central island formation is possible, just as in PRK.

Postprocedure Complications

Corneal flap displacement resulting from the lack of external flap sutures is a potential complication that is often discussed but infrequently seen in practice or described in clinical studies.[55,56] If the flap is displaced, it is usually seen within the first 12–24 hours and consists of flap movement of 1 mm or less. Immediate and frequent lubrication is the appropriate treatment until the flap can be lifted and repositioned. Replacement of the flap as soon as possible not only minimizes the risk of opportunistic infection but also minimizes the severity of flap striae or wrinkling and epithelial ingrowth into the exposed interface.[46]

Epithelial ingrowth has an incidence of approximately 2% and occurs when superficial corneal epithelial cells become implanted in the interface.[53,46] Because the normal epithelial disruption occurs at the flap margins during the microkeratome pass, epithelial ingrowth is generally a peripheral phenomenon, occurring more frequently when a frank epithelial defect is present or when poor flap adhesion or flap dislocation occurs. The ingrowth may migrate and advance toward the central cornea or the epithelial cells may become necrotic, leading to a flap melt,[57] or both complications may occur. Epithelial ingrowth has the potential to significantly affect corneal topography, producing regular or irregular astigmatism and ultimately reducing visual acuity. Not all instances of epithelial ingrowth are cause for concern, however. Peripheral epithelial ingrowth less than 2 mm in diameter without evidence of progression or alteration of topography or refractive error may not require treatment. Alternatively, aggressive cases of epithelial ingrowth require treatment by lifting the flap and mechanically clearing epithelial cells from the interface surfaces of the stromal bed and the underside of the flap. Stromal melts require similar treatment but have a poorer prognosis because the corneal flap is already damaged.

Nonspecific *diffuse intralamellar keratitis* is an early postprocedural granular haze occurring between the corneal flap and stromal bed. This interface haze is usually diffuse and has a powdery or sifted-sand appearance. Its cause has not been determined, and it is generally associated with uneventful intraoperative LASIK procedures. Speculation on various contaminants interacting within the interface have been proposed and a subsequent inflammatory reaction assumed primarily because this keratitis is responsive to a short but aggressive course of topical steroids.[58]

Central island formation is usually detected after the procedure, with associated symptoms of blurred vision, ghost images, or monocular diplopia. This abnormality is ablation related and may be defined topographically as a central region at least 2–3 mm in diameter showing a curvature 2 D or steeper than the surrounding cornea. Decreased best corrected visual acuity along with refraction measuring greater myopia than predicted by the corresponding uncorrected visual acuity are typically noted in patients with central islands. Prevention of central island formation is largely accomplished through algorithms incorporated into the software of the computer-controlled treatment profile. Lifting the flap and ablating in a manner similar to PTK may treat persistent islands. Topographic analysis is essential in planning treatment for central islands.

Residual Refractive Error

Ultimately, the final measure of success or failure with any corneal refractive procedure resides in the ability to provide adequate, functional vision with minimal dependence on optical aids. Therefore, even a procedure resulting in a perfect physiologic outcome falls short of the mark if residual refractive error remains relative to the intended correction. With RK, PRK, LASIK, and other techniques, an inaccurate preprocedural baseline refraction, perhaps owing to the lack of cycloplegia, can result in primary over- or undercorrection. Variable healing responses also can lead to residual refractive errors despite accurate preprocedural measurements. Differences in incisional scarring for RK patients, normal versus abnormal corneal haze formation for PRK patients, and variable flap healing and regression in LASIK patients all represent inescapable variation in individual biological systems. Each of these is associated with a corresponding refractive effect. RK incisions that heal minimally allow for greater myopic reduction or increased overcorrection toward hyperopia. PRK patients who maintain clear corneas throughout the early postprocedure period similarly show overcorrection, and aggressive haze formation is associated with greater regression into myopia. Normal LASIK recovery similarly shows mild regression during the first weeks after treatment; biological variation in this effect partially determines whether over- or undercorrection develops.

Management of primary residual refractive error generally involves consideration of surgical enhancement. However, many physiologic complications can create persistent decreased visual acuity and symptoms of vision disturbance, including glare, haloes, and shadows. For RK, any anomaly involving the incision, incision number or pattern, or the central clear zone relative to the pupil may have unwanted refractive or visual effects that create reduced vision or visual quality. Similarly, decentered ablations, development of persistent central islands, uneven healing and haze formation, LASIK flap wrinkling, and epithelial ingrowth may also result in reduced visual performance. In short, any corneal complication that creates a topographic disturbance can negatively affect refractive

error and vision quality. The development of such an irregular cornea may not be amenable to further surgical treatment. Corneal rehabilitation to improve residual refractive error and an irregular corneal surface may require the intervention of a corneal contact lens.

CONTACT LENS TREATMENT OPTIONS

Understandably, patients requiring supplemental optical correction after refractive procedures may be reluctant to return to contact lens wear. However, contact lenses are likely to remain preferable to glasses in this population, and optimal vision may require contact lens prescription, especially in light of corneal refractive complications.

Stable corneal physiology is a prerequisite for postprocedural contact lens fitting. Minimal intervals are 4 months after last incisional procedure, 6 months after LASIK, and 8–12 months after PRK. This period is necessary for physiologic reasons, to allow the corneal healing process to take place without the potentially detrimental influence of a contact lens. For example, corneal haze formation and refractive regression are likely if contact lens wear is resumed within the first 6 months after PRK. This period also allows the refraction to stabilize and be documented to form baseline measurements for controlled contact lens fitting. Furthermore, and not incidental to the clinical management of the case, this period allows the patient to become accustomed to the final surgical vision and residual symptoms. Patients may then better appreciate the subsequent necessity of partial or complete dependence on optical aids to restore optimal visual function.

Hydrogel Lenses

Contact lens fitting, including evaluation of ocular and corneal integrity, is performed as usual. In the post-RK eye, however, particular attention must be paid to the status of radial or arcuate incisions. Wound gape, epithelial plugs in the incisions, or corneal vascularization along the incisions should be carefully assessed. Practitioners have used standard hydrogel lenses with varying success. The soft material allows the lens to drape over the new corneal contour while the optical power corrects the residual ametropia. As such, thin lenses, including disposables, are preferred to the thicker conventional variety. Because of the new corneal profile, conventional hydrogel lenses may buckle as they vault over the flatter central cornea, creating visual fluctuation.

Higher water content increases the oxygen transmission, which is preferred to minimize hypoxia and the risk of subsequent corneal vascularization, particularly along the incisions. Extended-wear lens use is contraindicated for similar reasons. Hypoxia, vascularization, corneal distortion, and irregular astigmatism are risks of extended wear in the nonsurgical eye, and the potential for these complications are increased in the keratotomy eye.

Vascularization with hydrogels is more likely to occur in RK patients with older surgical techniques, in which the incisions start at the limbal vascular plexus. Newer techniques avoid beginning the incisions in this area, therefore, the risks of vascularization with daily-wear hydrogel lenses are greatly reduced.

Base curve selection should be made according to the flatter available parameters, corresponding to the flattened central corneal profile, and to avoid a tight-fitting lens, which may compromise corneal physiology, as in any other standard lens fitting. Astin has advocated a base curve trial chosen 1.50 D flatter than the flattest K reading after PRK.[59] Lens diameter of 14.0–15.0 mm is recommended for optimal lens centration.

Paragon Vision Sciences introduced the first approved hydrogel lens specifically designed for the correction of ametropia after corneal refractive procedures. The Flexlens *Harrison post refractive surgery lens* (Harrison PRS Lens) is a reverse-geometry soft lens, with the base curve having a flatter radius of curvature than the peripheral radius of the lens. The lens has an increased center thickness (0.28 mm at –1.00 D power) to achieve optical stability and minimize visual fluctuation with normal blinking. Peripheral lens thickness design is consistent with standard thin lenses to maximize oxygen permeability to the peripheral corneal and limbal tissues. Base curve selection is determined by trial fitting rather than central keratometric values. The manufacturer recommends the 8.7-mm base curve radius as a starting point. Subsequent evaluation of centration and movement, including over-refraction, is performed with appropriate modifications: steeper if edge lift is observed or flatter if the lens is judged to be tight on the manual push-up test. This spheric lens is available in 45% hefilcon and 55% methafilcon materials. Although little widespread experience exists with this first reverse-geometry hydrogel lens, it provides an alternative to standard lens designs, which have the potential for significant vaulting over the central cornea and subsequent visual fluctuation owing to optical zone buckling.

Rigid Gas-Permeable Lenses

RGP materials present the most flexible lens design to meet the needs of the individual patient. The superior optics inherent in a rigid lens modality may be the only method available to the postsurgical patient to restore crisp vision quality and visual acuity, especially where irregular astigmatism is concerned. Despite the initial comfort issue during adaptation, the clinician must be able to present the patient with RGP and hydrogel options and help the patient choose the one that is best for the patient's lifestyle. If visual acuity and quality of vision are the chief complaint, a gas-permeable design is the lens of choice.

After RK, standard RGP lens designs generally require a large diameter (10–11 mm) to achieve adequate centration and stability. Some have advocated that the most efficient base curve selection for RGP fitting after RK should be based on preincision keratometric readings.[60,61] However, such information is often not readily available. Ackley and coworkers suggest reliance on midperipheral keratometry readings obtained with fixation dots placed on the keratometer to determine the base curve and peripheral curve radii.[62] Studies have determined that pre-RK readings are not necessary for a successful RGP fit; lenses can be designed optimally based on flat postoperative keratometry.[63]

In a study of 10 patients fit with RGP lenses after PRK, Astin[64] found a base curve selection 0.1 mm steeper than the mean keratometric reading and an overall diameter between 9.2 and 10.0 mm to achieve an optimal fitting relationship. Although the RGP lenses provided optimal visual acuity in all cases and even improved best corrected visual acuity over glasses for those with irregular astigmatism, ultimately five of the 10 patients were refit with soft daily-wear lenses and four of the 10 eventually underwent PRK retreatment.[64]

Plateau lens designs, in which peripheral curves are steeper than the base curve, invert the normal prolate relationship and, therefore, better approximate the myopic postsurgical oblate cornea. The OK series (Contex, Inc., Sherman Oaks, CA), Plateau (Menicon USA, Clovis, CA), RK/Bridge (Conforma Labs, Norfolk, VA), and the RK Splint (Lexington[65]) use this reverse-geometry design, generally using large diameters (≥ 9.50 mm), small optical zone diameters (6.0 mm), and secondary curve radii, often 2–4 D steeper than the base curve. Good postmyopic refractive surgery contact lens fit normally displays obvious central fluorescein pooling. Because many of these reverse-geometry designs were intended for orthokeratology, some have advocated their use after refractive surgery as a means of further myopic reduction for residual myopia, as an alternative to enhancement surgery.[65] The growing availability of computer-assisted corneal topography along with contact lens design software and fluorescein pattern simulation further aid in fitting these postsurgical patients. Approval of hyperopic laser correction (in late 1998) means that, as with myopic correction, a subgroup of patients exists with residual refractive error or irregular astigmatism, necessitating optical and sometimes contact lens rehabilitation. These corneas maintain their prolate shape but have steeper-than-average curvature values. Standard lens designs but with steeper base curves or aspheric peripheral systems are required to adequately fit these postsurgical corneas.

A new lens design from C&H Contact Lenses (Dallas, TX) for patients with irregular and asymmetric corneas, particularly in cases of refractive surgery complications, is the MacroLens.[66] This semiscleral RGP lens ranges in diameter from 13.9 mm to 15.0 mm. The large size of the lens enables stable optics by masking of the corneal cylinder and improved centration, and it provides improvements in comfort from its scleral properties. The lens is fenestrated near the corneal limbus to facilitate tear flow under the lens and to prevent lens binding.

NEW TECHNOLOGIES AND PROCEDURES

The prevalence, severity, and impact of refractive errors on the vision of the world's population (Figs. 19-2–19-4), as well as the successes of the excimer laser for ophthalmic use, continue to stimulate further research into new techniques and innovative technology for the treatment of ametropia.

The *intrastromal corneal ring (ICR)* is a surgical but not a laser technique to implant a PMMA ring in the stroma between lamellae in the midperiphery of the cornea. A lamellar channel is surgically dissected within the corneal stroma in preparation for receiving the PMMA ring. Phase II clinical trials studied 99 eyes with myopic corrections between −1.00 and −6.00 D. Analysis of 3-month follow-up data revealed that 96% had ²⁰⁄₄₀ or better uncorrected visual acuity. Loss of two lines of best corrected visual acuity was seen in 1% (or one eye), and 67% of patients achieved an out-come within 1.00 D of the intended correction. Two eyes had the ring explanted owing to complications, and these eyes returned to within 0.75 D of their original manifest refraction.[67] Although the ring may be removed if necessary, the remaining lamellar channel seals itself by the apposition of the previously separated stromal fibrils (Fig. 19-5). Complications experienced with the ICR include tearing of Descemet's membrane, induced astigmatism, infiltrates, lamellar channel deposits, deep stromal vascularization, and pannus.[68] Further study will determine if the ICR develops as an alternative procedure in corneal refractive surgery.

SUMMARY

Rigid contact lenses have advanced from nonpermeable PMMA to initially limited gas-permeable materials with an oxygen permeability (Dk) of approximately 12. Advances in polymer technology now allow commercially available lens permeabilities with a Dk up to 250. Similarly, hydrogel lens materials first introduced in the early 1970s with Dk less than 9 now include materials such as lidofilcon B, with a Dk of 38. Silicone-based lenses have a Dk of 340 but have limited use because of problems with surface characteristics. However, it is possible that a truly safe extended-wear contact lens material will provide a non–tissue-altering corrective option. This, combined with advances in disposable lens technology, will meet the patient desire for clear, comfortable vision and exceptional convenience while preserving uncompromised corneal physiology. Meanwhile, ametropic correction options demand the discussion of glasses, hydrogel and RGP contact lenses (including orthokeratologic molding), and corneal refractive procedures such as PRK and LASIK.

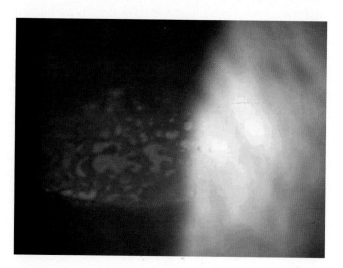

FIG. 19-2. *Flap striae or wrinkling. (Courtesy of Daniel Durrie, M.D.)*

FIG. 19-3. *Epithelial ingrowth. (Courtesy of Daniel Durrie, M.D.)*

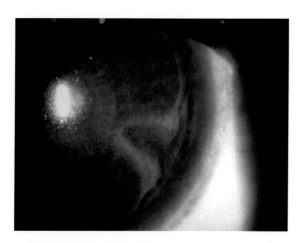

FIG. 19-4. *Flap melt. (Courtesy of Daniel Durrie, M.D.)*

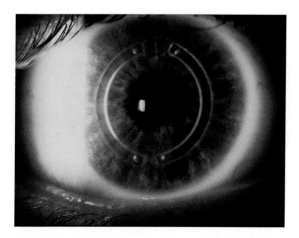

FIG. 19-5. *Intrastromal corneal ring. (Courtesy of Daniel Durrie, M.D.)*

REFERENCES

1. McDonald M, Shofner S, Klyce SD, et al: Clinical results of central photorefractive keratectomy (PRK) with the 193 nm excimer laser for the treatment of myopia: the blind eye study. Invest Ophthalmol Vis Sci (suppl.)30:216, 1989

2. McDonald M, Frantz JM, Klyce SD, et al: Central photorefractive keratectomy for myopia: the blind eye study. Arch Ophthalmol 108:799, 1990

3. Akiyama K, Shibata H, Kanai A, et al: Development of radial keratotomy in Japan, 1939–1960. p. 179. In Waring GO (ed): Refractive Keratotomy. Mosby, St. Louis, 1992

4. Akiyama K, Tanaka M, Kanai A, et al: Problems arising from Sato's radial keratotomy procedure in Japan. CLAO J 10:179, 1984

5. Waring GO: Development of radial keratotomy in the Soviet Union, 1960–1990. p. 222. In Waring GO (ed): Refractive Keratotomy. Mosby, St. Louis, 1992

6. Bores LD, Myer W, Cowden J: Radial keratotomy—an analysis of the American experience. Am J Ophthalmol 13:941, 1981

7. Waring GO, Lynn MJ, McDonnell PJ, et al: Results of the Prospective Evaluation of Radial Keratotomy (PERK) study 10 years after surgery. Arch Ophthalmol 112:1298, 1994

8. Ellingsen KL, Nizam A, Ellingsen BA, et al: Age-related refractive shifts in simple myopia. J Refract Surg 13:223, 1997

9. Waring GO, Lynn MJ, Fielding B, et al: Results of the Prospective Evaluation of Radial Keratotomy (PERK) study 4 years after surgery for myopia. JAMA 263:1083, 1990

10. Salz JJ, Maguen E, Nesburn AB, et al: A two-year experience with excimer laser photorefractive keratectomy for myopia. Ophthalmology 100:873, 1993

11. Barraquer JI: The history and evolution of keratomileusis. Int Ophthalmol Clin 36:1, 1996

12. Ruiz L, Slade SG, Updegraff SA: Excimer myopic keratomileusis: Bogota experience. p. 187. In Salz JJ (ed): Corneal Laser Surgery. Mosby, St. Louis, 1995

13. Pallikaris IG, Papatzanaki ME, Siganos DS, et al: A corneal flap technique for laser in situ keratomileusis; human studies. Arch Ophthalmol 109:1699, 1991

14. Gettes BC, Belmont O: Tropicamide: comparative cycloplegic effects. Arch Ophthalmol 66:336, 1961

15. Curtin BJ: The prevalence of myopia. p. 49. In Curtis BJ (ed): The Myopias. Harper & Row, Philadelphia, 1985

16. Rengstorff RH: Corneal rehabilitation. p. 7. In Bennett ES, Weissman BA (eds): Clinical Contact Lens Practice. Lippincott, Philadelphia, 1992

17. Koch DD, Husain SE: Corneal topography to detect and characterize corneal pathology. p. 159. In Gills JP, Sanders DR, Thornton SP, et al. (eds): Corneal Topography: The State of the Art. Slack, Thorofare, NJ, 1995

18. Maquire LJ, Bourne WM: Corneal topography of early keratoconus. Am J Ophthalmol 108:107, 1989

19. Maguire LJ, Lowry JC: Identifying progression of subclinical keratoconus by serial topography analysis. Am J Ophthalmol 112:41, 1991

20. Nesburn AB, Bahri S, Berlin M, et al: Computer assisted corneal topography (CACT) to detect mild keratoconus in candidates for photorefractive keratectomy. Invest Ophthalmol Vis Sci (suppl.)33:995, 1992

21. Wilson SE, Klyce SD: Screening for corneal topographic abnormalities before refractive surgery. Ophthalmology 101:147, 1994

22. Mandava N, Donnenfeld ED, Owens PL, et al: Ocular deviation following excimer laser photorefractive keratectomy. J Cataract Refract Surg 22:504, 1996

23. Waring GO, Casebeer JC: One-year results of a prospective multicenter study of the Casebeer system of refractive keratotomy. Casebeer Chiron Study Group. Ophthalmology 103:1337, 1996

24. Thompson KP, Steinert RF, Daniel J, et al: Photorefractive keratectomy with the Summit excimer laser: the Phase III U.S. results. In Salz JJ, McDonnell PJ, McDonald MB (eds): Corneal Laser Surgery. Mosby, St. Louis, 1995

25. Waring GO, Lynn MJ, Culbertson W, et al: Three-year results of the Prospective Evaluation of Radial Keratotomy (PERK) study. Ophthalmology 94:1339, 1987

26. Farah SG, Azar DT, Gurdal C, et al: Laser in situ keratomileusis: literature review of a developing technique. J Cataract Refract Surg 24:989, 1998

27. Jackson WB, Casson E, Hodge WG, et al: Laser vision correction for low hyperopia: an 18-month assessment of safety and efficacy. Ophthalmology 105:1727, 1998

28. Marmer RH: Radial keratotomy complications. Ann Ophthalmol 19:409, 1987

29. Sawelson H, Marks RG: Two-year results of radial keratotomy. Arch Ophthalmol 103:505, 1985

30. Arrowsmith PN, Marks RG: Visual, refractive and keratometric results of radial keratotomy: five-year follow-up. Arch Ophthalmol 107:506, 1989

31. Schanzlin DJ, Santos VR, Waring GO, et al: Diurnal change in refraction, corneal curvature, visual acuity, and intraocular pressure after radial keratotomy in the PERK study. Ophthalmology 93:167, 1986

32. Bourque LB, Cosand B, Drews C, et al: Reported satisfaction, fluctuation of vision and glare among patients one year after surgery in the Prospective Evaluation of Radial Keratotomy (PERK) study. Arch Ophthalmol 104:356, 1986

33. Deitz MR, Sanders DR: Progressive hyperopia with long-term follow-up of radial keratotomy. Arch Ophthalmol 103:782, 1985

34. Rashid ER, Waring GO: Complications of refractive keratotomy. p. 863. In Waring GO (ed): Refractive Keratotomy. Mosby, St. Louis, 1992

35. Geggel HS: Delayed sterile keratitis following radial keratotomy requiring corneal transplantation for visual rehabilitation. Refract Corneal Surg 6:55, 1990

36. Mandelbaum S, Waring GO, Forster RK, et al: Late development of ulcerative keratitis in radial keratotomy scars. Arch Ophthalmol 104:1156, 1986

37. Shivitz IA, Arrowsmith PN: Delayed keratitis after radial keratotomy. Arch Ophthalmol 104:1153, 1986

38. Darakjian NE, Marchese A: Assessment of corneal strength post radial keratotomy in rabbit eyes. Invest Ophthalmol Vis Sci (suppl.)22:26, 1982

39. Binder PS, Waring GO, Arrowsmith PN, et al: Traumatic rupture of the cornea after radial keratotomy. Arch Ophthalmol 106:1584, 1988

40. Machat JJ: PRK complications and their management. p. 192. In Machat JJ (ed): Excimer Laser Refractive Surgery Practice and Principles. Slack, Thorofare, NJ, 1996

41. Lin D: Corneal topographic analysis after excimer photorefractive keratectomy. Ophthalmology 101:1432, 1994

42. Uozato H, Guyton DL: Centering corneal surgical procedures. Am J Ophthalmol 103:264, 1987

43. Steinberg EB, Waring GO: Comparison of two methods of marking the visual axis on the cornea during radial keratotomy. Am J Ophthalmol 96:605, 1983

44. Maloney RK: Corneal topography and optical zone location in photorefractive keratectomy. Refract Corneal Surg 6:363, 1990

45. Doane JF, Cavanaugh TB, Durrie DS, et al: Relation of visual symptoms to topographic ablation zone decentration after excimer laser photorefractive keratectomy. Ophthalmology 102:42, 1995

46. Machat JJ: LASIK complications and their management. p. 385. In Machat JJ (ed): Excimer Laser Refractive Surgery Practice and Principles. Slack, Thorofare, NJ, 1996

47. Vrabec MP, Durrie DS, Chase DS: Recurrence of herpes simplex after excimer laser keratectomy. Am J Ophthalmol 116:101, 1992

48. Jaanus SD: Anti-inflammatory drugs. p. 177. In Bartlett JD, Jaanus SD (eds): Clinical Ocular Pharmacology. 2nd ed. Butterworth–Heinemann, Boston, 1989

49. Durrie DS, Lesher MP, Cavanaugh TB: Classification of variable clinical response after photorefractive keratectomy for myopia. J Refract Surg 11:341, 1995

50. Epstein D, Fagerholm P, Hamberg-Nystrom H, et al: Twenty-four–month follow-up of excimer laser photorefractive keratectomy for myopia. Ophthalmology 101:1558, 1994

51. Seiler T, Hoschbach A, Derse M, et al: Complications of myopic photorefractive keratectomy with the excimer laser. Ophthalmology 101:153, 1994

52. Slade SG, Updegraff SA: Lamellar refractive surgery. p. 343. In Azar DT (ed): Refractive Surgery. Appleton & Lange, Stamford, CT, 1997

53. Machat JJ: Preoperative LASIK patient evaluation. p. 300. In Machat JJ (ed): Excimer Laser Refractive Surgery Practice and Principles. Slack, Thorofare, NJ, 1996

54. Pallikaris IG, Siganos DS: Laser in situ keratomileusis to treat myopia: early experience. J Cataract Refract Surg 23:39, 1997

55. Perez-Santonja JJ, Bellot J, Claramonte P, et al: Laser in situ keratomileusis to correct high myopia. J Cataract Refract Surg 23:372, 1997

56. Buratto L, Ferrari M: Indications, techniques, results, limits and complications of laser in situ keratomileusis. Curr Opin Ophthalmol 8:59, 1997

57. Castillo A, Diaz-Valle D, Guteirrez AR, et al: Peripheral melt of flap after laser in situ keratomileusis. J Refract Surg 14:61, 1998

58. Machat JJ: Non-specific diffuse intralamellar keratitis. TLC Sharing the Vision 4:1, 1998

59. Astin CL: Refractive surgery and contact lenses. p. 363. In Hom MM (ed): Manual of Contact Lens Prescribing and Fitting. Butterworth–Heinemann, Boston, 1997

60. Aquavella JV, Shovlin JP, Pascucci SE, et al: How contact lenses fit into refractive surgery. Rev Ophthalmol 1:36, 1994

61. Shovlin JP, Kame RT, et al: How to fit an irregular cornea. Rev Optom 124:88, 1987

62. Ackley KD, Caroline PJ, Davis LJ: Retrospective evaluation of rigid gas permeable contact lenses on radial keratotomy patients. Optom Vis Sci (suppl.)70:32, 1993

63. Lee AM, Kastl PR: Rigid gas permeable contact lens fitting after radial keratotomy. CLAO J 24:33, 1998

64. Astin CL, Gartry DS, McG-Steele AD: Contact lens fitting after photorefractive keratectomy. Br J Ophthalmol 80:597, 1996

65. Koffler BH, Smith VM, Clements DC. Achieving additional myopic correction in under-corrected radial keratotomy eyes using the Lexington RK Splint design. CLAO J 25:21, 1999

66. Caroline PJ, Andre MP: Fitting after refractive surgery: Is there hope? Contact Lens Spectrum 14:56, 1999

67. Schanzlin DJ, Asbell PA, Burris TE, et al: The intrastromal ring segments. Phase II results for the correction of myopia. Ophthalmology 104:1067, 1997

68. Nose W, Neves RA, Burris TE, et al: Intrastromal corneal ring: 12-month sighted myopic eyes. J Refract Surg 12:20, 1996

20

Penetrating Keratoplasty

MICHAEL D. DEPAOLIS, JAMES V. AQUAVELLA, AND JOSEPH P. SHOVLIN

GRAND ROUNDS CASE REPORT

Subjective:
A 53-year-old man, presented with the chief complaint of blurred vision, especially at night. History of congenital cataract in the left eye (OS) with deep amblyopia, and chronic corneal edema in each eye (OU). The patient was in good general health and took no medications other than hypertonic saline drops OU twice a day.

Objective:
- Acuity: Best corrected entering acuities of the right eye (OD) $20/40$, and OS counting fingers at 1 ft
- Biomicroscopy: Grade 2+ Fuchs' dystrophy OU; Grade 2+ nuclear sclerosis with mild posterior subcapsular cataract (PSC) OD; Grade 4+ nuclear sclerosis OS

Assessment:
Reduced acuity of nonamblyopic eye from cataract and Fuchs' dystrophy; prognosis poor without surgical intervention.

Plan:
1. Lengthy discussion about the risks and benefits of surgery.
2. Patient consented to triple procedure of extracapsular cataract extraction, intraocular lens implantation, and corneal transplant OD.

Surgical Course:
Uncomplicated procedure with unremarkable short-term postoperative course.

Postoperative:
At 5 months after surgery, all interrupted corneal sutures were removed. At 14 months after surgery, best corrected acuity OD was $20/40^{-1}$ Corneal topography revealed significant amount of irregular astigmatism (Fig. 20-1). As a result, the final continuous suture was subsequently removed.

Follow-up:
After 1 week, the patient returned with complaint of monocular diplopia. Refraction gave best acuity of $20/70$. Topography confirmed increased irregular astigmatism as source of diplopia: A relaxing incision was placed in the graft-host junction from 4–6 o'clock, with immediate improvement in acuity to $20/40$.

One week later, patient presented for emergency follow-up owing to worsening of acuity OD ($^{20}/_{200}$). A wound separation was noted at the site of the relaxing incision. Three interrupted sutures were placed in the graft-host junction, centered around the 150-degree meridian.

Four months after wound repair, patient showed stable findings, with well-apposed graft-host junction. Interrupted sutures removed without complication. Final topography showed persistent irregular astigmatism (Fig. 20-2).

Keratometry: OD 41.50 @ 67 / 52.00 @ 157

Refraction: OD –5.75 = –5.00 × 75 ($^{20}/_{80}$)

Because of wound dehiscence associated with the relaxing incisions, further attempts at surgical intervention were discouraged and contact lens treatment initiated.

Contact Lens Treatment:

Diagnostic fitting with rigid gas-permeable (RGP) lenses of varying diameters (8.9–9.5) and base curve radii (7.60–7.00) were tried, with excessive edge lift and displacement with the blink, owing to inferior graft tilt (Fig. 20-3).

A piggyback system using a 55% water-content carrier lens of base curve 8.6, diameter 14.5 mm, and –1.00 D was used with optimal centration and movement. Overkeratometry and diagnostic fitting led to a fluoro-silicone/acrylate RGP lens of BC 7.00, diameter/optic zone (D/OZ), 9.5/8.5, and prescription of –9.50 D, which gave $^{20}/_{25}$ +3 acuity OD.

Patient now wears this system 12 hours daily with no symptoms. The RGP lens is central to inferior in position but does not eject (Fig. 20-4). Minimal debris exists between the two lenses and under the soft lens. The corneal transplant is clear, without edema, staining, or neovascularization.

For nearly 200 years, ophthalmic surgeons have attempted to address corneal structure and function in mediating benign refractive errors and potentially sight-threatening pathologies. Initial attempts at corneal surgery were quite rudimentary and fraught with complications.[1] Despite these early limitations, new technologies and an evolving body of knowledge have resulted in a tremendous expansion within the field of therapeutic and refractive corneal surgery.

Today's corneal surgeon uses a wide variety of procedures, including epikeratophakia, keratomileusis, penetrating keratoplasty, wedge resections, relaxing incisions, radial keratotomy, photorefractive keratectomy, phototherapeutic keratectomy, laser-assisted intrastromal keratomileusis, laser thermokeratoplasty, and intracorneal rings.

Despite these advances in corneal surgery, many concerns remain. Procedure accuracy and predictability, sta-

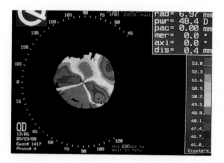

FIG. 20-1. *Corneal topography of patient in Grand Rounds Case Report 14 months after penetrating keratoplasty, before suture removal.*

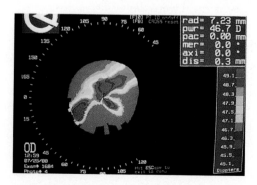

FIG. 20-2. *Corneal topography of patient in Grand Rounds Case Report 14 months after penetrating keratoplasty, after suture removal.*

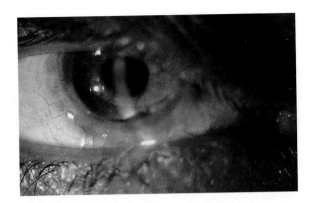

FIG. 20-3. *Fluorescein pattern of Grand Rounds Case Report patient's initial diagnostic rigid gas-permeable lens fitting over penetrating keratoplasty, with poor fluorescein pattern.*

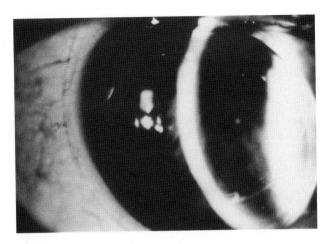

FIG. 20-4. *Grand Rounds Case Report patient with piggyback combination lens system.*

bility of results, corneal clarity, corneal physiology, and long-term safety require ongoing evaluation. Indeed, variability in individual patient healing might account for a poor visual response, thus obscuring an otherwise successful surgical procedure.

In light of the uncertainty accompanying corneal surgery, it is prudent to make provisions for postsurgical refractive care. Specifically, contact lenses remain a viable option in managing the corneal surgery patient, particularly when penetrating keratoplasty has been performed.

SHORT-TERM THERAPEUTIC CONTACT LENS APPLICATIONS

Regardless of the type of corneal surgery performed, a significant amount of short-term wounding can occur. For this reason, contact lenses have long served as therapeutic adjuncts for the corneal surgery patient. The potential benefits of a contact lens during the perioperative phase include protection (splint), pain relief, preserved wetting, improved vision, and medication delivery.[2] Most of these attributes are associated with hydrophilic bandage lenses.

The material's flexible nature and draping characteristics account for the hydrophilic bandage lens's ability to provide wound protection and improved healing. These attributes have been effective in managing postoperative wound dehiscence in penetrating keratoplasty patients[3] and postoperative pain related to exposed sutures after penetrating keratoplasty and epikeratoplasty.[4] By providing epithelial deturgescence and a smooth optical surface, a hydrophilic bandage lens can lead to improved visual performance.[5]

The ability of the hydrophilic bandage lens to deliver medication is largely limited by the polymer's inability to provide a gradual time release. Early studies demonstrated a material-dependent variation in pharmacologic delivery, with no specific material providing a sustained gradual release.[6] Material-specific responses have been identified and provide a clinical rationale for lens-assisted drug delivery.[7] Collagen bandage lenses have also demonstrated a drug delivery capability, including a sustained-release mechanism of up to 12 hours, particularly with aqueous-soluble drugs.[8] Furthermore, collagen bandages have proved beneficial in postoperative corneal wound healing. Applying a collagen bandage lens immediately after surgery can facilitate healing of radial keratotomy incisions[9] and in the re-epithelialization of penetrating keratoplasty.[10]

It is obvious that contact lenses play an instrumental role in the perioperative management of corneal surgery patients. These applications, however, must not be taken lightly because an altered corneal metabolism and topography can result in a challenging contact lens fit. The potential for neovascularization, edema, and infection must always be considered.[11] This chapter does not cover the specifics of fitting hydrophilic bandage lenses. This subject is covered in depth in Chapter 21.

KERATOREFORMATION TECHNIQUES

Today's refractive surgeon uses a host of procedures for keratoreformation, which can generally be categorized as surface-area techniques, surface-volume techniques, and full-thickness techniques. As these categories imply, each type of surgery uses a different strategy to achieve refractive change.

Surface-area techniques generally describe procedures in which incisions are made in the corneal surface. This strategy involves flattening the corneal meridian in which the incision is made, effectively lessening its refractive power. In radial keratotomy, the incisions are made in an equidistant radial fashion to symmetrically flatten the cornea and lessen myopia. The number and position of these incisions can alter the amount of myopia correction and astigmatic profile of the cornea.[12] In performing a relaxing incision, the refractive surgeon places an incision across the steep corneal meridian in a transverse fashion to lessen the amount of astigmatism. These incisions are usually arcuate or linear, placed in the midperiphery, and involve approximately 90% of the corneal thickness. The effect can be accentuated by the use of augmentation sutures orthogonal to the relaxing incision.[13]

Surface-volume techniques alter corneal refractive power by removing or adding corneal tissue. Barraquer was the first to describe a surface-volume technique when he introduced the procedure of keratomileusis.[14] The procedure was initially developed to address high myopia, high hyperopia, aphakia, and anisometropia. It is a technically difficult procedure that requires a microkeratome and a complex lathing apparatus. The surgeon first removes a section of corneal stroma with the microkeratome. The corneal tissue is cryolathed to the desired refractive outcome, reimplanted, and the insertion wound closed. Owing to the technically difficult nature of the procedure, the inordinate hardware requirements, and its limited efficacy, keratomileusis has not been well received by the ophthalmic community.[14]

Attempts to refine the concept of keratomileusis have led to procedures such as homograft keratoplasty and synthetic allograft keratoplasty. The indications for these procedures are essentially the same as for keratomileusis. In homograft keratoplasty, a lyophilized donor corneal lens is supplied for implantation. A microkeratome incision is made, the donor tissue is implanted, and the wound site is sutured. Although this procedure is more physician friendly, its outcomes are not significantly better than keratomileusis.[14] In synthetic allograft keratoplasty, corneal power is achieved by either changing curvature (hydrogel implant) or refractive index (polysulfone implant).[15] The success of allograft keratoplasty has been limited by inaccurate refractive results and problems with allograft rejection.[16]

In light of the limitations associated with allograft keratoplasty, Werblin et al.[17] developed the technique of epikeratoplasty to correct aphakia, anisometropia, high myopia, hyperopia, and keratoconus. In epikeratoplasty,

the surgeon removes the corneal epithelium and creates a circumferential trephination. A lyophilized prelathed corneal stromal lens is placed over the débrided recipient bed, with its edges in the trephination groove, and then anchored by interrupted sutures and allowed to epithelialize. This technique is often referred to as the *living contact lens* because it achieves refractive correction in much the same fashion as a corneal contact lens. Although heralded as a significant innovation in refractive surgery in the early 1980s, epikeratoplasty never fully realized its potential. Problems with donor button misalignment, interfacial haze, and refractive regression have limited its visual efficacy.[18] Furthermore, improved intraocular lenses for aphakia and alternate surgical strategies for myopia reduction have lessened the demand for epikeratoplasty. However, epikeratoplasty has shown encouraging results in the management of keratoconus.[19]

The most useful surface-volume techniques use the excimer laser. The use of the 193-nm excimer laser for *photorefractive* and *phototherapeutic keratectomy* has been well received.[20] In this procedure, the epithelium is either mechanically removed or lased and the underlying stroma is photoablated. The removal of stromal tissue is primarily responsible for the refractive error change. In fact, for a fixed optical zone size, the refractive change is directly proportional to the amount of tissue removed.[21] Excimer laser photoablative keratectomy has been successful in correcting myopia,[22] astigmatism,[23] and hyperopia.[24] A variation of photorefractive keratectomy, *laser in-situ keratomileusis* (LASIK) has become the procedure of choice for many refractive surgeons. This procedure combines microkeratome technology with the excimer laser. In LASIK, the surgeon uses a microkeratome to create an 8- to 9-mm-diameter corneal flap of approximately 165-μm thickness. The exposed stroma is then ablated with the excimer laser, and the flap is returned to its original position. Relative to PRK, LASIK often results in less postoperative inflammation and pain, requires fewer postoperative medications, and achieves a more rapid return to best corrected visual acuity. Consult Chapter 19 for more detailed information on PRK and LASIK procedures and their postoperative management with contact lenses.

Full-thickness techniques attempt to improve corneal refractive profile by replacing the diseased tissue. The most widely recognized full-thickness procedure is *penetrating keratoplasty*. Although not performed solely for cosmetic refractive purposes, penetrating keratoplasty often restores corneal integrity and vision. Patients with keratoconus, corneal leukoma, and bullous keratopathy, among others, often enjoy improved vision after penetrating keratoplasty. The elimination of corneal disease and the alteration in corneal curvature are largely responsible for the refractive effect.

Regardless of the type of corneal surgery, alterations in curvature, indices, or thickness are responsible for the attending refractive error change. Controlling these variables can be difficult. It is therefore not surprising that corneal surgery can result in residual refractive error. If the refractive error is mild and regular, intermittent use of spectacles may be all that is necessary. If the residual refractive error is significant or irregular, a contact lens is often the best option.

The surgically intervened cornea presents a rather interesting dichotomy. It is both in need of contact lens correction and in a condition least suited for these devices. The remainder of this chapter addresses contact lens management of the cornea undergoing penetrating keratoplasty, including unique prefit considerations, prescribing philosophies, and aftercare.

PENETRATING KERATOPLASTY: PROCEDURE AND POSTOPERATIVE CARE

Von Hippel is credited with the first successful corneal transplant in 1886.[25] In reality, Von Hippel's procedure is best described as a partial-thickness lamellar graft using non-human tissue. The first full-thickness corneal transplant using human donor tissue was actually performed later by Zirm.[26] Since these modest beginnings, corneal transplantation has become a highly refined surgical procedure. Today's tissue harvesting and transport techniques, micro-surgical instrumentation, and postoperative therapeutic agents have made penetrating keratoplasty one of the most successful transplantation procedures in medicine.

Penetrating keratoplasty is a full-thickness corneal surgery procedure. Although it is performed for a variety of reasons, the most common indications include bullous keratopathy, Fuchs' corneal dystrophy, keratoconus, and herpes simplex keratitis. Approximately 40,000 penetrating keratoplasties are performed in the United States annually (Eye Bank Association of America [EBBA] statistics, Washington, D.C.).

Corneal Transplantation: Procedure

To better understand the special considerations in prescribing contact lenses after penetrating keratoplasty, it is essential for the clinician to have a fundamental understanding of the actual procedure and postoperative care. Today, most penetrating keratoplasties are performed on an outpatient basis in an ambulatory surgical center. Anesthesia is accomplished by an intravenous sedation with rapid-acting pentothal, followed by a localized retrobulbar or peribulbar nerve block consisting of lidocaine and bupivacaine. The patient's contralateral eye is patched and the patient surgically draped. To ensure a stable surgical field, a lid speculum is placed in position and a bridle suture may be passed under the superior rectus, but often a fixation ring is applied to the sclera to maintain stability of the globe. The visual axis is marked for trephine centration. The actual trephination might be intentionally decentered in the case of a tectonic graft or a sagging keratoconus. The selected trephine diameter is actually 0.25–0.50 mm smaller than the intended donor button, depending on the existing pathology. This design ensures good wound coaptation, minimizes the likelihood of wound leakage, and reduces the incidence of postoperative glaucoma in aphakia. The actual trephination procedure involves approximately 90% of the corneal thickness. In some techniques, a diamond blade is used to deepen the initial trephination, and the remainder of the excision is performed with surgical scissors. This allows the surgeon to bevel the recipient bed so that the donor button does not sink through the recipient bed. Once in place, the donor button is anchored with four cardinal sutures. Quite a bit of controversy exists as to which type of suturing is best for minimizing postoperative astigmatism. Interrupted sutures, double continuous sutures, and combination (interrupted and continuous) sutures have been used with various degrees of success. Interrupted sutures offer the advantage of selective removal for better postoperative astigmatism control. Continuous sutures have traditionally been thought to ensure better wound apposition and, with postoperative adjustments, can also lessen postoperative astigmatism.[27] Many corneal specialists use interrupted and continuous suturing techniques for penetrating keratoplasty. Once suturing is completed, the surgeon may apply a bandage lens. Regardless of whether a bandage lens is used, the patient is patched under a protective shield.

Penetrating keratoplasty follow-up visits are conducted at 1 day, 7 days, 1 month, 2 months, and every other month for the first year. Additional visits may be necessary should complications arise. In the short term, the clinician must monitor visual acuity, intraocular pressure, re-epithelialization, and graft rejection. Hydrophilic bandage lenses can be used should a persistent epithelial defect or suture irritation occur. In the long term, graft rejection becomes less likely but must be considered. Here, the clinician monitors visual acuity, postoperative corneal topography, refractive findings, and intraocular pressure. Selective interrupted suture removal can take place as early as 1 month postoperatively, but the continuous suture often remains for 6–12 months and occasionally longer (see Figs. 20-1 and 20-2).

Refractive Contact Lens Considerations

Despite a successful surgical outcome, the penetrating keratoplasty patient often manifests residual refractive error. If the refractive error is reasonably mild and anisometropia is not a consideration, a spectacle prescription often suffices. Because of anisometropia and high refractive error, however, approximately 10–25% of all penetrating keratoplasty patients are fitted with contact lenses.[28,29] With the exception of a therapeutic hydrophilic bandage lens, postoperative contact lens fitting usually does not commence for 3–12 months after surgery. If the patient's immediate postoperative course is uncomplicated, a contact lens can be fitted over existing sutures. However, if the patient's postoperative course is marked by difficulties in re-epithelialization, poor wound apposition, high intraocular pressure, or graft rejection, contact lens fitting for visual restoration should be deferred. Ultimately, the clinician must decide which type of contact lens is most appropriate.

Many contact lens designs may be used for refractive error management involving penetrating keratoplasty patients. These include hydrogel, RGP, hybrid, combination (piggyback), and scleral lenses. The specific design selected depends on many considerations, including corneal graft physiologic status, corneal topography, refractive error, desired wearing schedule, and patient handling capabilities. Each variable must be weighed independently to ensure the greatest likelihood of contact lens success.

Prefitting Physiologic and Topographic Considerations

The penetrating keratoplasty patient presents with an unusual physiologic status. The patient's donor button is entirely repopulated with host epithelium, and keratocyte replacement has begun by the time contact lens fitting is initiated. Corneal innervation is permanently altered by penetrating keratoplasty,[30] however, and endothelial function may differ significantly from the preoperative status.[31] Whether these issues pose a specific threat to contact lens wear after penetrating keratoplasty is debatable, but the impact of contact lens wear on corneal innervation[32] and endothelial function[33] has been well documented. For this reason, it is prudent to select a lens design that minimally affects corneal physiology. In meeting this objective, ensuring adequate oxygen transmissibility is a major priority. The benefit of RGP lenses, by virtue of their direct oxygen transmission and adjunct tear pump, is obvious in this respect. Today, fluoro-silicone/acry-

lates are recommended because of their impressive oxygen transmission characteristics.[34] When a hydrogel lens is indicated, the clinician should consider an extended-wear material worn on a daily-wear basis. The limited oxygen profiles of hybrid and combination designs make each a less logical first choice. If these lens designs are indicated for other reasons, a limited wearing time may be recommended.

Another unique consideration for the penetrating keratoplasty patient involves corneal neovascularization. If the patient's pre-existing corneal disease is marked by severe inflammation, neovascularization may actually precede surgery. Additionally, neovascularization often develops during the postoperative healing phase. In either instance, the contact lens clinician must be aware of the consequences of corneal neovascularization. Indeed, aggressive corneal neovascularization can predispose an individual to or exacerbate a graft rejection episode.[35] In the contact lens population, neovascularization has been associated with intracorneal hemorrhage and lipid leakage, both of which can impair vision. Although the mechanism of contact lens–induced corneal neovascularization is not fully understood, the importance of adequate oxygenation and minimal inflammation is evident.[36] In an effort to address these needs, the clinician should use a gas-permeable lens design. Hydrogel, hybrid, and combination designs are less desirable for the vascularized corneal graft because they cover a larger portion of the peripheral cornea. This can result in a tight fit, hypoxia, and tear stagnation, inducing further vessel encroachment. Corneal neovascularization is not an absolute contraindication to these latter designs but must be monitored closely for progression.

Another important physiologic consideration of the penetrating keratoplasty patient involves corneal surface disease. In light of an altered corneal topography, penetrating keratoplasty patients often manifest an irregular tear film. This is most often evident at the graft-host junction and at the site of suture tracks. The compromised tear film may predispose these individuals toward ocular surface disease, including keratitis sicca, contact lens erosions, and infectious keratitis. Indeed, keratitis sicca is prevalent among older patients with eyelid laxity. Keratitis sicca management can be a perplexing problem because no single material or design is ideal for managing the dry eye. However, in selecting an RGP lens, it is prudent to avoid high–silicone content lenses.[34] With hydrogel lenses, high–water content lens options and ultrathin designs are usually contraindicated.[37] If the clinician has optimized contact lens material and design considerations, adjunct therapy may be necessary. Prophylactic lid hygiene, ocular surface lubricants, and punctal occlusion should be considered if the patient remains symptomatic. The potential for ocular surface erosion is greater if an RGP lens is prescribed for a highly irregular graft surface. Erosion often results from focal lens bearing and is often managed by altering lens design. If epithelial erosion persists despite lens design alterations, refitting into a hydrogel or combination design may be necessary.

The most dreaded consequence of ocular surface disease is infectious keratitis. The propensity of certain bacteria to colonize epithelial defects in contact lens wearers is well documented.[38] This is especially important among penetrating keratoplasty patients because the graft-host junction and suture tracks are more prone to infection and the eye may be immunocompromised from long-term steroid usage. Although infectious keratitis is most often associated with hydrogel extended wear, other lens modalities are not exempt.[39] The significance of epithelial erosion, loose sutures, improper contact lens hygiene, bacterial invasion, compromised host immunity, and delayed treatment is obvious when considering infectious keratitis. For this reason, the contact lens clinician must be sensitive to every aspect of contact lens wear.

Corneal Topography of the Corneal Transplant Patient

Besides the physiologic concerns of fitting the penetrating keratoplasty patient are obvious topographic considerations. Penetrating keratoplasty patients often manifest a topographic profile that differs considerably from the normal cornea (see Figs. 20-3 and 20-4). This has many factors, including preoperative corneal pathology, donor-recipient topographic discrepancies, surgical technique, and wound healing. To better understand how the penetrating keratoplasty patient differs, it is important to understand the topographic features of the normal cornea.

Today's clinician is fortunate to have computerized corneal topography to better understand the norm as well as its surgical variations. Most topographers function on the principle of reflective photokeratoscopy[40] and use a high-resolution, multiple-ring photokeratoscope for image acquisition. A real-time video image is scanned and digitized, the results of which are displayed in a multi-colored format for clinical interpretation. Although corneal topographies are quite varied among the population, some fundamental observations can be made. Figure 20-5 demonstrates corneal topography of a normal eye. It is *enantiomorphic* (mirror imagery with the fellow eye) and variably aspheric, with the nasal cornea flattening more rapidly than the temporal cornea. The center of the cornea has a bow-tie configuration and is oriented with the rule. Round, oval, or bow-tie optical configurations are com-

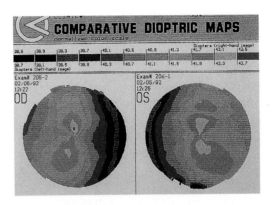

FIG. 20-5. *Normal corneal topography demonstrates enantiomorphism, variable asphericity, and a with-the-rule bow-tie configuration.*

mon among the population, whereas an irregular optic is fairly rare.[41] The with-the-rule profile is found in approximately two-thirds of the population, with the balance manifesting either against-the-rule or oblique configurations. Perhaps of greatest significance is that the corneal apex is in close proximity to the visual axis. This is thought to be almost universally expected[42] and is not always the case in postrefractive surgery patients.

With the penetrating keratoplasty patient, a significant discrepancy can exist between the donor and recipient topographies. The resultant cornea may manifest unusual asphericities, irregular optical zones, and a dramatically displaced apex. These topographies result in reduced vision and present as a challenge to the contact lens fitter. Figure 20-6 shows the topography of a penetrating keratoplasty patient. This particular patient manifests a rather steep central topography, consistent with a *proud* or protruding graft. Of course, the opposite topography can

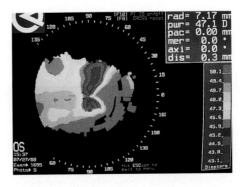

FIG. 20-6. *Post–penetrating keratoplasty corneal topography with a proud or protruding graft.*

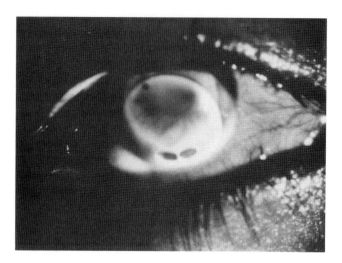

FIG. 20-7. *Fluorescein pattern. A fairly steep penetrating keratoplasty with inferior displacement of a rigid gas-permeable lens.*

occur in a patient with a sunken graft. Furthermore, this patient presents with a rather steep central topography and abrupt transition inferiorly, resulting in contact lens decentration and displacement (Fig. 20-7). This patient's apex is in proximity to his visual axis, but the optical zone is not symmetric. In this scenario, standard keratometry often implies a large amount of astigmatism. The contact lens clinician can erroneously assume symmetry and proceed with a back toric RGP design. The results are often disastrous, with a poor fitting relationship and reduced visual acuity. To avoid this situation, it is best to view the penetrating keratoplasty topography as a steep zone with two discrete hemimeridians.[43] One should not presume the highly astigmatic graft is symmetric unless topographic analysis confirms it.

Contact Lens Options

The fundamental goals of contact lens fitting after penetrating keratoplasty include refractive error correction, comfort commensurate with a reasonable wearing time, and maintenance of ocular health. It has long been accepted that such goals are achieved by using a variety of contact lens options and by using fitting techniques that are as much an art as a science. The authors of this chapter reviewed the files of 20 penetrating keratoplasty patients who were successfully wearing contact lenses. Although this sample is small, it is representative of the penetrating keratoplasty population from the standpoint of surgical indications and postoperative contact lenses worn. In this

sample, 65% wore RGP lenses, 15% wore hydrogel lenses, and 20% wore combination lenses. The sample did not include individuals fitted with either a hybrid or a scleral lens design.

Gas-Permeable Lenses
RGP lenses are appealing for a variety of reasons. Their ability to correct astigmatism and provide a sound physiologic environment is well understood, but the penetrating keratoplasty topography is often a challenge to fit with an RGP lens. To gain a better perspective on lens material and design considerations, each variable is examined here.

Lens Materials   In RGP materials, the fluoro-silicone/acrylate family of lenses offers the greatest margin of safety. These lens materials provide excellent oxygen transmission, improved surface characteristics, and acceptable flexure resistance relative to their predecessors. However, should an extremely thin design or a lower specific gravity be necessary, a low-Dk silicone/acrylate or PMMA lens might be acceptable.

Lens Diameter   Two theories on lens diameter have been advocated through the years. The concept of a small (7.0- to 8.0-mm) lens fitted inside the graft-host junction has largely been abandoned. Difficulties with lens position, poor comfort, and easy displacement accounted for this design's demise. Today, most clinicians agree that lenses with an overall diameter of at least 9.0 mm are indicated.[44] Larger overall diameters of 9.5–11.5 mm are often necessary if the corneal apex is grossly decentered and lens centration is a problem. These larger designs work by facilitating lid attachment.

Lens Optical Zone   Optical zone diameter should be modified according to overall lens diameter. Fundamentally, optical zone diameter should be as large as possible to facilitate lens centration and minimize glare but not so large as to create harsh bearing or result in lens binding.

Lens Base Curve   Most authors agree that a reasonable starting point is to straddle keratometric measurements.[45] Topography-based base curve selection has proved to be a valuable alternative.[46] Corneal topography not only facilitates base curve selection but also allows the fitter to classify topography shape, thereby assisting with lens design.[47] When using corneal topography data, sagittal maps are generally more appropriate. Once selected, the base curve should be adjusted to achieve a divided support fit (Fig. 20-8). In this strategy, the fitter strives for a lens-cornea fitting relationship in which approximately one-third surface-area bearing and two-thirds surface-area clearance exist.[48] Toric base curve options should be reserved for patients whose grafts are highly astigmatic and symmetric. Although most agree that approximately

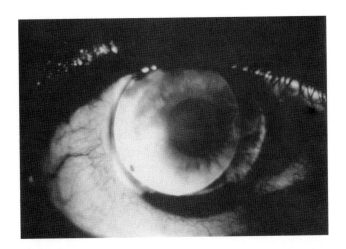

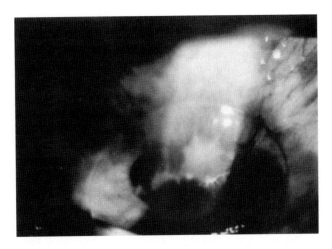

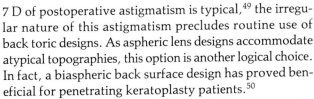

FIG. 20-8. *A fluorescein pattern demonstrating divided support of lens mass.*

FIG. 20-9. *A post–penetrating keratoplasty patient with rigid gas-permeable lens decentration and adherence.*

7 D of postoperative astigmatism is typical,[49] the irregular nature of this astigmatism precludes routine use of back toric designs. As aspheric lens designs accommodate atypical topographies, this option is another logical choice. In fact, a biaspheric back surface design has proved beneficial for penetrating keratoplasty patients.[50]

Lens Peripheral Curve Systems No clear consensus exists on the appropriate peripheral curve system for fitting the penetrating keratoplasty patient. As the central-peripheral corneal topography relationship is so dramatically altered, a traditional base curve–peripheral curve relationship may no longer be indicated. Indeed, peripheral curve systems play a secondary role in fitting most penetrating keratoplasty patients. One particular situation exists in which the peripheral curve system is of paramount importance. This involves the patient with a plateau graft and difficulty with lens centration. For this individual, an unusually steep peripheral curve system may be required. The development of RGP designs in which the secondary curve is actually steeper than the base curve has been beneficial in managing this dilemma. Referred to as *reverse-geometry* lenses, they are manufactured in a variety of RGP materials by several laboratories.

Lens Thickness The philosophy of fitting the lightest lens should prevail. Whenever possible, the thinnest design is used to enhance lens comfort, centration, and physiologic response. Thicker lenses should be reserved for problems with flexure, warpage, adherence, or frequent lens damage.

The penetrating keratoplasty patient may be prone to corneal edema, neovascularization, mechanical erosion, infection, and graft rejection. Although edema, neovascularization, and infection are fairly rare while wear-

ing RGP lenses, the potential for mechanical erosion is clearly evident. This is particularly true among those who experience lens adherence. Figure 20-9 shows one such patient. This individual had been successfully fitted with an RGP lens after penetrating keratoplasty for granular corneal dystrophy. Because of an irregular topography and a decentered RGP lens, she presented with asymptomatic lens adherence and an epithelial defect. Although the mechanism of this phenomenon is not fully understood, certain treatment protocols have been identified.[51]

Hydrogel Lenses

Although they are used less often in penetrating keratoplasty patients, hydrogel lenses offer distinct advantages in certain situations. An atypical graft-recipient topography with attending RGP lens instability is a strong indication for a hydrogel lens. In this case, the patient often enjoys greater contact lens stability and comfort. These individuals may also manifest significant astigmatism and require adjunctive spectacle correction. In addition, penetrating keratoplasty patients wearing hydrogel lenses must be monitored closely for neovascularization.

Lens Materials In prescribing for the penetrating keratoplasty patient, a balance between oxygen permeability and good surface characteristics is important. For myopic correction, this generally involves a nonionic, low–water content, thin-profile design. For moderate and high-plus correction, a medium–water content design is usually indicated. Although these lenses may be approved for extended wear, this option is rarely exercised. An exception may be the elderly, debilitated unilateral aphake. If this individual lives without reliable familial support and is unable to handle the lens daily, extended wear may be prescribed.[52]

Lens Thickness   Since the inception of hydrogel lenses, clinicians have embraced the concept of using standard-thickness designs to mask corneal astigmatism. This is not necessarily true in the nonsurgical population,[53] and little reason exists to believe it is a better strategy for the penetrating keratoplasty population. All other variables considered, it is advisable to prescribe a thinner, more oxygen-permeable design with an adjunct astigmatic spectacle correction. One exception to this strategy involves lens handling because a standard-thickness hydrogel lens is more appropriate for the patient with poor dexterity and a history of frequent lens damage.

Soft Toric Lenses   Clinicians may consider a toric hydrogel lens for the penetrating keratoplasty patient. This is an acceptable option if the patient achieves good vision with a standard refraction, but the clinician should be aware of irregular astigmatism. A diagnostic fitting with hydrogel toric lens, retinoscopy, and subjective over-refraction can identify patients in whom this type of lens is not successful.

The primary reason hydrogel lenses are not used more frequently for penetrating keratoplasty patients relates to poor vision. The potential for corneal neovascularization further relegates hydrogel lenses to a secondary status. Although most agree the potential for graft neovascularization in hydrogel extended wear is significant,[54] not everyone thinks this is an absolute contraindication. Certain authors have reported success in using extended-wear hydrogel lenses with concomitant use of topical steroids for suppression of neovascularization.[54] Clearly, the potential for secondary glaucoma and suprainfection must be carefully weighed if topical steroids are prescribed for prolonged periods. Fundamentally, if a hydrogel lens is indicated, daily wear and close professional supervision are necessary.

Although no implicit relationship exists between hydrogel lenses and infectious keratitis in the penetrating keratoplasty population, it is thought that if extended wear is prescribed, the risk of infectious keratitis increases.

Piggyback Lenses

When an RGP or hydrogel lens alone does not suffice, a combination of the two may be indicated. The concept of piggybacking a rigid contact lens over a hydrogel lens has gained acceptance in specialty lens applications.[55] The piggyback uses a hydrogel lens for surface smoothing and a rigid lens for visual restoration.

Materials   The potential for oxygen debt is significant with the simultaneous use of a hydrogel and rigid contact lens. Therefore, high–oxygen transmission materials

should routinely be prescribed. During lens adaptation, the clinician should carefully monitor biomicroscopy and adjust wearing time accordingly.

Design   The hydrogel lens type is individualized to each patient's needs. The two major determinants are corneal topography and prescription. If the patient manifests a flat or sunken graft, a mid–plus-range lens design is selected. This particular carrier lens accommodates the anticipated need for plus power correction while providing for a steeper topography on which to place the rigid lens. The hydrogel lens may even be a high-plus correction if the patient is aphakic as well. If the patient manifests a steep or proud graft, an ultrathin mid–minus-range lens design is indicated. This carrier lens lessens the amount of minus power necessary in the rigid lens while providing a flatter topography on which to fit the rigid lens. In either situation, the value of incorporating some of the refractive power into the hydrogel lens allows the use of a thinner, lighter rigid lens.

A hydrogel carrier lens specifically manufactured for piggyback applications has been available for years. Marketed as Flexlens (Paragon Vision Sciences, Mesa, AZ), this medium–water content hydrogel lens is available in a variety of base curves, diameters, and insert cuts.[56] The RGP lens is placed in the insert, thus ensuring adequate centration. Although conceptually sound, the Flexlens has yet to gain widespread acceptance. This is true, in part, because of its substantial overall thickness and attendant reduction in oxygen transmission.

Fitting and Evaluation   The actual fitting of a combination lens design begins with evaluation of the underlying hydrogel. The lens should be allowed to equilibrate and then be evaluated for centration and lens movement. Optimal to slightly excessive hydrogel lens movement is encouraged because once the rigid lens is placed on the hydrogel, its movement is almost certainly diminished. Once a satisfactory hydrogel lens fit is obtained, over-keratometry is performed, which serves as a starting point for rigid lens selection. The average of flat and steep over-keratometry is often a reasonable starting point for rigid lens selection. Final base curve, diameter, optical zone, peripheral curve, power, and thickness determinations are best accomplished by diagnostic fitting. High-molecular-weight fluorescein can be used to assess apical clearance of the rigid lens relative to its hydrogel carrier. Care must be taken to avoid a tightly fit rigid lens because this often traps interfacial debris (Fig. 20-10).

Complications   It is generally accepted that any complication that can occur with either a hydrogel or an RGP lens can occur when a piggyback system is used. This is not entirely true because peripheral corneal staining patterns common to RGP lenses do not occur in piggyback

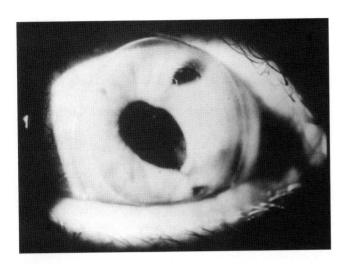

FIG. 20-10. *A piggyback contact lens combination with interfacial debris.*

combinations. However, edema, neovascularization, contact lens adherence, acute red-eye episodes, infectious keratitis, and graft rejection can occur with a piggyback combination.

Hybrid Lenses

A relatively new entry in the contact lens management of penetrating keratoplasty is hybrid design, introduced to satisfy the demands for comfort and acceptable optics. Initially developed by Precision-Cosmet and marketed as the Saturn lens, the first hybrid lens offered a styrene rigid lens center molecularly bonded to a low–water content hydroxyethyl-methacrylate skirt.[57] Because of performance limitations, this lens has been redesigned and is currently marketed by Wesley-Jessen (Des Plaines, IL) as the SoftPerm lens. Although it is made of the same material, the SoftPerm features significant design improvements. The larger overall diameter, in conjunction with the larger RGP insert and a transition curve between materials, provides for a wider range of applications.[57]

Considerable debate exists on the benefits of a hybrid design for penetrating keratoplasty. The limited oxygen transmission of each material justifies concerns about an edematous response. The tendency toward lens binding can lead to neovascularization, epithelial erosion, acute red eye, infiltrative keratitis, and graft rejection. Indeed, early work with the Saturn confirmed the clinical limitations of this design.[58] However, the ability of a hybrid lens to perform as a combination lens should be considered. Hybrid lenses offer excellent centration and stability, as well as correction of modest amounts of

astigmatism. Experiences with SoftPerm have been more favorable; however, certain precautions must be taken. The proper base curve must be selected by diagnostic fitting, with each trial lens allowed to equilibrate for a minimum of 15 minutes. Regardless of how comfortable and clear the lens is, adequate movement is essential. If adequate movement is not obtainable with a diagnostic lens fitting, an alternate lens option should be selected. Once an adequate fit is obtained, the patient must be closely monitored for an unacceptable edematous response.

REFERENCES

1. Binder PS: Optical problems following refractive surgery. Ophthalmology 93:739, 1986
2. Aquavella JV: Therapeutic uses of hydrophilic lenses. Invest Ophthalmol 13:484, 1974
3. Mannis MJ, Zadnik K: Hydrophilic contact lenses for wound stabilization in keratoplasty. CLAO J 14:199, 1988
4. Plotnik RD, Mannis MJ, Schwab IR: Therapeutic contact lenses. Int Ophthalmol Clin 31:35, 1991
5. Bence BG, Blaze PA: Therapeutic soft contact lenses. Contact Lens Spectrum 3:52, 1988
6. Waltman SR, Kaufman HE: Use of hydrophilic contact lenses to increase ocular penetration of topical drugs. Invest Ophthalmol 9:250, 1970
7. Lesher GA, Gunderson GG: Continuous drug delivery through the use of disposable contact lenses. Optom Vis Sci 70:1012, 1993
8. Sawusch MR, O'Brien TP, Dick JD, Gottsch JD: Use of collagen corneal shields in the treatment of bacterial keratitis. Am J Ophthalmol 106:279, 1988
9. Aquavella JV, del Cerro M, Ueda S, DePaolis M: The effect of a collagen bandage lens on corneal wound healing: a preliminary report. Ophthalmic Surg 18:570, 1987
10. Ruffini JJ, Aquavella JV, LoCascio JA: Effect of collagen shields on corneal epithelialization following penetrating keratoplasty. Ophthalmic Surg 20:21, 1989
11. Dohlman CH, Boruchoff A, Mobilia EF: Complications in use of soft contact lenses in corneal disease. Arch Ophthalmol 90:367, 1973
12. Sanders DR, Hoffman RF (eds): Refractive Surgery: A Text of Radial Keratotomy. Slack, Thorofare, NJ, 1985
13. Arffa RC: Results of a graded relaxing incision technique for post keratoplasty astigmatism. Ophthalmic Surg 19:624, 1988
14. Swinger CA: Comparison of results obtained with keratophakia, hypermetropic keratomileusis, intraocular lens implantation, and extended-wear contact lenses. Int Ophthalmol Clin 23:59, 1983
15. Shovlin JP: The use of alloplastics: a new realm of refractive surgery? Int Contact Lens Clin 16:304, 1989
16. Beekhuis WH, McCarey BE, Van Rij G, et al: Complications of hydrogel intracorneal lenses in monkeys. Invest Ophthalmol Vis Sci 105:116, 1987

17. Werblin TP, Kaufman HE, Friedlander MH, Granet N: Epikeratophakia: the surgical correction of aphakia. III. Preliminary results of a prospective clinical trial. Arch Ophthalmol 99:1957, 1981

18. Binder PS, Zavala EY: Why do some epikeratoplasties fail? Arch Ophthalmol 105:63, 1987

19. Dietze TR, Durrie DS: Indications and treatment of keratoconus using epikeratophakia. Ophthalmology 95:236, 1988

20. Seiler T, Kahle G, Kriegerowski M: Excimer laser (193 nm) myopic keratomileusis in sighted and blind human eyes. Refract Corneal Surg 6:165, 1990

21. Steinert RF, Puliafito CA: Laser Corneal Surgery. Little, Brown and Company, Boston, 1988

22. Aron-Rosa DS, Colin J, Aron B, et al: Clinical results of excimer laser photorefractive keratectomy: a multicenter study of 265 eyes. J Cataract Refract Surg 21:644, 1995

23. Dausch D, Klein R, Landesz M, Schroder E: Photorefractive keratectomy to correct astigmatism with myopia or hyperopia. J Cataract Refract Surg 20:252, 1994

24. Dausch D, Klein R, Schroder E: Excimer laser photorefractive keratectomy for hyperopia. Refract Corneal Surg 9:20, 1993

25. Von Hippel A, Albrecht V: Graefes Arch Ophthalmol 34:108, 1888

26. Zirm E, Albrecht V: Graefes Arch Ophthalmol 64:580, 1906

27. Van Meter WS, Gussler JR, Soloman KD, Wood TO: Post-keratoplasty astigmatism control. Ophthalmology 98:177, 1991

28. Jensen AD, Maumenee AE: Refractive error following keratoplasty. Trans Am Ophthalmol Soc 72:123, 1970

29. Buxton JM: Contact lenses in keratoconus. Cont Intraocular Lens Med J 4:74, 1978

30. Ruben M, Colebrook E: Keratoconus, keratoplasty curvatures, and lens wear. Br J Ophthalmol 63:268, 1979

31. Brown NAP, Bron AJ: Endothelium of the corneal graft. Trans Ophthalmol Soc UK 94:863, 1974

32. Millodot M: Effect of the length of wear of contact lenses on corneal sensitivity. Acta Ophthalmol 54:721, 1976

33. Holden BA, Sweeney DF, Vannas A, et al: Contact lens induced endothelial polymegethism. Invest Ophthalmol Vis Sci (suppl.)26:275, 1985

34. Tomlinson A: Choice of materials—a material issue. Contact Lens Spectrum 5:27, 1990

35. Lemp MA: The effect of extended-wear aphakic hydrophilic contact lenses after penetrating keratoplasty. Am J Ophthalmol 90:331, 1980

36. McMonnies CW: Etiology of contact lens induced corneal vascularisation. Int Contact Lens Clin 11:287, 1984

37. Helton DO, Watson LS: Hydrogel contact lens dehydration rates determined by thermogravimetric analysis. CLAO J 17:59, 1991

38. Reichert R, Stern G: Quantitative adherence of bacteria to human corneal epithelial cells. Arch Ophthalmol 102:1394, 1984

39. Chalupa E, Swarbrick HA, Holden BA, Sjostrand J: Severe corneal infections associated with contact lens wear. Ophthalmology 94:17, 1987

40. Gormley D, Gerston M, Koplin RS, Lubkin V: Corneal modeling. Cornea 7:30, 1988

41. Bogan SJ, Waring GO, Ibrahim O, et al: Classification of normal corneal topography based on computer-assisted videokeratography. Arch Ophthalmol 108:945, 1990

42. Dingeldein SA, Klyce SD: The topography of normal corneas. Arch Ophthalmol 107:512, 1989

43. Maguire LJ, Bourne WM: Corneal topography of transverse keratotomies for astigmatism after penetrating keratoplasty. Am J Ophthalmol 107:323, 1989

44. Zadnik K: Post-surgical contact lens alternatives. Int Contact Lens Clin 15:211, 1988

45. Daniel R: Fitting contact lenses after keratoplasty. Br J Ophthalmol 60:263, 1976

46. Wicker D, Bleckinger P, Kowalski L, Wisniewski K: Gaining efficiency in fitting the post-penetrating keratoplasty patient. Contact Lens Spectrum 12:45, 1997

47. Szotka LB: Contact lenses for the irregular cornea. Contact Lens Spectrum 13:21, 1998

48. Shovlin J, Kame R, Weissman B, DePaolis M: How to fit an irregular cornea. Rev Optom 124:88, 1987

49. Genvert GI, Cohen EJ, Arentsen JJ, Laibson PR: Fitting gas-permeable contact lenses after penetrating keratoplasty. Am J Ophthalmol 99:511, 1985

50. Weiner B: Contact lens correction of the post-penetrating keratoplasty patient. Contact Lens Update 8:61, 1989

51. Kenyon E, Mandell RB, Poise KA: Lens design effects on rigid lens adherence. J Br Contact Lens Assoc 12:32, 1989

52. Cowden JW: Continuous wear aphakic soft contact lenses following keratoplasty. Ann Ophthalmol 12:579, 1980

53. Wechsler S, Ingraham T, Sherill D: Masking astigmatism with spherical soft lenses. Contact Lens Forum 11:42, 1986

54. Lemp MA: The effect of extended-wear aphakic hydrophilic contact lenses after penetrating keratoplasty. Am J Ophthalmol 90:331, 1980

55. Soper JW, Paton D: A piggy-back contact lens system for corneal transplants and other cases with high astigmatism. Contact Lens Intraocular Lens Med J 6:132, 1980

56. Caroline PJ, Doughman DJ: A new piggyback lens-design for correction of irregular astigmatism—a preliminary report. Contact Lens Intraocular Lens Med J 5:40, 1979

57. Edwards GL: Birth of a new lens ... SoftPerm. Contemp Optom 8:10, 1989

58. Zadnik K, Mannis M: Use of the Saturn II lens in keratoconus and corneal transplant patients. Int Contact Lens Clin 14:312, 1987

VIII

*Therapeutic Aspects
of Contact Lens Wear*

21

Therapeutic Bandage Lenses

BARRY M. WEINER

GRAND ROUNDS CASE REPORT

Subjective:
A 69-year-old woman presents with a history of bilateral recurrent corneal erosions over past 2 years. Prior treatment with ocular lubricants and antibiotic drops during abrasion episodes was unsuccessful. Patient denies prior trauma. Medical history includes hypertension and taking metoprolol (Lopressor), disopyramide (Norpace), and ranitidine (Zantac).

Objective:
- Best corrected acuity: right eye (OD) $^{20}/_{20}$; J-1 @ 16 in., left eye (OS) $^{20}/_{20}$; J-1 @ 16 in.
- Biomicroscopy: OS small epithelial defect at 12 o'clock, 2 mm × 1 mm, 2 mm inside the limbus; each eye (OU) map-dot-fingerprint dystrophy; 1+ corneal guttata.
- Ophthalmoscopy: 1+ nuclear sclerosis OU; retinal vasculature shows mild hypertensive changes.

Assessment:
Recurrent corneal erosion secondary to epithelial basement membrane dystrophy; mild Fuchs' dystrophy.

Plan:
1. Hyperosmotic therapy initiated with 5% saline drops four times a day OU.
2. Erythromycin ointment OS twice a day until erosion heals.

Follow-up:
One-week follow-up: No trace abrasion; discontinue antibiotic.

Five-week follow-up: Patient presented with recurrence of erosion OS; given 5% saline drops and 5% hypertonic ointment plus antibiotic; ocular lubricants four times a day.

Symptoms recurred twice over next 3 months.

Plan:
Therapeutic bandage lens OS only. Lens was 38% water content, for continuous wear; 5% saline drops to be used four times a day with lens.

Follow-up at 1, 2, and 4 weeks unremarkable, with good comfort and lens tolerance. A fresh lens was provided at 4 weeks and at regular 4-week intervals.

After 16 weeks, lens use was discontinued, with hypertonic saline used OU during day and hypertonic ointment at night; also, ocular lubricants OU.

Patient has remained free of symptoms for many months with no sign of recurrence of corneal erosion.

Comment:
Use of a contact lens protects the cornea from the shearing forces of the upper lid, allowing a more secure hemidesmosomal attachment of epithelium to Bowman's membrane.

HISTORY

The concept of an eye bandage was attributed to Celsus in the first century A.D. when he was reported to have applied a honey-soaked linen bandage to an eye to prevent the formation of symblepharon after removal of a pterygium.[1] Leonardo Da Vinci first mentioned the theoretical use of a contact lens–like device for improvement of vision in 1508. René Descartes in 1637, Thomas Young in 1801, and Sir John Herschel in 1823 also contributed to the theoretical basis of the bandage contact lens.[1]

In 1887, at the suggestion of a physician, F.A. Muller developed a thin, glass-blown shell to protect an eye from the drying effects of lagophthalmos, thus using a contact lens as a therapeutic device. In 1888, Dr. Eugene Kalt of Zurich began using a glass corneal lens design to correct the irregularity caused by keratoconus.[2] Scleral lenses, first made of glass and later of polymethylmethacrylate, came into use for advanced keratoconus, corneal transplant irregularity, and irregular corneas after trauma.[3]

Kaufman and Gasset[4] experimented with a contact lens glued to a de-epithelialized Bowman's membrane with cyanoacrylate glue. This epikeratoprosthesis was found to be of some value in selected cases of bullous keratopathy, keratoconus, and dry eye syndromes, but the technique has not gained widespread acceptance.[4]

The development of hydroxyethyl methacrylate by Professor Otto Wichterle began the modern soft lens era and widened the application of contact lenses as a therapeutic modality. Hydrophilic contact lenses have found use as protective devices for the cornea, as pressure bandages to relieve pain, to promote corneal healing, to improve vision during the healing process, and to serve as a delivery mechanism for pharmaceutical agents.

PRESCRIPTION OF A THERAPEUTIC CONTACT LENS

Selecting an appropriate therapeutic contact lens depends on patient characteristics and the disorder for which the lens is being prescribed. Patient characteristics may include age, any physical deformity (e.g., arthritis), a physical or mental handicap, and patient comprehension and motivation to use a contact lens. Concomitant conditions, such as dry eye, blepharitis, and meibomian gland dysfunction, may also influence lens selection and suitability.

High–water content hydrogel lenses, in general, are best used when minimal disturbance to the underlying epithelium is the first priority. They are contraindicated when a dry eye condition is evident as a primary or concomitant condition. High–water content lenses are better tolerated in eyes with corneal or anterior segment inflammation.[5] Medium–water content or low–water content lenses are used when little lens movement is desirable, as in splinting procedures used in treatment of corneal perforations and descemetocele. Low–water content lenses are best suited for eyes that show little or no inflammation or in which a dry eye condition exists.[6] Medium–water content lenses are recommended when significant corneal or limbal irregularity exists.

Collagen shield lenses, which were developed by Fyodorov and made from porcine or bovine scleral collagen, were introduced to protect corneas after radial keratotomy. They have found use as short-term protective and lubricating devices after corneal surgery and as delivery vehicles for topical application of drugs, such as antibiotics and glaucoma medications.

INDICATIONS FOR THERAPEUTIC CONTACT LENSES

Corneal Epithelial Abnormalities and Defects

Recurrent Corneal Erosion
Therapeutic contact lens application lends itself well to the treatment of recurrent corneal erosion when standard hypertonic saline therapy alone is not successful. The patient often experiences a foreign-body sensation with pain and photophobia, usually occurring immediately on arising in the morning. Recurrent corneal erosion may be

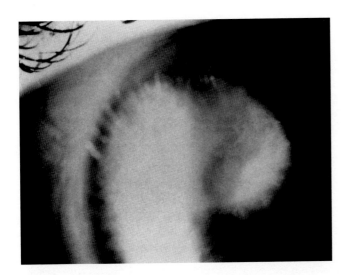

FIG. 21-1. *Recurrent corneal erosion.*

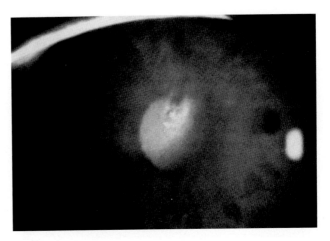

FIG. 21-2. *Recurrent corneal erosion.*

accompanied by mild conjunctival injection, lacrimation, and blepharospasm.

The patient usually relates a history of previous corneal trauma. If no such history is elicited, careful slit-lamp evaluation may reveal an anterior basement membrane dystrophy (Cogan's microcystic dystrophy, map-dot-fingerprint dystrophies, or Reis-Buckler's superficial dystrophy).

Epithelial breakdown frequently occurs after trauma, when an abnormal basement membrane does not permit secure hemidesmosomal adhesion between the basal epithelium and Bowman's membrane.[7] Bandage hydrogel contact lenses protect the epithelium from being separated from Bowman's membrane by the mechanical action of the lids. This allows time for adequate hemidesmosomal attachment to develop[8] (Figs. 21-1 and 21-2).

Application of a therapeutic lens is governed by the severity of the patient's symptoms. Initial therapy is ocular lubricants with a corneal desiccant regimen of hypertonic saline drops or hypertonic saline ointment, or both. Bandage lenses are used when this initial therapy is deemed unsuccessful.[9] A bandage lens is commonly used on an extended-wear basis for 2–3 months, with removal and replacement only as necessary. Concurrent hypertonic saline drops should also be used, along with nonpreserved ocular lubricants. Hyperosmotic ointments are not indicated because of their effect on the wettability of the lens as well as their blurring effect.

Recalcitrant corneal erosion may also be addressed using anterior stromal puncture or with excimer laser phototherapeutic keratectomy. Anterior stromal puncture for post-traumatic nonaxial erosions may be attempted if standard therapy proves ineffective but is contraindicated for erosions secondary to corneal dystrophic changes.

Phototherapeutic keratectomy has proved effective in eliminating recurrent corneal erosion.[10] Treatment technique requires the removal of the epithelium in the affected area along with 5 μm of Bowman's membrane.[11] A therapeutic contact lens is used for 3–4 days after the procedure along with concomitant antibiotic treatment to protect the healing epithelium and to palliate pain.

Filamentary Keratitis

Filamentary keratitis is characterized by the presence of filaments of twisted epithelium attached at their base to the surrounding corneal epithelium.[12] The patient may experience severe pain as the filament is detached from the underlying epithelium by action of the lids. Visual acuity may also be affected secondary to induced irregular corneal astigmatism (Figs. 21-3 and 21-4).

Dry filamentary keratitis can be treated with artificial tears and ocular lubricants. Secondary as well as idiopathic wet filamentary keratitis does not respond to lubricant therapy and may continue to recur after the filaments are mechanically removed. Use of a hydrophilic bandage lens with concomitant use of corticosteroids and atropine often relieves this condition within 7 days, without recurrence.[13] A bandage lens protects the epithelium from exogenous trauma from the lids and allows time for the epithelium to heal. The pressure-bandage effect of the lens also may help to relieve the pain associated with this condition.

Thygeson's Superficial Punctate Keratitis

Thygeson's punctate keratitis is characterized by multiple discrete opacities, which usually are found in the pupillary area but in fact may involve all areas of the cornea. The lesions, which may number from three to 20 or more, are often observed as a conglomeration of small punctate

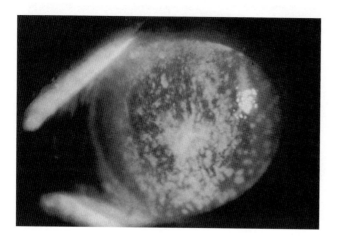

FIG. 21-3. *Filamentary keratitis.*

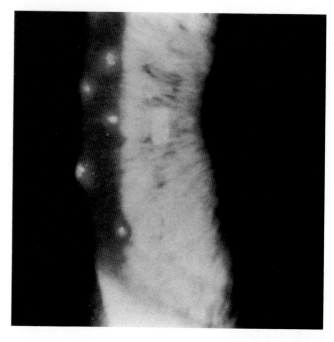

FIG. 21-5. *Thygeson's superficial punctate keratitis.*

opacities (Figs. 21-5 and 21-6).[14] This condition is usually bilateral and can last from 6 months to 4 years, with some reported instances lasting up to 24 years.[15] Patients experience intermittent episodes of tearing, photophobia, and foreign-body sensation.[16] The etiology of Thygeson's punctate keratitis is unknown, although a viral etiology is suspected.[17]

The epithelial opacities distort the epithelial surface and reduce visual acuity. Therapeutic soft lenses smooth out the distorted surface, improving visual acuity, and act as a pressure bandage to relieve pain and foreign-body sensation.

Several therapeutic regimens have been described for this condition, but no single regimen seems to be a true cure. Symptomatic relief with short-term use of topical cor-

ticosteroids and ocular lubricants can be provided during the active phase of the condition, along with the use of a bandage contact lens. Long-term use of steroids may be counterproductive, however, and prolong the condition. Using a therapeutic contact lens gives the patient visual and palliative relief from pain and allows normal functioning, with minimal disruption to the patient's daily routine.

The lesions gradually become less pronounced and may become subepithelial. The patient should use an extended-wear schedule with the bandage lens when symptoms are

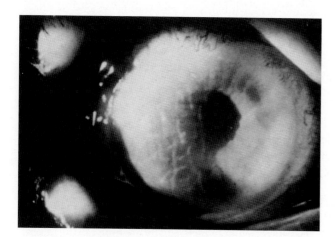

FIG. 21-4. *Filamentary keratitis in a patient with bullous keratopathy.*

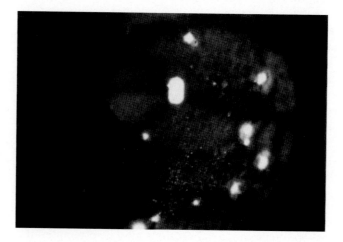

FIG. 21-6. *Thygeson's superficial punctate keratitis.*

acute, changing to a daily-wear schedule when asymptomatic, with a return to extended wear as needed.[18]

Superior Limbic Keratoconjunctivitis

Superior limbic keratoconjunctivitis (SLK) is a chronic bilateral condition, more prevalent in middle-aged women, that is characterized by inflammation of the superior tarsal and superior bulbar conjunctiva. Positive fluorescein and rose bengal staining of the superior limbal area are usually seen in SLK. Approximately one-third of patients have an associated thyroid condition, and appropriate referral and treatment should be made.[18] The patient experiences burning, pain, photophobia, blepharospasm, and a foreign-body sensation.

Traditional treatment often entails application of a 0.5% silver nitrate solution to the upper palpebral conjunctiva, but recurrence of the condition after treatment is common. Pressure patching to relieve the initial discomfort, followed by the use of a bandage soft lens, has proved to be highly successful in eliminating the mechanical effects of the lids on the globe during the blink.[19] Patching helps to relieve the blepharospasm and inflammatory signs associated with SLK and makes the subsequent use of a therapeutic lens more effective in preventing recurrences.[8]

Persistent Corneal Ulcer

Patients with persistent corneal ulcers that do not respond to conventional medical intervention can achieve relief from pain through the use of a bandage contact lens.[20] Persistent corneal ulcers that do not respond to medical intervention may lead to full-thickness corneal scarring, corneal melt, or perforation. It is not known whether the persistence of this condition results from some active microbial agent or is a healing problem with poor hemidesmosomal attachment between Bowman's membrane and the epithelium (Fig. 21-7).

Conventional intervention for persistent ulcers may include patching, tarsorrhaphy, or conjunctival flap procedures, but these treatments do not allow the patient use of the eye during therapy and also hide the eye from the view of the attending physician. Medicating the eye is also difficult.[21] The use of a therapeutic contact lens, therefore, allows the eye care practitioner to observe the effects or consequences of treatment while relieving the patient's pain and allowing the patient some degree of useful vision.

Treatment of persistent stromal ulcers depends on the location of the ulcer. Ulcers respond well to low–water content lenses that show little lens movement. The low permeability and lack of movement encourage the limbal vessels to invade the ulcerated area and help promote healing.

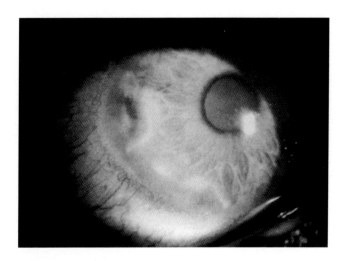

FIG. 21-7. *Persistent corneal ulcer.*

Central stromal ulcers with extreme tissue loss are more readily treated surgically. If less than 80% thinning exists, a conjunctival flap minimizes the possibility of corneal perforation. Penetrating keratoplasty is called for if the stroma is more than 80% thinned. If an active inflammatory response exists, a high–water content lens and topical medication can be used until the eye quiets enough to allow the keratoplasty to be performed.[22]

Collagen shield lenses soaked in topical medications have been used to promote healing in persistent corneal ulceration. Studies have shown that a system of collagen lenses soaked in antibiotics can increase corneal penetration of certain drugs up to 30-fold.[23] Collagen shields maintain contact of the medication against the eye and in the tear film much longer than with conventional drops or ointments.

Mooren's Ulcer

Mooren's ulcer is a progressive ulceration of the peripheral cornea, which begins with an elevated, de-epithelialized leading edge at the corneal periphery and may progress centrally and circumferentially. If untreated, it may progress to involve the central cornea. As it progresses, a vascularized pannus forms in its wake, and corneal perforation may result (Fig. 21-8). The basic etiology of Mooren's ulcer is unknown, but it is usually preceded by corneal trauma, surgery, or inflammation. An autoimmune process may also play a role.

This condition usually responds to corticosteroid therapy, but if the defect persists, application of a low- or medium–water content therapeutic lens along with corticosteroids may be necessary. The lens acts as a splint to allow epithelial healing and as a pressure bandage.[24]

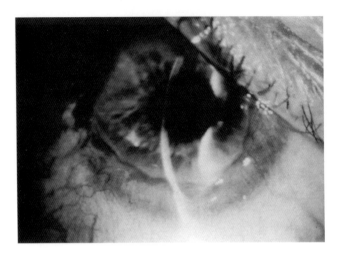

FIG. 21-8. *Mooren's ulcer.*

Pellucid Marginal Degeneration

Pellucid marginal degeneration bilaterally affects the inferior peripheral cornea. Unlike Mooren's ulcer, usually no scarring or vascularization exists. Pellucid marginal degeneration may cause marked irregular astigmatism or high amounts of against-the-rule astigmatism, which is difficult to correct with spectacles. The etiology of this condition is unknown, but a strong genetic factor exists, and it has much in common with keratoconus.

Rigid contact lenses can be used to improve acuity, but fitting rigid lenses is difficult because of the high degree of astigmatism and the marked cylindrical protrusion of the inferior portion of the affected cornea. It may be necessary to use a therapeutic soft lens as the base for a piggyback system with a rigid lens to increase patient acuity

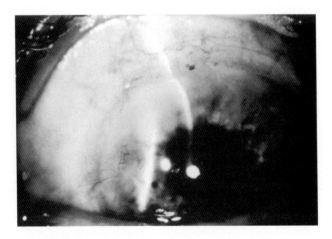

FIG. 21-9. *Terrien's marginal degeneration.*

and comfort when the condition is severe and when vision cannot be corrected by other means.[25]

Terrien's Marginal Degeneration

Terrien's marginal degeneration is a slowly progressive, marginal thinning and ectasia of unknown etiology. It most often occurs in men between 20 and 30 years of age and is usually bilateral (Fig. 21-9).

High degrees of against-the-rule astigmatism may occur as this condition progresses. Using a therapeutic soft lens as a base with an RGP contact lens in a piggyback system may be necessary to restore usable acuity. Surgical intervention may include annular full-thickness keratoplasty, crescentic lamellar keratoplasty, or large eccentric penetrating grafts, and may be necessary when the contact lens system can no longer be tolerated.[26]

Herpes Simplex Keratitis

Primary herpes simplex infection of the eye is usually characterized by vesicles on the skin of the lids, follicular conjunctivitis, and occasionally punctate keratitis. Recurrent infections usually take the form of dendritic ulceration of the cornea. The incidence of corneal ulceration and perforation in persistent herpes simplex keratitis is very high. A study by Cavanagh[27] showed that 68% of the studied patients had corneal ulcers and 40% progressed to corneal perforation.

A therapeutic soft lens, in conjunction with minimal levels of corticosteroids and topical antiviral medication, is the treatment regimen of choice. The therapeutic contact lens protects the healing epithelium and acts as a drug reservoir to enhance penetration of the antiviral agents, whereas drops used alone show very poor corneal penetration. The therapeutic lens reduces patient discomfort and may improve visual performance.[28]

A 1975 study reported that during an 18-month period, herpetic ulcers accounted for 46% of all corneal epithelial defects reported (52 of 114 patients) in the Cornea Service of the Massachusetts Eye and Ear Infirmary.[29] The defects occurred after the viral infection subsided and may have been exacerbated by excessive use of steroids or antiviral medication.

The epithelial defects are usually centrally located and have ragged, raised edges. New epithelial cells tend to heap at the margins of the defect, poorly covering the affected area, making healing very slow. In one study, the average healing time was 15 weeks when no therapeutic contact lens was used and 8–10 weeks when a bandage contact lens was used along with the medications.

Incorporating a therapeutic lens into the medical regime, along with antiviral medications, helps to relieve pain, improve the patient's vision, and speed the healing process.

The lens should be applied early in the treatment process and remain in place until healing is complete.[27] Topical steroids, if and when prescribed, should only be given with a concurrent antiviral cover.[28]

Corneal Lacerations, Perforations, and Descemetocele

Trauma to the eye may result in corneal abrasions, laceration, or perforation. Concussive injury or direct contact injury to the epithelium may result in abrasions and localized or generalized edema, with folds present at the level of Bowman's or Descemet's membrane. Corneal erosion may be of late onset and should be anticipated. This recurrent erosion after trauma can be treated with a therapeutic contact lens if desiccation therapy with hypertonic saline is not effective.

Corneal Laceration

Partial-thickness corneal lacerations involving the stroma, where the wound edges are well appositioned, can be treated by using a bandage soft lens along with concomitant antibiotic therapy. Thin, low–water content lenses are the modality of choice.

Penetrating corneal lacerations can have major consequences, including loss of the anterior chamber, lenticular penetration and subsequent opacification, vitreous hemorrhage, uveal prolapse, iris incarceration, corneal opacification, and intraocular infection. Full-thickness lacerations larger than 3 mm require surgical intervention, usually under general anesthesia, to repair the wound, reform the anterior chamber, and deal with other complications.

Small, full-thickness wounds can be treated with a therapeutic contact lens and the appropriate antibiotic treatment. Leibowitz[30] treated five penetrating corneal wounds with a therapeutic contact lens and copious antibiotics. The lenses were worn continuously for up to 7 days. All five patients healed completely, with only small scars left at the entrance sites.

Use of bandage lenses is limited to small lacerations with well-appositioned wound edges. Wound gape, malpositioned wound edges, and incarceration of iris or uveal tissue are all contraindications for a contact lens.

Bandage lenses, when appropriate, have advantages over surgery. Application of a lens is technically easy and requires little or no instrumentation or equipment. The lens reduces pain by acting as a pressure bandage. Other treatment, if necessary, is not compromised by contact lens application, such as suturing or the use of cyanoacrylate glue.[30]

Some clinicians advocate the use of cyanoacrylate glue as the treatment of choice. The application of glue is tech-

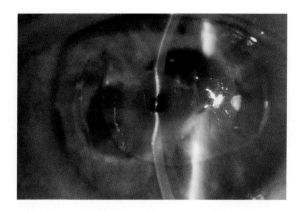

FIG. 21-10. *Corneal perforation and descemetocele.*

nically simple and can be repeated as necessary in uninfected eyes. The adhesive is covered by a thin, low–water content therapeutic lens to protect it from the shearing effects of the lid and to increase patient comfort.[31]

Corneal Perforation and Descemetocele

Corneal perforation or descemetocele may result from complications of corneal infection or corneal melt. Perforation can cause a flat anterior chamber, anterior synechia, secondary glaucoma, chronic iridocyclitis, cataract, or endophthalmitis.[32] Treatment may include conjunctival flap procedures, patch grafts, penetrating keratoplasty, tissue adhesive, or bandage contact lenses (Figs. 21-10–21-12).

Descemetocele secondary to trauma, infection, exposure, or chemical burn constitutes an ocular emergency that must be treated as soon as possible. The lens acts as a splint to reinforce Descemet's membrane and to prevent distention until more permanent treatment, such as penetrating keratoplasty or patch grafting, can be performed.[31]

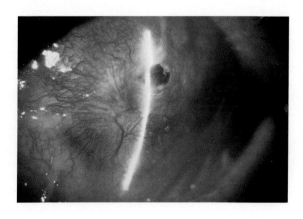

FIG. 21-11. *Descemetocele.*

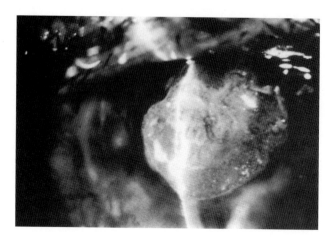

FIG. 21-12. *Descemetocele.*

Thick, high-water content lenses are the materials of choice in this situation.

Contact lenses are simple in comparison with other therapies and are reversible, if complications arise, without prejudicing other treatment modalities.

Endothelial Disorders

Bullous Keratopathy

Bullous keratopathy is caused by the failure of the corneal endothelium to regulate the fluid balance of the cornea. It is most often seen in severely diseased eyes, most commonly with long-standing glaucoma or after perforating wounds or corneal surgery. The influx of fluid causes corneal edema, seen as a loss of corneal transparency, corneal thickening, and folds at Descemet's membrane (Fig. 21-13).

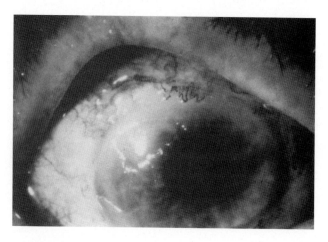

FIG. 21-13. *Bullous keratopathy.*

As the epithelium becomes edematous, fluid begins to accumulate within the basal cells and then settles between the cells and finally subcellularly, lifting the epithelium and forming the characteristic bullae. Bullae induce irregular corneal astigmatism and produce pain as the patient blinks across them or when they rupture. Patient symptoms include pain, irritation, redness, and photophobia. Therapeutic, high-water content, thick lenses improve acuity and relieve pain. Many investigators have found that hydrophilic lenses give almost immediate relief of pain and substantial improvement in visual acuity.[33-36]

The use of a therapeutic lens must be accompanied by other concomitant therapy. Because iritis is often associated with bullous keratopathy, instillation of a cycloplegic on lens insertion is usually necessary and continues until the epithelium heals. Antibiotics for prophylaxis may also be used. Use of a therapeutic contact lens can delay the need for more radical intervention, such as penetrating keratoplasty. In many instances, the marked improvement of the cornea after this therapeutic regimen allows periodic discontinuation of lens wear until such time as the patient may experience the renewal of symptoms. In this event, the therapeutic bandage lens and concomitant therapy can be resumed.

Fuchs' Endothelial Dystrophy

Fuchs' endothelial dystrophy is an inherited autosomal dominant condition affecting the corneal endothelium, producing corneal guttata as well as stromal and epithelial edema. It is four times as common in women as in men and usually occurs after menopause.[37] It is usually bilateral but asymmetric, and symptoms usually do not manifest before age 50 years.[38]

Fuchs' dystrophy begins with minor posterior corneal manifestations of irregularly distributed guttata. As the condition progresses, patients experience decreasing acuity and increasing glare as corneal edema increases. Advanced Fuchs' dystrophy causes the cornea to take on a ground-glass appearance, with distinct folds noted at Descemet's membrane (Fig. 21-14).

Treatment in early stages may entail the use of hypertonic drops or ointment to reduce edema and blowing warm air across the cornea on awakening to increase tear evaporation and help reduce the edema.[39]

Therapeutic lenses are best suited for patients who report blurred vision or pain. The lens smoothes the irregular astigmatism induced by the bullae and acts as a pressure bandage to relieve the pain.

Posterior Polymorphous Dystrophy

Posterior polymorphous dystrophy is an inherited autosomal dominant dystrophy. It is usually bilateral but may

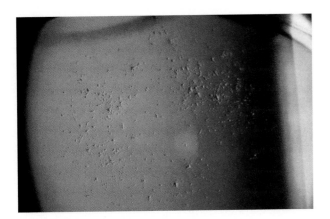

FIG. 21-14. *Guttata in Fuchs' endothelial dystrophy.*

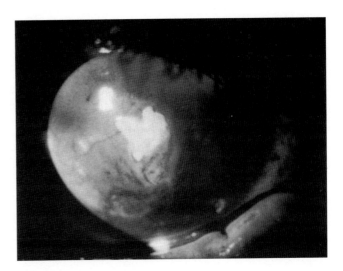

FIG. 21-15. *Corneal abrasion.*

be asymmetric or unilateral. It is a slowly progressive congenital condition characterized by small grouped vesicles and large, geographically shaped blisterlike lesions in broad bands that appear as a thickening of Descemet's membrane.[40]

Patients with posterior polymorphous dystrophy who also have mild stromal or epithelial edema can be treated with a thick, high–water content lens and concomitant hypertonic saline. As in Fuchs' dystrophy, the lens smoothes the anterior surface of the cornea to increase visual acuity.

Congenital Hereditary Endothelial Dystrophy

Congenital hereditary endothelial dystrophy can be inherited as either an autosomal dominant or an autosomal recessive trait. The autosomal recessive condition is usually present at birth and remains stationary and asymptomatic. The dominant form appears in the first or second year of life and manifests symptoms of tearing and photophobia. It may progress over the next 5–10 years and cause epithelial and stromal edema involving the entire cornea.[41] A gray thickening can be noted at the level of Descemet's membrane.

As in other endothelial dystrophic conditions, this condition may reduce the patient's acuity by inducing irregular astigmatism. Application of a therapeutic, thick, high–water content lens may improve the patient's vision.

TRAUMA

Corneal Abrasions

A large percentage of eye care problems presenting for emergency treatment are the result of traumatic corneal abrasions (Fig. 21-15).[42] The traditional treatment for a corneal abrasion consists of a topical antibiotic, combined with instillation of a topical cycloplegic, and pressure patching for 24–48 hours. An alternative treatment may be the application of a therapeutic bandage contact lens.

Acheson et al.[42] divided presenting corneal abrasion patients at the St. Joseph's Hospital in London into two groups, with group 1 receiving conventional antibiotic–pressure patch therapy and group 2 receiving a bandage contact lens with antibiotic drops administered before lens placement. Group 2 patients had less pain and more rapid epithelial healing. The mean healing time for group 1 was 2.57 days, whereas for group 2, it was 1.85 days.[42] Another study evaluated the use of a pressure patch, a bandage contact lens, and a bandage contact lens with concomitant use of ketorolac tromethamine (Acular). The group using a pressure patch showed more rapid healing than did the other two groups, but the patients receiving the bandage contact lens and the group with the bandage lens along with Acular were able to return to normal activity more quickly (1.23 and 1.37 days, respectively, compared to 1.93 days with pressure patching alone).[43] A study by Salz et al. showed significant pain relief using a bandage lens in conjunction with antibiotic drops and diclofenac (Voltaren) nonsteroidal anti-inflammatory drops in patients with corneal abrasions and recurrent corneal erosions.[44] Enhanced corneal healing requires protection of the abraded area from lid-induced trauma. It also requires a normal precorneal tear film and an intact basement membrane. Hydrophilic bandage lenses fulfill all these criteria. In addition, they allow direct observation of the healing

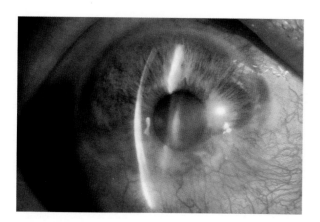

FIG. 21-16. *Alkali chemical burn.*

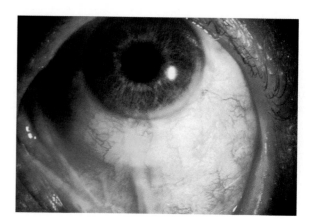

FIG. 21-17. *Symblepharon secondary to alkali burn.*

cornea without the need to remove the patch as in conventional therapy.

Corneal Burns

Corneal surface burns can result from exposure to chemicals, acids, or alkaline solutions. They may also result from exposure to ultraviolet radiation, electric shock, direct thermal contact, or radiation. All these can cause severe corneal damage and lead to corneal distortion and opacity. Bandage soft lenses, along with supportive medical therapy, reduce pain and protect the re-forming corneal epithelium.

Acid Burns

Acid burns are usually less traumatizing to the cornea than alkali burns because of the almost immediate coagulation and opacification of the corneal epithelium on contact with acids, which slows their penetration into the corneal structure.

Treatment includes copious irrigation with sterile saline solutions if available (or tap water, if not), application of topical antibiotics, cycloplegia to minimize posterior synechiae, and topical corticosteroids to control anterior uveitis. Re-epithelialization can be aided by using a therapeutic soft lens. High–water content lenses seems to be the most effective modality.

Alkali Burns

Alkali corneal burns are more traumatic to the cornea than acid burns because of rapid penetration and persistence of the alkaline material in corneal and scleral tissue. Prolonged exposure may produce lysis of cell membranes in all anterior segment structures, including the cornea, sclera, iris, ciliary body, and lens. Alkali-burned corneas

are extremely susceptible to corneal ulceration owing to persistent epithelial defects (Fig. 21-16).

Treatment includes copious irrigation for up to 2 hours after exposure, topically applied antibiotics, and cycloplegia. Antibiotics are continued as long as an epithelial defect is present. The use of collagenase inhibitors, such as cysteine and acetylcysteine, started 7 days after exposure, has reduced the incidence of corneal ulcers.[45]

Bandage soft lenses facilitate re-epithelialization of the cornea by protecting the new tissue from lid-induced trauma and exposure. Rewetting drops should be used frequently during the healing process.

Totally burned corneas healed up to 5 weeks earlier in contact lens–protected eyes than in alkali burns treated without contact lens application.[45] In partially burned eyes, healing took approximately 4 weeks, but recurrent corneal erosion was frequently noted after removal of the eye dressing. Fitting a therapeutic lens after a first episode of corneal erosion is effective in reducing the incidence of recurrences.[45]

The use of collagen shield lenses after an alkali burn is contraindicated. An experimental study by Wentworth et al.[46] showed that use of a collagen shield in alkali-burned rabbit corneas resulted in earlier corneal ulceration than was noted in control eyes. The possible etiology for this was not conclusively shown.

Symblepharon is common when the conjunctiva has also been involved. Kaufman and Thomas[47] applied a therapeutic soft lens with a doughnut-shaped methylmethacrylate former 20–26 mm in diameter inserted into the fornices, thus preventing symblepharon formation (Fig. 21-17).

High–water content therapeutic lenses are the modality of choice for alkaline burns if a lens is to be used in the treatment regimen.

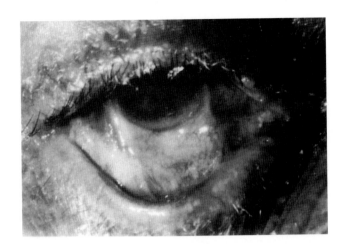

FIG. 21-18. *Ocular cicatricial pemphigoid.*

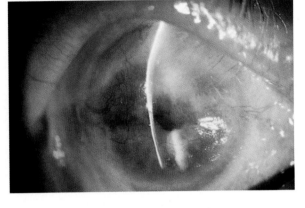

FIG. 21-19. *Ocular cicatricial pemphigoid.*

Ultraviolet Radiation Burns

The cornea readily absorbs ultraviolet radiation. Exposure may occur from a welding flash, from sun-tanning or ultraviolet lamps, or from snow blindness. Pain, photophobia, and a foreign-body sensation usually appear 3–6 hours after exposure to the ultraviolet source. Therapeutic contact lenses can be used to relieve pain if other therapy is ineffective.

Thermal Burns

Thermal burn patients may escape eye damage even where severe facial burns occur because of protection from the lids and from Bell's phenomenon. Treatment depends on the severity of exposure, with eye damage usually resulting from direct contact with flame or hot gases, exposure to released toxic chemicals, or exposure to molten metal or hot liquids.

Direct thermal injuries cause vascular necrosis and symblepharon. The first priority for rehabilitation is re-epithelialization of the injured cornea and conjunctiva. Lid scarring secondary to the injury may cause ectropion or spastic entropion. Therapeutic lenses protect the eye from drying caused by exposure, protect the cornea from scarring by in-turned cilia, and promote epithelial healing.[48]

CONJUNCTIVAL ABNORMALITIES

Ocular Cicatricial Pemphigoid

Ocular cicatricial pemphigoid is a relatively rare condition that primarily affects the mucous membranes. It is more common after age 60 years and is more predominant in women.[49] Ocular involvement begins with conjunctivitis accompanied by subepithelial fibrosis. The fibrosis progresses, causing cicatrization of the conjunctiva, more markedly in the lower fornix.

This condition, also called *progressive essential shrinkage of the conjunctiva*, causes drying of the eye because scarring interferes with proper lacrimal tear flow and production. Severe drying or xerosis of the cornea then results. Entropion and symblepharon may occur and if not treated, may opacify the cornea (Figs. 21-18 and 21-19).

Treatment in early-to-moderate disease consists of systemic corticosteroids. Rapidly developing cases are treated more aggressively by combining steroids with immunosuppressive drugs. A therapeutic contact lens of low water content protects the cornea. Concomitant use of ocular lubricants, instilled frequently during waking hours, is necessary to prevent lens adhesion to the cornea.[33]

Stevens-Johnson Syndrome (Erythema Multiforme)

Erythema multiforme is an acute inflammatory polymorphic skin condition of multiple or undetermined origin. Drugs, radiation therapy, or environmental contaminants are implicated in adults, whereas infectious causes are suspected in juvenile cases.[50] The highest incidence is in the first three decades of life, with the syndrome having a higher prevalence in males.[51]

Erythema multiforme affecting the eye is known as *Stevens-Johnson syndrome*. It manifests as bilateral catarrhal, purulent, or pseudomembranous conjunctivitis. Corneal ulceration and perforation may occur.[50]

A thick, low– or medium–water content therapeutic contact lens reduces pain and increases visual acuity and hastens re-epithelialization.

DRY EYE

Use of contact lenses for marginal to severely dry eyes is controversial.[7,48,52,53] Low–water content thick lenses have been used successfully with the marginally dry eye but have had limited success as a treatment of last resort for the true corneal sicca patient.

Marginal Dry Eyes

The marginal dry eye shows somewhat reduced findings in office tear testing, such as tear breakup time or Schirmer's test. Lysozyme testing of the tears may reveal underactive lacrimal or accessory lacrimal glands.[53]

The marginally dry eye patient with no other contact lens contraindication can be fitted with contact lenses, although success rates are not high. The lens of choice is usually a thick, low–water content hydrogel lens because this combination generally retains hydration more effectively. Additionally, an RGP lens may also be considered and has the advantage of having no polymer-containing fluids to lose through evaporation. Careful follow-up procedures and the use of lubricating drops with or without punctal occlusion are mandatory.

Patients who report discomfort with lenses should discontinue lens wear if reducing wearing time or increasing the frequency of lubricating drops does not alleviate the symptoms.

Therapeutic contact lenses for the marginally dry eye are not recommended and may prove to be counterproductive.

Keratoconjunctivitis Sicca

Deficient tear production is the essential cause of keratoconjunctivitis sicca (KCS). It is diagnosed by abnormally low Schirmer's test results, rapid tear breakup time, and pathologic rose bengal staining of the cornea and conjunctiva.

Sjögren's Syndrome

Sjögren's syndrome combines KCS with systemic disorders, such as dryness of the oral cavity, rheumatoid arthritis, and other connective tissue disease. Patient symptoms include a feeling of ocular dryness, stinging, foreign-body sensation, photophobia, and blurred vision. Standard therapy includes frequent (up to hourly) instillation of tear substitutes, hypotonic saline, or punctal occlusion, either surgically or with punctal plugs.

Application of a therapeutic soft lens in KCS or in Sjögren's syndrome has shown varied results.[6,48,52–54] A therapeutic lens may improve visual acuity and relieve pain. Careful patient control is essential because of increased risks of contact lens–related complications. Dehydration of the lens causes it to tighten and may cause hypoxia-related complications, such as edema, striae, neovascularization, corneal staining, and infections.

Use of therapeutic lenses in the true dry eye, as in KCS and Sjögren's syndrome, must be approached with caution and is usually reserved as the therapy of last resort. If used at all, lenses should be used strictly on a daily-wear basis. Because of decreased protective aqueous components in the tears, there may be less corneal protection against pathogens. Therefore, clinicians electing to prescribe a soft therapeutic lens for KCS should consider the concomitant use of antibiotic eye drops.

Review Chapter 10 for an in-depth discussion of dry eye–related matters and contact lens wear.

CONTACT LENSES AND DRUG DELIVERY

The ability of soft hydrogel lenses to absorb and release fluids is well known.[55,56] A contact lens can act as a reservoir when soaked in topically administered medications.

Administration of topical medications by a contact lens has two advantages: The lens can act to protect the corneal surface, and the efficacy of the drug is enhanced while dosage of the medication is decreased.[57] Available studies have shown that the effect of a soft contact lens on the pharmacokinetics of topical medications can be reasonably predicted.[58]

Antibiotic therapy is enhanced when used in conjunction with a contact lens. Matoba and McCulley[58] found significantly higher levels of tobramycin in rabbit corneas at 1, 2, 4, and 6 hours after instillation than in control eyes not using a contact lens. Increased corneal penetration of the drug was found to be approximately the same, whether a low–water content lens (38%) or a high–water content lens (71%) was used.

A study by Kaufman et al.[59] reported on the application of a Griffin soft lens with pilocarpine drops in the glaucomatous eye. They found that 2 drops of 1% pilocarpine with a soft lens had significantly greater and more prolonged pupillary effect than did 8% pilocarpine instilled in a non–lens-wearing eye.[59]

Podos et al.[60] found that soft lenses soaked in 0.5% pilocarpine diminished intraocular pressure for up to 23 hours while a lens was being worn. The same dosage instilled three times per day over a lens that had not been presoaked in this medication showed little effect on the same eye.

Use of antibiotics for prophylaxis with therapeutic hydrogel lenses in compromised eyes is controversial. It is known that antibiotics instilled with a soft lens in place increase their concentrations in the cornea for up to 4 hours after instillation.[58] The effects on normal ocular flora are negligible.[61] Binder and Worthen[61] found that the use of a contact lens does not significantly increase or decrease the bacteria or fungi found in normal ocular cultures. Use of prophylactic antibiotic drops (combined neomycin sulfate/polymyxin B sulfate/gramicidin) did not alter the normal ocular flora.[61]

Binder et al.[62] also found no reduction in normal bacterial flora when 0.5% chloramphenicol was used three times per day in patients with soft contact lenses.

The use of preserved (benzalkonium chloride) antibiotics in conjunction with a contact lens was found by Lemp[63] to have no adverse effects on the cornea. He found no increase in corneal staining, edema, or evidence of endothelial damage using antibiotics or artificial tears preserved with benzalkonium chloride.

Topical prophylactic antibiotics with a therapeutic contact lens may be of benefit in the patient at high risk for corneal infection. The risk-benefit ratio in these high-risk patients leans toward concomitant use of the drugs because the consequences of use are minimal.[61]

Read Chapter 22 for an in-depth discussion of therapeutic medications and contact lens wear.

LASER REFRACTIVE SURGERY

Laser photorefractive keratectomy by the very nature of the procedure induces a large 6 mm plus corneal epithelial defect that without some form of palliative intervention would cause intense pain.

Therapeutic contact lens application immediately after the procedure along with the use of topical nonsteroidal anti-inflammatory drugs greatly reduces the discomfort after photorefractive keratectomy. The lens is worn continuously for 3–4 days or until complete re-epithelialization of the cornea has occurred.[64]

Although generally unnecessary, a bandage lens can also be used after laser in situ keratomileusis for 1 day to speed flap margin re-epithelialization and to protect the flap from lid-induced postoperative trauma. Use of a therapeutic lens after laser in situ keratomileusis decreases postoperative pain but delays visual rehabilitation.[65]

COMPLICATIONS ASSOCIATED WITH THERAPEUTIC LENS USE

Complications of extended wear of a therapeutic contact lens are similar to those of a cosmetic extended-wear lens. The compromised nature of the eye needing therapeutic application does not seem to increase or decrease the incidence of lens complications.[66] The complications may be mechanical in nature, including discomfort from a poorly fitting lens or damage to the lens from patient handling. Physiologically induced complications may include epithelial edema, stromal edema, superficial punctate staining, or neovascularization. Minor brush-type abrasions may be found on surgically altered corneas with irregular corneal surfaces. Solution sensitivity reactions and giant papillary conjunctivitis have been reported.[66,67] In addition, sterile infiltrates and sterile hypopyon secondary to uveitis have also been observed.[67]

Bacterial ulcers are potentially the most serious of lens-related complications. Patients must be cautioned to immediately report any pain, redness, abnormally blurred vision, or discharge. The possibility of bacterial or fungal infection is higher in corneas that are compromised enough to require a therapeutic lens than in uncompromised eyes.[67]

The primary reason for therapeutic lens application may complicate the detection of lens-related complications. Stromal edema, which is usually present in such conditions as bullous keratopathy, herpetic disease, or anterior segment necrosis, makes detection of lens-related edema difficult. Significant increases in edema indicate lens-related hypoxia, which must be addressed by changing the lens material or lens fit.[67]

Neovascularization, which is an unwanted complication in cosmetic lens wear, may be beneficial in certain therapeutic lens applications. Increased vascularization in chemical burns, stromal ulceration, or ocular surface disease is a sign of healing and can be encouraged by deliberately using a lens that induces hypoxia, such as a low–water content, tight-fitting lens (Fig. 21-20).[67]

Superficial vascularization rarely invades the pupillary axis. It is usually very slow to progress and may not necessarily require cessation of lens wear. Often, the underlying pathology that necessitated lens use ceases to exist before the vascularization becomes a problem.[66]

Dryness commonly associated with compromised eyes may cause rapid deposition on the lens surface. Frequent

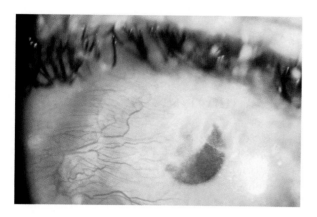

FIG. 21-20. *Corneal vascularization in a chemical burn.*

TABLE 21-1. *U.S. Food and Drug Administration–Approved Therapeutic Lenses*

Company	Trade Name	Water Content (%)
Bausch & Lomb, Inc. (Rochester, NY)	B, O, U Series, Plano T	38
CIBA Vision (Duluth, GA)	Protek	55
Cooper Vision (Fairport, NY)	Permalens Therapeutic	71
Kontur Kontact Lens (Richmond, CA)	Kontur Custom	55
United Contact Lens (Everett, WA)	UCL Bandage	55
Wesley-Jessen (Des Plaines, IL)	CSI-FW	38.6

lens replacement may be necessary. These deposits may be lipids, proteins, or calcium-lipid. Lens surface contamination reduces comfort and vision and may lead to autoimmune reactions, such as giant papillary conjunctivitis.[66]

Temporary wrinkling of corneas fitted with ultrathin therapeutic contact lenses was reported by Mobilia et al.[68] After 48 hours of continuous wear, 16 of 87 patients demonstrated a rippled pattern on the lens surface. When the lenses were removed, the corneal surface also was found to be rippled. The corneas returned to normal within 4 hours after the lens was removed.[68]

The ability to accurately measure intraocular pressure is important when steroid therapy accompanies bandage lens use and in patients with pre-existing glaucoma.

Studies have proved the accuracy of pneumotonometry and the Tono-Pen tonometer (Mentor O & Q, Inc., Norwell, MA) when used while a therapeutic lens is in place. Pneumotonometry did provide more reliable intraocular pressure readings than did the Tono-Pen in eyes with elevated pressure. Pneumotonometry overestimated intraocular pressure at low levels of pressure, whereas the Tono-Pen was shown to be more accurate at these levels.[69] Lenses with center thicknesses greater than 0.45 mm affect the accuracy of these instruments.[70]

LENS MATERIALS

Hydrogel Lenses

As with cosmetic hydrophilic lenses, therapeutic lenses can be high-, low-, or medium–water content. The lens type adopted depends on the condition for which the lens is being prescribed (Table 21-1). Epithelial trauma is minimized by high–water content lenses. Eyes being treated

for anterior segment inflammation seem to do better with high–water content lenses. Medium–water content lenses are more appropriate when significant corneal or limbal irregularities exist. Medium- or low–water content lenses are well suited for corneal splinting (e.g., in corneal perforations, lacerations, or descemetocele) when minimal lens movement is beneficial. Low–water content lenses are best suited to dry eye conditions when minimal inflammation is present.[6]

Collagen Shield Lenses

Collagen shield lenses are used for short-term corneal protection, to promote epithelial healing after surgery, for lubrication, and to deliver topical drugs to the cornea and conjunctiva. Current collagen lenses are made of porcine scleral collagen or bovine corium collagen and are designed to dissolve in 12, 24, or 72 hours. The lenses are purchased in a dehydrated state and can be hydrated with balanced saline or in medications when they are used as drug delivery vehicles. On application, the lens acts as a therapeutic bandage lens to protect the healing corneal epithelium. Contact with the tears causes proteolytic and hydrolytic effects that begin to degrade the lens. This produces a thick, mucuslike film. As the lens further dissolves, the material has a lubricating effect.[71]

Collagen lenses can be used as drug reservoirs that passively release the intended medication. This passive release becomes more rapid as the lens dissolves. Aquavella et al.[71] concluded that collagen shield lenses soaked in tobramycin, gentamicin, pilocarpine, dexamethasone, or flurbiprofen sodium are useful for protection, lubrication, and drug delivery to the cornea, with minimal adverse results.

The efficacy of antibiotics has been shown to increase with the use of medication-impregnated collagen lenses. In a study by Clinch et al.,[72] collagen shields impregnated with tobramycin and supplemented with topical tobramycin drops reduced bacterial colony-forming units significantly more than topical drops alone in an experimentally induced *Pseudomonas* keratitis in rabbit corneas. A similar response was shown with collagen shields impregnated with tobramycin and *Staphylococcus aureus* as the infective agent.[73] Collagen shields soaked in 0.5% amphotericin B with supplemented application of 0.25% amphotericin B every 2 hours has been shown to be an effective treatment for *Aspergillus* keratomycosis.[74] The use of collagen shield lenses impregnated with gentamicin and dexamethasone has no significant adverse effects on the cornea and delivers drug concentrations similar to those of antibiotic-corticosteroid injections, with the added benefit of being less invasive.[75] It has also been noted that these patients experience less pain, less conjunctival injection, and less aqueous flare.[76] Presoaked collagen shields have not been shown to prevent endophthalmitis because aqueous concentration of the drugs did not approach minimum inhibitory concentrations for common ocular pathogens.[77]

Numerous studies have shown the bolus effect of hydrogel lenses soaked in antibiotics without a sustained-release effect. Collagen lenses soaked in gentamicin, tobramycin, or vancomycin produce levels of antibiotics in the aqueous, corneal stroma, and tears greater than or equal to topical installation of fortified antibiotics or subconjunctival injection.[78]

Collagen shield lenses have been shown to enhance epithelialization after corneal surgical procedures, such as penetrating keratoplasty,[71,79] radial keratotomy,[80] epikeratophakia,[79] and cataract extraction.[71] Collagen lenses are not suitable, however, for long-term application for chronic ocular surface diseases.[81] Other applications may include treatment of corneal abrasions,[79] recurrent corneal erosion,[79] promotion of healing of leaking glaucoma-filtering blebs,[81] wound healing,[80] and bacterial keratitis.[23]

Disposable Hydrogel Lenses

Disposable hydrogel lenses used as therapeutic devices have been shown to be effective in numerous studies. To date, the U.S. Food and Drug Administration has approved no commercially marketed disposable lens for therapeutic application.

The use of disposable contact lenses is cost and time effective because these lenses are readily available in most contact lens–oriented practices. Use of disposable contact lenses in conditions that require short-term therapeutic

contact lenses, such as postoperative wound leak, corneal abrasions, or keratorefractive surgery, is more cost effective and more convenient for the patient than using conventional therapeutic bandage lenses. Conditions that require long-term use of bandage lenses, such as bullous keratopathy, may be better treated with conventional therapeutic lenses because frequent replacement of the disposable lens may be more costly and time consuming.[82] Complications of disposable hydrogel contact lenses used for therapeutic application are similar to those encountered with standard therapeutic lenses (i.e., lens loss, discomfort, tight lens syndrome, sterile and infectious ulcer, and corneal neovascularization).[83]

REFERENCES

1. Arrington GE: A History of Ophthalmology. MD Publishers, New York, 1959
2. Bailey N: Neal Bailey's contact lens chronicles. Contact Lens Spectrum 7:6, 1987
3. Mandell RB: Contact Lens Practice. 3rd ed. Thomas, Springfield, IL, 1981
4. Kaufman HE, Gasset AR: Clinical experience with the epikeratoprosthesis. Am J Ophthalmol 67:38, 1969
5. Plotnik RD, Mannis MJ, Schwab IR: Therapeutic contact lenses. Ophthalmol Clin 31:2, 1991
6. Thoft RA: Therapeutic soft contact lenses. p. 477. In Smolin G, Thoft RA (eds): The Cornea. Little, Brown and Company, Boston, 1983
7. McDermott ML, Chandler JW: Therapeutic uses of contact lenses. Surv Ophthalmol 33:381, 1989
8. Hayworth NAS, Asbell PA: Therapeutic contact lenses. CLAO J 16:137, 1990
9. Williams R, Buckley RJ: Pathogenesis and treatment of recurrent erosion. Br J Ophthalmol 69:435, 1985
10. Rapuano CJ, Laibson PR: Excimer laser phototherapeutic keratectomy for anterior corneal pathology. CLAO J 20:4, 1994
11. Rapuano CJ: Excimer laser phototherapeutic keratectomy: long term results and practical considerations. Cornea 16:2, 1997
12. Bloomfield SE, Antonio RG, Forstot SL, et al: Treatment of filamentary keratitis with the soft contact lens. Am J Ophthalmol 76:978, 1973
13. Leibowitz HM, Rosenthal P: Hydrophilic contact lenses in corneal disease: superficial, sterile, indolent ulcers. Arch Ophthalmol 85:163, 1971
14. Thygeson P: Superficial punctate keratitis. JAMA 114:1544, 1950
15. Tabbara KF, Ostler HB, Dawson C, Oh J: Thygeson's superficial punctate keratitis. Am Acad Ophthalmol 88:75, 1981
16. Forstot SL, Binder PS: Treatment of Thygeson's superficial punctate keratopathy with soft contact lenses. Am J Ophthalmol 88:186, 1979

17. Tantum LA: Superficial punctate keratitis of Thygeson. J Am Optom Assoc 53:985, 1982

18. Ehlers WH, Suchecki J, Donshik PC: Therapeutic contact lenses. Ophthalmol Clin North Am 2:2, 1989

19. Mondino BJ, Zaidman GW, Salamon SW: Use of pressure patching and soft contact lenses in superior limbic keratoconjunctivitis. Arch Ophthalmol 100:1932, 1982

20. Hovding G: Hydrophilic contact lenses in corneal disorders. Acta Ophthalmol 62:566, 1984

21. Kaufman HE: Therapeutic use of soft contact lenses. p. 461. In Dabezies OH (ed): Contact Lenses, the CLAO Guide to Basic Science and Clinical Practice. Grune & Stratton, Orlando, FL, 1984

22. Bodner BI: Selection of therapeutic lenses. p. 471. In Dabezies OH (ed): Contact Lenses, the CLAO Guide to Basic Science and Clinical Practice. Grune & Stratton, Orlando, FL, 1984

23. Sawusch MR, O'Brien TP, Dick JD, Gottsch JD: Use of collagen corneal shields in the treatment of bacterial keratitis. Am J Ophthalmol 106:279, 1988

24. Wood TO, Tuberville AW: Mooren's ulcer. p. 424. In Fraunfelder FT (ed): Current Ocular Therapy. Saunders, Philadelphia, 1990

25. Dresner MS, Schanzlin DJ, Fraunfelder FT: Pellucid Marginal Corneal Degeneration. In Fraunfelder FT (ed): Current Ocular Therapy. Saunders, Philadelphia, 1990

26. Mannis MJ: Terrien's marginal degeneration. p. 426. In Fraunfelder FT (ed): Current Ocular Therapy. Saunders, Philadelphia, 1990

27. Cavanagh HD: Herpetic ocular disease: therapy of persistent epithelial defects. Int Ophthalmol Clin 15:67, 1975

28. Aquavella JV: The treatment of herpetic stromal disease. EENT Monthly 51:15, 1972

29. Cavanagh HD, Pihlaja D, Thoft RA, Dohlman CH: Pathogenesis and treatment of persistent epithelial defects. Trans Am Acad Ophthalmol Otolaryngol 81:754, 1976

30. Leibowitz HM: Hydrophilic contact lenses in corneal disease. Arch Ophthalmol 88:602, 1972

31. Hirst LW, Smiddy WE, Stark WJ: Corneal perforations. Changing methods of treatment, 1960–1980. Am Acad Ophthalmol 89:630, 1982

32. Rehim MHA, Shafik MAA, Samy M: Management of corneal perforations by therapeutic contact lenses. Contact Lens J 18:4, 1990

33. Gasset AR, Kaufman HE: Therapeutic uses of hydrophilic contact lenses. Am J Ophthalmol 69:252, 1969

34. Gasset AR, Kaufman HE: Bandage lenses in the treatment of bullous keratopathy. Am J Ophthalmol 72:376, 1971

35. Wilson M, Leigh E: Therapeutic use of soft contact lenses. Proc Soc Med 68:55, 1975

36. Andrew NC, Woodward EG: The bandage lens in bullous keratopathy. Ophthal Physiol Opt 9:66, 1989

37. Cross HE, Maumenee AE, Cantolino SJ: Inheritance of Fuchs' endothelial dystrophy. Arch Ophthalmol 85:125, 1967

38. Waring GO III, Rodrigues MM, Laibson PR: Corneal dystrophies. II. Endothelial dystrophies. Surv Ophthalmol 23:147, 1978

39. Devoe AG: The management of endothelial dystrophy of the cornea. Am J Ophthalmol 61:1084, 1966

40. Cibis GW, Kratchmer JA, Phelps CD, Weingeist TA: The clinical spectrum of posterior polymorphous dystrophy. Arch Ophthalmol 95:1529, 1977

41. Judisch GF, Maumenee IH: Clinical differentiation of recessive congenital hereditary endothelial dystrophy and dominant endothelial dystrophy. Am J Ophthalmol 85:606, 1978

42. Acheson JF, Joseph J, Spalton DJ: Use of soft contact lenses in an eye casualty department for the primary treatment of traumatic corneal abrasions. Br J Ophthalmol 71:285, 1987

43. Donnenfeld ED, Selkin BA, Perry HD, et al: Controlled evaluation of a bandage lens and a topical nonsteroidal anti-inflammatory drug in treating traumatic corneal abrasions. Ophthalmol 102:6, 1995

44. Salz JJ, Reader AL, Schwartz LJ, et al: Treatment of corneal abrasions with soft contact lenses and diclofenac. J Refract Corneal Surg 10:6, 1994

45. Brown SI, Tragakis MP, Pearce DB: Treatment of the alkali-burned cornea. Am J Ophthalmol 74:316, 1972

46. Wentworth JS, Paterson CA, Wells JT, et al: Collagen shields exacerbate ulceration of alkali burned rabbit corneas. Arch Ophthalmol 111:3, 1993

47. Kaufman HE, Thomas EL: Prevention and treatment of symblepharon. Am J Ophthalmol 88:419, 1979

48. Wilson M, Leigh E: Therapeutic use of soft contact lenses. Proc R Soc Med [Sect Ophthalmol] 68:55, 1975

49. Morrison LH, Swan KC: Cicatricial pemphigoid. p. 403. In Fraunfelder FT (ed): Current Ocular Therapy. Saunders, Philadelphia, 1990

50. Levy B: Bandage lenses in atypical erythema multiforme. Am J Optom Physiol Opt 61:552, 1984

51. Howard GM: Erythema multiforme. p. 177. In Fraunfelder FT (ed): Current Ocular Therapy. Saunders, Philadelphia, 1990

52. Gasset AR, Kaufman HE: Hydrophilic lens therapy of severe keratoconjunctivitis sicca and conjunctival scarring. Am J Ophthalmol 71:1185, 1971

53. Mackie IA: Contact lenses in dry eyes. Trans Ophthalmol Soc UK 104:477, 1985

54. Morrison R, Shovlin JP: A review of the use of bandage lenses. Metab Pediatr System Ophthalmol 6:117, 1981

55. Wichterle O, Lim D: Hydrophilic gels for biological use. Nature 185:117, 1960

56. Waltman SR, Kaufman HE: Use of hydrophilic contact lenses to increase ocular penetration of topical drugs. Invest Ophthalmol 9:250, 1970

57. Krejci L, Brettschneider I, Praus R: Hydrophilic gel contact lenses as a new drug delivery system in ophthalmology and as a therapeutic bandage lens. Acta Univ Carolina Med 21:387, 1975

58. Matoba AY, McCulley JP: The effect of therapeutic soft contact lenses on antibiotic delivery to the cornea. Ophthalmology 92:97, 1985

59. Kaufman HE, Uotila MH, Gasset AR, et al: The medical uses of soft contact lenses. Trans Am Acad Ophthalmol Otolaryngol 75:361, 1971

60. Podos SM, Becker B, Asseff C, Hartstein J: Pilocarpine therapy with soft contact lenses. Am J Ophthalmol 73:336, 1972
61. Binder PS, Worthen DM: A continuous-wear hydrophilic lens: prophylactic topical antibiotics. Arch Ophthalmol 94:2109, 1976
62. Binder PC, Abel RA, Kaufman HE: The effect of chronic administration of a topical antibiotic on the conjunctival flora. Arch Ophthalmol 7:1429, 1975
63. Lemp MA: Bandage lenses and the use of topical solutions containing preservatives. Ann Ophthalmol 10:1319, 1978
64. Cherry PMH: The treatment of pain following excimer laser photorefractive keratectomy: additive effect of local anesthetic drops, topical diclofenac and bandage soft contact. Ophthalmic Surg Lasers (suppl.)27(S):477, 1996
65. Montes M, Chayet AS, Castellanos A, et al: Use of bandage contact lenses after in situ keratomileusis. J Refract Surg (suppl.)13:5, 1997
66. Nesburn AB: Complications associated with therapeutic soft contact lenses. Ophthalmology 86:1130, 1979
67. Thoft RA, Mobilia EF: Complications with therapeutic extended wear soft contact lenses. Int Ophthalmol Clin 21:197, 1981
68. Mobilia EF, Yamamoto GK, Dohlman CH: Corneal wrinkling induced by ultra-thin soft contact lenses. Ann Ophthalmol 12:371, 1980
69. Scibilia GD, Ehlers WH, Donshik PC: The effects of therapeutic contact lenses on intraocular pressure measurement. CLAO J 22:4, 1996
70. Mark LK, Asbell PA, Torres MA, et al: Accuracy of intraocular pressure measurements with two different tonometers through bandage contact lenses. Cornea 11:4, 1992
71. Aquavella J, Ruffini J, LoCascio J: Use of collagen shields as a surgical adjunct. J Cataract Refract Surg 14:492, 1988
72. Clinch TE, Hobden JA, Hill JM, et al: Collagen shields containing tobramycin for sustained therapy (24 hours) of experimental Pseudomonas keratitis. CLAO J 18:4.1992
73. Callegan MC, Engel LS, Clinch TE, et al: Efficacy of tobramycin drops applied to collagen shields for experimental staphylococcal keratitis. Curr Eye Res 13:12, 1994
74. Mendicute J, Ondarra A, Eder F, et al: The use of collagen shields impregnated with amphotericin B to treat *Aspergillus* keratomycosis. CLAO J 21:4, 1995
75. Mencini U, Lanzetta P, Ferrari E, et al: Efficacy of collagen shields after extracapsular cataract extraction. Eur J Ophthalmol 4:3 1994
76. Rennard G, Bennani N, Lutaj P, et al: Comparative study of a collagen shield and a subconjunctival injection at the end of cataract surgery. J Cataract Refract Surg 19:48, 1993
77. Taravella M, Stepp P, Young D: Collagen shields delivery of tobramycin to the human eye. CLAO J 24:3, 1998
78. Nilsson L, Soren L, Radberg G: Frequencies of variants resistant to different aminoglycosides in *Pseudomonas aeruginosa*. J Antimicrob Chemother 20:255, 1987
79. Poland DE, Kaufman HE: Clinical uses of collagen shields. J Cataract Refract Surg 14:489, 1988
80. Aquavella J, del Cerro M, Musco P, et al: The effect of a collagen bandage lens on corneal wound healing: a preliminary report. Ophthalmic Surg 18:570, 1987
81. Mondino BJ: Collagen shields. Am J Ophthalmol 112:587, 1991
82. Gupta S, Arora R, DasSota L, et al: An alternative approach to bandage contact lenses. CLAO J 24:2, 1998
83. Bouchard CS, Trimble SN: Indications and complications of therapeutic disposable ACUVUE contact lenses. CLAO J 22:2, 1996

ADDITIONAL SUGGESTED READINGS

Aasuri MK, Sreedhar MS: Bandage contact lenses in ocular disorders. Int Contact Lens Clin 24:6, 1997

Ajamian PC, Winski F: The management of filamentary keratitis and dry eye using bandage contact lenses and punctal occlusion. Clin Eye Vision Care 2:2, 1990

Amos DM: The use of soft bandage lenses in corneal disease. Am J Optom Physiol Opt 52:524, 1975

Aquavella J, Norton S, Barsoumian K: Conjunctival bandage. Ophthalmic Surg 11:847, 1980

Aquavella J, Shaw E: Hydrophilic bandages in penetrating keratoplasty. Ann Ophthalmol 8:1207, 1976

Arentsen JJ, Tasman W: Using a bandage contact lens to prevent recurrent corneal erosion during photocoagulation in patients with diabetes. Am J Ophthalmol 92:714, 1981

Beckman RL, Sofinski SJ, Greff LJ, et al: Bandage contact lens augmentation of 5-fluorouracil treatment in glaucoma filtration surgery. Ophthalmic Surg 22:563, 1991

Beekhuis WH, van Rij G, Eggink FAGJ, et al: Contact lenses following keratoplasty. CLAO J 17:27, 1991

Bence BG, Blaze PA: Therapeutic soft contact lenses. Contact Lens Spectrum 3:52, 1988

Blok MDW, Kok JHC, van Mil C, et al: Use of the Megasoft bandage lens for treatment of complications after trabeculectomy. Am J Ophthalmol 110:264, 1990

Bouchard CS, Lemp MA: Tight lens syndrome associated with a 24-hour disposable collagen lens: a case report. CLAO J 17:141, 1991

Braun D: Use of a therapeutic contact lens in treatment of radiation keratopathy. Int Contact Lens Clin 14:4, 1987

Cakanac CJ: Managing recalcitrant disease: how to break the cycle of recurrent corneal erosion. Rev Opt 134:3, 1997

Callizo J, Cervello I, Mayayo E, et al: Inefficacy of collagen shields in the rabbit cornea wound-healing process. Cornea 15:3, 1996

DePaolis MD: Can we really use hydrophilic disposable lenses for therapeutic purposes? Contact Lens Spectrum 5:8, 1991

Dohlman CH: Complications in therapeutic soft lens wear. Trans Am Acad Ophthalmol Otolaryngol 78:399, 1974

Dunnebier EA, Kok JHC: Treatment of an alkali burn-induced symblepharon with a Megasoft bandage lens. Cornea 12:1, 1993

Farris RL, Stuchell RN, Nisengard R: Sjögren's syndrome and keratoconjunctivitis sicca. Cornea 10:207, 1991

Fontana FD: Soft lenses to protect the cornea after Fasanella ptosis surgery. J Am Optom Assoc 49:316, 1978

Forstot SL, Damiano RE: Trauma after radial keratotomy. Ophthalmology 95:833, 1988

Gasset AR, Lobo L: Simplified soft contact lens treatment in corneal diseases. Ann Ophthalmol 9:843, 1977

Goldberg DB, Schanzlin DJ, Brown SI: Management of Thygeson's superficial punctate keratitis. Am J Ophthalmol 89:22, 1980

Groden LR, White W: Porcine collagen corneal shield treatment of persistent epithelial defects following penetrating keratoplasty. CLAO J 16:95, 1990

Harkins T: Managing corneal abrasions. Clin Eye Vision Care 8:4, 1996

Harrison KW: Collagen corneal shields, an important therapeutic modality. J Ophthal Nursing Technol 8:97, 1989

Henahan JF: Soft contact lens may treat postoperative glaucoma problems. Ophthalmol Times 16:65, 1991

Hovding G: Conjunctival and contact lens bacterial flora during continuous bandage lens wear. Acta Ophthalmol 60:439, 1982

Jackson AJ, Sinton JE, Frazer DG, et al: Therapeutic contact lenses and their use in the management of anterior segment pathology. J Br Contact Lens Assoc 19:1, 1996

Johnston WH, Wellish KL, Beltran F, et al: Collagen shields. Int Ophthalmol Clin 33:4, 1993

Kanpolat A, Batioglu F, Yilmaz M, et al: Penetration of cyclosporin A into the rabbit cornea and aqueous humor after topical drop and collagen shield administration. CLAO J 20:2, 1994

Karambelas D, Bahr RL, Dowling JL: Therapeutic and extended wear. Contact Lens Forum 9:8, 1984

Kaufman HE, Gasset AR: Therapeutic soft bandage lenses. Int Ophthalmol Clin 10:379, 1970

LeBourlais C, Acar L, Zia H, et al: Ophthalmic drug delivery systems—recent advances. Prog Retinal Eye Res 17:1, 1998

Lesher GA, Gunderson GG: Continous drug delivery through the use of disposable contact lenses. Optom Vis Sci 70:12, 1993

Levinson A, Weissman BA, Sachs U: Use of the Bausch & Lomb Soflens Plano T contact lens as a bandage. Am J Optom Physiol Opt 54:97, 1977

Levy B, Nguyen N: Therapeutic utilization of disposable lenses. Int Contact Lens Clin 20:9, 1993

Lindahl KJ, DePaolis MD, Aquavella JV, et al: Applications of hydrophilic disposable contact lenses as therapeutic bandages. CLAO J 17:4, 1991

Mannis MJ, Zadnik K: Hydrophilic contact lenses for wound stabilization in keratoplasty. CLAO J 14:199, 1988

Milani JK, Verbukh I, PleyerU, et al: Collagen shields impregnated with gentamicin-dexamethasone as a potential drug delivery device. Am J Ophthalmol 116:5, 1993

Mobilia EF, Dohlman CH, Holly FJ: A comparison of various soft contact lenses for therapeutic purposes. Contact Lens 3:9, 1977

Mobilia EF, Kenyon KR: A new bandage lens for treatment of corneal disease: Softcon XT. CLAO J 10:353, 1984

Novak PH, Kuchar A, Ergun E, et al: Indications for therapeutic contact lenses after cataract and glaucoma surgery. Orbit Suppl 16:3, 1997

Reidy JJ, Gebhardt BM, Kaufman HE: The collagen shield. Cornea 9:196, 1990

Ros FE, Tijl JW, Faber JAJ: Bandage lenses: collagen shield vs. hydrogel lens. CLAO J 17:187, 1991

Rubinstein MP: Disposable contact lenses as therapeutic devices. J Br Contact Lens Assoc 18:3, 1995

Ryan RA: When contact lenses promote corneal healing. Rev Opt 131:4, 1994

Saini JS, Rao GN, Aquavella JV: Post-keratoplasty corneal ulcers and bandage lenses. Acta Ophthalmol 66:99, 1988

Simsek NA, Manav G, Tugal-Tutkun I, et al: An experimental study on the effect of collagen shields and therapeutic contact lenses on corneal wound healing. Cornea 15:6, 1996

Smiddy WE, Hamburg TR, Kracher GP, et al: Therapeutic contact lenses. Ophthalmology 97:291, 1990

Spraul CW, Lang GK: Contact lenses and corneal shields. Curr Opin Ophthalmol 8:4, 1997

Srur M, Dattas D: The use of disposable contact lenses as therapeutic lenses. CLAO J 23:1, 1997

Tanner JB, DePaolis MD: Disposable contact lenses as alternative bandage lenses. Clin Eye Vision Care 4:4, 1992

Tripathi RC, Sharath R, Tripathi BJ: Prospects for epithelial growth factor in the management of corneal disorders. Surv Ophthalmol 34:457, 1990

vanSetten GB: The clinical use of contact lenses and collagen shields. Curr Opin Ophthalmol 7:4, 1996

Wedge CI, Rootman DS: Collagen shields: efficacy, safety and comfort in the treatment of human traumatic corneal abrasion and effect on vision in healthy eyes. Can J Ophthalmol 27:6, 1992

Weiner BM: How and when to prescribe bandage contact lenses. Rev Opt 133:10, 1996

Yamamoto GK, Pavan-Langston D, Stowe GC, Albert DM: Fungal invasion of a therapeutic soft contact lens and cornea. Ann Ophthalmol 11:1731, 1979

Zadnik K: Post-surgical contact lens alternatives. Int Contact Lens Clin 15:201, 1988

Zadnik K: Contact lenses in the geriatric patient. J Am Optom Assoc 65:3, 1994

22

Medications and Contact Lens Wear

Jimmy D. Bartlett

GRAND ROUNDS CASE REPORT

Subjective:
A 52-year-old woman presents with sudden-onset pain and discomfort in the right eye (OD) for 1 week. Ocular discomfort is continuous throughout the day. Patient has good acuity but notices slight redness in the temporal aspect OD. History of successful monovision rigid gas-permeable contact lens wear for presbyopia over the past 2 years. She has been asymptomatic until last week. Patient reports that she started taking chlorpheniramine maleate 4 mg orally q6h several days before onset of symptoms. Patient takes no other oral or topical medications.

Objective:
- Entrance acuities with contact lenses: OD $^{20}/_{20}$, left eye (OS) 0.4 M @ 40 cm
- Pupils equal, reactive, no afferent defect. Contact lenses position centrally. Optimal lens movement and tear flush in each eye (OU), with aligned fluorescein pattern.
- Biomicroscopy: Large, thin dellen at 9:30 o'clock at limbus OD, staining heavily with fluorescein, with slight bulbar conjunctival injection temporal to dellen. All other structures are normal.

Assessment:
Acute corneal dellen formation OD associated with anticholinergic properties of the oral antihistamine chlorpheniramine maleate.

Plan:
1. Patient is instructed to discontinue contact lens wear immediately.
2. Aggressive artificial tear therapy q2h while awake on first day, and subsequently q6h for 1 week.

Other:
Patient seen in follow-up 1 week later with dellen formation completely resolved. Normal corneal thickness observed at limbal area, with absence of sodium fluorescein staining. Patient is advised to resume contact lens wear but to avoid oral medications with anticholinergic side effects that might precipitate dry eye signs or symptoms.

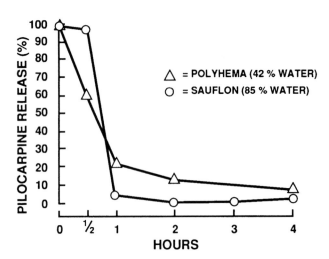

FIG. 22-1. *Pilocarpine release (percentage) from soft contact lenses with different water contents. (Modified with permission from M Ruben, R Watkins: Pilocarpine dispensation for the soft hydrophilic contact lens. Br J Ophthalmol 59:455, 1975.)*

The efficacy of many topically applied medications is determined, in part, by the delicate relationships among tear film volume, amount of drug instilled, and the pharmacokinetics of drug absorption across the cornea. The presence of a contact lens, either rigid or hydrogel, can influence the rate of drug absorption across the cornea or otherwise interfere with drug delivery to the intended target site.[1] It is therefore important for the ophthalmic practitioner to know how contact lens materials can influence ocular drug delivery, particularly as it relates to potential side effects and complications of locally applied compounds. On the other hand, systemic medications used for nonocular reasons can sometimes adversely affect the success of contact lens wear.[1] This chapter discusses how the efficacy of topically applied medications can be enhanced by application of contact lenses and how systemically administered drugs can limit successful contact lens wear. Guidelines are provided to facilitate the development of management strategies to prevent untoward complications or to permit successful resolution of clinical problems as they arise.

TOPICAL MEDICATIONS

The use of topical ocular medications with rigid lenses is permissible in some cases because these lens materials do not absorb the drugs. A rigid lens, however, may prevent a drug from reaching the cornea or, once under the lens, may be kept in contact with the cornea for longer than normal periods. Because contact lenses may compromise the corneal epithelium, reduce the blink rate, and impair tear circulation, topically applied drugs are likely to penetrate the cornea in greater quantity. Moreover, topically applied ointments cause blurred vision if instilled during rigid contact lens wear. Therefore, as a rule, it is best to instill topical medications without contact lenses in place.

Hydrogel lenses, however, absorb water-soluble compounds. If this type of lens is placed in a drug solution, the drug usually concentrates in the lens. This characteristic of hydrogel lenses has been used clinically to treat various ocular conditions.

Contact Lenses as Drug Delivery Devices

One of the significant problems with the delivery of drugs in solution is that the drug administration is pulsed, with an initial period of overdosage followed by a period of relative underdosage. The use of hydrogel contact lenses as drug delivery devices represents an attempt to overcome this disadvantage. In the United States, the use of hydrogel lenses for drug delivery was initially proposed by Waltman and Kaufman in 1970.[2] The use of hydrogel lenses to prolong drug contact with the eye and to promote drug penetration into the eye seems to be effective for several medications that have been studied.[3-5]

Drugs penetrate hydrogel lenses at a rate that depends on the pore size between the cross-linkages of the three-dimensional lattice structure of the lens, concentration of drug in the soaking medium, soaking time, water content of the lens, and molecular size of the drug. Lenses with higher water content absorb more water-soluble drug for later release into the precorneal tear film.[6-9] For example, the polyHEMA lens, consisting of 42% water, releases approximately 62% of impregnated pilocarpine after 30 minutes of wear, whereas the Sauflon lens, consisting of 85% water, releases approximately 95% of impregnated pilocarpine (Fig. 22-1).[10] It may not be practical, however, to equate the percentage of pilocarpine released in vivo with the concentration actually available in the precorneal tear film because of variables such as amount of water lost from the lens by evaporation and temperature changes and the rate of tear flow into the lens. The rates of drug entry into the polymer and the subsequent passage of drug into the cornea depend on the specific physical properties of the drug as well as those of the polymer used.[9] Drugs with molecular weights greater than 500 usually have difficulty entering the substance of the polymer.[9]

The degree of permeability is also related to lens thickness. A thinner lens allows a greater amount of topically applied drug to pass into the lens-cornea interface, whereas a thicker lens stores a greater amount of the drug without immediately releasing it to the cornea.[9]

Maximal drug delivery is usually obtained by presoaking the lens.[2,11-14] This procedure produces a more sustained high yield of drug.[11,15] In addition, prolonged soaking to a state of equilibrium before clinical use produces a more standardized form of presoaked lens. In addition to pilocarpine,[8,11,12] many other drugs have been studied for their usefulness in hydrogel contact lens delivery systems. The release of antibiotics, including chloramphenicol, ciprofloxacin, tetracycline, bacitracin, gentamicin, tobramycin, and polymyxin B, has been studied.[3,5,15-17] Bacitracin is released from the lens somewhat more rapidly than polymyxin B, but after 5 hours, the content of both antibiotics in the contact lens is about the same, approximately 40% of the original amount. Chloramphenicol and tetracycline are easily released from hydrogel lens materials, chloramphenicol more rapidly than tetracycline. Approximately 50% of the tetracycline and 75% of the chloramphenicol is released during the first 3 hours. Ciprofloxacin is released at a rate that provides higher drug concentrations than achieved with topically instilled eyedrops.[5]

Other drugs have also been delivered with hydrogel lenses, including ethylenediaminetetraacetic acid (EDTA) for alkali burns.[16] In some cases, 48 hours of intensive treatment with EDTA using hydrogel contact lenses may be more effective than more traditional methods of treating severe chemical burns. Other drugs used in conjunction with soft contact lenses have included cysteine hydrochloride,[16] acetylcysteine,[18] lubricating solutions,[19] normal saline,[20] mitomycin C,[4] idoxuridine,[20] corticosteroids,[20-22] and hyperosmotic solutions.[23] Disposable soft contact lenses have even been used as piggybacks on medicated corneal collagen shields to promote postoperative corneal epithelial healing and to provide sustained delivery of medications after corneal surgery.[24]

Lubricating, comfort, or rewetting solutions are commonly used to provide increased comfort when hydrogel lenses are worn. Occasionally, contact lens surfaces become dry, especially in low-humidity or windy environments. Lubricants are designed to rewet the surface and, in some cases, to help prevent and remove surface deposits. Such solutions may make the lenses temporarily more comfortable and extend wearing time. Solutions with high viscosity tend to provide a coating on the lens surface and remain on the lens until mechanically wiped or washed away by lid action and tearing. Because these solutions are inert, however, no chemical interaction occurs between the lubricant and the lens surface.[25]

The most common lubricants used in contact lens solutions are the substituted cellulose ethers, including methylcellulose and its derivatives, hydroxyethylcellulose, and hydroxypropylcellulose.[26] Solutions of these compounds form a thicker film on the lens than does polyvinyl alcohol, but no correlation exists between contact angle and film thickness.[27] Increased film thickness may be detrimental because a thick film can cause blurred vision and a sticky sensation. As thick films dry, they may form a white coating on the lids.

Early in the use of hydrogel contact lenses as a drug delivery system, it was recommended never to soak lenses in solutions containing preservatives because the prolonged delivery of relatively high concentrations of preservatives might be toxic to the eye, producing ocular irritation as well as superficial punctate corneal erosions.[28] Lemp,[19] however, found no evidence of benzalkonium chloride (BAK) concentration in hydrogel lenses used as drug delivery devices. He also did not find clinical evidence of corneal toxicity associated with the preservative. Therefore, the use of ophthalmic medications containing BAK in conjunction with hydrogel contact lenses appears to be a clinically acceptable practice, especially in conjunction with disposable or frequent-replacement soft contact lenses.

At present, therapeutic soft contact lenses for drug delivery appear to be of greatest clinical value in the treatment of bullous keratopathy, dry eye syndromes, and corneal conditions requiring protection.[6,24,29] The most significant disadvantage of this mode of therapy, however, is the rapid loss of most drugs from the lens. Because drug-impregnated hydrogel lenses are characterized by first-order kinetics,[14] in which peaks and valleys of drug concentration occur over time, they only occasionally offer any significant advantage over topically applied solutions or ointments. Therefore, this method of drug administration has not become popular. Moreover, because the most advantageous way to use soft contact lenses as drug delivery devices is to soak them with medication before fitting, this poses some potential logistic problems for the patient as well as for the practitioner.[30] Despite these limitations, however, bandage soft contact lenses are especially useful today to reduce the pain associated with corneal abrasions[31,32] or excimer laser photorefractive keratectomy[21,22,33] when used to deliver topical nonsteroidal anti-inflammatory drugs, such as diclofenac or ketorolac.

Mast Cell Stabilizers

Cromolyn sodium has become an important therapeutic agent for mast cell–mediated ocular disease, including giant papillary conjunctivitis (GPC) associated with contact lens wear.[34] Cromolyn acts primarily by stabilizing the mast cell,[35] but other mechanisms may also account for its clinical effectiveness. In a study of 60 patients with noninfectious inflammatory reactions, Felius and van Bijsterveld[36] reported that cromolyn was effective, although several patients had neither laboratory evidence nor history of atopic disease. They proposed that cromolyn protects the tear film against abnormal rupture. These investigators reported that the mean tear breakup time increased from 5.95 seconds to 9.9 seconds with cromolyn administration. In addition, Mikuni[37] reported that cromolyn also prevents the change in refractive index of tears seen in untreated eyes challenged with cedar pollen.

Ophthalmic drug disposition studies have been conducted to determine the amount of ocular and systemic absorption after cromolyn administration to the eye.[38,39] When multiple dosages of cromolyn sodium 4% were instilled into healthy rabbit eyes, less than 0.07% of the administered dose was absorbed into the systemic circulation. Less than 0.01% was present in the aqueous humor. In human studies, analysis of drug distribution indicates that approximately 0.03% of cromolyn applied topically is absorbed into the eye.[38] Iwasaki et al.[40] have shown that topical ocular application of cromolyn does not result in accumulation of drug in either daily-wear or extended-wear contact lenses. Moreover, Lesher and Gunderson[5] showed that cromolyn is released from disposable contact lenses at rates higher than those obtained with topical application alone, which suggests that cromolyn can be safely used in combination with continued contact lens wear in patients with GPC. However, the 4% preparation should be discarded within 4 weeks of opening, and the formulation should be protected from direct sunlight and stored below 30°C.[39]

Corticosteroids

Although many clinicians use a variety of topically applied corticosteroids for treatment of contact lens–associated GPC, only loteprednol etabonate has been documented to be effective for this condition.[41–43] Bartlett et al.,[43] in a phase II study, were the first to show statistically significant effects on reduction of papillae when loteprednol was compared with placebo. Patients also discontinued lens wear during the 4 weeks of steroid treatment. Loteprednol was well tolerated and did not elevate intraocular pressure during the study.

Two identical phase III studies were reported by Friedlaender and Howes[41] and Asbell and Howes.[42] The studies were double masked and placebo controlled, and patients with contact lens–associated GPC were randomized to receive loteprednol or its vehicle four times daily for 6 weeks. Papillae, itching, contact lens intolerance, and other signs and symptoms of GPC were assessed.

It is of interest that all patients continued to wear the offending contact lenses during the study. In both studies, loteprednol demonstrated a rapid and more effective therapeutic response, relative to placebo, for all signs and symptoms of GPC. This rapid therapeutic response, combined with the transient nature of any intraocular pressure elevations, suggests that loteprednol is an appropriate treatment for contact lens–associated GPC.

Decongestants

Ocular decongestants, such as phenylephrine or naphazoline, are occasionally used with contact lens wear. In some cases, their use may be justified, but ocular decongestants should not be used routinely because they may mask irritation or signs of a poorly performing lens. It is important that the underlying cause of persistent redness and irritation be diagnosed and properly corrected.

Phenylephrine 0.12% or 0.125% is found in several over-the-counter collyria designed to cause vasoconstriction and thereby "whiten the eye."[44] These agents may be administered indiscriminately by the user and, because phenylephrine can induce pupillary dilation even at low concentrations, it should be used sparingly in eyes predisposed to angle-closure glaucoma. Corneal trauma, including the effects of daily- or extended-wear contact lenses, can promote increased drug penetration across the cornea. This can potentially lead to increased risk of angle-closure glaucoma when phenylephrine is used to soothe an eye irritated from contact lens wear. Chronic use of phenylephrine at low concentrations for ocular vasoconstriction can also result in rebound congestion of the conjunctiva, in which the eye appears to be even more inflamed as a result of phenylephrine use.[45]

Naphazoline, tetrahydrozoline, and oxymetazoline are known collectively as the imidazole decongestants.[46–49] Rebound congestion has not been reported after ophthalmic use of naphazoline[50] or tetrahydrozoline.[48,49] Peyton and associates[51] conducted a clinical trial in which 16 subjects were fitted with Cibasoft clear daily-wear contact lenses and were instructed to use 2 drops of tetrahydrozoline 0.05% twice daily for 4 months in only one eye. Visual acuity, lens coloration, and slit-lamp findings were compared with baseline data between the test and the control eye of each subject. Visual acuity and lens coloration results showed statistically insignificant changes from baseline. However, clinically important changes in corneal integrity were noted in 46.7% of the tetrahydrozoline-treated eyes. The induced lesions were in the form of epithelial punctate staining observed with sodium fluorescein. The investigators attributed this effect to the BAK preservative. The authors concluded that tetrahydrozoline should not be used on a daily basis while

TABLE 22-1. *Lubricating and Rewetting Solutions*

Trade Name	Manufacturer	Ingredients
Solutions for rigid gas-permeable lenses		
Boston Rewetting Drops	Polymer Technology (Wilmington, MA)	Chlorhexidine gluconate 0.006%, EDTA 0.05%, cationic cellulose derivative polymer as wetting agent
Wet-N-Soak	Allergan (Irvine, CA)	Borate buffered, isotonic, hydroxyethyl cellulose
Solutions for soft lenses		
Blairex Lens Lubricant	Blairex Laboratories (Columbus, IN)	Sorbic acid 0.25%, EDTA 0.1%, borate buffer, NaCl, hydroxyproplymethyl cellulose, glycerin
Clerz 2	Alcon Laboratories, Inc. (Fort Worth, TX)	NaCl, KCl, hydroxyethyl cellulose, poloxamer 407, sodium borate, boric acid, sorbic acid, EDTA
Lens Lubricant	Bausch & Lomb, Inc. (Rochester, NY)	Thimerosal 0.004%, EDTA 0.1%, povidone, polyoxyethylene
Lens Plus Rewetting Drops	Allergan (Irvine, CA)	Buffered, isotonic; NaCl, boric acid, preservative-free
Opti-Tears	Alcon Laboratories, Inc. (Fort Worth, TX)	Isotonic, EDTA 0.1%, polyquaternium, dextran, NaCl, KCl, hydroxypropylmethyl cellulose
Sensitive Eye Drops	Bausch & Lomb, Inc. (Rochester, NY)	Buffered, sorbic acid 0.1%, EDTA 0.025%, NaCl, boric acid, sodium borate
Soft Mate Comfort Drops	Wesley-Jessen (Des Plains, IL)	Borate-buffered, potassium sorbate 0.13%, EDTA 0.1%, NaCl, hydroxyethyl cellulose, octylphenoxyethanol
Lens Drops	CIBA Vision (Duluth, GA)	Buffered, isotonic, NaCl, poloxamer 407, EDTA 0.2%, sorbic acid 0.15%

EDTA = ethylenediaminetetraacetic acid.

low–water content daily-wear hydrogel lenses are worn, but that occasional use of tetrahydrozoline should induce no serious compromise of corneal integrity or of the contact lenses themselves.

Lubricants

Occasionally, patients wearing contact lenses experience dehydration of the lens surface, causing blurred vision or drying of the peripheral cornea and conjunctiva. This can lead to symptoms of burning, stinging, conjunctival hyperemia, and ocular discomfort. It is important for the practitioner to find and alleviate the underlying cause, which might include a poorly fitted lens, inadequate lens oxygen permeability, or a poorly shaped or thick lens edge that causes infrequent blinking. If none of these problems exists and the signs and symptoms appear to result from low humidity or a dry eye, lubricating solutions may be used temporarily to alleviate symptoms.

Lubricating solutions used with contact lenses (Table 22-1) are usually isotonic or slightly hypertonic to enable water to be removed from the cornea in cases of edema.[52] It has been suggested that a 1% NaCl solution alone provides a longer effect than the usual lubricating solutions.[53] Lubricating solutions usually contain a viscosity or wetting agent to keep the eye moist as long as possible between drug instillations. Most of the solutions also contain preservatives to prevent bacterial contamination.

These preparations should not be used excessively owing to the potential detrimental effects of preservatives and other compounds on the cornea.[54] Moreover, the patient may have or may develop a sensitivity to an ingredient in the solution. The practitioner should determine if the patient is using such drops when other solutions are changed in response to a suspected solution reaction. If the patient continues to use the lubricating drops after discontinuing other contact lens solutions, the adverse signs and symptoms may continue unabated.

Ocular lubricants also play a role in the therapeutic management of many other conditions often seen in the contact lens wearer. These include pingueculae, exposure keratoconjunctivitis, acne rosacea, and superior limbic keratitis. It is usually prudent to discontinue lens wear during treatment of these conditions to enable a more rapid response to treatment and to minimize patient frustration with lens wear. In these instances, the preserved ocular lubricants present little risk to the patient or to the lens materials, because the lubricants are not used in conjunction with lens wear. Many patients, however, may continue lens wear with use of a nonpreserved artificial tear substitute several times daily.[55] As an alternative, use of a preservative system that is rapidly inactivated by tear film enzymes is acceptable clinical practice. Sodium perborate, the active preservative in GenTeal (CIBA Vision, Duluth, GA), is rapidly metabolized to oxygen and water when instilled into the eyes. This solution is compatible with most soft contact lens

TABLE 22-2. *Topical Ocular Antihistamine/Decongestants*

Trade Name	Manufacturer	Antihistamine	Decongestant
Naphcon-A	Alcon Laboratories, Inc. (Fort Worth, TX)	Pheniramine 0.3%	Naphazoline 0.025%
Opcon-A	Bausch & Lomb, Inc. (Rochester, NY)	Pheniramine 0.315%	Naphazoline 0.027%
Vasocon-A	CIBA Vision (Duluth, GA)	Antazoline 0.5%	Naphazoline 0.05%
Livostin	CIBA Vision (Duluth, GA)	Levocabastine 0.05%	—
Emadine	Alcon Laboratories, Inc. (Fort Worth, TX)	Emedastine 0.05%	—
Patanol	Alcon Laboratories, Inc. (Fort Worth, TX)	Olopatadine 0.1%	—

materials, especially those intended for use as disposables or frequent-replacement lenses.

Antihistamines

H_1 antihistamines are indicated for the relief of symptoms of mild-to-moderate allergic conjunctivitis or GPC, in which the symptoms are largely caused by mast cell degranulation and release of histamine. Several commercially available antihistamines are used for the topical treatment of ocular allergic disease (Table 22-2).[56] Most of these agents are commercially available only in combination with a vasoconstrictor, either phenylephrine or naphazoline. Therefore, such antihistamine combinations have the same potential for adverse ocular effects as the topical decongestants previously discussed in the Decongestants section. Mydriasis[57] with angle-closure glaucoma is a potential side effect of the vasoconstrictor and the antihistamine. In addition, long-term use may lead to local hypersensitivity reactions, attributable mainly to the antihistamine component.[58]

Topically applied antihistamines can be used alone or in conjunction with other therapeutic agents, such as lubricants, cromolyn sodium, or steroids, for treatment of mild-to-moderate allergic conjunctivitis or GPC. It is usually more productive to discontinue contact lens wear while these conditions are being treated. This usually helps to improve symptoms and hastens resolution of the disease process. In addition, potential drug-induced contact lens complications are avoided. In patients, however, who cannot or do not discontinue lens wear during treatment, topical levocabastine (Livostin) and its preservative BAK accumulate only slightly in soft contact lens materials and are safe to use concurrently for at least 1 week.[59]

Local Anesthetics

To evaluate the eye's normal physiologic responses to contact lens wear, contact lenses should be fitted without topical anesthesia. Certain limited circumstances, how-

ever, may justify use of topical anesthetics in contact lens evaluations. These include determining the effect of a rigid lens on monocular diplopia when the cornea is suspected to be the source. Topical anesthesia allows the rigid lens to be easily placed on the eye and to be readily tolerated by the patient during the initial diagnostic evaluation. Topical anesthetics can also be used when infants and very young children are fitted with rigid contact lenses. The molding of scleral lenses is facilitated by topical anesthesia, as is the fitting of rigid lenses to certain mentally retarded patients or other patients whose inability to cooperate precludes the necessary evaluation procedures. The practitioner, however, should avoid the use of topical anesthetics in conjunction with hydrogel lenses. These lenses absorb the anesthetic and act as a drug reservoir by gradually releasing the drug to the eye, with the potential complications associated with long-term anesthesia.[60]

Topical anesthetics are commonly used for tonometry during routine ocular and vision examinations. Patients who wear contact lenses should wait at least 60 minutes after application of the anesthetic before resuming lens wear.[61] This is necessary because topical anesthetics render the eye vulnerable to accidental damage during the period of anesthesia. The protective blink reflex is inhibited and abnormal drying of the cornea can occur.

When the use of sodium fluorescein, lissamine green, or rose bengal is anticipated for staining of ocular tissues, such as for evaluation of suspected dry eye syndromes or of patient complaints suggesting anterior segment involvement, the practitioner must avoid instilling an anesthetic until after the vital staining and evaluation procedures have been performed. This is necessary because the topical anesthetic itself can induce corneal epithelial changes that may mask or otherwise confound the corneal or conjunctival signs. In addition, the anesthetic-induced corneal epithelial changes can significantly alter the results obtained during evaluation of the tear breakup time.[62]

Contact lens patients who present with infectious corneal ulcers should have culture specimens taken from the lid margins or conjunctiva without the prior instillation of an anesthetic.[63,64] Topical anesthetics contain preservatives with antibacterial and antifungal properties. Moreover, the anesthetic agent itself is often toxic to micro-organisms. Tetracaine 0.05% has been shown to inhibit the growth of *Staphylococcus aureus* and *Monilia*.[65] In a concentration of 0.5%, tetracaine is toxic to *Pseudomonas*.[66] Kleinfeld and Ellis[64] showed that proparacaine, when used without preservative, does not inhibit the growth of *Staphylococcus albus, Pseudomonas aeruginosa*, and *Candida albicans*. These investigators, accordingly, have suggested that proparacaine, in single-dose containers without preservative, should be used when topical anesthesia is desired before obtaining culture specimens. Proparacaine appears to be the best topical anesthetic for use before obtaining culture material.

When an acute corneal lesion is evaluated in a contact lens wearer, the practitioner may be tempted to prescribe a topical anesthetic for pain relief at home by the patient. This practice, however, is extremely dangerous and has led in many instances to severe infiltrative keratitis and even loss of the eye from anesthetic misuse or abuse by the patient.[67–69] Topical anesthetics must be used only for obtaining initial relief of ocular pain and never as part of a prolonged therapeutic regimen. The potential corneal toxicity of topical anesthetics precludes their use as self-administered drugs.

Sodium Fluorescein

Sodium fluorescein can be topically applied to the eye in the form of a solution or by fluorescein-impregnated filter paper strips. When formulated in solution, fluorescein is highly susceptible to bacterial contamination, especially by *P. aeruginosa*.[70] This organism thrives in the presence of fluorescein. Several methods have been devised to reduce the possibility of bacterial growth. Kimura[71] developed fluorescein-impregnated filter paper strips. When the strip is wetted with sterile saline or irrigating solution, the dye is released and can be applied to the eye. Commercially available fluorescein strips are clinically useful for contact lens fitting and for evaluation of corneal epithelial integrity while minimizing the risk of bacterial contamination of the eye.

It has been suggested that Goldmann applanation tonometry can be performed without fluorescein.[72,73] This might have the advantage of avoiding possible contamination of the eye or hydrogel contact lens with fluorescein. Several investigators,[74–76] however, have compared ocular pressure measurements with Goldmann applanation tonometry in the presence and absence of fluorescein. The results indicate that readings using white light without fluorescein are significantly lower than those obtained using cobalt blue light with fluorescein. Roper[74] found an underestimation of 5.62 mm Hg when fluorescein was not used.

Bright and associates[76] found that readings without fluorescein were lower by an average of 7.01 mm Hg. The lower readings observed in the absence of fluorescein can be attributed to difficulty in viewing the applanated area of the cornea. The apex of the tear film meniscus, which defines the applanated area, is not clearly visible without fluorescein.[77] Although there could be definite advantages to the hydrogel lens wearer by performing Goldmann tonometry without fluorescein, the differences in readings at higher intraocular pressure levels can present potentially important clinical problems in the diagnosis or monitoring of glaucoma.

Because topically administered dyes discolor hydrogel contact lenses, the lenses should not be reinserted until the dye has left the eye, usually after 30–60 minutes. Alternatively, the lenses can be reinserted immediately after irrigation of the dye from the eye. Accidental staining of hydrogel lenses with sodium fluorescein can be remedied by purging the lenses, using frequent long-term soaks in normal saline or disinfecting solution normally used with the lenses.

Because sodium fluorescein can penetrate hydrogel contact lenses, the lenses become discolored, which is cosmetically objectionable. Moreover, the boundary between lens and tears becomes obscured, which precludes the use of sodium fluorescein in hydrogel lens fitting. Fluorexon, a high-molecular-weight solution similar to fluorescein, is less readily absorbed by the hydrogel lens material and has been suggested as a more useful dye in fitting and evaluating hydrogel lenses.[78] Fluorexon can be applied to the eye with the hydrogel lens in place, but it is more effective when placed in the posterior bowl of the lens before insertion. Fluorexon stains the hydrogel lens if it remains in contact with the lens for more than a few minutes. However, repeated rinsing with saline usually removes the dye from the lens. Fluorexon is not recommended for use with highly hydrated hydrogel lenses (water content $\geq 60\%$) because, in such cases, absorption of dye by the lens is much more difficult to rectify. In clinical use, fluorexon has proved to be nontoxic to ocular tissue. However, this agent has not been widely used because the observation of dye-stained tears in the evaluation of hydrogel lens fitting is not significantly more effective than simple evaluation of the lens without dye. In addition, a special yellow filter is required to enhance observation of the fluorescence, which makes the procedure more cumbersome.

Toxicity of Preservatives

BAK is present in many solutions used with polymethylmethacrylate contact lenses. This surface-active agent is a cationic detergent and acts against micro-organisms by adsorbing on the cell membrane and increasing its permeability. It is used in concentrations of 1 in 100,000 to 1 in 10,000.[79] As with any preservative, there must be a high enough concentration to prevent microbial growth without causing significant ocular toxicity. Several studies[80,81] have shown that BAK can cause corneal damage in concentrations as low as 0.005%, although it may require a longer exposure time than would normally occur with a solution used on a rigid contact lens.[82,83] At concentrations of 0.0075–0.01%, significant corneal epithelial damage can occur within several minutes of continuous exposure. Moreover, because hydrogel lenses readily absorb and concentrate significant amounts of BAK,[84,85] it cannot be used in soaking solutions for these lenses. Although BAK is still widely used in contact lens solutions, its use is declining because of its incompatibility with new lens materials, especially hydrogel lenses, and because of its detrimental effect on the cornea.[1]

Chlorobutanol is a preservative that has been incorporated into some solutions for use with polymethylmethacrylate lenses. This compound is easily deactivated by heat, and because of its instability and slow kill rate, it is seldom used. However, it is sometimes used in combination with other preservatives, such as BAK, but chlorobutanol is incompatible with hydrogel lenses.[26]

Thimerosal is an organic mercury compound used in rigid and hydrogel lens solutions. It does not bind significantly to hydrogel lens materials.[86] Thimerosal is usually used in concentrations of 0.001–0.2% in combination with other preservatives, such as EDTA or chlorhexidine. It is not chemically compatible with BAK. The most clinically significant problem with thimerosal is the development of sensitivity to the compound, which occurs in as many as 25–50% of patients wearing hydrogel lenses.[87,88] Thimerosal may be absorbed into the corneal epithelium, at least under some conditions, causing corneal damage.[89] Signs and symptoms vary with each patient, as do the time course of allergic or toxic reactions to thimerosal. Patients who have previously been sensitized to thimerosal can develop a very injected and irritated eye within minutes after a lens soaked in the solution is placed on the eye. A relatively severe reaction can also occur in these patients by irrigating the eye with a thimerosal-preserved solution. A more common history, however, is that the patient seems to do well with the lenses for weeks or months, and then the eyes become injected and irritated immediately on inserting the lenses. The patient had not been previously sensitized to the thimerosal but developed the typical delayed hypersensitivity response during use. In such cases, skin patch testing is often positive to thimerosal.[88,90,91] The other type of reaction is characterized by gradual and progressive worsening of signs and symptoms. In addition to the conjunctival inflammation, there may be corneal subepithelial infiltrates, punctate epithelial keratitis, or

swollen eyelids.[92] With long-term use, neovascularization can occur. The patient may complain of itching, burning, dryness, photophobia, pain, and decreased visual acuity. When any of these signs or symptoms occurs with a well-fitted lens, the patient's contact lens care system should be changed to unpreserved saline or to a solution without thimerosal, such as sorbic acid–preserved saline or hydrogen peroxide.[52]

Chlorhexidine is used as a preservative in hydrogel lens solutions. Chlorhexidine digluconate and chlorhexidine diacetate have been used, the former causing less ocular irritation. Chlorhexidine binds to hydrogel lens materials and is only slowly released.[93,94] It also binds to proteins and other tear film substances, enhancing hypersensitivity reactions to the compound. This preservative can cause corneal epithelial damage but not to the extent demonstrated by BAK.[83]

Sorbic acid or its salt, sorbate, is a preservative commonly used in hydrogel contact lens solutions. This preservative is associated with a very low incidence of allergic or toxic reactions.

Tris (2-hydroxyethyl) tallow ammonium chloride has been used in conjunction with thimerosal as a hydrogel lens disinfecting solution. The solution contains other polymeric compounds to aid in the formation of micelles, large groups of molecules that minimize absorption of the preservatives into the lens and thus decrease allergic or toxic reactions.

Polyquad is a high-molecular-weight quaternary compound that is not absorbed into most hydrogel lenses. Therefore, toxic or allergic reactions are rare. However, the initial formulation containing this preservative did cause some toxic reactions when used with high–water content ionic lenses.[26]

Polyaminopropyl biguanide (Dymed) was developed for use with hydrogel lenses to avoid the toxic and allergic reactions common with solutions containing thimerosal and chlorhexidine. This preservative is from the same group of compounds as chlorhexidine, but polyaminopropyl does not have the parachloroaniline end group that may degrade, causing the toxic problems occasionally encountered with chlorhexidine.

Drugs That Have Adverse Effects on Lens Materials

With high–water content hydrogel lenses, sorbic acid– or sorbate-preserved solutions may cause slight lens yellowing or discoloration. If a higher concentration (0.3% or greater) of sorbate or sorbic acid is used, discoloration is common. Discoloration apparently results from the breakdown of sorbic acid to aldehydes, which in turn react with amino acids from proteins coating the lens.[95]

Chlorhexidine can cause hydrogel lens surfaces to become hydrophobic, which increases adherence of lipids to the lens surface.[96] Decomposition of these lipids may turn the lens yellow to yellow-green.

Soaking lenses in or repeated instillation of epinephrine, phenylephrine, or related oxidizable adrenergic drugs can stain hydrogel lenses gray, black, or brown. This adverse effect, known as *adrenochrome staining*, results in diffuse pigment deposits throughout the lens.[97,98] Such staining of hydrogel lenses with epinephrine can occur within 2–6 weeks of initial topical epinephrine therapy for glaucoma. Therefore, the glaucoma patient wearing hydrogel lenses and using topical epinephrine should remove the lenses before instillation of the epinephrine and should wait at least 15 minutes before reinserting the lenses after epinephrine instillation. Once such lens staining has occurred, however, hydrogen peroxide or another oxidizing agent may be useful to clear the lens.[52]

In contrast to epinephrine preparations, dipivefrin can be used in patients wearing hydrogel lenses, without significant risk of adrenochrome staining.[98] The addition of two pivalyl groups to form the dipivalyl epinephrine molecule may render the drug less subject to oxidation and, therefore, may prevent the formation of breakdown products that stain the contact lens. Thus, this epinephrine prodrug may be useful for treatment of glaucoma in patients who must also wear hydrogel contact lenses.

Macsai et al.[99] reported deposition of opaque deposits of ciprofloxacin, prednisolone acetate, and prednisolone phosphate in contact lenses of patients with persistent epithelial defects who were using SeeQuence (Bausch & Lomb, Inc., Rochester, NY) disposable contact lenses. High-performance liquid chromatography revealed the deposits to be precipitates of ciprofloxacin and prednisolone, formed when ciprofloxacin was combined with either prednisolone acetate or prednisolone phosphate.

An interesting observation is that tears can become discolored after the use of systemic rifampin.[100] The tears usually become orange but may also be pink or red. Hydrogel lenses may also stain, and it has therefore been suggested that lens wear may have to be curtailed during rifampin therapy in patients who secrete this drug into the tears.[101] Other drugs reported to discolor hydrogel lenses after excretion into the tear film include phenazopyridine, tetracycline, phenolphthalein, and nitrofurantoin.[102]

SYSTEMIC MEDICATIONS

Many systemic medications can affect contact lens wear, usually by causing changes in the tear film. Dry eye is an especially important complication of systemic medication use that can adversely affect the contact lens wearer.[1] In other instances, topically applied contact lens solutions may adversely interact with certain systemic medications. For example, disulfiram (Antabuse), a drug used in the management of chronic alcoholism, has been reported to cause a reaction with rigid lens wear similar to that which occurs if alcohol is imbibed. The reaction, related to polyvinyl alcohol in the wetting solution, consisted of flushing, dry mouth, prickly sensation, dizziness, nausea, vomiting, and weakness.[103]

Several classes of drugs can affect aqueous tear secretion, influence tear constituents, or appear in the tears after systemic administration. These medications can induce watery or dry eyes and other symptoms relating to drug action on the tears. Among the agents that frequently reduce tear secretion are the anticholinergics and antihistamines. Both classes of drugs are present in many over-the-counter products, such as sedatives, sleep aids, cold preparations, antidiarrheals, and nasal decongestants.

Drugs That Cause Dry Eye

Anticholinergics
Dryness of mucous membranes is a common side effect of anticholinergic medications because atropine and related drugs inhibit glandular secretion. In one study,[104] oral administration of atropine caused tear secretion to fall from 15 μl to 3 μl per minute. A similar dose of atropine given subcutaneously induced a nearly 50% reduction in lacrimal secretion.[105] Scopolamine, 1–2 mg orally, reduced tear secretion from 5 μl to 0.8 μl per minute.[104] Similarly, when used to prevent motion sickness, transdermal scopolamine can lead to symptoms of dry eye and dry mouth. Therefore, a careful medication history is important to determine the specific etiology of sometimes elusive patient complaints.

Antihistamines
In addition to their receptor-blocking effects, H_1 antihistamines have various degrees of atropinelike actions, including the ability to alter tear film integrity.[105,106] Koeffler and Lemp[107] administered 4 mg daily of chlorpheniramine maleate to healthy volunteers. Tear secretion was measured using the Schirmer's test. A significant reduction in tear flow was observed on the days when chlorpheniramine was taken. Systemic use of antihistamines can aggravate an underlying condition of keratitis sicca.[108] Use of 200 mg daily of diphenhydramine has resulted in the recurrence of filamentary keratitis in a woman with arthritis. When the medication was discontinued, the symptoms disappeared. This observation suggests that patients with a compromised tear film may aggravate the condition by using antihistamines. The patient illustrated in the Grand Rounds Case Report that begins this chapter is an excellent example of this effect.

Isotretinoin

Dry eye symptoms have been reported as a side effect of systemic isotretinoin therapy for cases of severe, recalcitrant acne. The prevalence has been estimated to be as high as 20%, and approximately 8% of patients wearing contact lenses have lens intolerance.[109] Isotretinoin decreases tear breakup time,[109,110] and it is also possible that lipid secretion by the meibomian glands is reduced, decreasing the lipid layer and thereby increasing evaporation rate of the aqueous tears.

Analysis of lacrimal gland fluid of rabbits and human tears of subjects treated with isotretinoin has shown the presence of this vitamin derivative in tears. Therefore, isotretinoin in tear fluid could decrease stability of the lipid layer of the tear film, thus enhancing the formation of dry spots. This effect could be responsible, in turn, for the dry eye symptoms, contact lens intolerance, and conjunctival irritation that accompany isotretinoin therapy.[111]

β-Adrenergic Blocking Agents

Reduced tear secretion is a reported side effect of oral β-blocking drugs. Although most reported cases involve practolol,[112] other β-blockers, such as propranolol and timolol, have also been implicated in dry eye syndrome.[113,114] Ocular side effects of practolol have been described as an "oculomucocutaneous syndrome," in which patients develop symptomatic lesions of the ocular surface.[112] Other β-blocking agents have been implicated in patients with dry eye symptoms.[114,115]

Oral Contraceptives

Oral contraceptives have been implicated in contact lens wearing problems.[116] Possible etiologic mechanisms include changes in tear production and corneal thickness or curvature. Although oral contraceptives have been suspected to cause reduced tear production and problems associated with lens wear, the scientific and medical literature is devoid of well-documented studies showing a definite relationship between oral contraceptive use and contact lens intolerance.[117-119]

Miscellaneous Agents

Other drugs with possible anticholinergic actions, such as the phenothiazines, anxiolytics, and tricyclic antidepressants, have been associated with dry eye syndromes. Diuretics, such as hydrochlorothiazide, can also reduce tear production.[120]

Drugs That Cause Increased Aqueous Tears and Tear Film Constituents

Several studies have indicated that systemic administration of certain cholinergic, adrenergic, and antihypertensive agents can stimulate lacrimation.[104,121] Subcutaneous pilocarpine can increase tear production in normal eyes, and neostigmine, given subcutaneously or intramuscularly, also induces lacrimation. Several antihypertensive agents can increase tear production, including reserpine, hydralazine, and diazoxide.

Drug penetration into tears has been reported with certain antimicrobial agents and aspirin. Sulfonamides, tetracyclines, erythromycin, and rifampin have been detected in tears of human subjects.[122] Ampicillin and penicillin penetrate into tears very poorly, and important bioactive concentrations are not obtained. In contrast, erythromycin levels in tears have been determined to be higher than the serum concentration, implying active transport of this antibiotic into tears after systemic administration.[122] After oral administration, 36–88% of the daily erythromycin dosage is present in tears, potentially resulting in surface irritation to the eye or contact lens intolerance.

Aspirin taken orally is excreted into the tears.[123] This drug might also be absorbed into a hydrogel lens and cause corneal epithelial irritation because aspirin is known to be an irritant.[124]

Table 22-3 summarizes the important effects on aqueous tears of systemically administered medications.[125]

TABLE 22-3. *Drugs That Can Affect Aqueous Tear Secretion*

Drug Class	Example
Agents causing dry eye	
Anticholinergics	Atropine, scopolamine
Antihistamines	Chlorpheniramine, diphenhydramine
Vitamin A analogues	Isotretinoin
β-Adrenergic blockers	Propranolol, timolol
Phenothiazines	Chlorpromazine, thioridazine
Antianxiety agents	Chlordiazepoxide, diazepam
Tricyclic antidepressants	Amitriptyline, doxepin
Agents causing lacrimation	
Adrenergic agonists	Ephedrine
Antihypertensives	Reserpine, hydralazine
Cholinergic agonists	Neostigmine

Source: Modified with permission from SD Jaanus, JD Bartlett, JA Hiett: Ocular effects of systemic drugs. p. 957. In JD Bartlett, SD Jaanus (eds): Clinical Ocular Pharmacology. 3rd ed. Butterworth–Heinemann, Boston, 1995.

REFERENCES

1. Silbert JA: A review of therapeutic agents and contact lens wear. J Am Optom Assoc 67:165, 1996
2. Waltman SR, Kaufman HE: Use of hydrophilic contact lenses to increase ocular penetration of topical drugs. Invest Ophthalmol Vis Sci 9:250, 1970

3. Jain MR: Drug delivery through soft contact lenses. Br J Ophthalmol 72:150, 1988

4. Meitz H, Distelhorst M, Rump, et al: Ocular concentration of mitomycin C using different delivery devices. Ophthalmologica 212:37, 1998

5. Lesher GA, Gunderson GG: Continuous drug delivery through the use of disposable contact lenses. Optom Vis Sci 70:1012, 1993

6. Fraunfelder FT, Hanna C: Ophthalmic drug delivery systems. Surv Ophthalmol 18:292, 1974

7. Scullica L, Squeri CA, Ferreri G: "Minor" applications of soft contact lenses. Trans Ophthalmol Soc UK 97:159, 1977

8. Ruben M, Watkins R: Pilocarpine dispensation for the soft hydrophilic contact lens. Br J Ophthalmol 59:455, 1975

9. Aquavella JV: New aspects of contact lenses in ophthalmology. Adv Ophthalmol 32:2, 1976

10. Fraunfelder FT, Hanna C: Ophthalmic ointments. Trans Am Acad Ophthalmol Otolaryngol 77:467, 1973

11. Hillman JS: Management of acute glaucoma with pilocarpine-soaked hydrophilic lenses. Br J Ophthalmol 58:674, 1974

12. Podos SM, Becker B, Asseff C, et al: Pilocarpine therapy with soft contact lenses. Am J Ophthalmol 73:336, 1972

13. Maddox YT, Bernstein HN: An evaluation of the Bionite hydrophilic contact lens for use in a drug delivery system. Ann Ophthalmol 4:789, 1972

14. Lamberts DW: Solid delivery devices. Int Ophthalmol Clin 20:63, 1980

15. Busin M, Spitznas M: Sustained gentamicin release by presoaked medicated bandage contact lenses. Ophthalmology 95:796, 1988

16. Krejci L, Brettschneider I, Praus R: Hydrophilic gel contact lenses as a new drug delivery system in ophthalmology and as a therapeutic bandage lens. Acta Univ Carol [Med] 21:387, 1975

17. O'Brien TP, Sawusch MR, Dick JD, et al: Use of collagen corneal shields versus soft contact lenses to enhance penetration of topic tobramycin. J Cataract Refract Surg 14:505, 1988

18. Shaw EL, Gasset AR: Management of an unusual case of keratitis mucosa with hydrophilic contact lenses and *N*-acetylcysteine. Ann Ophthalmol 6:1054, 1974

19. Lemp MA: Bandage lenses and the use of topical solutions containing preservatives. Ann Ophthalmol 10:1319, 1978

20. Wilson M, Leigh E: Therapeutic use of soft contact lenses. Proc R Soc Med 68:55, 1975

21. Sher NA, Frantz JM, Talley A, et al: Topical diclofenac in the treatment of ocular pain after excimer photorefractive keratectomy. Refract Corneal Surg 9:425, 1993

22. Arshinoff SA, Mills MD, Haber S: Pharmacotherapy of photorefractive keratectomy. J Cataract Refract Surg 22:1037, 1996

23. Jaanus SD: Anti-edema drugs. p. 369. In Bartlett JD, Jaanus SD, (eds): Clinical Ocular Pharmacology. 3rd ed. Butterworth–Heinemann, Boston, 1995

24. Palmer RM, McDonald MB: A corneal lens/shield system to promote postoperative corneal epithelial healing. J Cataract Refract Surg 21:125, 1995

25. Schnider CM: Dyes. p. 389. In Bartlett JD, Jaanus SD (eds): Clinical Ocular Pharmacology. 3rd ed. Butterworth–Heinemann, Boston, 1995

26. Lowther GE: Contact lens solutions and care systems. p. 409. In Bartlett JD, Jaanus SD (eds): Clinical Ocular Pharmacology. 3rd ed. Butterworth–Heinemann, Boston, 1995

27. Benedetto D, Shah D, Kaufman H: The dynamic film thickness of cushioning agents on contact lens materials. Ann Ophthalmol 10:437, 1978

28. Kaufman HE, Uotila MH, Gasset AR, et al: The medical uses of soft contact lenses. Trans Am Acad Ophthalmol Otolaryngol 75:361, 1971

29. Andrew NC, Woodward EG: The bandage lens in bullous keratopathy. Ophthal Physiol Opt 9:66, 1989

30. Bartlett JD: Ophthalmic drug delivery. p. 47. In Bartlett JD, Jaanus SD (eds): Clinical Ocular Pharmacology. 3rd ed. Butterworth–Heinemann, Boston, 1995

31. Salz JJ, Reader AL, Schwartz LJ, VanLe K: Treatment of corneal abrasions with soft contact lenses and topical diclofenac. J Refract Corneal Surg 10:640, 1994

32. Donnenfeld ED, Seldin BA, Perry HD, et al: Controlled evaluation of a bandage contact lens and a topical non-steroidal anti-inflammatory drug in treatment of traumatic corneal abrasions. Ophthalmology 102:979, 1995

33. Cherry PM: The treatment of pain following excimer laser photorefractive keratectomy: additive effect of local anesthetic drops, topical diclofenac, and bandage soft contact. Ophthalmic Surg Lasers (5 suppl.)27:S477, 1996

34. Kruger CJ, Ehlers WH, Luistro AE, Donshik PC: Treatment of giant papillary conjunctivitis with cromolyn sodium. CLAO J 18:46, 1992

35. Perkins ES, MacFaul PA: Indomethacin in the treatment of uveitis; a double-blind trial. Trans Ophthalmol Soc UK 85:53, 1965

36. Felius K, van Bijsterveld OP: Effect of sodium cromoglycate on tear film break-up time. Ann Ophthalmol 17:80, 1987

37. Mikuni I: Efficacy of two percent DSCG ophthalmic solution for allergic conjunctivitis from Japanese cedar pollinosin. Jpn J Clin Ophthalmol 34:1655, 1980

38. Lee VHL, Swarbrick J, Stratford RE, Morimoto KW: Disposition of topically applied sodium cromoglycate in albino rabbit eye. Int J Pharmaceut 16:163, 1983

39. Ross RW: Opticrom 4% in Clinical Practice. A monograph. Fisons Corporation, Bedford, MA, 1984

40. Iwasaki W, Kosaka Y, Momose T, et al: Absorption of topical disodium cromoglycate and its preservatives by soft contact lens. CLAO J 14:155, 1988

41. Friedlaender MH, Howes J: A double-masked, placebo-controlled evaluation of the efficacy and safety of loteprednol etabonate in the treatment of giant papillary conjunctivitis. Am J Ophthalmol 123:455, 1997

42. Asbell P, Howes J: A double-masked, placebo-controlled evaluation of the efficacy and safety of loteprednol etabonate in the treatment of giant papillary conjunctivitis. CLAO J 23:31, 1997

43. Bartlett JD, Howes JF, Ghormley NR, et al: Safety and efficacy of loteprednol etabonate for treatment of papillae in

contact lens–associated giant papillary conjunctivitis. Curr Eye Res 12:313, 1993

44. Weiss DI, Shaffer RN: Mydriatic effects of one-eighth percent phenylephrine. Arch Ophthalmol 68:727, 1962

45. Meyer SM, Fraunfelder FT: Phenylephrine hydrochloride. Ophthalmology 87:1177, 1980

46. Babel J: Action of 2-(1-naphthylmethyl) imidazoline hydrochloride on the eye. Schweiz Med Wochenschr 71:561, 1941

47. Hurwitz P, Thompson JM: Use of naphazoline (Privine) in ophthalmology. Arch Ophthalmol 43:712, 1950

48. Grossmann EE, Lehman RH: Ophthalmic use of tyzine. Am J Ophthalmol 42:121, 1956

49. Menger HC: New ophthalmic decongestant, tetrahydrozoline hydrochloride. JAMA 170:178, 1958

50. Abbott WO, Henry CM: Paredrine (β-4-hydroxyphenylisopropylamine): a clinical investigation of a sympathomimetic drug. Am J Med Sci 193:661, 1937

51. Peyton SM, Joyce RG, Edrington TB: Soft contact lens and corneal changes associated with Visine use. J Am Optom Assoc 60:207, 1989

52. Lowther GE: Contact lens solutions and care systems. p. 424. In Bartlett JD, Jaanus SD (eds): Clinical Ocular Pharmacology. 3rd ed. Butterworth–Heinemann, Boston, 1995

53. Poster MG: Optical efficacy of rewetting and lubricating solutions. Contact Lens Forum 6:25, 1981

54. Zand ML: The effect of non-therapeutic ophthalmic preparations on the cornea and tear film. Aust J Optom 64:44, 1981

55. Caffery BE, Josephson JE: Is there a better "comfort drop"? J Am Optom Assoc 61:178, 1990

56. Bartlett JD, Jaanus SD: Antiallergy and decongestant agents. p. 59. In Bartlett JD, Fiscella RG, Ghormley NR, et al. (eds): Ophthalmic Drug Facts. Facts and Comparisons. St. Louis, 1999

57. Williams TL, Williams AJ, Enzenauer RW: Case report: unilateral mydriasis from topical Opcon-A and soft contact lens. Aviat Space Environ Med 68:135, 1997

58. Jaanus SD, Hegeman SL, Swanson MW: Antiallergy drugs and decongestants. p. 337. In Bartlett JD, Jaanus SD (eds): Clinical Ocular Pharmacology. 3rd ed. Butterworth–Heinemann, Boston, 1995

59. Momose T, Ito N, Kanai A, et al: Adsorption of levocabastine eye drops by soft contact lenses and its effects in rabbit eyes. CLAO J 23:96, 1997

60. Talley DK, Bartlett JD: Topical and regional anesthesia. p. 463. In Bartlett JD, Jaanus SD (eds): Clinical Ocular Pharmacology. 3rd ed. Butterworth–Heinemann, Boston, 1995

61. Hill RM: Anesthetic impact. Int Contact Lens Clin 7:199, 1980

62. Bartlett JD, Jaanus SD: Local anesthetics. p. 117. In Bartlett JD, Jaanus SD (eds): Clinical Ocular Pharmacology. 3rd ed. Butterworth–Heinemann, Boston, 1995

63. Havener WH: Ocular Pharmacology. Mosby, St Louis, 1983

64. Kleinfeld J, Ellis PP: Effects of topical anesthetics on growth of microorganisms. Arch Ophthalmol 76:712, 1966

65. Erlich H: Bacteriologic studies and effects of anesthetic solutions on bronchial secretions during bronchoscopy. Ann Rev Respir Dis 84:414, 1961

66. Murphy JT, Allen HF, Mangiaracine AB: Preparation, sterilization, and preservation of ophthalmic solutions: experimental studies and a practical method. Arch Ophthalmol 53:63, 1955

67. Henkes HE, Waubke TN: Keratitis from abuse of corneal anesthetics. Br J Ophthalmol 62:62, 1978

68. Epstein DL, Paton D: Keratitis from misuse of corneal anesthetic. N Engl J Med 279:369, 1968

69. Michaels RH, Wilson FM, Grayson M: Infiltrative keratitis from abuse of anesthetic eyedrops. J Indiana State Med Assoc 72:51, 1979

70. Vaughan DG: The contamination of fluorescein solutions—with special reference to *Pseudomonas aeruginosa*. Am J Ophthalmol 39:55, 1955

71. Kimura SJ: Fluorescein paper; a simple means of insuring the use of sterile fluorescein. Am J Ophthalmol 34:446, 1951

72. Smith R: Applanation tonometry without fluorescein. Am J Ophthalmol 87:583, 1979

73. Weinstock FJ: Applanation tonometry without fluorescein. Ophthalmology 94:797, 1979

74. Roper DL: Applanation tonometry with and without fluorescein. Am J Ophthalmol 90:668, 1980

75. Rosenstock T, Breslin CW: The importance of fluorescein in applanation tonometry. Am J Ophthalmol 92:741, 1981

76. Bright DC, Potter JW, Allen DC, Spruance RD: Goldmann applanation tonometry without fluorescein. Am J Optom Physiol Opt 58:1120, 1981

77. Moses RA: Fluorescein in applanation tonometry. Am J Ophthalmol 49:1149, 1960

78. Refojo MF, Miller D, Fiore AS: A new fluorescent stain for soft hydrophilic lens fitting. Arch Ophthalmol 87:275, 1972

79. Mullen W, Shepherd W, Labovitz J: Ophthalmic preservatives and vehicles. Surv Ophthalmol 17:469, 1973

80. Dabezies DH: Contact lenses and their solutions: a review of basic principles. EENT Monthly 45:39, 1966

81. Burstein NL: Preservative alteration of corneal permeability in humans and rabbits. Invest Ophthalmol Vis Sci 25:1453, 1984

82. Burstein NL, Klyce SD: Electrophysiologic and morphologic effects of ophthalmic preparations on rabbit corneal epithelium. Invest Ophthalmol Vis Sci 18:899, 1977

83. Burstein NL: Preservative cytotoxic threshold for benzalkonium chloride and chlorhexidine digluconate in cat and rabbit corneas. Invest Ophthalmol Vis Sci 19:308, 1980

84. MacKeen DG, Bulle K: Buffers and preservatives in contact lens solutions. Contacto 21:33, 1977

85. Lumbroso P, Nhamias M, Nhamias S, Tranche P: A preliminary study of the adsorption and release of preservative by contact lenses and collagen shields. CLAO J 22:61, 1996

86. Sibley MJ, Young G: A technique for the determination of chemical binding to soft contact lenses. Am J Optom Physiol Opt 50:710, 1973

87. Kline LN, DeLuca TJ: Thermal vs. chemical disinfection. Int Contact Lens Clin 5:23, 1978

88. Tosti A, Tosti G: Thimerosal: a hidden allergen in ophthalmology. Contact Dermatitis 18:268, 1988

89. Winder AF, Astbury NJ, Sheraidah GAK, et al: Penetration of mercury from ophthalmic preservatives into the human eye. Lancet 2:237, 1980

90. Molinari JF, Nash R, Badham D: Severe thimerosal hypersensitivity in soft contact lens wearers. Int Contact Lens Clin 9:323, 1982

91. Gordon A: Prospective screening for thimerosal hypersensitivity: a pilot study. Am J Optom Physiol Opt 65:147, 1988

92. Baines MG, Cai F, Backman HA: Ocular hypersensitivity to thimerosal in rabbits. Invest Ophthalmol Vis Sci 32:2259, 1991

93. Kaspar H: Binding characteristics and microbiological effectiveness of preservatives. Aust J Optom 59:4, 1976

94. Refojo M: Reversible binding of chlorhexidine gluconate to hydrogel contact lenses. Contact Intraocul Lens Med J 2:47, 1976

95. Sibley M, Chu V: Understanding sorbic acid preserved contact lens solutions. Int Contact Lens Clin 9:531, 1984

96. Kleist FD: Appearance and nature of hydrophilic contact lens deposits. II. Inorganic deposits. Int Contact Lens Clin 6:177, 1979

97. Sugar J: Adrenochrome pigmentation of hydrophilic lenses. Arch Ophthalmol 91:11, 1974

98. Mahmood MA, Pillai S: Epinephrine staining of soft contact lens. Arch Ophthalmol 105:1021, 1987

99. Macsai MS, Goel AK, Michael MM, et al: Deposition of ciprofloxacin, prednisolone phosphate, and prednisolone acetate in SeeQuence disposable contact lenses. CLAO J 19:166-168, 1993

100. Fraunfelder FT: Orange tears. Am J Ophthalmol 89:752, 1980

101. Lyons RW: Orange contact lenses from rifampin. N Engl J Med 300:372, 1979

102. Wartman RH: Contact lens related side effects of systemic drugs. Contact Lens Forum 12:42, 1987

103. Newson SR, Hayer BS: Disulfiram alcohol reactions caused by contact lens wetting solutions. Contact Intraocul Lens Med J 6:407, 1980

104. Balic J: Effect of atropine and pilocarpine on the secretion of chloride ion into the tears. Cesk Oftalmol 14:28, 1958

105. Erickson OF: Drug influences on lacrimal lysozyme production. Stanford Med Bull 18:34, 1960

106. Crandall DC, Leopold IH: The influence of systemic drugs on tear constituents. Ophthalmology 86:115, 1979

107. Koeffler BH, Lemp MA: The effect of an antihistamine (chlorpheniramine maleate) on tear production in humans. Am J Ophthalmol 12:217, 1980

108. Seedor JA, Lamberts D, Bermann RB, et al: Filamentary keratitis associated with diphenhydramine hydrochloride (Benadryl). Am J Ophthalmol 101:376, 1986

109. Fraunfelder FT, Baico JM, Meyer SM: Adverse ocular reactions possibly associated with isotretinoin. Am J Ophthalmol 100:534, 1985

110. Ensink BW, Van Voorst Vader PC: Ophthalmological side effects of 13-*cis*-retinoic therapy. Br J Dermatol 108:637, 1983

111. Ubels JL, MacRae SM: Vitamin A is present as retinol in tears of humans and rabbits. Curr Eye Res 3:815, 1984

112. Felix FH, Ive FA, Dahl MGC: Cutaneous and ocular reactions with practolol administration. Oculomucocutaneous syndrome. BMJ 1:595, 1975

113. Scott D: Another beta blocker causing eye problems. BMJ 2:1221, 1977

114. Mackie IA, Seal DV, Pescod JM: Beta-adrenergic receptor blocking drugs: tear lysozyme and immunological screening for adverse reactions. Br J Ophthalmol 61:354, 1977

115. Almog Y, Monselise M, Almog CH, et al: The effect of oral treatment with beta blockers on tear secretion. Metab Pediatr Syst Ophthalmol 6:343, 1983

116. Koetting RA: The influence of oral contraceptives on contact lens wear. Am J Optom Physiol Opt 43:268, 1966

117. Chizek DJ, Franceschetti AT: Oral contraceptives: their side effects and ophthalmological manifestations. Surv Ophthalmol 14:90, 1969

118. Verbeck B: Augenbufende und Stoffwechselverhalten bei Einnahme von Ovulation-schemmern. Klin Monatsbl Augenheilkd 162:612, 1973

119. Frankel SH, Ellis PP: Effect of oral contraceptives on tear production. Ann Ophthalmol 10:1585, 1978

120. Berman MT, Newman BL, Johnson NC: The effect of a diuretic (hydrochlorothiazide) on tear production in humans. Am J Ophthalmol 99:473, 1985

121. De Haas EBH: Lacrimal gland response to parasympathomimetics after parasympathetic denervation. Arch Ophthalmol 64:34, 1960

122. Melon J, Reginster M: Passage into normal salivary, lacrimal and nasal secretions of ampicillin and erythromycin administered intramuscularly. Acta Otorhinolaryngol Belg 30:643, 1976

123. Valenic JP, Leopold IH, Dea FJ: Excretion of salicylic acid into tears following oral administration of aspirin. Ophthalmology 87:815, 1980

124. Miller D: Systemic medications. Int Ophthalmol Clin 21:177, 1981

125. Jaanus SD, Bartlett JD, Hiett JA: Ocular effects of systemic drugs. p. 957. In Bartlett JD, Jaanus SD (eds): Clinical Ocular Pharmacology. 3rd ed. Butterworth–Heinemann, Boston, 1995

23

Contact Lenses for Cosmetic Disfigurement

Michael R. Spinell

Cosmetic is a term that has been defined as "correcting physical defects" or "decorative or superficial rather than functional." Historically, in the context of contact lenses, this word has referred to the routine fitting of a contact lens to improve vision without the use of spectacles. Years ago, when the wearing of spectacles was considered less than desirable, contact lenses were promoted to improve the cosmetic appearance of an individual. Therefore, over the years, the word *cosmetic* has come to refer to routine lens fitting. In fact, the term is used by insurance companies to describe the standard contact lens services and remuneration associated with a particular vision plan. The term *medical necessity* was then introduced to differentiate situations in which it was felt that an individual could benefit from wearing contact lenses for noncosmetic purposes. This includes such conditions as aphakia, irregular astigmatism, keratoconus, and postoperative corrections.

Another important reason for wearing contact lenses actually makes the current use of the term *cosmetic* seem inappropriate or, at least, ill defined. For example, many people can use various types of specialty contact lenses to improve their cosmetic appearance but in an entirely different context. This includes individuals with physical defects, either congenital or acquired, as may occur from trauma or accidents, or as the result of a pathologic or degenerative process. These patients have a true cosmetic need or desire to wear contact lenses because their problem or deformity cannot be resolved by wearing spectacles. In some instances, vision can be improved simultaneously, although this may not always be the primary objective.

Frequently, busy health care practitioners start to take their own abilities and contributions for granted. They may forget the influence they have on the quality of life experienced by others. This can range from refracting

patients to enable them to see efficiently at distance or near to removing cataracts to enable people to see dramatically better. An extension of this type of contribution occurs when the clinician begins to work with people who have some form of cosmetic disfigurement. It does not take very long to comprehend their sensitivity about their problems, and it is a blessing to be able to help these people and share in their success and happiness.

The circumstances involving such patients often vary so widely that it is important for the practitioner to obtain and assess baseline information before deciding on a course of action. In the next four sections of this chapter are questions that should be asked in the hope of eliminating any future misunderstandings.

WHAT IS THE EXACT PROBLEM THE PATIENT WANTS TO IMPROVE?

Some patients have multiple problems but may be interested in correcting only one of them. An example of this might be a patient who has a very noticeable corneal scar covering one pupil, which creates a cosmetic and a vision problem. The patient may realize that vision in that eye will never be useful, so the primary motivation for seeking help is to correct the cosmetic defect. Other patients with multiple problems may believe that correcting one problem automatically makes the others improve or disappear. An example of this might be a patient with leukocoria who has lost all ability for that eye to fixate on the same target as the fellow eye, and a very noticeable tropia may also be present. These patients may believe, naively, that covering up the white pupil also makes the eye appear straight. In actuality, tropias can sometimes be camouflaged by using special prism-ballasted cosmetic lenses with decentered irides and pupils.[1] This requires caution, however, because in some cases it may sacrifice some degree of peripheral or central vision.

Some patients may also be extremely sensitive to something that others may even find amusing or an attribute that can become the topic of many interesting conversations. Examples of this include patients with heterochromia. Some patients are extremely upset by the fact that their eyes are noticeably different in color or that one eye has some form of a sectoral heterochromia in which only a single area appears different. The practitioner should make a careful assessment of the patient's goals, address these concerns, and evaluate what is feasible and realistic. The patient's primary goal may be to eliminate the heterochromic appearance, even though this may be a minor issue from the practitioner's standpoint. Yet, addressing this patient concern may make the difference between a lens that is used regularly and one that is rarely worn.

Sometimes, a patient may have multiple problems in which vision and cosmesis are involved. It may be possible in some instances to improve both problems simultaneously. An example of this is a person who has had some form of ocular trauma that resulted in a corectopia and dislocated crystalline lens. The use of a special iris-imagery lens that forms a more natural pupil and simultaneously corrects the refractive error improves cosmesis and acuity. The important thing is to ensure that the patient has reasonable expectations because some internal ocular damage may also have occurred to make pretrauma acuity levels impossible to achieve.

WHAT ARE THE PATIENT'S EXPECTATIONS?

It is helpful for the practitioner to know exactly what expectations the patient has for correcting the problem. Some patients believe that because they have taken the initiative to seek help from someone with experience with their type of problem, complete resolution and restoration will occur. Others are more than grateful if any type of cosmetic or vision improvement takes place. After careful assessment of the problem, the practitioner should present the options honestly, with a sense of optimism but not losing sight of what is realistic and practical. Never promise something that may be difficult to achieve.

WHAT EXPECTATIONS DO PEOPLE WHO ARE CLOSE TO THE PATIENT HAVE?

At times, a patient's relatives or close friends may influence the patient's perceptions about what can be done and what the results will be. It is therefore wise to have some-

one close to the patient present during the consultation so that a better understanding of the situation can be achieved. This may later help to reinforce the points that were discussed. During a consultation visit, a great deal of testing and conversation may take place. Under these circumstances, it is very easy to understand how an apprehensive and hopeful patient may forget or confuse something that was said. It is also advisable to keep detailed records that fully document what was discussed.

WHAT MODALITIES ARE AVAILABLE TO ADDRESS THE PATIENT'S PROBLEM?

Once the patient's problem has been identified, the practitioner must decide on a course of action that can improve or resolve it. It is helpful to have thorough knowledge of the various lens designs available. It is also helpful to be imaginative and to discuss the patient's particular needs with some of the laboratories that fabricate these unique lenses.

Practitioners should understand that many people do not fully appreciate just how specialized some of these lenses are. Consequently, it is highly recommended that every effort be made to inform the patient about anticipated costs, lens fabrication time, and the number of office visits that may be necessary. Patients may have to travel great distances to see a practitioner who offers these specialized services. Therefore, it is helpful to learn as much as possible about a patient's problem before the actual consultation, thus increasing efficiency. Sometimes, taking a case history over the phone, consulting with a colleague who has previously seen the patient, and evaluating photographs that illustrate the exact problem can save a great deal of time. This preliminary evaluation may also provide the opportunity to discuss lens design options with various fabricating laboratories before the patient's fitting visit.

Many types of ocular problems can be helped with the use of standard or *stock* lenses in addition to special custom-designed lenses. Sometimes, nothing more than a little ingenuity is necessary to address such situations. For example, better results can be obtained in monocular situations when two stock lenses are used instead of one very expensive custom lens.

GENERAL COMMENTS ON LENS PERFORMANCE

Regardless of the type of lens design being considered, certain basic criteria must be met in evaluating the performance of the lens on the eye. These include evaluation of lens movement, position, comfort, vision when applicable, and postwear health of the eye. The practitioner must address each factor from the perspective that there may be features that distinguish them from the criteria used for healthy eyes.

Lens Movement

Any lens placed on an eye must demonstrate some amount of movement. This is necessary to avoid limbal compression, which in itself creates physiologic problems (from post-lens tear debris that may become trapped behind the lens and from poor circulation). However, in fitting cosmetic lenses, it is important that the lenses move minimally so that the cosmetic effect does not look unnatural.

Lens Position

Lenses must position centrally to maintain a natural appearance. If an opaque cosmetic lens is decentered or changes position, the cosmetic effect is compromised.

Lens Comfort

As with any lens, it is important that the patient experiences an acceptable level of comfort. If, for some reason, a lens is not comfortable, the practitioner must rapidly determine the cause of the problem. Reasons for lens discomfort may include the following:

- The lens is ripped.
- The lens is inside out.
- Dirt or tear debris is trapped behind the lens.
- The surface of the lens is dirty.
- The eye is dry or irritated.
- The lens is too loose and moving excessively.
- Edge standoff is occurring.
- The lens has been inaccurately manufactured.

Vision

It is necessary to determine whether an eye being fitted with a cosmetic lens has useful vision. If vision is to be corrected, it is important that the fabricating laboratory does nothing to encourage further loss of vision by providing a lens with good cosmetic effect but inferior optics. It should also be noted that an eye may have a significant refractive error but still be amblyopic under the best of conditions. Sometimes, including prescriptive power in the contact lens improves the overall quality of vision, even though the actual Snellen acuity may not have changed.

Postwear Health

As with any contact lens placed on an eye, it is imperative that these special types of lenses do not cause adverse physiologic changes to the ocular tissues. Some of these lenses may be manufactured with thicknesses that do not permit as much oxygen to permeate the lens matrix as is required for proper corneal physiology. It is important, therefore, to carefully monitor postwear health to ensure that complications are not overlooked. This can sometimes happen with nonseeing eyes when the practitioner focuses attention primarily on the cosmetic aspect of the evaluation. Consequently, routine postwear biomicroscopy with sodium fluorescein should be done. Often, an eye that is being fitted already has some pre-existing problems, such as neovascularization, scarring, or epithelial staining. It becomes a matter of professional judgment as to just how much staining or vascularization is acceptable. This decision can be influenced by the amount of staining or vascularization routinely present before a lens has been worn, if the eye in question is a seeing or nonseeing eye, and if the patient is experiencing any discomfort. It is always a good idea to review with patients the well-known triad popularized by Dr. Stanley Yamane: If the eye doesn't "feel good, look good, or see good," the patient should take the lens out and call his or her practitioner.

Perhaps the best way to illustrate the various ocular problems and their solution is to start at the anterior segment of the eye and then systematically work backward. Representative case histories in the well-known subjective, objective, assessment, plan (SOAP) system are used along with color photographs. Keep in mind that the exact method used in each example is often based on whether the affected eye or eyes have absolutely no vision (not even light perception) or whether some degree of useful vision remains.

CORNEA

Corneal Scarring

Severity
Many victims of trauma or disease processes develop various degrees of corneal scarring. Minor scars can often be ignored because they are difficult to see and, unless they are located in the immediate vicinity of the visual axis, do not usually interfere with vision. In many instances, however, a very noticeable scar may be present, making the patient very self-conscious. It is not unusual to find

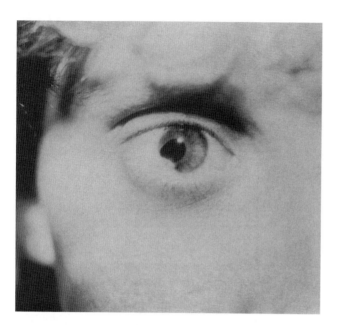

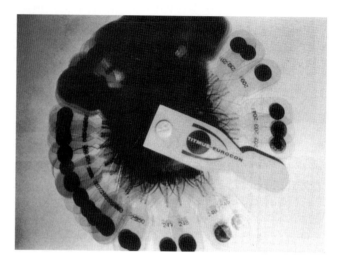

FIG. 23-2. *Color template wheel for iris matching.*

FIG. 23-1. *An inferotemporal scar out of the line of sight. The scar and the irregular pupil are noticeable.*

these patients wearing sunglasses or even a hat pulled down slightly over their eyes to hide the deformity.

Location
The exact location of the scar is important because the practitioner must know whether the scar must be masked by an opaque lens with a clear pupil (functional vision assumed) or one with the pupil blocked (no useful vision) (Fig. 23-1).

Iris Color and Iris Architecture
It is important to consider the color of the iris because the iris acts as a backdrop for the corneal scar. Some scars can be adequately hidden simply by using basic transparent tinted lenses that are actually designed to enhance or modify eye color in healthy eyes. This is sometimes possible when a patient has a blue iris and the scarring is not severe. However, when the iris is brown or the scarring is more prominent, the necessity for some type of opaque lens becomes much more probable.

One should also consider the details of iris appearance when deciding what type of lens to use. It is helpful to take high-quality color photographs of the healthy eye and send them to the fabricating laboratory to provide a good idea of the iris details desired. The color of the iris in the photograph should be compared with the true iris color because color photographs are not always accurate. Some practitioners send the laboratory a sample of a colored template that is used to determine the required lens color (Fig. 23-2). Other practitioners use old prosthetic eyes for this type of comparison (Fig. 23-3). From expe-

rience, it becomes obvious that light irides, such as blue and hazel green, require more accurate color matches than do brown irides, especially dark ones.

Pupil Size
Pupil size should be matched as accurately as possible. This measurement varies from patient to patient and within the same patient owing to effects of illumination. Therefore, the possibility that the specialized lens may create an appearance of anisocoria must be considered. It may be advisable to use a pupil size that is something of a compromise rather than have it appear perfect only some of the time. Again, this measurement becomes less critical when brown irides are involved because, in these eyes, it is often difficult to see the pupils.

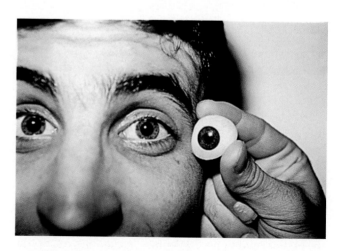

FIG. 23-3. *Old artificial eyes make excellent templates to use for matching iris color and architecture of the healthy eye.*

GRAND ROUNDS CASE REPORT 1

Subjective:
A 41-year-old accountant had had a serious ocular injury to the right eye in an automobile accident 7 years earlier. Eventually, retinal detachment occurred, requiring surgery in which a scleral buckle was used in an attempt to save some vision. Further complications developed, resulting in severe corneal scarring and loss of vision (Fig. 23-4). The patient was interested in being fitted with a lens that would hide the obvious scarring and improve her appearance.

Objective:
The healthy eye had a 5-mm pupil in room illumination. The iris was dark brown. Because of this, pupillary size was taken using the Burton lamp and a pupil template. The ultraviolet light made the pupils appear purple so that the pupillary size could be more accurately measured. Realistically, this measurement was not very critical because the extremely dark irides would mask any anisocoria, but pupillary size was necessary for fabrication. It was a nonseeing eye, so no correction for refractive error was involved. An attempt to take a keratometric reading to obtain some idea of the corneal contour resulted in a deceptive reading, showing 8 D of astigmatism. In actuality, the reading was taken over part of the corneal scar, so little pertinent information was really gained. The patient had a visible iris diameter of 11 mm.

Several commonly used spheric soft lenses were used to help determine what overall lens diameter could be used and whether lenses were able to center properly and move adequately. In this case, it was not difficult to get good positioning and movement with the lenses tried.

Assessment and Plan:
The patient's information was sent to the Narcissus Foundation (now part of the new Wesley-Jessen Special Eyes Foundation), which would be making the actual lens. A sample artificial eye was enclosed to act as a template for matching the iris color. Several weeks later, a preliminary lens arrived. This lens was entirely opaque white (Fig. 23-5). If it positioned and moved properly, it would be sent back to have the iris architecture imprinted on it. Consequently, a lens with a base curve of 8.0 mm and a diameter of 14 mm was used. A dark-brown 11-mm iris was imprinted on the lens along with a 5-mm black pupil. The 1.5-mm annular area located peripherally around the lens would be opaque white, which would blend nicely with the patient's own sclera (Fig. 23-6).

Several weeks after the opaque white lens was returned to the manufacturer, the final lens arrived (Fig. 23-7). This lens nicely covered the underlying scarred area. Lens movement was minimal but sufficient to avoid compressing the underlying tissues. The patient was educated in the overall care of the lens as well as placement and removal techniques and given a conventional wearing schedule. She was cautioned to watch for any unusual redness or lens awareness and remove the lens and call us if any such sign or symptom did occur. At a 1-week check-up visit, corneal physiology would be evaluated.

Arcus Senilis or Arcus Juvenilis

A common corneal problem that can frequently be improved with the use of contact lenses is arcus senilis, correctly termed *arcus juvenilis* when it occurs in a younger population. Basically, this involves the deposition of lipids in the periphery of the cornea. In patients younger than age 40 years, systemic conditions, such as hypercholesterolemia or hyperlipidemia, should be investigated. It is considered a normal age-related change in older patients. Although many consider this particular cosmetic prob-lem minor, it is still considered a cosmetic detraction. Sometimes, it is possible to fit these patients with stock tinted lenses (a yellow-amber or light green transparent tint often works best) that are actually designed to enhance iris color and not to hide corneal opacities (Figs. 23-8 and 23-9). It should be kept in mind that enhancing eye color too much sometimes actually draws attention to the eyes, when the initial intent was to take attention away from the eyes by camouflaging the problem. An example of this might be the wearing of an aqua or turquoise lens on a

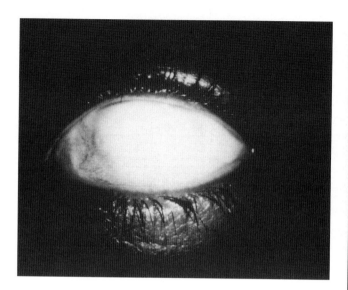

FIG. 23-4. *Grand Rounds Case Report 1 patient. Note heavily scarred cornea.*

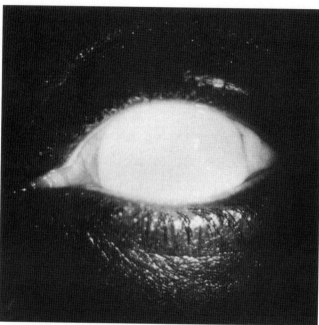

FIG. 23-5. *Grand Rounds Case Report 1 patient wearing an opaque white Narcissus (Wesley-Jessen, Des Plaines, IL) lens before iris color imprinting.*

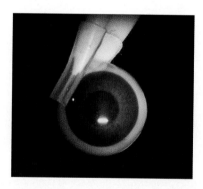

FIG. 23-6. *The finished Narcissus lens (Wesley-Jessen, Des Plaines, IL) with iris imprint in Grand Rounds Case Report 1.*

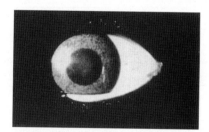

FIG. 23-7. *Grand Rounds Case Report 1 patient wearing the finished Narcissus lens (Wesley-Jessen, Des Plaines, IL).*

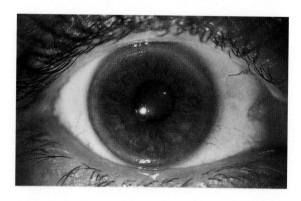

FIG. 23-8. *Arcus senilis. (Courtesy of CIBA Vision, Duluth, GA.)*

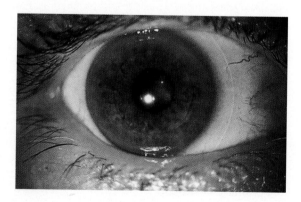

FIG. 23-9. *Same eye as in Fig. 23-8 with amber transparent tinted lens, reducing the prominent arcus. (Courtesy of CIBA Vision, Duluth, GA.)*

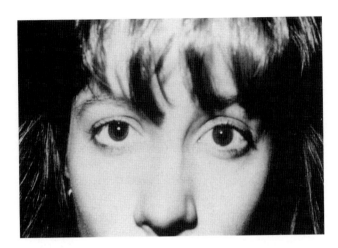

FIG. 23-10. *A "flat" brown opaque lens (no iris detail) worn on the left eye.*

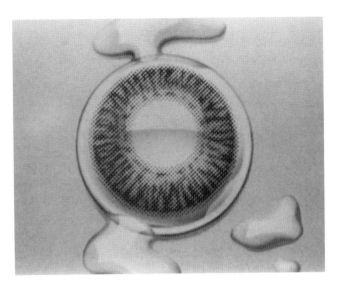

FIG. 23-11. *The Wesley-Jessen opaque lens design with a clear pupil and a 12.5-mm colored dot-matrix pattern. The pattern can be double printed for greater density. (Courtesy of Wesley-Jessen Corp., Des Plaines, IL.)*

light-colored iris. This combination frequently results in a cosmetic effect that some people may find flattering, but others may find shocking.

IRIS AND PUPIL

Even though separate problems are associated with the iris and pupil, they are discussed together because they are intimately related.

Heterochromia

Perhaps one of the most interesting cosmetic problems involves various forms of heterochromia. In some cases, the entire iris color of one eye may differ from the iris color of the fellow eye. In others, a segment of one iris may differ in color from the rest of the iris and from the iris color of the fellow eye. This is sometimes referred to as *sectoral heterochromia* because a sector of the iris is involved. For some patients, this unique abnormality can become an interesting conversation item. For others, it may be viewed as an undesirable distraction. These people often ask their eye-care practitioners if anything can be done. Historically, the answer has been yes, but the solution was frequently more expensive than desired. Special custom-made cosmetic lenses, complete with realistic irides imprinted on them, were required. These lenses are similar to the ones described in Grand Rounds Case Report 1. New options have become available that, in many cases, make the solution more economical. For example, any conventional opaque tinted lenses can now be considered. These lenses are available in two general designs. Some have opaque colors that change the underlying iris color

but are "flat" and, therefore, do not appear as realistic as some people would like (Fig. 23-10). These lenses can be obtained from a number of companies, including Adventure in Color in Colorado, White Ophthalmics in Canada, Alden Contact Lenses in New York, Crystal Reflections in Arizona, and Specialty Tint in California. Others have unique iris-colored prints designed to give a more realistic appearance. Depending on how one wishes to categorize things, six lens designs that can alter the appearance of the iris are available.

Wesley-Jessen Opaque Lens Design (Durasoft Colors)

The Wesley-Jessen (Des Plaines, IL) opaque lens design was the first commercially available lens for changing eye color that could be referred to as a *stock* lens because it was inventoried and readily available. It works on the principle of an opaque dot-matrix pattern, coloring areas of the underlying iris with transparent spaces interspersed and helping to give the illusion of depth. The opaque pattern is applied to the outer surface of the lens (Fig. 23-11). A great deal of research went into the final design so that a proper proportion of spaces and dots was used to achieve the color change. For example, many irides display a spokelike pattern and have variable intensities of color along their different axes. Therefore, the exact color change achieved is a function of the lens color and the patient's own underlying iris color and architecture. It is thus possible that the same color of lens worn by one brown-eyed person may look different on another brown-eyed per-

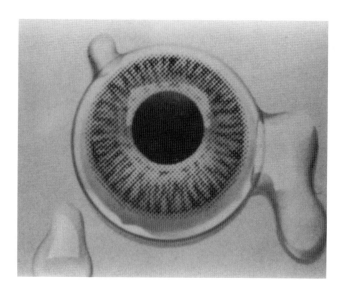

FIG. 23-12. *The Wesley-Jessen pupillary block lens. The pupil zone is opaque black. An overlay of any opaque color, single or double printed, is available. (Courtesy of Wesley-Jessen Corp., Des Plaines, IL.)*

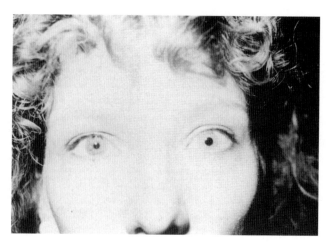

FIG. 23-13. *A Wesley-Jessen prosthetic lens with blue overlay worn on a blue iris.*

son. A modification of this design has been introduced and is referred to as the *Complements* series. It differs from the original design in that a different pattern of opaque dots in a complementary color is placed around the pupillary area, thus creating a more natural transition between the new iris color, the underlying iris color, and the black pupil.

An extension of this type of opaque lens technology has taken place. Based on the theory that the natural color of the eye is often a blend of several different shades of color, a colorblend pattern was developed. In this technology, three colors are blended on each lens, thereby creating an appearance that is supposed to be more natural. The use of this lens design for cosmetic disfigurements seems quite possible. It could be used on only one eye to match the fellow eye or on both eyes in the hope of creating an excellent binocular match while using less expensive stock lenses.

Wesley-Jessen Prosthetic Lens

The Wesley-Jessen prosthetic lens is a special series of custom-made lenses made available to the ophthalmic professions that encompasses several types of tinting for prosthetic cases. The availability of these designs in a hydrogel material has helped many patients with more severe deformities with lenses that are comfortable to wear. The practitioner and the patient should be aware that fabrication time can take 3–8 weeks, depending on the type of lens. The simplest lens in this set is a basic pupillary block lens,[2] which can be made with 3- to 8-mm opaque black pupils (Fig. 23-12). The

single print design is essentially the same lens as the regular Wesley-Jessen opaque lens, but it can have an opaque black pupil added if desired (Fig. 23-13). A double iris print lens is also available. This design uses twice the amount of ink as the regular opaque lens and, therefore, has a denser dot-matrix pattern, providing a greater amount of masking. Various iris colors can be imprinted over it. The final lens design available in this set is the most opaque lens and is referred to as the *underprinted iris lens.* The black or light meshline underprintings can have various iris colors, including the new colorblends imprinted over them. The lens is available with either clear or occluder black pupils that can be from 3.0 to 5.0 mm in diameter. It is more appropriate for corneas that have dense scars or for eyes with aniridia (Fig. 23-14).

The CIBA ILLUSIONS Lens

The CIBA ILLUSIONS (Duluth, GA) lens uses a slightly different approach to changing eye color. It was thought that a better three-dimensional effect could be achieved by placing the opaque material deeper into the lens matrix instead of on the front surface of the lens. Therefore, an opaque white iris pattern incorporating a unique reflective pigment is embedded within the lens matrix and is covered by a transparent tint on the front surface. The transparent tint is basically the same process that is used on the front surfaces of CIBA Softcolor lenses. Thus, a combined effect of color masking and color mixing exists. Special attention was also given to the iris pattern to simulate the crypts, striations, and pupillary frill. The final colors now available were determined by adjusting the mixture of opaque and transparent pigments until popular colors were achieved.

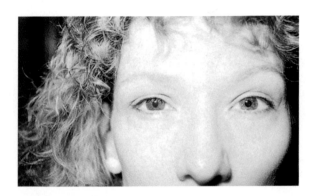

FIG. 23-14. *A Wesley-Jessen underprinted chestnut brown lens with a clear pupil. This lens is effective for aniridia or for hiding dense scars.*

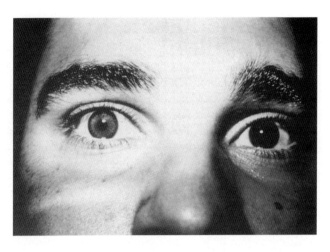

FIG. 23-15. *A blue opaque Narcissus lens (Wesley-Jessen, Des Plaines, IL) used over a brown iris.*

Cooper Vision Natural Touch Lens

The Cooper Vision *Natural Touch* (Fairport, NY) lens is another type of stock opaque cosmetic lens. Like the lenses described in the CIBA ILLUSIONS, this lens can be used to provide a color change for healthy eyes and for special cosmetic problems. It differs in appearance from the other lens designs in that it has a dark peripheral ring that is said to give the lens a more natural appearance, resembling the peripheral iris and limbal area more accurately. A unique aspect of this lens is that during fabrication, the color of the lens is blended with the polymer during the actual molding process.

Narcissus Lens Designs

Narcissus lens designs (Wesley-Jessen, Des Plaines, IL) come in translucent and opaque imprinted forms. The translucent tinted lens modifies the color of light irides and is available with power, so it can be used on seeing eyes. The opaque imprinted lens is very useful on nonseeing eyes because it can be manufactured to mask an injury and to closely match

the appearance of the fellow eye. It is not available with corrective powers and, therefore, cannot be used on seeing eyes (Fig. 23-15). These lenses have been discontinued as of August 1999.

Iris Colobomas

Another abnormality of the iris occurs when a portion of the iris is missing or damaged. This can result from a congenital defect, surgery, or injury, disease, or a degenerative process.[3] Early methods of cataract surgery also produced a coloboma of the iris, usually positioned at approximately 12 o'clock. Although this form of surgery is now seldom, if ever, performed, many patients are still alive today who display this form of coloboma. The flaccid superior lid often droops down over this area, so glare may become a lesser problem than was first anticipated.

GRAND ROUNDS CASE REPORT 2

Subjective:
A 35-year-old woman was seen for a contact lens examination. Her history was unremarkable except that she had worn soft daily-wear lenses for approximately 13 years. Her present lenses were approximately 2 years old and were not providing the comfort and vision she desired.

Objective:
The patient had low-grade compound myopic astigmatism. Biomicroscopy revealed no abnormal findings. The only unusual observation was that her right eye was heterochromatic, showing a section of the iris that was different in color from the remainder of the iris and the entire iris of the fellow eye (Fig. 23-16). It was not until a

casual comment was made about it that the patient volunteered that she was somewhat annoyed by this situation. She knew that lenses were available to correct this condition but assumed that they were expensive. She was then informed about an innovation in contact lenses that enabled brown eyes to be changed to another color without the use of expensive custom lenses. Because diagnostic fitting lenses were available, it would be relatively easy to see if the desired effect could be obtained. The lens to be used was the Wesley-Jessen Durasoft Colors (Des Plaines, IL) opaque lens. The immediate question that had to be answered clinically was whether this lens with its dot-matrix design would provide a uniform color over all areas of the iris. In theory, this lens could change the eye color but in a manner that might not eliminate the color differences, thereby possibly providing only another form of heterochromia. Opaque blue lenses were consequently tried at the patient's request.

Assessment:
After adaptation, the lenses moved adequately, positioned centrally, were comfortable, and provided good, consistent vision. In this case, the additional evaluation of eye color also was favorable because both eyes appeared uniformly blue. A close biomicroscopic view revealed a difference in underlying iris color, but this was not apparent to the naked eye (Fig. 23-17). This is an important point to remember. Viewing some of these lenses under extremely bright illumination or high magnification may reveal minor differences that are not visible to the naked eye.

Plan:
Because of the favorable results, lenses in the proper power were ordered, dispensed, and subsequently evaluated. This case illustrates how an economical solution was found for a patient with an interesting form of heterochromia.

Regardless of the exact etiology, the end result is the same. Because more light enters the eye than desired, loss of visual clarity and visual efficiency exists. These patients are usually bothered by glare and have difficulty with certain visual tasks that require good resolution.

Several lens designs can be used to improve this condition. The design chosen is often based on the location of the coloboma, its size, and the color of the healthy iris.[4] The darker the iris, the more options exist and the less perfect in match the colored lens must be. This is true because it is frequently difficult to see a black pupil adjacent to a dark brown iris even under good illumination.

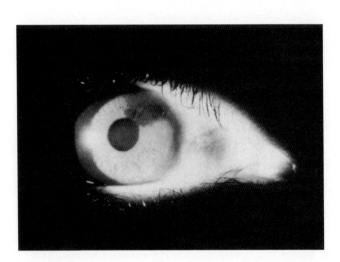

FIG. 23-16. *Grand Rounds Case Report 2 patient with sectoral heterochromia of the iris.*

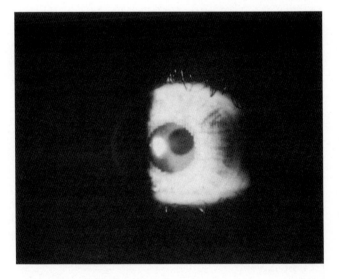

FIG. 23-17. *Grand Rounds Case Report 2 patient wearing a standard Wesley-Jessen opaque blue lens to hide the heterochromia and to change iris color.*

GRAND ROUNDS CASE REPORT 3

Subjective:
A 35-year-old nurse made an appointment to be fitted with a special contact lens that she knew would reduce some of the glare that she was experiencing. She had had a severe injury to her right eye 30 years earlier when a lawnmower propelled a rock into her eye. The eye eventually developed glaucoma and a cataract that had been removed 3 years before this appointment. Other internal ocular problems developed that resulted in retinal detachment and subsequent loss of vision. The end result was a scarred eye with a coloboma, causing glare and an unappealing cosmetic appearance. She had previously been fitted with a lens to improve the cosmesis, but that lens was now old and had even ripped. At the time of this appointment, patient was still taking timolol maleate ophthalmic solution (Timoptic) 0.5% twice a day and pilocarpine 1% four times a day in this eye (Fig. 23-18).

Objective:
Refractively, the patient had no useful vision in this eye. Keratometry showed a flat meridian reading of 37.00 D that was distorted because it was measured over part of the scar. She now had a microcornea in this eye, which measured 9 mm in diameter, in contrast to her other cornea, which measured 11 mm in diameter. Her pupil in the healthy eye was 4 mm in room illumination. A traumatic iris coloboma was also present.

The patient was advised of several options available at that time. Because cost was important, it was decided to use a soft lens with a 14-mm diameter and an 11-mm diameter opaque chocolate-brown annulus containing no clear pupillary area. Based on a routine diagnostic lens-fitting procedure, the lens used had a base curve of 8.7 mm and plano power. The diameter of the opaque area was important in this case because the appearance of the right eye needed to be enlarged so that it matched the size of the healthy left eye (Fig. 23-19).

Assessment:
Several weeks after the lens was ordered, it was placed on the affected eye, given time to equilibrate, and then evaluated. The lens positioned centrally and moved sufficiently so that no peripheral binding was present. Equally important, the ghost imagery and glare previously present were now absent. Cosmetically, the lens looked very natural because of the dark-brown iris. Subsequent visits confirmed that this relatively simple lens design had reduced the glare, improved cosmesis, and provided a good physiologic response.

Plan:
Routine check-up visits were to be scheduled. The patient was also informed that because soft lenses have a certain life expectancy, good hygiene must be practiced so that replacement lenses would not have to be ordered sooner than necessary.

Options for Coloboma

The simplest form of lens design to cover a coloboma is a soft lens with a doughnut-shaped opaque black or brown ring surrounding the pupillary area. The size of the ring can vary depending on the exact location of the coloboma but is often approximately 10–12 mm in diameter. Similarly, the pupil can vary in size, depending on the size of the pupil of the other eye and the required width of the opaque ring. Although quite suitable for patients with dark brown irides, this specific type of lens is definitely not recommended for patients with light iris color because the cosmetic effect is so poor. These patients are much better cared for with one of the more sophisticated lens types.

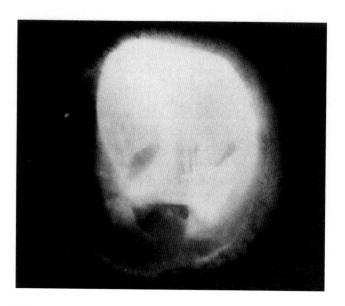

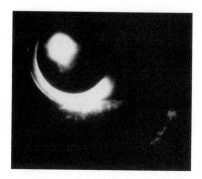

FIG. 23-19. *Grand Rounds Case Report 3 patient wearing a White Ophthalmic Design B (Calgary, Alberta, Canada) opaque chocolate brown lens.*

FIG. 23-18. *Grand Rounds Case Report 3 patient. Note severe scarring, traumatic coloboma, and vascularization.*

GRAND ROUNDS CASE REPORT 4

Subjective:
A patient was seen for a special contact lens consultation after experiencing trauma to his left eye in a tennis accident. The injury left him with a subluxated lens and a displaced pupil, resulting in poor acuity and annoying glare (Fig. 23-20).

Objective:
The refractive error in the left eye was $+10.00$ D, which gave him $^{20}\!/_{40}{}^-$ acuity. It was thought that this might improve even more if the glare could be reduced. The astigmatic component in his prescription could be placed in a spectacle overcorrection that would also incorporate the necessary add for near vision. Because of the light brown color of the irides and the superior location of his pupil, it was thought that the best lens design would be an artificial iris-imagery annulus lens incorporating a clear pupillary area. If this lens positioned properly, it was hoped that the superior portion of the new pupil would coincide with the inferior portion of the displaced pupil sufficiently to allow light rays in the visual axis to reach the macula and maximize acuity. Proper power would be supplied by the combination of the soft lens power and the spectacle overcorrection. The horizontal visible iris diameter, pupillary size, and iris color and appearance were assessed and information furnished to the fabricating laboratory (Fig. 23-21).

Assessment:
The initial lens was placed on the eye and allowed to equilibrate. It was comfortable and positioned reasonably well. The displaced pupil was covered by the opaque annulus, resulting in an immediate decrease in glare. Vision also improved. An overcorrection would improve this even more. Cosmetically, the lens was an improvement. A further modification in design would be required to make things even more realistic because correction for the arcus senilis present in both eyes was not initially incorporated into the lens, resulting in a less-than-perfect match. It should also be mentioned that the picture presented here actually looks worse than the naked-eye view

because the camera and lens used make it look as though the underlying iris is easily visible behind the printed iris on the contact lens. This was not the case (Fig. 23-22).

Plan:
A final lens was ordered that incorporated the suggestions. A modified back vertex power was ordered, incorporating the results of the diagnostic lens over-refraction.

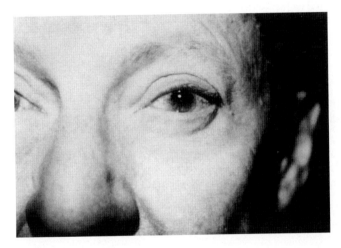

FIG. 23-20. *Subluxated lens and displaced pupil secondary to a tennis injury (Grand Rounds Case Report 4).*

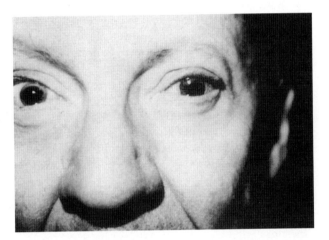

FIG. 23-22. *Grand Rounds Case Report 4 patient wearing iris-imagery lens. Note arcus senilis present in the healthy eye, not yet matched in the prosthetic lens.*

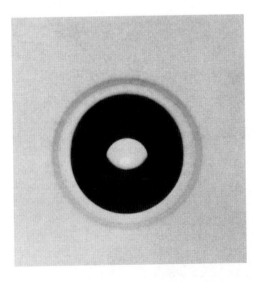

FIG. 23-21. *Iris-imagery annulus lens (Grand Rounds Case Report 4).*

GRAND ROUNDS CASE REPORT 5

A slight variation on the problem in Grand Rounds Case Report 4 illustrates the use of another type of lens design, a prism-ballasted opaque annulus lens with decentered pupil.

Subjective:

A 41-year-old man experienced a traumatic injury to his left eye in 1963 from a pencil point. Eventually, his crystalline lens had to be removed, and iris atrophy subsequently developed. He was experiencing monocular diplopia from the polycoria (Figs. 23-23 and 23-24).

Objective:

After an initial assessment with a diagnostic lens, it was decided to try an opaque prism-ballasted aphakic lens with a 3-mm decentered clear pupil to match the location of the patient's own pupil. Two and one-half prism diopters of base-down prism was also used to help keep the lens in the proper position. The iris diameter was 10.5 mm, and a photographic slide was sent to the laboratory (Narcissus Foundation) to try to match the dark-brown iris color.

Assessment:

This lens did not prove satisfactory for dispensing but became an excellent diagnostic lens to use for the final ordered lens. This lens positioned inferiorly and temporally. A water-insoluble marking pen was used to dot the position of the new pupil to more accurately describe its location. Consequently, the new lens was to have the pupil now located 2 mm superiorly and nasally from its previous position. An over-refraction was also done to refine the final lens power.

The second lens ordered had a base curve of 8.6 mm, an overall diameter of 15 mm, a back vertex power (BVP) of +11.25 D, and 2.5 D of base-down prism. The opaque brown annulus was 10.5 mm in diameter and had a 3-mm clear pupil. The entire annulus was decentered superiorly and nasally so that when it was placed on the eye, the clear pupil would align with the patient's own displaced pupil. This lens moved approximately 0.5–1.0 mm and provided ²⁰⁄₅₀ acuity, which was quite acceptable considering the condition of the eye (Fig. 23-25).

Plan:

The lens was dispensed and routine check-up visits were scheduled. The patient was cautioned about properly caring for this lens owing to the lengthy fabrication time for replacement lenses.

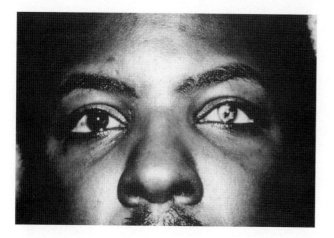

FIG. 23-23. *Frontal view of Grand Rounds Case Report 5 patient, showing the scarred and atrophic iris in the left eye.*

Aniridia

An extreme form of iris or pupil problem occurs in aniridia, a significant absence of iris tissue (Fig. 23-26). These cases are usually congenital, although other causes, such as trauma or disease, are possible. The congenital form of this condition is usually accompanied by lens opacities, macular hypoplasia, and a predisposition to glaucoma. Vision is frequently poor or at least reduced, and a searching type of nystagmus may be present. The afflicted individual is bothered greatly by glare and ghostlike images and sometimes reports a form of diplopia caused by some of the light entering the eye being deviated by the lens opacities. Lenses incorporating artificial irides and clear pupils can be very advantageous in reducing the glare, in correcting any ametropia that might be present, and in improving cosmesis. The result is an individual who looks

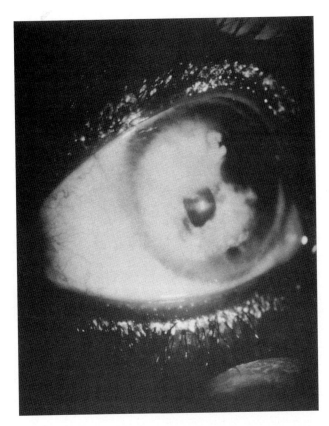

FIG. 23-24. *Magnified view (stereo) of Grand Rounds Case Report 5 patient, demonstrating polycoria.*

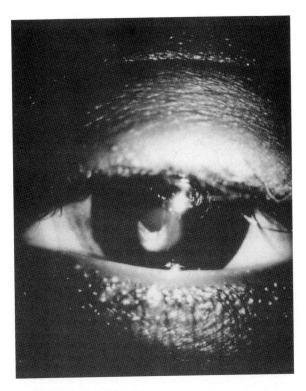

FIG. 23-25. *Grand Rounds Case Report 5 patient with prism-ballasted opaque annulus lens using a decentered pupillary zone.*

better, sees better, and feels better. Many years ago, the only lens design available for these patients was a special custom-made lens incorporating an artificial iris image with a clear pupil. Other lens designs have since become available that provide alternatives that may be more affordable and may give satisfactory results. These include the opaque black or brown annulus with clear pupil and a stock opaque lens with iris images, available through a number of manufacturers.

Leukocoria

Occasionally, a patient presents with a problem involving the crystalline lens of the eye, an intraocular tumor, or other etiology creating a noticeable leukocoria (white pupil). In the case of dense cataract, these eyes usually have very poor vision and often have other internal problems that make routine cataract surgery and intraocular lens implantation ill advised. Laser interferometry as well as A and B scan ultrasound can provide useful information in confirming a prognosis for surgery. It is also possible that surgery may improve vision but that the patient's

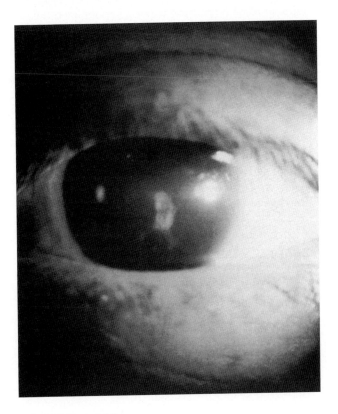

FIG. 23-26. *Aniridia.*

general health is so poor that it is not recommended. Occasionally, a patient refuses surgery because of religious beliefs, lack of information, fear of anesthesia, or simply fears of surgery in general. In many cases, the appearance of the eye is dramatic because an obvious white mass is present centrally. These individuals often wear sunglasses or hats with brims to cover up their deformity.

If the situation becomes a detriment to the individual's interactions with others, a relatively simple contact lens design is advised. A soft lens with an opaque black pupil can be used to hide the underlying leukocoria. The lens is fitted in a routine manner to provide good centration and minimal movement. As previously discussed in the Iris Color and Iris Architecture section, light irides present more of a problem than dark-brown irides because the size of the opaque black pupillary area is more obvious. It is quite possible that, depending on the background illumination, anisocoria may be present and visible at different times. It is necessary to ensure that the opaque black pupil is large enough to cover the underlying white pupil and to provide some degree of tolerance for decentration because the lens may not center perfectly all the time and moves a bit during a blink or eye movement.

GRAND ROUNDS CASE REPORT 6

Subjective:

A 25-year-old student was referred for a special cosmetic contact lens evaluation. Her history revealed that she had bilateral congenital aniridia and was having trouble passing the visual acuity requirements for operating a motor vehicle, especially at night. This was an important factor in her ability to advance in her professional career.

Objective:

The patient was currently wearing spheric soft lenses that gave her $^{20}/_{40}{}^-$ acuity in the right eye and $^{20}/_{50}{}^+$ in the left eye. Despite borderline driving acuity, she was unable to remove the night driving restriction from her license. Her refraction was interesting in that she was a relatively high hyperope who, when refracted, showed a significant amount of with-the-rule cylinder, yet obtained the same objective and subjective acuity with her previous spheric soft lenses regardless of whether the cylinder was incorporated. This often occurs when amblyopes are refracted because they have not developed a keen enough ability to discriminate for incorporation of the cylinder. If necessary, an overcorrection with spectacles could be used to refine the final results. The keratometric readings were 39.25 axis 005/41.75 axis 095 and left eye 39.50 axis 005/41.25 axis 095. The refraction in the right eye was +5.75 = –4.25 cx 180, which gave $^{20}/_{40}{}^-$ acuity, and in the left eye +4.75 = –3.75 cx 015, which gave $^{20}/_{50}{}^+$ acuity. Binocular vision was still $^{20}/_{40}{}^-$. A cycloplegic refraction also showed several diopters of latent hyperopia. At the time of this initial encounter, the only designs available were the iris-imagery lenses from the Narcissus Foundation and the annulus type of lens design. However, the Wesley-Jessen opaque lens was being introduced for routine cosmetic use, designed for dramatically changing eye color. This lens design incorporates a dot matrix and uses the patient's own iris to obtain an individualized cosmetic effect.[5] The hope was to reduce the amount of light entering the eye by providing a smaller pupillary opening. Even though this could not be considered a true pinhole effect, it was hoped that the final result would be less visual confusion and a slight increase in acuity. The big question was if a lens designed to use the underlying iris would function advantageously when no iris was present. Initially, blue opaque lenses were tried but proved to be too much of a cosmetic change, but they did enable an evaluation of the optical system to see if any visual improvement would occur. Results were encouraging enough that Wesley-Jessen was eventually able to provide a special pair of brown lenses (Figs. 23-27 and 23-28).

Assessment and Plan:

The special brown opaque lenses were placed on the eyes and evaluated for movement, position, comfort, and acuity. Both lenses were plano in power so that our patient was able to use her own spectacles as an overcorrection. Cosmetically, they provided a rather nice appearance that was not too dramatic a change from her normal appearance. Equally important, vision was improved sufficiently to have the night-driving restriction removed. Because of these results, no other lens designs were tried at that time. The lenses were dispensed and subsequent follow-up visits were scheduled.

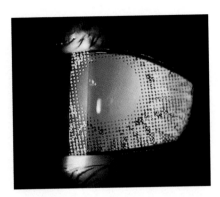

FIG. 23-27. *Retroillumination of brown opaque lenses, showing absence of underlying iris in aniridia (Grand Rounds Case Report 6).*

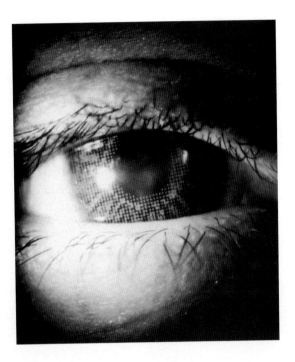

FIG. 23-28. *Grand Rounds Case Report 6 patient wearing Wesley-Jessen opaque lens for aniridia.*

GRAND ROUNDS CASE REPORT 7

Subjective:
A 16-year-old was seen for a routine examination, primarily because of a progressing cataract in his left eye that was becoming noticeable (Fig. 23-29). He had not been in this country very long and was shy and quite sensitive about his condition. He had recently been diagnosed as having an old, fully detached retina so that the prognosis for useful vision in that eye was poor. He adamantly refused to consider surgery.

Objective:
Vision in his healthy right eye was 20/20, with no significant refractive error. Vision in his left eye was barely light perception. The pupillary diameter was 5 mm in dim illumination. He had dark brown irides; therefore, this measurement was taken with the Burton lamp because the pupils appeared purple and were easy to compare against pupillary templates. The opaque black pupillary diameter of the occluder lens to be ordered would be made slightly larger to ensure adequate coverage.[6] For the patient, this would not present any real cosmetic problem because his irides were so dark that it was unlikely anyone would notice the induced anisocoria.

An Aquaflex Standard Vault II lens (Wesley-Jessen, Des Plaines, IL) was initially tried. Because of some initial tearing, this lens initially positioned too low and did not cover a portion of the patient's superior pupil. After adaptation, the situation improved slightly, but a small area of the superior pupil was still exposed, revealing the white cataract beneath (Fig. 23-30). An Aquaflex Standard Vault III lens was then tried in the hope of reducing lens movement and improving centration.

Assessment:
The Vault III lens positioned nicely, moved minimally, and because of the 6-mm opaque black pupil, completely hid the underlying leukocoria (Fig. 23-31). The patient was given the usual dispensing visit instructions on lens

handling and care and was given a conservative wearing schedule. On several follow-up visits, the lens continued to perform well and created no adverse physiologic problems. This was especially monitored around the limbus because lens movement was purposely kept minimal and a standard-thickness lens (approximately 0.15-mm center thickness) was used.

Plan:
Routine check-up visits were scheduled every 6 months, although the patient has habitually returned only when a replacement lens was required. He has continued to do well with this lens design.

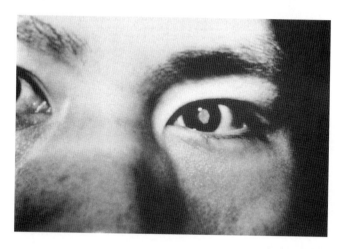

FIG. 23-29. *Grand Rounds Case Report 7 patient with leukocoria in the left eye.*

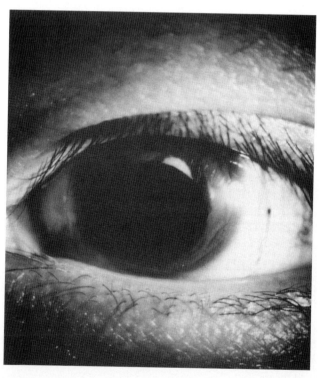

FIG. 23-30. *Grand Rounds Case Report 7 patient with slightly loose Vault II Wesley-Jessen (Des Plaines, IL) Aquaflex standard lens with pupillary block tinting.*

UNIQUE SITUATIONS

Situations exist in which the ingenuity and resourcefulness of the practitioner become important in customizing a lens design that meets the specific needs of a patient. For example, a patient who has one type of visual handicap may be helped in other ways by using a lens design that first appears to exaggerate the initial problem. This is exemplified in Grand Rounds Case Report 8, in which the lens that was dispensed reduced vision in a partially sighted individual but gave an overall improvement in visual function and efficiency.

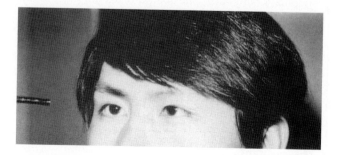

FIG. 23-31. *Grand Rounds Case Report 7 patient with the leukocoria well masked, using a Vault III Wesley-Jessen (Des Plaines, IL) Aquaflex standard lens with a 6-mm black pupil.*

GRAND ROUNDS CASE REPORT 8

Subjective:

A 25-year-old business administrator was diagnosed 10 years earlier as having Stargardt's disease. Despite poor acuity, this remarkable individual was able to earn a master's degree and successfully participate in a responsible position in the business world. Various forms of visual aids were used, including soft lenses for refractive correction. Her chief complaint was that she was experiencing unacceptable amounts of glare, especially from the lighting at work. Changing the lighting was not a practical solution and would naturally not solve the problem when it occurred at other times. The main concern was how to reduce glare sufficiently to alleviate the daily headaches she was getting, without further compromising her already reduced acuity.[7]

Objective:

Her private practitioner had determined that vision was improved when she wore lenses with –2.00 D of power, which gave her Snellen acuity of $^{10}/_{350}$. It was finally decided to try some of the opaque soft lenses currently available to see if any improvement was noted. Several different types of Wesley-Jessen opaque lenses were evaluated, including lenses from their Prosthetic Fitting Set. These special lenses incorporated double-density dot matrices and a black underlying meshwork, and offered varying pupillary diameters that were either opaque or clear. Some improvement was noted but not enough to really solve the patient's problem.

The next attempt was to evaluate regular Wesley-Jessen opaque lenses but to piggyback them with pupillary block lenses with varying amounts of light absorption values in different pupillary diameters. These lenses were supplied by Adventure in Color, Inc. (Golden, CO) (Fig. 23-32). Once again, some degree of improvement was noted. In this cumbersome arrangement of piggyback diagnostic lenses, a small area of normal pupil was always left slightly uncovered by the overlying, somewhat opaque pupillary block lens so that more light was allowed through than would later occur when both lens designs would be combined into a final, single lens.

The CIBA ILLUSIONS opaque lens (CIBA Vision, Duluth, GA) was also evaluated with the pupillary block lenses. The pupillary block lenses aligned nicely with the pupillary opening of the ILLUSIONS lens so that no extraneous light entered the eye (Fig. 23-33).

On the basis of these preliminary results, the patient had to decide whether the results seemed favorable enough to send the CIBA ILLUSIONS lenses to Adventure in Color. That firm would apply the black pupillary tint in the same absorption (approximately 75%) as the sample that she thought gave her the best overall results.

Assessment:

The modified ILLUSIONS lenses were tried and dispensed to our patient. Less glare was reported, even when her working conditions were simulated. A surprising advantage was that she did not think that she had any significant loss of vision despite her wearing an elaborate lens system that was designed to cut out light.

Plan:

A check-up visit was scheduled for approximately 1 week later. This would give the patient sufficient time to use the lenses under her normal wearing conditions and provide some time for adaptation. This unique arrangement did give the desired results and continues to be well tolerated.

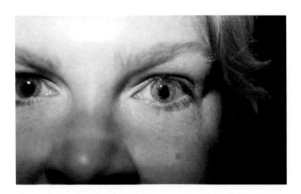

FIG. 23-32. *Grand Rounds Case Report 8 patient wearing a pupillary block lens piggybacked over a Wesley-Jessen (Des Plaines, IL) opaque lens.*

OTHER SPECIAL USES OF TINTED CONTACT LENSES

Amblyopia

The secondary advantages of contact lenses can sometimes be used to assist a patient who really had no intention of wearing a contact lens. This is illustrated by cases of amblyopia in which the traditional method of occluding or patching the good eye for some period is not acceptable to the patient. A soft contact lens with a high-plus fogging correction can be used on the healthy eye.[8] These lenses are a viable alternative because they are very comfortable to wear and can be worn on a periodic wearing schedule without any significant adaptive problems. The availability of planned replacement lenses makes them even more economically advantageous to use.

Another possibility is the opaque black pupillary block lens. This lens also serves as an occluder on the healthy eye by preventing light from reaching the retina. The end result is that the amblyopic eye is now forced to work because vision in the healthy eye is so greatly reduced. If the opaque pupil is made too small, however, the patient may be able to see around it, which negates the intended effect of the lens.

Color Deficiency

Unusual lens designs and optical systems are sometimes helpful for other visual problems as well. Although such problems may not be present in a great percentage of the population, they can still be helpful to the individual involved.

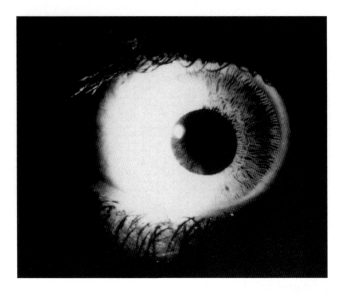

FIG. 23-33. *Grand Rounds Case Report 8 patient wearing final lens incorporating pupillary block tinting (Adventure in Color, Golden, CO) of a CIBA ILLUSIONS (CIBA Vision, Duluth, GA) opaque lens.*

A good example is that of people with a color vision deficiency. Various degrees of this problem exist. However, approximately 8% of the male population and 0.5% of the female population have some form of color vision problem. Abnormalities involving color vision are generally classified into two categories: anomalous trichromats and dichromats. Anomalous trichromatism is less severe and more common. People with this problem can match colors with red, green, or blue, but they require more of one color than is normally needed. If they are *green weak*, the condition is called *deuteranomaly*. Approximately 5% have this problem. If they are *red weak*, the condition is called *protanomaly*. Approximately 1% have this problem. *Tritanomaly* is the third form of anomalous trichromatism and is characterized by a blue weakness. It is a very rare condition. Dichromatism is the other form of color vision abnormality. Basically, two stimuli are used to match all colors. In deuteranopia, severe problems exist with discriminating red and green colors, and brightness is approximately 50% reduced. With protanopia, a substantial loss of sensitivity to red occurs, and brightness is also substantially reduced. Regardless of classification, most people who have a color vision problem would be more than happy not to have it. Depending on the severity, these people must be careful about

how they dress and about giving their opinion on something relating to color discrimination. Most people take
color vision for granted. However, color deficiency can
sometimes be very embarrassing, may present barriers
to certain occupations, and may even be potentially
dangerous.

In 1971, Zeltzer published the original paper on a
new contact lens called the X-CHROM lens, which he
had been using on patients with color deficiencies.[9] This
dark red lens transmits light essentially only in the red
zone from approximately 590 μ to 700 μ. When used
monocularly, it can improve color perception remarkably in some individuals. It does not cure the condition
but simply changes color perception so that they are
much better able to discriminate colored objects. A frequently heard comment is that X-CHROM lens wearers think that they see things more "vividly" or
"vibrantly" than before. Best results are obtained with
anomalous trichromats, although dichromats are also
helped to some degree. The lens is usually fitted on the
nondominant eye, which seems to be less bothersome
to most individuals. However, it can also be tried on
the dominant eye. The actual mechanism of why or
how this lens works is not well understood. A common
theory is that if a binocular individual is wearing an X-
CHROM lens on one eye, the brain receives some new
and very confusing information from the two eyes. Perhaps, by alternating this information from the two eyes
through the process of retinal rivalry, a new perception of color occurs that is advantageous. With time,
even better color enhancement may occur as the patient
learns to use the new information that is being
processed.

A red rigid-gas permeable contact lens is now available. At one time, only a polymethylmethacrylate version of this lens was available, but a rigid gas-permeable
(RGP) material (Transaire Ex, Amsilfocon, Rand Scientific Research, Sacramento, CA) can now be obtained
from various rigid lens laboratories. Fitting rigid red lenses
is basically the same as fitting conventional rigid lenses,
using the usual criteria for proper lens performance. Many
of these lens wearers do not wear their lenses all day but
use them only when they think that the lenses are needed.
Lens thickness is important because a lens that is made
too thick may reduce the amount of light transmission
to such a degree that the improvement in color perception is greatly reduced. Consequently, the rigid lens fitter may have to consider modifying such aspects as the
overall lens diameter or switching to a lenticular design
(especially if higher plus powers are required) to keep the
center thickness optimal. Because these lenses are red,

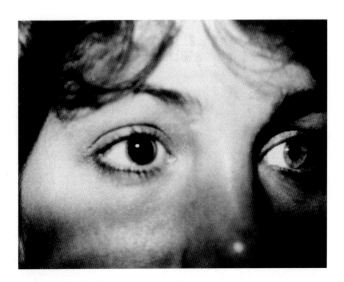

FIG. 23-34. *An X-Chrom red lens is quite noticeable when placed on a blue iris.*

the lens wearer may take approximately 0.50 D less minus
power than anticipated.

Many people with some form of color vision problem
may try these lenses and be very favorably impressed but
do not necessarily order a lens for personal use. It seems
that they merely wanted to confirm rumors they may
have heard about a special contact lens for color enhancement but were actually satisfied with their habitual situation. This sometimes leaves the contact lens practitioner
in a mild state of bewilderment, especially if the patient
seemed favorably impressed with the improvement in
color vision.

Several companies now make hydrophilic versions
of this lens so that lens wearers can more easily adapt
to a lens that is initially more comfortable and transmits more oxygen. This can be especially advantageous
when the lens is worn only for limited periods. It is
extremely important when a soft lens is ordered that
the size of the red pupillary zone be made large enough
to cover the pupil during different types of illumination, so that no peripheral light rays sneak in and reduce
its effectiveness.

As with anything else, some definite disadvantages are
associated with this lens. For one thing, not everyone
appreciates an improvement in color vision. In addition,
the lens can be annoying when worn in reduced illumination or at night. Cosmetically, the lens is not very noticeable in individuals with dark brown irides, but with light
irides, the red lens is very apparent and even resembles
an anisocoria (Fig. 23-34).

GRAND ROUNDS CASE REPORT 9

Subjective:

A 14-year-old girl was born with congenital cataracts, which were surgically removed soon after birth. She also had bilateral microcorneas and aniridia. No implants were used. It was thought that if a suitable contact lens could be designed, many visual, psychological, and emotional advantages would follow (Fig. 23-35).

Objective:

Her refractive error was right eye +19.00 = –1.25 cx 85 and left eye + 16.00 = –1.25 cx 75, which enabled her to see approximately ¹⁰⁄₃₀ in each eye. A slight nystagmus was also noted in each eye. Each cornea measured only 6 mm in diameter. Her keratometric readings were difficult to measure but showed approximately 3 D of with-the-rule astigmatism, with the flat meridians being approximately 46.25 D. To add to the difficulty, her vertical palpebral apertures measured 5 mm in the right eye and 6 mm in the left eye. A computerized topographic corneal plot showed that both corneas were actually steeper than first thought.

Assessment:

This patient had numerous ocular problems, any one of which could be considered challenging to handle. To add to the problem, lens effectiveness required her contact lens prescription to be higher in plus power than the manifest refraction, further adding to the weight and thickness of the lenses. The small apertures also could present practical problems during the lens placement and removal procedures. The fact that her corneas were steep was a minor help, in that these lenses would be a little less apt to gravitate inferiorly than they would on flat corneas. It was thought that if relatively steep and small high-powered aphakic lenses could be made, significant cosmetic and visual improvements would occur. These lenses would be similar to those sometimes required for pediatric aphakic use in which small and very high plus-powered lenses are necessary, especially during a baby's first year of life. An opaque dark-brown or black annulus lens with a 3- to 4-mm clear pupil would be considered if early results were promising. On the basis of the preliminary information, an initial diagnostic lens was designed that had a base curve of 8.3 mm, a diameter of 10 mm, and a back vertex power (BVP) of +19.00 D.

This lens proved to be much too loose and positioned inferiorly on both corneas. Although somewhat disappointing in performance, it still provided valuable information: When digitally moved onto the cornea with the lower lid margin, a better assessment of visual potential was obtained and it was apparent that a steeper and slightly larger lens would also be required. On the basis of these preliminary results, two new diagnostic lenses were designed. The first lens had an 11-mm diameter, a 7.0-mm base curve, and a BVP of +23.00 D. This lens was placed on the steeper right cornea and produced markedly better centration. However, it also produced an air bubble caused by excessive vaulting of the cornea.

The second diagnostic lens also had an 11-mm diameter but a flatter 7.4-mm base curve. The BVP was +22.00 D. This lens proved to be very valuable when evaluated on both eyes. Eventually, a lens was designed for the right eye that had a 7.4-mm base curve, a 12-mm diameter, and a BVP of +22.00. A 10-mm dark-brown opaque iris was also ordered, with a 4-mm clear pupil. The left eye also had a 7.4-mm base curve but an 11.5-mm diameter and a +19.00 BVP. The opaque annulus and pupil were made the same for both lenses. The final order was based on the fact that the 7.4-mm/11-mm diagnostic lens was slightly loose on both eyes but more so on the right eye. The slightly larger diameters would provide better stabilization, especially considering that the eyes had nystagmoid movement. The final lens powers were determined by over-refraction using freely held trial lenses. Loose trial lenses are best used in such situations because they better simulate real-world environments compared with having a patient hidden behind a phoropter in a dark room.

The lenses took several weeks to fabricate. They were then placed on each eye and given time to stabilize. Each lens moved 0.5–1.0 mm with the blink, positioned centrally, and provided vision that was at least equal to her spectacle prescription. The patient also found the lenses to be quite comfortable. Her subjective responses indicated that she actually thought that she saw better than with her glasses. The brown annulus portion of the lenses also gave the eye a more normal-sized appearance and cut down on the extraneous light that was entering the eye (Fig. 23-36).

Because of the high prescription, a conservative wearing schedule was used until a postwear check-up could be scheduled. Although these lenses were made from a 60%–water content material, they still had a rather thick center (0.37 mm). Therefore, the possibility existed of unacceptable vertical striae indicating corneal swelling.

The idea of using a silicone elastomer lens with a high permeability (Dk) value was considered. However, these lenses cannot be tinted in the manner desired. Some dyeing processes actually alter the lens parameters, whereas other dyeing processes do not work because silicone material contains virtually no water.

Plan:
The lenses were dispensed and the patient was allowed to build up wearing time slowly. A progress evaluation visit was purposely scheduled within the week. This visit confirmed the initial findings and showed that with a little perseverance, several problems could be addressed and improved. The patient was now able to see better than with her heavy, unattractive spectacle glasses, glare was greatly reduced, objects appeared more lifelike, and her eyes appeared more natural in size.

OTHER LENS DESIGNS

From the previous discussion in Grand Rounds Case Report 9, one might assume that soft hydrogel lenses are the only lens designs available for use in people with the types of problems the patient had. This is definitely not true. In fact, because hard lenses were available many years before soft lenses, they were frequently used for these purposes.[10–12]

Several reasons exist why soft lenses have largely replaced hard lenses for these specialized cases. Soft lenses are larger, so they cover a greater area of the cornea. They also move less and are therefore not as obvious on the eye. For example, the painted iris-imagery lens and the pupillary block lens are very noticeable and can also lose their intended effectiveness if they move too much after each blink. Soft lenses are also much more comfortable initially and, therefore, have some subjective advantages. Physiologically, soft lenses can be advantageous because they usually can be made thin enough to

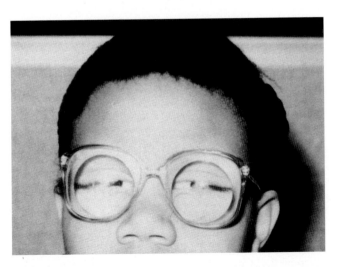

FIG. 23-35. *Grand Rounds Case Report 9 patient had congenital cataracts (surgically removed), aniridia, and microcorneas.*

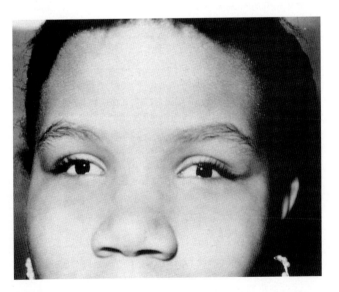

FIG. 23-36. *Grand Rounds Case Report 9 patient wearing small, custom-made aphakic hydrogel lenses with dark brown opaque irides.*

allow good oxygen transmission. However, this must be carefully monitored because different lenses in different designs and powers can vary in the actual amount of oxygen reaching the cornea.

Most of the hard lenses used have been fabricated from polymethylmethacrylate, which requires a very good tear pump to avoid the commonly seen edematous responses in the cornea. Therefore, lens size must be kept relatively small and lens movement must be sufficient to facilitate a good tear exchange mechanism. Because of the way these special lenses are fabricated, they are often thicker than normal and, therefore, are more prone to positioning inferiorly, or causing excessive movement. Hard lenses, however, do have some advantages. In some cases, they may provide a better visual response than any soft lens design. Consequently, some patients with minor cosmetic problems may be better off with hard lenses. If future advances enable good-quality RGP materials to be used in these unique designs, their frequency of use may increase dramatically. This would be especially true if RGP scleral lenses were made easily available. It would be important for the lens to be made of a material that permitted acceptable oxygen transmission without sacrificing wettability, machinability, and the opportunity to add a cosmetic design when necessary.[13]

As with soft lenses, ingenuity on the part of the lens designer can often help to solve some inherent hard lens problems. For example, in some cases, a lenticular minus edge carrier design can be used to improve lens positioning and movement problems by attaching the lens to the superior lid and having the lens move with the lid.[14] Larger lens diameters may also be used. It may take several modifications in lens design to achieve acceptable results. Consequently, the practitioner and the patient must be aware of the difficult challenges that may be faced and of the accompanying financial responsibilities. Many times, misunderstandings can be eliminated by discussing the particular options with the fabricating laboratory while the patient is still in the office. Sometimes, the laboratory can say immediately if a contemplated design is physically possible to manufacture. Frequently, loaner or library lenses can be obtained that are invaluable in helping to determine the final lens design and thereby facilitate the fitting procedures.

REFERENCES

1. Meshel L: Prosthetic Contact Lenses: CLAO Guide to Basic Science and Clinical Practice. Grune & Stratton, New York, 1984

2. Putz J, McMahon T: Dot matrix opaque black pupil: a modification for use on disfigured eyes. Contact Lens Spectrum 5:59, 1990

3. Cutler S, Sando R: Contact lens correction for the post-operative large pupil. Contact Lens Forum 14:23, 1989

4. Wodak G: Soft artificial iris lenses. Contacto 21:4, 1977

5. Spinell M, Haransky E: The use of the new Wesley-Jessen opaque lens for a congenital aniridia patient. Int Contact Lens Clin 14:489, 1987

6. Spinell M, Bernitt D: Cosmetic occluder lens. Optom Monthly 76:21, 1985

7. Spinell M, Santilli J: An unusual contact lens design for a patient with Stargardt's disease. Contact Lens Spectrum 7:17, 1992

8. Greenspoon M, Silver R: Applying contact lens expertise to patients with disfigured corneas. Optom Today Jan/Feb:35, 1992

9. Zeltzer H: The X-Chrom lens. J Am Optom Assoc 42:933, 1971

10. Amos DM, Robinson JT, Smith G: Case report: use of cosmetic contact lens for heterochromia, iris atrophy, and opaque cataract. J Am Optom Assoc 48:105, 1977

11. Scheid T, Langer P: Therapeutic applications of cosmetic iris rigid lenses. Optom Monthly 73:610, 1982

12. Zadnik K: Prosthetic hard contact lens for postsurgical, enlarged pupil. Contact Lens Forum 12:24, 1987

13. Berkowitsch A: Cosmetic haptic contact lenses. J Am Optom Assoc 55:277, 1984

14. Armitage B: A cosmetic PMMA lens for a congenital defect. Int Eyecare 2:631, 1986

SUGGESTED READINGS

Bailey CS, Buckley RJ: Ocular prostheses and contact lenses. Cosmetic devices. BMJ 302:1010, 1991

Cannon WM: Putting the promises into practice. Contact Lens Spectrum 5:65, 1990

Comstock T: The use of tinted hydrogel prosthetic lenses. Contact Lens Spectrum 12:54, 1988

Creighton C: An improved fitting system. Alden Optical Laboratories, Alden, NY, 1988

Farkas P, Kassalow T, Farkas B: Use of a pupillary lens in aphakia. J Am Optom Assoc 47:61, 1976

Fontana A: Coping with the nystagmoid albino: lens designs that really work. Rev Optom 116:36, 1979

Gienesk N: W-J opaque lens provides aphakic power, matching tint. Rev Optom 126:103, 1989

Greenspoon MK: History of the cinematic uses of contact lenses. Am J Optom Arch Am Acad Optom 46:63, 1969

Greenspoon M: Optometry's contribution to the motion picture industry. J Am Optom Assoc 58:983, 1987

Key J, Mobley C: Cosmetic hydrogel lenses for therapeutic purposes. Contact Lens Forum 12:18, 1987

Koetting RA: Cosmetic contact lens in the care of the child. J Am Optom Assoc 50:1245, 1979

McMahon T, Krefman R: A four year retrospective study of prosthetic hydrogel lens use. Int Contact Lens Clin 11:146, 1984

Meshel L: Tinted lenses: new "life" for dead eyes. Contact Lens Forum 3:13, 1978

Moss H: A minimum clearance molded scleral cosmetic-refractive contact lens. J Am Optom Assoc 49:277, 1978

Narcissus Foundation Bulletin. Narcissus Medical Foundation. Daly City, CA

Oleszewski S, Wood J: Painted iris lens improves cosmetic appearance. Rev Optom 123:56, 1986

Scheid T: Reverse piggy-back for cosmetic change in RGP wearers. Contact Lens Forum 14:21, 1989

Schlanger J: Enhancing color vision with new hydrogel lens. Contact Lens Forum 13:57, 1988

Zack M: The cosmetic treatment of Adie's tonic pupil using selectively tinted hydrophilic soft contact lenses. Contact Lens J 12:14, 1984

Appendix 23-1

U.S. Companies Providing Cosmetic Lenses

Alden Optical Laboratories, Allen, NY	(800) 232-4747
Adventure in Color, Inc., Golden, CO	(800) 537-2845
CIBA Vision Corporation, Duluth, GA	(800) 241-5999
Cooper Vision Inc., Fairport, NY	(800) 341-2020
Crystal Reflections Inc., Green Valley, AZ	(800) 407-8722
Specialty Tint Inc., La Jolla, CA	(800) 748-5500
Wesley-Jessen Corporation, Des Plaines, IL	(800) 488-6859

IX

Corneal Topography

24

Corneal Topography and Contact Lens Complications

KENNETH A. LEBOW

Contact lenses (both rigid and soft) can change the shape of the cornea by physiologic or mechanical forces. Chronic corneal hypoxia and anoxia cause microcystic formations,[1,2] polymegethism,[3] and stromal acidosis[4,5] on a microscopic level. The resultant corneal edema[6] produces a steepening of or distortion in keratometry values and potential structural tissue changes.[7] Mechanical pressure owing to increased lens mass from rigid lenses,[8] base curve-to-cornea fitting relationships,[9,10] post-lens tear film depletion,[11] and wearing patterns[12] can also induce keratometric changes and produce corneal distortion. Although edematous corneal changes are generally considered a physiologic complication of contact lens wear, lens adherence is thought to be a mechanically induced problem.[13] Nevertheless, both conditions can change the corneal curvature from its prefitting state.[14] The role of the eye care practitioner is to detect these changes before they become severe and irreversibly alter vision.

KERATOMETRY

Traditionally, the keratometer has been used to measure corneal curvature and document its changes over time.[15] Although keratometric corneal curvature measurements are useful, they are inherently limited. The keratometer presumes the cornea to be a normal spherocylindrical surface, although it is generally accepted that the actual corneal shape is best described as an asymmetric toroid asphere[16] that flattens from its apex to the periphery.[17-19] The measured corneal zone is limited to approximately 3 mm from the corneal apex, and no information is available describing the curvature inside or outside of this zone.[20] Moreover, small amounts of astigmatism often distort keratometric mires, making accurate measurements impossible.[21]

CORNEAL TOPOGRAPHY

Corneal topography (CT) provides a more comprehensive and detailed analysis of the corneal curvature and a greater surface area for measurement than does keratometry.[22] Contemporary corneal topographers using placido disk technology measure 8–12 mm of the corneal surface using thousands of data points. With these points, they mathematically reconstruct a two- or three-dimensional representation of corneal shape using color-coded maps.[23] Some systems claim the ability to map the corneal surface from limbus to limbus. Most contemporary CT systems (Zeiss Humphrey Systems, Dublin, CA; Tomey Technology, Inc., Cambridge, MA; and EyeSys Technologies, Houston, TX) use reflective placido ring technology to analyze and map the corneal surface. Other corneal topographers use rasterstereographic images (PAR Vision Systems, New Hartford, NY),[24-28] projected slit-lamp beams with triangulation (Bausch & Lomb Orbtek, Rochester, NY),[29] and Fourier Profilometry (Euclid System Corp., Herndon, VA)[30] to capture corneal images. Rasterstereography provides limbus-to-limbus corneal coverage and can be used with a nonreflective corneal surface, such as those encountered in corneal surgery.[26,31] Projected slit-lamp beams also provide limbus-to-limbus corneal coverage and can determine corneal thickness.[29] All systems use cool colors (blues) to represent flat corneal curvatures or depressions below a reference surface and warm colors (reds) for steep corneal curvatures and elevations above a reference surface. A variety of mapping (axial versus tangential) and scaling (absolute versus autoscale) strategies are available for all systems, but it is not the purpose of this chapter to describe or differentiate them.

Studies evaluating manufactured spheric and nonrotationally symmetric toroid aspheric surfaces have demonstrated a high degree of accuracy and reproducibility in comparing CT measurements with those obtained using the keratometer.[32–34] When healthy and diseased corneas were measured with the PAR and EyeSys CT systems and those results were compared with the Javal keratometer, the PAR values most closely matched the keratometer values, with EyeSys reporting lower values for flat and steep curvatures as well as less total corneal astigmatism.[35] Other studies found statistically significant differences between videokeratography and either the radiuscope or keratometer when measuring the toric surface of contact lens buttons (i.e., the amount of toricity was underestimated by as much as 25%).[36] Some variability in CT measurements depends on the nature of the surface measured[37] and other issues, such as smoothing problems, the inability to read large transitions, loss of accuracy in the periphery, and poor central coverage.[38] In a comparison of several systems, the Humphrey MasterVue system (Zeiss Humphrey Systems, Dublin, CA) was most accurate centrally but had errors in the periphery, whereas the Alcon EyeMap (Alcon Laboratories, Inc., Fort Worth, TX) demonstrated moderate smoothing. TMS (Tomey Technology, Inc., Cambridge, MA) and Keratron (Alliance Medical Marketing, Inc., Jacksonville Beach, FL) had poor or inaccurate central coverage, and EyeSys and Topcon (Tokyo, Japan) produced excessive smoothing of data.[38] A study comparing several topography systems also reported the Humphrey Atlas to be the most accurate topographer, although there were statistically significant differences in dioptric values at corresponding corneal points among all units tested.[39] In another study, the TMS-1 in dioptric values at corresponding corneal points was found to be more accurate in detecting astigmatism, whereas the EyeSys Corneal Analysis System underestimated surface astigmatism owing to excessive smoothing, and the Visioptic EH-270 demonstrated central zone errors resulting from ring localization problems.[34] Despite these limitations, CT has increased our understanding of corneal shape dramatically. New information includes the following:

- The arbitrary division of the cornea into central and peripheral zones is too simplistic because the shape of the normal cornea is so highly variable.[40]
- A more clinically practical separation of the cornea may be central, paracentral, peripheral, and limbal zones.[16]

- A definable exact apical region cannot be confirmed.[18]
- Normal cornea shape can be classified as round (22.6%), oval (20.8%), symmetric bow tie (17.5%), asymmetric bow tie (32.1%), or irregular (7.1%), based on videokeratoscopic patterns.[41]
- By combining CT analysis and ultrasound pachymetry, it appears that the healthy adult corneal structure may be characterized as a highly ordered, three-dimensional architecture with symmetry.[42] A specific distribution of corneal thickness and the radius of curvature of the anterior corneal surface along the principle meridians may be essential for the refractive function of the human cornea in vivo.[42]

NORMAL CORNEAL SHAPE

Although the shape of the normal cornea is highly variable and unique, it is generally accepted to be a radially asymmetric, toroid surface that flattens from its apex to the periphery.[43–45] The rate of flattening varies along every meridian, but clinically it is useful to think of the corneal surface as a section of an ellipse with a rate of flattening along its flattest meridian.[46] The rate of flattening of an ellipse is termed its *eccentricity* and is described by the following equation: $(1 - {}^{b^2}/_{a^2})^{1/2}$. Several other conic shape parameters (i.e., p, Q, and e) have also been used to describe the general shape of the cornea.[47] However, by using the term *shape factor* (SF), which approximately represents the square of the eccentricity (SF $= 1 - p$, where p represents an aspheric constant), a single numeric value can be used to describe the shape of the cornea.[48] In most normal corneas, this value is positive and describes a prolate ellipse where the radius of curvature is steeper in the center than the periphery. Conversely, an oblate ellipse is a negative value and describes a corneal flattening pattern, where the steeper curvature is in the periphery rather than the center.[49] An SF or eccentricity of 0.0 mathematically defines a circle and, by definition, has no peripheral flattening. Values more than 0.0 but less than 1.0 describe increasingly greater rates of peripheral flattening and a less spheric shape. When the SF or eccentricity equals 1.0, a parabola is defined, whereas values more than 1.0 define hyperbolic shapes (Fig. 24-1). Normal spheric topography maps show a uniform curvature gradient centrally with progressively flatter peripheral curvatures in the periphery (Fig. 24-2). Normal symmetric astigmatic topography maps clearly demonstrate a steep and flat corneal axis, evidenced by the presence of a vertical (with-the-rule astigmatism), horizontal (against-the-rule astigmatism), or oblique (oblique astigmatism) bow-tie pattern (Fig. 24-3).

FIG. 24-1. *Terminology used in describing corneal configuration topography for spheric and aspheric surfaces. (Reprinted with permission from GO Waring: Making sense of keratospeak II: proposed conventional terminology for corneal topography. Refract Corneal Surg 5:362, 1989.)*

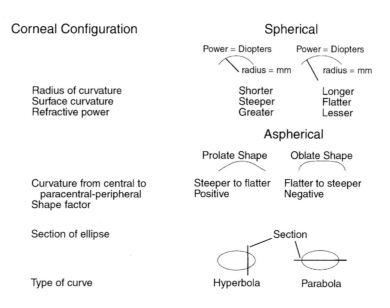

Asymmetric astigmatic topography maps have patterns similar to symmetric astigmatic maps except that the steepest corneal curvature is displaced from the geometric center of the cornea (Fig. 24-4). However, an asymmetric or angled bow-tie appearance of a corneal map suggests a decentered corneal apex rather than corneal asymmetry and may lead to a misdiagnosis of the type or magnitude of corneal toricity, keratoconus, or other corneal irregu-larity.[50] As more patients are evaluated for refractive surgery procedures and more practitioners routinely use CT, the incidence of abnormal topography patterns has also increased.[51] The frequency of appearance of abnormal CT patterns, especially with regard to refractive surgery screenings, has caused some practitioners to anecdotally estimate an increase in the incidence of keratoconus in the general population to as high as 5.7–10%.[51]

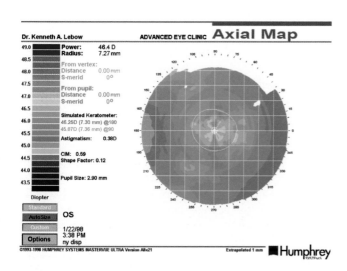

FIG. 24-2. *Axial corneal topography map demonstrating a normal spheric corneal topography. (CIM = corneal irregularity measure.)*

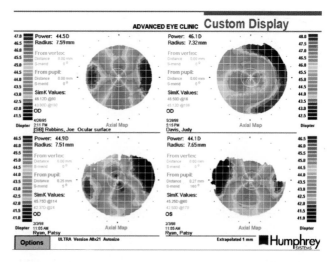

FIG. 24-3. *Composite axial corneal topography map demonstrating various forms of symmetric corneal astigmatism: symmetric with-the-rule (upper left), asymmetric against-the-rule (upper left), and symmetric oblique (lower left and right). (SimK = simulated K reading.)*

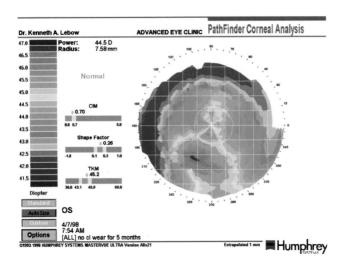

FIG. 24-4. *Corneal analysis and axial corneal topography map demonstrating a displaced corneal apex with asymmetric corneal astigmatism. (CIM = corneal irregularity measure; TKM = toric mean reference curvature.)*

FIG. 24-5. *Corneal analysis and axial corneal topography map demonstrating true keratoconus with a high shape factor, greatly increased corneal irregularity measure. (CIM = corneal irregularity measure; TKM = toric mean referemce curvature.)*

CORNEAL COMPLICATIONS

Normal CT can be altered in one of three ways[52]:

1. Inflammatory or noninflammatory abnormalities of the corneal epithelium
2. Central or peripheral changes in the stromal thickness
3. External compressive (mechanical) forces from the lid, surgery, trauma, or contact lenses

Contact lens wear can create topographic complications in all these categories, and unique CT patterns may be associated with a variety of corneal complications. For example, qualitative CT maps of keratoconus typically demonstrate superior flattening and marked inferior steepening of the corneal curvature (Fig. 24-5).[53]

Other conditions, including contact lens–induced corneal warpage,[52,54-60] subclinical (forme fruste) keratoconus,[61-63] displaced corneal apex,[64] soft contact lens wear,[65] and pellucid marginal degeneration,[66] can mimic the clinical topographic appearance of keratoconus. It is extremely important for the practitioner to be able to differentiate these conditions. Refractive surgery[67] and orthokeratology[68] CT maps are unique in that they usually demonstrate an area of central corneal flattening surrounded by an area of peripheral steepening characterized by an oblate corneal ellipse (negative SF).

STATISTICAL INDICES

Qualitative evaluation of CT maps is necessary to visually recognize unique topographic patterns. However, quantitative analysis provides the mathematic basis for determining various geometric corneal shapes, and aids in the identification and differentiation of similar qualitative patterns as well as the quantification of progressive changes for patterns, thereby minimizing clinical subjectivity in data interpretation.[69,70] Currently, the EyeSys Technologies Eye-Sys 2000 Corneal Analysis System, Computed Anatomy TMS-2 Topographic Modeling System, and Humphrey Systems Atlas Corneal Topography System offer statistical packages that analyze and evaluate topographic data using different maps and statistical variables (Table 24-1). The Holladay diagnostic summary for the EyeSys 2000 Corneal Analysis System offers a combination of refractive power (standard and AutoScale), a profile difference, and distortion maps (Fig. 24-6) to quantify CT data. It is designed to give the clinician in a single report information about the true refractive power of the cornea, the shape of the measured cornea compared to a normal cornea, and the optical quality of the corneal surface.[71] It also provides 15 additional corneal parameters used in intraocular lens calculations.[71] Table 24-2 summarizes the key variables used in the Holladay diagnostic summary. This analysis program demonstrates changes in the maps and various indices that enable practitioners to recognize and monitor corneal disease and refractive surgery, and to correlate those changes with patient symptoms.[72] Using this program and analyz-

TABLE 24-1. *Comparison of Various Keratoconus Detection Software Programs Available with Corneal Topography (CT) Systems*

CT System	Keratoconus Detection Program	Indices Included
EyeSys 2000 Corneal Analysis System	Holladay diagnostic summary[71]	Standard refractive power map Autoscale refractive power map Profile difference map Distortion map 15 corneal and refractive parameters
TMS-1 Topographic Modeling System	Rabinowitz test[75]	Simulated keratometry value Inferior-superior value
	Rabinowitz-McDonnell test[76]	Steepness of the central corneal curvature (>47 D) Degree of asymmetry between the superior and inferior corneal curvatures (>3 D) Asymmetry between the central corneal power of fellow eyes in excess of 1 D
	Klyce/Maeda test[77]	Average corneal power Opposite sector index Corneal eccentricity index Center-surround index Standard deviation of power Irregular astigmatism index Differential sector index Analyzed area
	Classification Neural Network[79]	Differential sector index Opposite sector index Center-surround index Analyzed area Cylinder Irregular astigmatism index Steep axis-simulated keratometry Surface regularity index Surface asymmetry index Standard deviation of corneal power
Atlas Corneal Topography System	Pathfinder Corneal Analysis Module[85]	Shape factor Corneal irregularity measure Toric mean reference curvature

ing 132 pre- and post–photorefractive keratectomy (PRK) patients, greater amounts of positive central corneal asphericity (the central cornea changed from a prolate shape [negative asphericity] to an oblate shape [positive asphericity]) were correlated with higher refractive errors.[73] (Note: In this example, asphericity, which is defined as the Q value and is negative, should not be confused with either eccentricity or SF, which are other measures of peripheral corneal flattening and are generally considered positive in prolate corneas.) Unique to this program is the ability to calculate and print intraocular lens (IOL) powers using second-generation lens implant power formulas[74] and potential visual performance owing to surface irregularities in the cornea.[71] However, the Holladay diagnostic summary was not intended to identify or quantify corneal disease based on the parameters measured.

The Rabinowitz and Klyce/Maeda keratoconus detection programs used with the Computed Anatomy TMS-1 Topographic Modeling System represents the first attempt to detect keratoconus with CT patterns. Several

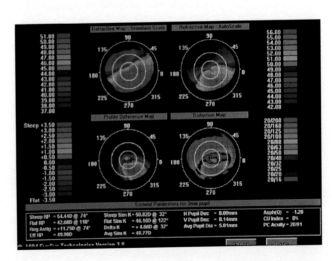

FIG. 24-6. *The Holladay diagnostic summary demonstrating refractive (standard and AutoScale), profile difference, and distortion maps as well as 15 specific corneal parameters used in intraocular lens calculations (EyeSys Technologies [Houston, TX] 2000 Corneal Analysis System).*

TABLE 24-2. *Summary Description of Various Corneal Indices Used with the Holladay Diagnostic Summary on the EyeSys 2000 Corneal Analysis System*

Index	Description
Refractive power (RP) measurements	
Steep RP	*Steep RP* is the strongest RP in any single meridian of the cornea expressed in diopters with the axis of that meridian.
Flat RP	*Flat RP* is the weakest RP in any single meridian of the cornea expressed in diopters with the axis of that meridian. Note that the steep RP and flat RP are not necessarily 90 degrees apart and that when this occurs, oblique irregular astigmatism is present.
Total astig	The *total astigmatism* of the cornea is represented by the difference between the steep RP and the flat RP expressed in plus cylinder and therefore referenced at the steep RP.
Eff RP	The *effective RP* is the RP of the corneal surface within the 3-mm pupil zone, taking into account the Stiles-Crawford effect. It is commonly known as the *spheroequivalent power of the cornea* and is the value used for the power of the cornea for intraocular lens calculations and for refractive surgery procedures.
Simulated keratometry (SimK) measurements	
Steep SimK	The *steep SimK reading* is the steepest meridian of the cornea using only the points along the 3-mm pupil perimeter, not the entire zone.
Flat SimK	The *flat SimK reading* is the flattest meridian of the cornea using only the points along the 3-mm pupil perimeter.
Delta K	*Delta K* is the difference between the steep SimK and the flat SimK expressed in diopters at the axis of the steep SimK.
Ave SimK	The *average SimK* is the average of the steep and flat SimKs. The difference between the eff RP and the ave SimK is another measure of the degree of irregular astigmatism. Although the eff RP should always give a more reliable value for the corneal power than the ave SimK, the discrepancy indicates that one should expect a higher degree of variability in the results of an intraocular lens calculation than with a normal cornea.
Pupil Parameters and Regular Astigmatism	
H Pupil Dec	*Horizontal pupil decentration* is the horizontal decentration in millimeters from the center of the map to the centroid of the pupil, where *out* (temporal) means the pupil is out with respect to the center of the map and *in* (nasal) means the pupil is in with respect to the center of the map. This value is commonly referred to clinically as *angle Kappa* and is nominally 0.2 mm out in the human.
V Pupil Dec	*Vertical pupil decentration* is the distance in millimeters from the center of the map to the centroid of the pupil. *Up* (superior) means the pupil is up with respect the center of the pupil and *down* (inferior) means the pupil is down with respect to the center of the maps. The nominal value for the human is approximately zero.
Avg Pupil Dia	*Average pupil diameter* is the average of the pupil at the time of the photograph. Because the photograph is taken under bright light conditions, without dilation, the pupil diameter is usually less than 3.0 mm.
Reg Astig	*Regular astigmatism* is the amount and axis of the astigmatism that can be neutralized with a spherocylindrical correction. Regular astigmatism often provides a good starting point refraction and is always less than the total astigmatism because total astigmatism includes irregular as well as regular astigmatism. The disparity in the two values represents a measure of the degree of irregular astigmatism.
Miscellaneous Measurements	
Asph (Q)	*Asphericity* is a measure of the rate of flattening of the cornea from the apex to the periphery. This is the only corneal parameter that uses an area other than the 3-mm pupillary zone for the value. A pupil of 4.5 mm is used to calculate asphericity. The Q measurement allows positive values to describe *oblate* surfaces, which are steeper in the periphery than the center, and negative values to describe *prolate* surfaces, which are steeper centrally and flatten toward the periphery. The normal human asphericity (Q) is –0.26.
CU Index	*Corneal uniformity index* is a measure of the uniformity of the distortion of the corneal surface within the 3-mm pupil expressed as a percentage. A CU index of 100% indicates that the optical quality of the cornea is almost perfectly uniform over the central 3-mm pupil. A CU index of 0% indicates that the optical quality of the cornea is nonuniform over the central 3-mm pupil. This does not indicate that the cornea has good optical quality but simply describes the uniformity of the surface. This index is useful in the differentiation of corneal pathology where generalized or localized characteristic patterns are present.
PC Acuity	*Predicted corneal acuity* provides a single value in units of Snellen acuity of the optical quality of the corneal surface within the 3-mm zone ranging from 20/10 to 20/200. The PC acuity estimates the predicted acuity if the cornea is the limiting factor in the visual system and is helpful in characterizing corneal abnormalities and monitoring changes over time.

Source: Reprinted with permission from JT Holladay: Understanding Corneal Topography: The Holladay Diagnostic Summary, User's Guide and Tutorial Version 3.30-3.11. EyeSys Technologies, 1995.

other methods have been reported. The Rabinowitz criterion for keratoconus detection is based solely on the simulated keratometry (SimK) and inferior-superior values.[75] The steeper the SimK value and the greater the disparity between the inferior and superior curvatures, the greater the likelihood of detecting a keratoconuslike topography pattern. Although this analysis provides a relative sensitivity for keratoconus detection, it is not as specific for keratoconus and requires that both eyes be mapped for a true analysis.[80] The modified Rabinowitz-McDonnell test analyzes the steepness of the central corneal curvature (greater than 47 D), the degree of asymmetry between the superior and inferior corneal curvatures (greater than 3 D at points 3 mm superior and inferior to the corneal center), and asymmetry between the central corneal power of fellow eyes in excess of 1 D, thus creating a more sensitive measure of the probability that keratoconuslike patterns are present.[76] When high sensitivity is required, this criterion for keratoconus screening is more sensitive than keratometry, although the expert system classifier (Klyce/Maeda) is even more appropriate than either keratometry or the modified Rabinowitz-McDonnell test when high specificity is needed.[58] The Klyce/Maeda index uses an automated keratoconus detection program that combines a classification tree with a linear discriminant function derived using various indices obtained from TMS-1 videokeratoscope data to differentiate keratoconus patterns from other conditions.[77] The Klyce/Maeda index reports the keratoconus index (KCI), which estimates the presence of keratoconuslike patterns from 0% (no keratoconuslike pattern) to 1–95% (some degree of keratoconuslike pattern).[78] The latest approach to keratoconus detection uses computer-enhanced artificial intelligence programming with neural networks that are capable of learning qualitative and quantitative keratoconus topography patterns. These achieve higher levels of accuracy and specificity when distinguishing keratoconus patterns from keratoconus suspects compared to previous detection tests.[79] The Smolek/Klyce Method actually reports the keratoconus severity index (KSI), which is derived from a combination of neural network models and decision tree analysis. Unlike KCI, KSI increases in a more or less linear fashion with the progression of keratoconus and is therefore thought to be capable of tracking the natural history of the disease.[79] For example, when the KSI reaches 0.15, a keratoconus suspect is indicated, whereas values of 0.30 and greater indicate clinical keratoconus. Figure 24-7 demonstrates a keratoconus patient with a KCI of 79.8% and a KSI of 35.8%, which strongly suggest a keratoconuslike pattern. Figure 24-8, representing an eye with corneal warpage, demonstrates a KCI of 0% (implying no similarity to ker-

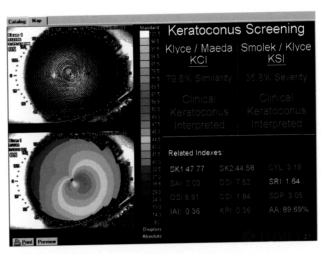

FIG. 24-7. *The Klyce/Maeda and Smolek/Klyce keratoconus screening indices, indicating the similarity and severity with which a topography map appears like keratoconus (Computed Anatomy TMS-2 and TMS-3 Topographic Modeling Systems). (AA = area analyzed; CSI = center/surround index; CYL = simulated keratometric cylinder change; DSI = differential sector index; IAI = irregular astigmatism index; KCI = keratoconus index; KPI = keratoconus predication index; KSI = keratoconus severity index; OSI = opposite sector index; SAI = surface asymmetry index; SDP = standard deviation of corneal power; SK1 = simulated keratometry 1; SK2 = simulated keratometry 2; SRI = surface regularity index.)*

atoconus) and a 15.8% KSI (suggesting the possibility of a keratoconuslike pattern).

These and other studies using the inferior-superior asymmetry index, surface asymmetry index (SAI), surface regularity index (SRI), and various combinations of indices have reported the potential for detecting and differentiating keratoconus from other normal and abnormal CT maps.[76,77,79-84] Each index describes differences in surface powers across the cornea. The inferior-superior asymmetry index measures the difference in mean superior and inferior powers from rings 14–16, where values between 1.4 and 1.9 represent suspected keratoconic patterns. The SAI measures the difference between the corneal powers at every ring (180 degrees apart) over the entire corneal surface; values more than 5.0 may indicate moderately advanced keratoconus. The SRI, like the SAI, is a quantitative measure that attempts to correlate the optical quality of the corneal surface with potential visual acuity. The SRI is derived from the local regularity of corneal surface over that area of the cornea enclosed by an approximate average virtual pupil of 4.5 mm. Hence, the TMS-2 and TMS-3 Modeling System uses differences in corneal curvature over the surface of the eye rather than a geomet-

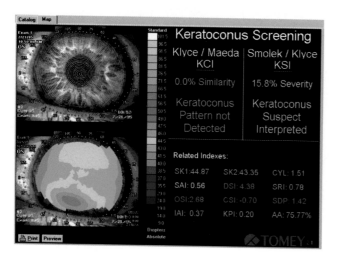

FIG. 24-8. *The Klyce/Maeda and Smolek/Klyce keratoconus screening indices indicating the similarity and severity with which a topography map appears to show keratoconus but actually manifests corneal warpage (Computed Anatomy TMS-2 and TMS-3 Topographic Modeling Systems). (AA = area analyzed; CSI = center/surround index; CYL = simulated keratometric cylinder change; DSI = differential sector index; IAI = irregular astigmatism index; KCI = keratoconus index; KPI = keratoconus predication index; KSI = keratoconus severity index; OSI = opposite sector index; SAI = surface asymmetry index; SDP = standard deviation of corneal power; SK1 = simulated keratometry 1; SK2 = simulated keratometry 2; SRI = surface regularity index.)*

ric model of the cornea to identify keratoconuslike patterns. Table 24-3 summarizes the various parameters that are used with the TMS-2 and TMS-3 CT systems.

The Pathfinder Corneal Analysis Module for the Humphrey Systems Atlas Corneal Topographer is the newest keratoconus/pathology detection software module (Fig. 24-9).[80] Unlike previous keratoconus detection programs, this software algorithm differentiates keratoconus on the basis of geometric shape using three key variables: SF, corneal irregularity measure (CIM), and toric mean reference curvature (TKM).[81] Table 24-4 summarizes the parameters that are used with the Pathfinder Corneal Analysis Module.

SF is a single numeric value that represents peripheral corneal flattening and describes the shape of the cornea. It was originally introduced by Bibby in 1976[48] and describes the square of the eccentricity of a corneal meridian. In the MasterVue system, SF is equal to 1 −p, where p (an aspheric constant) is a value often used as a conic section parameter. Because the SF is always associated with a meridional curve, the MasterVue system reports the SF of the flattest meridian of the best-fit toric surface.

Traditionally, high eccentricity values (0.9 or greater) are nearly always associated with keratoconus.[18] Even in the absence of objective slit-lamp findings, abnormally high eccentricity values (e = 0.8) were diagnostic of early keratoconus with 98% specificity and 97% sensitivity.[82] The Pathfinder Corneal Analysis nomogram targets any SF in excess of 0.6 as a potential suspect. The mean SF in the normal distribution of the population is 0.24, with 96% of the population falling between 0 and 0.46.[85] (Although SF is mathematically related to eccentricity, SF is used here because its sign has the advantage of differentiating prolate surfaces [positive SF] from oblate surfaces [negative SF]) (Fig. 24-10).

CIM is a statistical index that describes the cornea's irregularity compared to a best-fit computer-generated toric surface. This value is obtained by taking elevation differences between the actual corneal surface and the ellipsoid found at each point for the inner 10 rings and calculating the variance of those differences. It is equal to the square root of the variance between the measured elevation values for the central cornea and the elevation values of the best-fit quadric surface. Ellipsoids (quadric surfaces) fit normal corneal surfaces quite well but do not fit abnormal corneal shapes, such as keratoconus and contact lens–induced corneal warpage, nearly as well. The CIM provides a numeric quantification of the fitting relationship between the actual corneal surface and the best-fit ellipse. The lower the CIM, the better an ellipsoid matches the corneal curvature. Conversely, larger CIM values imply greater difficulty matching an ellipse to the corneal curvature. Also, the higher the CIM, the more irregular or uneven the surface is optically. The mean CIM value for the human population is 0.63 μ; 67% of the population falls between 0.03 and 0.64 μ.[85] CIM values of 1.0 or higher are indicative of distorted or suspect corneal shapes (Fig. 24-11). The surface irregularity map graphically displays the elevation differences used to calculate CIM.

Toric mean reference curvature (TKM) is the mean or average curvature at the apex of the toric surface that best fits the measured corneal surface. This value is important because most cones have significant toricity at the cone apex, although it may not always be detected with CT.[131] TKM is different from traditional keratometer values in that keratometer values represent central curvatures taken with normal fixation and do not necessarily represent the curvature at the corneal apex. More likely, keratometer values are roughly centered at the corneal vertex, an area tangent to a plane normal to the line of sight that is usually not coincident with the corneal apex (i.e., the surface location with the highest mean curvature). Although the separation between these two points

TABLE 24-3. *Summary Description of Various Corneal Indices Used with Klyce/Maeda and Smolek/Klyce Methods of Keratoconus Detection Using the Computed Anatomy Inc. TMS-2 and TMS-3 Topographic Modeling Systems*

Index	Description
SK1	*Simulated keratometry 1* is obtained from the powers observed in the corneal surface with an average of rings 6–8 along every meridian. *SimK1* is the power and axis of the meridian with the highest power.
SK2	*Simulated keratometry 2* is the power of the meridian 90 degrees from SK1.
CYL	*Simulated keratometric cylinder change* is obtained from the SimK1 (SK1 minus SK2) readings. Higher than normal values of CYL are associated with severe pathologies, trauma, and surgery.
SAI	*Surface asymmetry index* measures the difference in corneal powers at every ring 180 degrees apart over the entire corneal surface. The SAI is often higher than normal in keratoconus, penetrating keratoplasty, decentered myopic refractive surgery procedures, trauma, and contact lens warpage. Adequate spectacle correction is often not achieved when SAI is high.
DSI	*Differential sector index* is the area-corrected greatest difference between any two of the eight sectors of the cornea. It is higher than normal for a keratoconuslike pattern.
SRI	*Surface regularity index* is a correlate to potential visual acuity and is a measure of local fluctuations in central corneal power. When the SRI is elevated, the corneal surface ahead of the entrance pupil is irregular, leading to a reduction in best spectacle-corrected visual acuity. High SRI values are found with dry eye, contact lens wear, trauma, and penetrating keratoplasty.
OSI	*Opposite sector index* is the maximum difference in area-corrected corneal powers between any two opposite sectors of the cornea. It is high for keratoconuslike patterns.
CSI	*Center/surround index* is the area-corrected difference in average corneal power between the central 3 mm of analyzed area and an annulus surrounding the central area from an inner radius of 1.5 mm to an outer radius of 3 mm.
SDP	*Standard deviation of corneal power* is calculated from the distribution of all corneal powers in a videokeratograph. SDP is often high for keratoconus, transplants, and trauma, all situations in which a wide range of powers occurs in the measured topography.
IAI	*Irregular astigmatism index* is an area-compensated average summation of inter-ring power variations along every meridian for the entire corneal surface analyzed. IAI increases as local irregular astigmatism in the corneal surface increases. IAI is high in corneal transplants shortly after surgery. Persistence often heralds suboptimal best spectacle-corrected vision.
KPI	*Keratoconus predication index* is calculated from a discriminant analysis equation and is used with a decision tree to calculate KCI, the final interpretation for the presence of clinical keratoconus.
AA	The *area analyzed* gives the fraction of the corneal area covered by the mires that could be processed by the AutoTopographer. AA is lower than normal for corneas with gross, irregular astigmatism, which causes the mires to break up and not be resolved. A lower than normal AA is found with early postoperative corneal transplants, advanced keratoconus, and trauma. AA can also be artificially low when the eyes are not opened wide.

Source: Reprinted with permission from Tomey Manual. AutoTopographer (TMS-3) Operator Manual, Version 2.1, 10:8, 1998.

may be small, the mean curvature at the apex is thought to be a better indicator of keratoconus than the mean curvature at the corneal vertex. In addition, the TKM is the surface that is used to find the CIM, to generate the irregularity map, and to give the SF. The greater the difference between the two toric K values used to calculate the TKM, the greater the astigmatism at the corneal apex. Once the toric reference surface is determined (usually an ellipse), the curvature or K values at the apex are known. The maximum and minimum values are displayed to give the TKM. The meridian associated with the minimum K value is, by definition, the flattest meridian. Because one of the principal characteristics of keratoconus is high surface curvature in local areas of the affected cornea, the mean curvature at the apex is thought to be a valuable criterion for differentiating keratoconus. The mean value for TKM is 44.5 D; 96% of the population falls between 41.25 and 47.25 D (Fig. 24-12).[85] The

normal, borderline, and abnormal values for SF, CIM, and TKM are listed in Table 24-5.

The Humphrey Pathfinder Corneal Analysis system, using SF, CIM, and TKM, approaches the detection of keratoconus differently than do the Rabinowitz or Klyce/Maeda algorithms. By deriving a mathematic model of a general ellipse and a toroid surface that most closely fit the individual CT pattern, the Pathfinder systems attempt to reconstruct a geometric shape. Keratoconic eyes have high SFs, extremely high CIM values, and steep TKMs. Almost spheric (prolate) to negative (oblate) SFs, elevated CIM values, and normal TKMs characterize contact lens–induced pseudokeratoconic shapes.[83] Using the TMS-1 videokeratoscope to measure the central asphericity for normal eyes and eyes with contact lens–induced warpage from rigid gas-permeable (RGP) lenses, a statistically significant reduction in central asphericity has been reported.[84] From analysis of these geometric data,

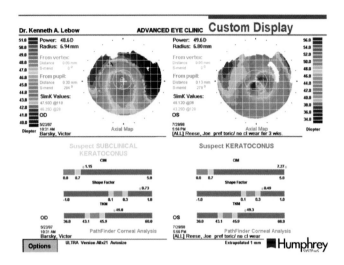

FIG. 24-9. *Pathfinder (Humphrey Systems) software module showing subclinical and true keratoconus detection using corneal irregularity measure, shape factor, and mean toric K value. (CIM = corneal irregularity measure; SimK = simulated K reading; TKM = toric mean reference curvature.)*

similar shapes can be readily identified and differentiated by their unique geometry. The use of these indices represents a new approach to the detection and differentiation of keratoconus and contact lens–induced warpage. No comparisons between Pathfinder and other keratoconus detection programs have been reported. Table 24-6 represents the relative sensitivity and specificity of various keratoconus detection programs.

CORNEAL EDEMA

Increased corneal edema has been associated with changes in corneal curvature,[85,86] but concomitant CT pattern changes are difficult to correlate with areas of increased corneal thickening, especially when edema is induced with nitrogen chamber goggles.[87] This phenomenon may result from the inherent difference in swelling characteristics between polymethylmethacrylate (PMMA), RGP, and soft contact lenses. Hypoxia-induced curvature changes with PMMA and RGP lenses are not uniform across the corneal surface, causing localized curvature changes.[88,89] Because edema with soft lenses (and probably from nitrogen chamber goggles) is more uniformly spread across the entire corneal surface, topographic changes are less apparent.[90,91] When topographic changes in corneal thickness are measured by ultrasound pachymetry over the corneal surface in response to 2 hours' wear of a thick hydrogel

TABLE 24-4. *Summary Description of Various Corneal Indices Used with the Pathfinder Corneal Analysis Module for the Humphrey Systems Atlas Corneal Topographer*

Index	Description
SF	The *shape factor* is a measure of the asphericity of the cornea and a derivative of eccentricity. The SF index can be used to determine whether the cornea is more oval or elliptical in shape. SF is unique and different from eccentricity in that it is possible to calculate a negative, or oblate, shape, as well as a positive, or prolate, shape. Normal human SFs vary from 0.13 to 0.35; borderline SFs vary from 0.02 to 0.12 and 0.36 to 0.46; abnormal SFs vary from –1.0 to 0.01 and 0.47 to 1.0.
CIM	*Corneal irregularity measure* is a number or index assigned to represent the irregularity of the corneal surface. The higher the irregularity index, the more uncorrectable or uneven the surface is optically. High CIM values call attention to irregular astigmatism that often results in visual distortion. Mathematically, CIM represents the standard deviation of the difference in height between the perfect model of the patient's cornea and the actual cornea measured in micrometers. Normal human CIM values vary from 0.03 to 0.68 μ; borderline CIM values vary from 0.69 to 1.0 μ; abnormal CIM values vary from 1.1 to 5.0 μ.
TKM	*Mean toric keratometry* value is derived using elevation data from the best fit toric reference surface compared to the actual cornea. Two values are calculated at the apex of the flattest meridian and their mean is determined. This is described as the mean value of the apical curvature. The higher the TKM index becomes, the greater the likelihood that excessive corneal toricity exists, a condition that often is associated with keratoconus. By fitting the topography of the patient's cornea to the best-fit toric reference, all the correctable sphere and cylinder can be accounted for in the topographic data. Normal human TKM values vary from 43.1 to 45.9 D; borderline TKM values vary from 41.8 to 43.0 D and 46.0 to 47.2 D; abnormal TKM values vary from 36.0 to 41.7 and 47.3 to 60.0 D.

Source: Reprinted with permission from DW Doughman: Corneal edema. In TD Duane, EA Jaeger (eds): Clinical Ophthalmology. Harper & Row, Philadelphia, 1985.

lens, a complex and dynamic process begins in which the greatest amount of edema occurs in the central and midperipheral temporal cornea.[92] This is directly influenced by local and regional lens thickness profiles.[93] Hence, diffuse areas of central corneal steepening are often associated with the overnight wear of hydrogel lenses. It may also result from hydrogel lens adherence to the cornea because of on-eye lens dehydration causing a steeper base curve–to-cornea fitting relationship, thereby producing

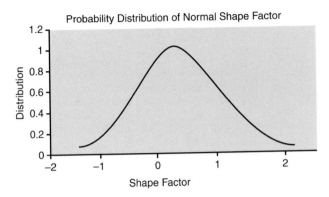

FIG. 24-10. *The distribution of normal corneal shape factor in the human population appears as a bell-shaped curve in which the mean value is 0.24 and 96% of the population falls between 0 and 0.46.*

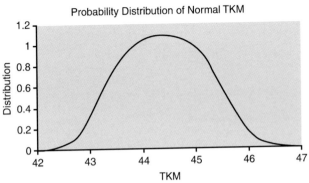

FIG. 24-12. *Normal probability distribution for toric mean reference curvature in the general population. The toric mean reference curvature distribution appears as a bell-shaped curve in which the mean value is 44.5 and 96% of the population falls between 41.25 and 47.25 D. (TKM = toric mean reference curvature.) (Courtesy of Humphrey Systems.)*

corneal edema.[94] Owing to the lack of significant slit-lamp findings, however, this subtle edema is visible only with a detailed topographic analysis of CT. Qualitative CT analysis of hydrogel-induced corneal edema is also quite subtle and may demonstrate only minor areas of central corneal steepening. Only when edematous maps are compared with pre-fitting baseline findings does the zone of corneal steepening become more apparent (Fig. 24-13).

Quantitatively, one would expect a relative increase in the SF because a steeper central curvature with flatter peripheral curvature increases corneal eccentricity.[95] Actually, a stable-to-slightly increased CIM value occurs because hydro-

gel-induced edema is uniformly dispersed over the corneal surface and corneal smoothness is not meaningfully altered. These values generally remain within normal limits. The patient depicted in Fig. 24-13 had been sleeping in daily-wear hydrogel lenses; the magnitude of the changes in such a situation gives practitioners a critical scale to detect corneal edema and monitor its resolution.

CORNEAL TOPOGRAPHY CHANGES ASSOCIATED WITH CONTACT LENS WEAR

Rigid[96-100] and soft[99,100] contact lenses are known to be able to change the corneal curvature. Initial adaptation to PMMA lenses usually causes increased corneal steepening,[102,108] which gradually returns to baseline levels as

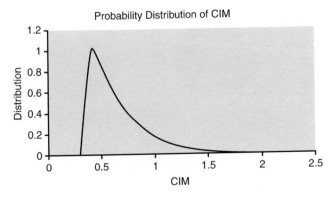

FIG. 24-11. *The distribution in the human population with a mean corneal irregularity measure value of 0.63 μ and 67% of the population falls between 0.03 and 0.64 μ. A bell-shaped distribution curve is not seen because negative numbers cannot be calculated using corneal irregularity measure, thus resulting in a skewed distribution plot. (CIM = corneal irregularity measure.)*

TABLE 24-5. *Normal, Borderline, and Abnormal Values for Shape Factor, Corneal Irregularity Measure, and Toric Mean Reference Curvature*

	Shape Factor	Corneal Irregularity Measure	Toric Mean Reference Curvature
Normal	0.13–0.35	0.03–0.68 μ	43.1–45.9 D
Borderline	0.02–0.12	0.69–1.0 μ	41.8–43.0 D
	0.36–0.46		46.0–47.2 D
Abnormal	−1.0–0.01	1.1–5.0 μ	36.0–41.7 D
	0.47–1.0		47.3–60.0 D

Source: Reprinted with permission from DW Doughman: Corneal edema. In TD Duane, EA Jaeger (eds): Clinical Ophthalmology. Harper & Row, Philadelphia, 1985.

TABLE 24-6. *Relative Sensitivity and Specificity of Various Keratoconus Detection Systems*

Detection Procedure	Key Criteria for Keratoconus Detection	Sensitivity Analysis	Specificity Analysis
Holladay diagnostic summary[71]	Not applicable	Not applicable	Not applicable
Rabinowitz test[57,75,76]	Central keratometry threshold = 48.7 D Inferior-superior value threshold = 1.9	High sensitivity (+ + + +)	Moderate specificity (+ +)
Simulated keratometry values	Mean average simulated keratometry threshold = 45.57 D	Least sensitive (+)	Least specific (+)
Klyce/Maeda keratoconus prediction index[57,78]	Discriminant analysis of eight corneal indices	Higher sensitivity (+ + +)	Higher specificity (+ + +)
Klyce/Maeda keratoconus index[57,77]	Logic-based rules to evaluate the similarity of topography pattern to that of typical kerato-conus (100%) or no detectable keratoconus (0%)	High sensitivity (+ + + +)	Moderate specificity (+ +)
Classification Neural Network keratoconus severity index[57,79]	Ten topographic indexes	Most sensitive (+ + + +)	Most specific) (+ + + +
Pathfinder Corneal Analysis Module[85]	Shape factor Corneal irregularity Index Toric mean reference curvature	High sensitivity (+ + + +)	High specificity (+ + + +)

adaptation is achieved and, after approximately 1 year of lens wear, actually flattens the corneal curvature beyond baseline values.[102,108] Ultimately, the corneal contour grows more spheric and symmetric with well-fit, aligned, or nearly aligned rigid lenses.[100] However, corneal molding by the back surface of a spheric base curve can occur with mild-to-moderate corneal toricity, resulting in spheri-calization of the corneal curvature (Fig. 24-14).[101] The upper left axial map demonstrates no contact lens wear and shows symmetric with-the-rule corneal toricity of

1.75 D; the upper right map shows the influence of RGP lens wear, which reduces toricity to 1.00 D. The difference map on the bottom demonstrates the central flattening and sphericalization of the cornea from the lenses. Because the SF (not shown) reduced from 0.40 before lens wear to 0.04 after lens wear, this contact lens not only induced some sphericalization but also created slight corneal warpage and an orthokeratologic effect.

Normal curvature changes associated with RGP lenses are related to contact lens oxygen transmissibility per-

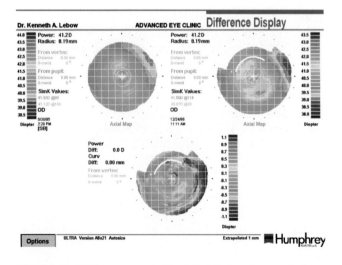

FIG. 24-13. *Difference map of hydrogel-induced corneal edema comparing baseline (upper left) with edematous (upper right) corneal maps in a patient using daily-wear lenses overnight. (SimK = simulated K reading.)*

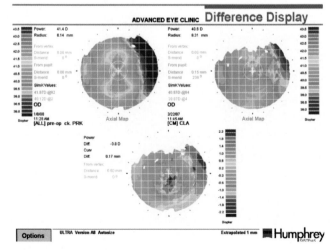

FIG. 24-14. *Corneal topographic map demonstrating corneal sphericalization resulting from rigid contact lens wear. (SimK = simulated K reading.)*

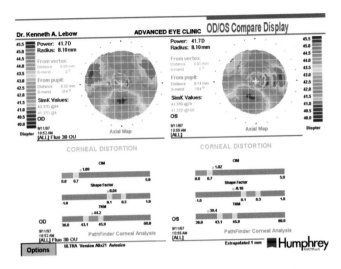

FIG. 24-15. *Left and right eye comparison axial corneal topographic maps demonstrating contact lens–induced corneal warpage, as demonstrated by superior corneal flattening and inferior corneal steepening, associated with a high-riding, flat-fitting rigid gas-permeable lens. (CIM = corneal irregularity measure; SimK = simulated K reading; TKM = toric mean reference curvature.)*

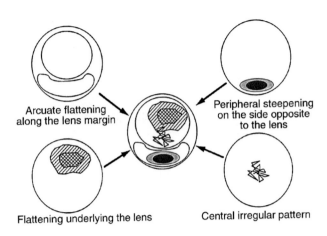

FIG. 24-16. *Composite topographic patterns of contact lens–induced warpage associated with superiorly decentered rigid contact lens fit. (Reprinted with permission from N Maeda, SD Klyce, H Hamano: Alteration of corneal asphericity in rigid gas permeable contact lens induced warpage. CLAO J 20:27, 1994.)*

formance resulting in minimal, insignificant keratometric changes.[102] Even with RGP extended-wear lenses, corneal curvature changes are minimal and typically result in post–lens wear curvatures flatter than baseline readings.[103,104] However, using aspheric, highly oxygen-permeable RGP lenses has been shown to create significant changes in corneal curvature, especially in the vertical meridian.[105] Soft lenses also demonstrate an initial corneal flattening with adaptation[106] followed by corneal steepening, but the likelihood of finding large curvature changes secondary to soft lens wear is low.[106,107] The majority of these reports, however, relied solely on the keratometer to measure curvature variations. Using CT to assess corneal curvature changes in normal asymptomatic rigid and soft lens wearers demonstrates that corneal topographic alterations are common in asymptomatic contact lens wearers and frequently are only detectable with computer-assisted topographic analysis.[108] Rigid contact lenses, presumably owing to their increased lens mass, produce more frequent and severe topographic abnormalities than do daily- or extended-wear soft lenses, but soft lenses can also change the CT.[65,108,109] Although these curvature changes are considered adaptive and "normal," alterations in CT from contact lenses should be limited to changes in simulated keratometry readings and not abnormal CT pattern development or significant changes in the statistical indices. Problems such as corneal molding, distor-

tion, warpage, and contact lens adhesion are capable of significantly changing the corneal geometry, altering normal CT, and ultimately affecting visual acuity.

CONTACT LENS DISTORTION OR WARPAGE

Corneal distortion owing to prolonged hypoxia occurs in approximately 30% of PMMA lens wearers[110] and is evidenced by distorted keratometric mires with or without irregular astigmatism and decreased postwear refraction visual acuity.[111] Corneal warpage syndrome is associated with PMMA, RGP, and soft lens wearers and is topographically characterized by central irregular astigmatism, loss of radial symmetry, and reversal of the normal progressive flattening of the corneal contour from the apex to the periphery.[56] Qualitatively, this results in an abnormal CT pattern demonstrating superior corneal flattening with inferior steepening on the side opposite the lens that may be difficult to differentiate from true keratoconus (Fig. 24-15).[55] Compared to normal eyes, thinner inferotemporal corneas can offer additional confirmation of the presence of keratoconus, although this phenomenon has not be investigated in eyes with contact lens–induced warpage.[112] Moreover, combining ultrasound pachymetry and CT may allow for a potentially more sensitive classification of the severity of keratoconus.[113] Other videokeratographic patterns of contact lens–induced corneal warpage include central irregular patterns and arcuate flattening along the lens margin (Fig. 24-16).[114]

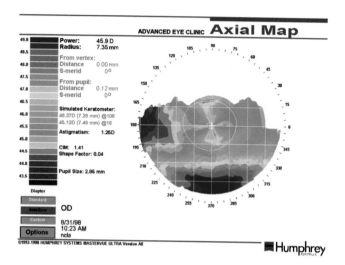

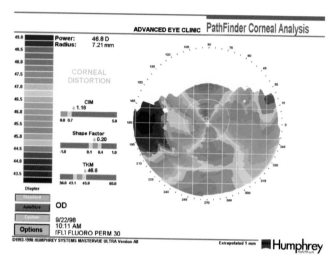

FIG. 24-17. *Axial map demonstrating contact lens–induced corneal distortion with radial asymmetry, superior flattening, inferior steepening, increased irregularity, and a relatively oblate corneal shape owing to a poorly fitting rigid gas-permeable contact lens. (CIM = corneal irregularity measure.)*

FIG. 24-18. *Same eye as in Fig. 24-17, showing improved symmetry in with-the-rule toricity, less irregularity, and a more normal prolate corneal shape after refitting with a flatter-fitting base curve-to-cornea relationship. (CIM = corneal irregularity measure; TKM = toric mean reference curvature.)*

Quantitatively, contact lens–induced corneal warpage is described by an extremely low prolate to moderately oblate SF, relatively flat TKM, and slightly elevated CIM.[86,88] Orthokeratology and refractive surgery CT maps produce a similar qualitative appearance with significantly different quantitative findings.[68] For rigid lenses, the most significant risk factor associated with corneal topographic change appears to be lens decentration, resulting in relative flattening of the corneal curvature under the resting position of the lens.[54,56] Moreover, refitting PMMA-warped corneas with RGP lenses may not alter or improve this abnormal topographic pattern.[27]

REFITTING CORNEAL DISTORTION

The goal of refitting a distorted cornea is to return the postfitting refraction, keratometry, corneal shape, and best corrected visual acuity to prefitting levels. Corneal distortion is typically manifest in CT with superior flattening, inferior steepening, and radial asymmetry associated with an increase in corneal irregularity and an oblate or just slightly prolate shape. The proper base curve–to-cornea fitting relationship is the key variable required to reverse corneal distortion patterns. Remember, astigmatic corneas, when sphericalized, are just as distorted as spheric corneas that manifest superior flat-

tening, inferior steepening, and radial asymmetry. Figure 24-17 shows a cornea that has been flattened superiorly and centrally with significant inferior steepening and radial asymmetry as a result of a steep-fitting RGP contact lens. The CIM value is elevated (1.41) and the SF (0.04), although not oblate, is greatly reduced and relatively oblate based on a normal population distribution. There was no apparent distortion of topography rings, but the best corrected visual acuity immediately after the removal of contact lenses was ²⁰/₄₀. A flatter-fitting base curve was applied in an attempt to achieve an alignment fitting relationship and allow the cornea to return to its prefitting curvature. Subsequent CT shows the formation of symmetric with-the-rule toricity with a reduction in corneal irregularity to 1.18 and an increase in corneal shape to 0.20, representing a more normal prolate shape (Fig. 24-18). Postfitting refractive changes also returned the patient's vision to ²⁰/₂₀. Although statistically this CT pattern is considered to represent a normal corneal shape (symmetric with-the-rule astigmatism), elevated CIM values and increased TKM still define this eye as distorted. The overall changes in corneal shape as a result of achieving the proper fitting relationship are clearly seen in the difference map comparing pre- and postfitting topography patterns (Fig. 24-19). Based on this analysis, it appears that this cornea was depressed centrally as a result of the original lens fit, and refitting allowed the central cornea to steepen or pop back into a more normal shape, allowing the reformation of the apparently pre-existing corneal toricity.

KERATOCONUS

Keratoconus is a bilateral disorder of corneal shape with gradual progression of central corneal steepening, corneal thinning (ectasia), and Vogt's striae that is generally thought to be irreversible.[115] Topographically, steepening of the cornea curvature produces a highly irregular surface, resulting in a high CIM value. With a more rapid rate of flattening than normal from the corneal apex to the periphery measured along the flattest corneal meridian, a large prolate SF (high eccentricity) is also present. Finally, excessive apical toricity results in a steep TKM value (see Fig. 24-5).

Keratoconus is presumed to be caused by a functional loss of the structural elements and reduced tensile strength of the cornea, which results in an overall stretching of the tissue, producing increased curvature and a protruding surface area.[116] Although the normal corneal stroma is characterized by two preferred collagen fibril orientations orthogonal to each other, alteration of this regular arrangement in keratoconus may be related to the biomechanical instability of the tissue.[117] The stromal matrix of edematous corneas reveals wavy lamellae and collagen-free zones rather than decreases in the quantity of corneal lamellae.[118] Theoretically, when corneal fibrils lengthen and surface area increases, as in the case of keratoconus, regions of high curvature surrounded by transition zones of lower curvature are created. This would result in high TKM and SF values. When compared to a normal cornea with progressive peripheral flattening (prolate SF), rearranging the corneal fibrils, as occurs with contact lens–induced warpage, results in a decrease in the central curvature with a concomitant increase in the peripheral curvature. This causes low TKM and SF values with possible oblate SFs. Although true keratoconus and contact lens–induced warpage produce shapes that are dissimilar, their increased irregularity (high CIM value) implies that neither shape approximates that of the normal cornea. Moreover, the substantially greater irregularity associated with keratoconus may be associated with increased epithelial distortion and stromal scarring. Thus, contact lens–induced warpage and keratoconus are structural corneal irregularities that may have distinctly unique etiologies in spite of visually similar CT patterns. Because the literature has several references to contact lenses causing keratoconus,[56,60,119,120] it is important for practitioners to distinguish between these two conditions.

The location of and power at the apex of a cone are important considerations in CT, and they vary depend-

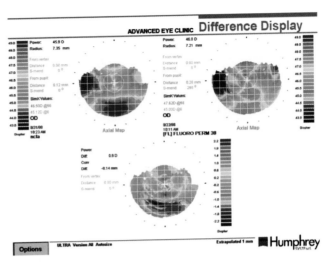

FIG. 24-19. *Difference map for the eye shown in Figs. 24-17 and 24-18, demonstrating the appropriate refitting topography changes obtained when the proper base curve–to–cornea fitting relationship is achieved. (SimK = simulated K reading.)*

ing on the map display (e.g., axial, tangential, or elevation). In keratoconic eyes, axial and instantaneous maps differ significantly in apical position and apex curvature; in the instantaneous map, the corneal apex is consistently located closer to the center.[121] Although axial power maps are less sensitive to noise than refractive, instantaneous, or position power maps, instantaneous power maps provide the most sensitive measure of local curvature changes, such as those occurring in keratoconus or refractive surgery.[122,123] Although instantaneous radius may better represent actual corneal shape, axial curvatures better predict the final RGP base curve in keratoconus patients.[131] However, elevation maps are currently thought to provide the best indication for the location of the corneal apex in keratoconus. Figure 24-20 demonstrates the difference in curvature and apex location when a keratoconic eye is mapped using these different strategies. The steepest curvature (58.1 D) on the axial map is located 1.77 mm at 284 degrees from the vertex position, whereas on the tangential map, the steepest curvature (60.9 D) is located closer to the corneal apex at 1.45 mm and 284 degrees. The elevation map shows the highest point over the reference sphere to be located slightly between the axial and tangential locations at 1.59 mm and 324 degrees from the corneal vertex.

Axial maps—and to a greater degree, instantaneous maps—are capable of demonstrating optically significant shape asymmetries, but they can also misrepre-

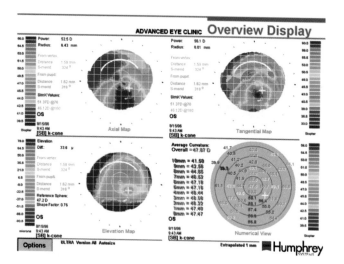

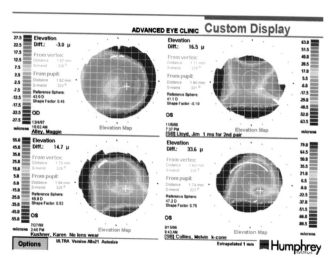

FIG. 24-20. *Overview display with axial, tangential, elevation, and numeric maps of a keratoconic eye demonstrating different locations and curvatures for the presumed apex location of the cone. The white plus sign in the elevation map shows the presumed location of the corneal apex based on elevation data and the differences seen in both the axial and tangential maps. (SimK = simulated K reading.)*

FIG. 24-21. *Custom display of elevation maps comparing normal elevation (upper right), corneal warpage (upper left), subclinical keratoconus (lower left), and keratoconus (lower right) demonstrating a marked elevation of corneal apex of the keratoconic eye over the reference sphere.*

sent refractive power away from the apex.[124] Normal decentration of the corneal apex in keratoconus itself causes significant power errors, but even without proper alignment at the cone apex, instantaneous power maps are more accurate than standard (sagittal) power maps.[125] However, although keratoconic eyes less than 55 D at the apex provided reasonably valid measurements, cones exceeding 55 D have greater errors in measurements with some CT systems, even assuming that proper (apex) alignment was achieved.[126] Elevation maps show true CT,[133] and when the height of a cone exceeds that of the reference curvature, the location of the apex becomes readily apparent (Fig. 24-21).[127]

CT also gives the practitioner the ability to map and observe the progression of keratoconus (i.e., areas of corneal steepening) and to distinguish its various types. One study found a marginally increased sensitivity in detecting and quantifying keratoconus based on inferior-superior asymmetry thickness measurements (pachymetry) compared to inferior-superior asymmetry videokeratometric measurements.[123] However, controversy exists about the exact location of the apex of the cone in keratoconus. It is generally believed that the cone apex is most frequently located in the inferonasal paracentral corneal quadrant because this is the location of the most senile epithelial cells.[128] Nasal, supe-

rior, and central areas of corneal steepening have also been identified as possible cone locations.[129] Initially, steepening occurs midperipherally, below the corneal midline, but as the severity of keratoconus progresses, steepening can spread more nasally to include the inferior 6 o'clock position and inferonasal cornea. Ultimately, this causes rotation at and above the midline along a path that includes temporal, superior temporal, and 12 o'clock corneal areas (Fig. 24-22).[130] This may explain the various locations of steepest curvature reported in the literature, and it was confirmed with pachymetry measurements.

Because most of the significant changes in keratoconus occur beyond the 3-mm area measured by the keratometer, various keratoconic shapes have been identified using CT.[131,140] Originally, *nipple, oval*, and *globus* cones were described,[132] but a bow-tie–shaped cone has also been reported, although the bow-tie pattern appears to be more gaze dependent than the other patterns (Fig. 24-23).[141] It is possible that alterations in the amount of corneal asphericity through simple manipulation of the cornea SF are responsible for the bow-tie pattern observed in CT power maps.[133] Although keratoconus is generally accepted as a contraindication to refractive surgery, the concept of a physiologically "displaced apex syndrome" may allow positive refractive surgery results in some patients whose maps appear to demonstrate true keratoconus.[64]

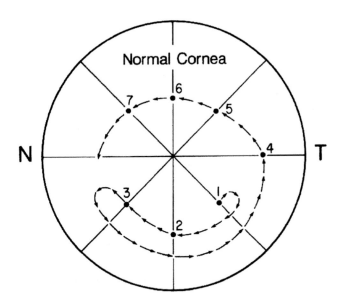

FIG. 24-22. *Quadrantal pattern of keratoconus progression, with initial steepening in the inferior temporal quadrant. (N = nasal; T = temporal.) (Reprinted with permission from PJ Caroline, MA Andre, C Norman: Corneal topography in keratoconus. Contact Lens Spectrum 12:36, 1997.)*

SUBCLINICAL KERATOCONUS

Subclinical keratoconus consists of mild topographic changes occurring on CT maps in the absence of associated visual, refractive, biomicroscopic, or keratometric changes.[62] This apparently abortive form of keratoconus may demonstrate autosomal dominant and recessive inheritance patterns with incomplete penetrance.[134] Members of the immediate family of individuals with keratoconus may have increased corneal steepening and astigmatism,[135] although other members may exhibit no topographic changes.[63] These findings are usually less severe than those found in true keratoconus and may represent the variable expression of a gene contributing to the development of keratoconus.[136] Moreover, videokeratography has confirmed the presence of early keratoconus in the apparently unaffected eye among patients who were originally diagnosed with unilateral keratoconus, suggesting that keratoconus is almost always bilateral with genetic influences in the pathogenesis of the disease.[137,138]

Although subclinical keratoconus qualitatively resembles true keratoconus, the geometric indices used to describe the cornea are not as severe. Because of its similarity with keratoconus and corneal warpage, subclinical keratoconus is often hard to differentiate clinically and topographically. Using Humphrey Systems' Pathfinder Corneal Analysis software, the CIM and TKM

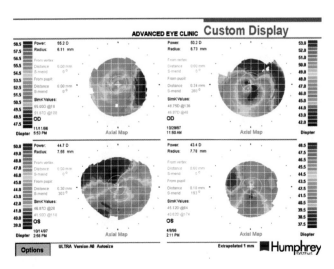

FIG. 24-23. *Custom display showing axial maps of nipple (upper left), oval (upper right), globus (lower left), and bow-tie (lower right) keratoconus patterns. (SimK = simulated K reading.)*

may be moderately abnormal, whereas the SF remains normal to slightly abnormal (Fig. 24-24).[139] By using serial CT measurements, however, the progression of subclinical keratoconus to true keratoconus can be documented.[61] A difference map clearly shows the progression of subclinical keratoconus from one visit to another (Fig. 24-25).

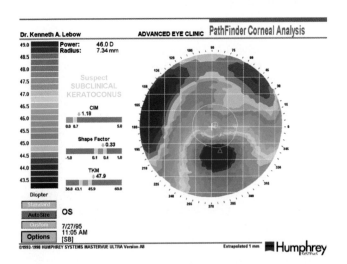

FIG. 24-24. *Corneal analysis map showing subclinical keratoconus with abnormal corneal irregularity measure and toric mean reference curvatures with normal to slightly abnormal shape factor value. (CIM = corneal irregularity measure; TKM = toric mean reference curvature.)*

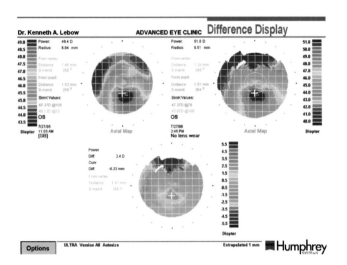

FIG. 24-25. *Difference map showing the progression of a subclinical keratoconus to true keratoconus with greater inferior steepening. (SimK = simulated K reading.)*

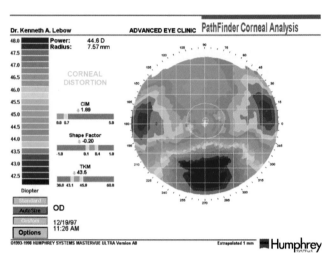

FIG. 24-26. *Corneal analysis map demonstrating radial asymmetry associated with a displaced corneal apex mimicking true keratoconus in a case of contact lens–induced pseudokeratoconus (warpage or distortion). (CIM = corneal irregularity measure; TKM = toric mean reference curvature.)*

PSEUDOKERATOCONUS

Pseudokeratoconus is a term generally applied to videokeratographs that demonstrate radially asymmetric bowtie patterns but without clinical biomicroscopic signs or symptoms of true keratoconus (Fig. 24-26).[50] This term has also been used to describe subclinical keratoconus and contact lens–induced corneal warpage, which has resulted in some confusion.

Frequently, pseudokeratoconus results from a misalignment of the videokeratograph from the corneal apex and the algorithm used for the calculation of corneal power.[50,140] Misalignment deviations as small as 5 degrees can produce videokeratographs demonstrating inferior corneal steepening, which mimics true keratoconus with increased inferior-superior values.[141] Often, proper alignment over the corneal apex produces increased symmetry, which indicates that a decentered apex may be the cause of the radial asymmetry. However, early keratoconus or subclinical keratoconus with excellent spectacle visual acuity, minimal distortion of keratometer mires, and relatively normal apical curvatures can produce similar topographic patterns.[142,143]

CONTACT LENS ADHESION

When either rigid or soft contact lenses stop moving on the eye, the lens is said to adhere. Generally, lens adhesion occurs with extended wear,[144,145] although the problem can also occur when lenses are removed overnight[146] and, for rigid lens wearers, adhesion appears to be a patient-dependent phenomenon.[147] Estimates of the frequency of lens adhesion vary from 30% to 100% of extended-wear patients.[11,12] Because the observation of lens binding most frequently occurs immediately on awakening, blink-induced lens movements may initiate lens movement and obscure any biomicroscopic evidence of lens adhesion. Rigid lenses produce more and greater sequelae than do hydrogel lenses, including corneal staining and a compression or indentation ring in the midperipheral cornea (Fig. 24-27).[148]

In the absence of obvious slit-lamp evidence of rigid lens adhesion (i.e., central staining and indentation ring), analysis of videokeratoscopic images and CT maps provides valuable information on the presence and severity of lens binding. The most direct indication of lens binding can be seen in the actual videokeratoscopic image. Normally, no deflection or obstruction of the reflected placido ring image implies the absence of lens adhesion (see Fig. 24-28A). When a contact lens adheres to the corneal surface, the placido rings are displaced in an S-shaped fashion (see Fig. 24-28B–24-28D). With increasingly greater severity of lens adhesion, a greater number of adjacent rings demonstrates a deflection from their normal path, and based on the severity of the indentation ring, some rings actually lose their normal visibility and continuity. Depending on the severity of lens binding, observation of videokeratoscopic images can be used to

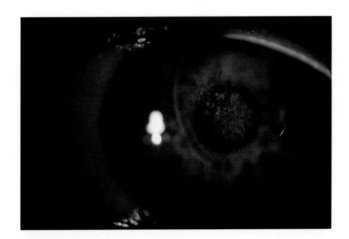

FIG. 24-27. *Photograph of central corneal staining and midperipheral compression or indentation, or both, secondary to rigid gas-permeable lens adhesion to the ocular surface.*

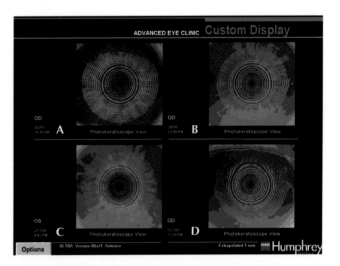

FIG. 24-28. *Custom display demonstrating videokeratoscopic images of no lens compression (**A**), mild (**B**), moderate (**C**), and severe (**D**) lens compression. The images show various S-shaped displacements in the placido ring contour, wavelike distortions, increasing ring involvement, and deterioration of ring visibility and continuity.*

categorize lens adhesion as mild, moderate, or severe (Table 24-7 and Fig. 24-28).

Axial and tangential (instantaneous) maps have demonstrated the ability to represent *micro* (mild and moderate) and *macro* (severe) distortions, but only elevation maps can measure the depth of the indentation ring (relative to a reference sphere), thus offering a more accurate method to classify the severity of lens binding. Although definitive studies of this analysis have not yet appeared, comparing the elevation maps represented by the videokeratoscopic images in Fig. 24-29 demonstrates the principle that greater depression on the corneal surface is associated with more severe lens binding.

PELLUCID MARGINAL DEGENERATION

Pellucid marginal degeneration is a noninflammatory corneal thinning disorder that can mimic keratoconus

CT maps. Although histopathologically, pellucid marginal degeneration is considered a variant of keratoconus, it differs from keratoconus in that the marked corneal steepening occurs more inferiorly (usually between 4 and 8 o'clock) and above a narrow band (1–2 mm) of corneal stromal thinning concentric to the inferior limbus.[149] Also, a 1- to 2-mm wide region of uninvolved normal cornea exists between the thinned region and the limbus. This often results in high against-the-rule corneal astigmatism and minimal central corneal distortion, producing gull-winged areas of inferior corneal steepening.[150] Much larger and more diffuse areas of steepening are associated with this corneal degeneration (Fig. 24-30).

TABLE 24-7. *Classification of the Severity of Contact Lens Adhesion Based on the Observation of Placido Ring Deflection and Clarity*

Classification	Ring Deflection	Ring Clarity
No lens compression	Normal ring appearance	Normal ring clarity
Mild lens compression	Peripheral S-shaped displacement 2–3 rings involved	Normal ring clarity
Moderate lens compression	Peripheral S-shaped displacement Wavelike distortion 4–5 rings involved	Slight obliteration of ring quality and continuity
Severe lens compression	Peripheral S-shaped displacement Wavelike distortion 7–8 rings involved	Complete obliteration of ring quality and continuity

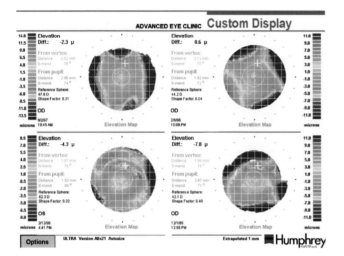

FIG. 24-29. *Custom display demonstrating elevation maps of no lens compression (upper left), mild (upper right), moderate (lower left), and severe (lower right) lens compression showing "micro" and "macro" (see text) corneal compression and the amount the indented surface falls below the calculated reference sphere.*

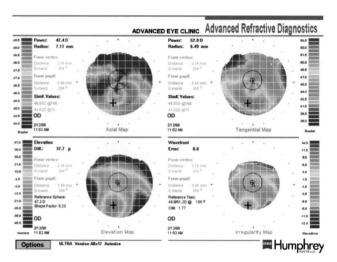

FIG. 24-30. *Advanced refractive diagnostic map of pellucid marginal degeneration showing axial (upper left), tangential (upper right), elevation (lower left), and irregularity (lower right) maps. Pellucid marginal degeneration demonstrates a topography pattern that mimics keratoconus, with superior flattening and inferior flattening vertically (against-the-rule astigmatism) but with a larger, more diffuse zone of inferior steepening. Marked peripheral elevation over the reference sphere inferiorly and a relatively low corneal irregularity measure can also be seen. (CIM = corneal irregularity measure; SimK = simulated K reading.)*

CHANGES IN ORTHOKERATOLOGY

Orthokeratology is the deliberate attempt to modify the corneal curvature to produce a reduction or elimination of the refractive anomaly by programmed application of contact lenses.[151] Initially, central keratometry values were used to monitor the progress of corneal changes, but they were quite limited in their ability to describe the changes that occurred to the overall corneal geometry.[68] CT analysis facilitates the selection of appropriate candidates for this procedure, demonstrates the effect of progressive base curve flattening on the corneal geometry, aids in the determination of a stopping point in the treatment, and monitors the process for the development of abnormal surface changes.

Early attempts to select appropriate orthokeratology candidates involved the evaluation of peripheral corneal flattening using the general formula (flat central K reading) – (peripheral K reading) (2) + (1 D) to predict the maximum potential myopic reduction.[152] If the refractive error equaled or was less than the dioptric value calculated by the peripheral flattening formula, emmetropization was possible. Positive correlation between corneal eccentricity and changes in subjective refraction was found to be a good predictor of improvement in visual acuity in orthokeratology.[153,154] CT can provide peripheral curve and eccentricity (SF) values more easily and consistently than

keratometry, thereby providing an excellent screening tool for evaluating candidates for this procedure. Although no orthokeratology contact lens fitting nomograms are part of a topography system, the data provided by CT make it a logical programming sequence for manufacturers.

The typical post-orthokeratology CT pattern mimics that of refractive surgery, with central flattening, reduced SF, and slightly increased CIM values (Fig. 24-31).

Application of orthokeratology lenses flattens the central corneal curvature while steepening the peripheral curvature, resulting in a sphericalization of the corneal geometry.[161,162] Mathematically, the SF approaches zero as the cornea becomes more spheric, changing its normal prolate shape to a more oblate shape. Analysis of changes in the SF as it varies from prolate (positive) to spheric (zero) to oblate (negative) correlates with the treatment regimen of progressively flatter base curve–to-cornea relationships. Theoretically, orthokeratology is limited to creating minimally oblate surfaces compared to refractive surgery procedures that produce significantly larger negative SFs. Although it is often difficult to directly observe corneal flattening on the axial map, the use of a difference map clearly demonstrates this effect (Fig. 24-32).

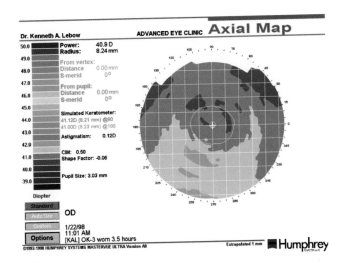

FIG. 24-31. *Axial map demonstrating central corneal flattening over the line of sight in an orthokeratology patient after wearing a flat-fitting contact lens. (CIM = corneal irregularity measure.)*

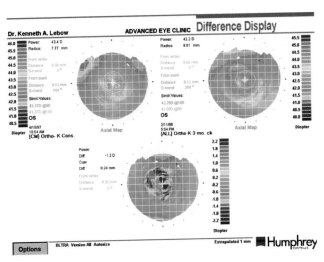

FIG. 24-32. *Difference map comparing baseline (upper left) and postorthokeratology fitting (upper right) demonstrating central corneal flattening positioned directly over the patient's line of sight. (SimK = simulated K reading.)*

Successful orthokeratology patients demonstrate uniform flattening over the line of sight, but lens decentration can create complications similar to those experienced with decentered ablation zones in refractive surgery.

The endpoint of the orthokeratology process has always been difficult to define. One approach is based on reversing the entire refractive error irrespective of corneal curvature. Users of another approach think that a contact lens may not be capable of flattening sufficient corneal curvature to correct all the refractive error. Long-term contact lens decentration can induce curvature changes, including the development of increased corneal astigmatism,[155] which can mimic the corneal distortion syndrome[156] and, in more severe situations, can produce keratoconuslike changes (Fig. 24-33).[157] The application of *reverse-geometry* lenses for *accelerated orthokeratology* has produced new topography patterns. More dramatic zones of central corneal flattening develop, surrounded by a marked ring of midperipheral steepening that corresponds to the reverse peripheral curve on the base curve of the lens (Fig. 24-34).

CONTACT LENS FITTING MODULES

Rigid Gas-Permeable Lenses

Contemporary RGP contact lens fitting requires a delicate balance of many corneal shape and lens design variables. With the increased use of soft lens fitting in the marketplace, clinicians apply these intricate fitting relationships less frequently. Practitioners still use simple central keratometry readings rather than CT maps to fit RGP lenses. The goal of fitting RGP lenses with computer-driven artificial intelligence software is to achieve an appropriate base curve–to-cornea fitting relationship with

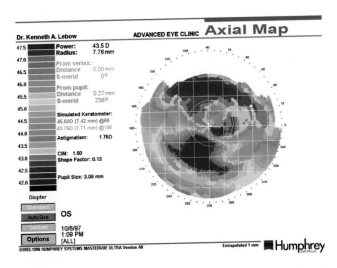

FIG. 24-33. *Axial map showing a superiorly decentered corneal flattening zone owing to a high-riding, flat-fitting spheric base curve orthokeratology contact lens. (CIM = corneal irregularity measure.)*

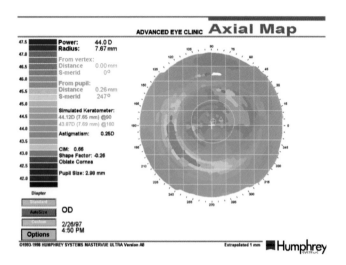

FIG. 24-34. *Axial map showing central corneal flattening surrounded by a midperipheral zone of steepening owing to a reverse-geometry contact lens for orthokeratology. (CIM = corneal irregularity measure.)*

the correct lens power, overall diameter, optical zone, and peripheral curve configuration.

Contact lens base curve selection in computerized topography software uses either axial, tangential, or elevation mapping strategies. Because axial or power maps provide

a running average of the analyzed data for a given peripheral location and are spherically biased, they are more appropriate for base curve selection than are instantaneous mapping strategies. Instantaneous maps, similar in appearance, but smaller than axial maps, provide more accurate localized curvature information and may depict a more accurate fluorescein pattern.[88] Table 24-8 summarizes the similarities and differences between radius of curvature–based (ROC-D) and axial distance–based (AD-D) topography maps.[158]

Topography systems capable of generating elevation data may be more accurate in locating an exact corneal position and hence generate more precise tear film thickness profiles, which are critical for accurate base curve selection and subsequent lens power calculations.[159] Elevation maps represent relative height differences between a computer-generated spheric representation of the corneal surface (reference sphere) and the actual surface.[134] Red or warm colors denote higher elevations relative to the reference surface. These areas displace (touch) fluorescein, whereas blue or cool colors represent areas below the specified reference sphere and pool (clearance) fluorescein (Fig. 24-35). Tear layer thickness models generate fluorescein patterns so that areas of pooling represent greater tear layer thickness. When the mapped area of the cornea has an elevation below the reference sphere (blue or cool colors), it implies that a greater tear layer thickness is present, as demonstrated by pooling in the fluo-

TABLE 24-8. *Differences and Similarities between Radius of Curvature–Based and Axial Distance–Based Topographic Maps*

	ROC-D Shape Representation	AD-D Shape Representation
Numerator	337.5	337.5
Denominator	Radius of curvature (mm)	Axial distance (mm)
Plane of intersection with cornea	Meridional	Meridional
Reference axis	Axis independent	Tied to central reference axis
Curvature	Scaled curvature	Running average of scaled curvature
Pattern	Qualitatively similar to AD	Qualitatively similar to ROC
	Smaller pattern	Bigger pattern
	Features (i.e., cone) are more centrally located	Features (i.e., cone) are pushed toward periphery
Numeric value	Qualitatively different from AD	Qualitatively different from ROC
	Depicts local detail	Average
	Extreme values may be present	Extreme values averaged out
Comparison to refraction	Not appropriate	Not appropriate
Units in diopters	Not power or function	Not power or function
	Shape only	Shape only
Application to clinical practice	Local detail important (i.e., postrefractive surgery)	Global representation needed (i.e., contact lens fitting)
Current terminology	Instantaneous	Axial
	Tangential	Color map
	Local	Default
	Ture	Sagittal

AD = axial distance–based; ROC-D = radius of curvature–based.
Source: Reprinted with permission from B Soper, J Shovlin, E Bennett: Evaluating a topography software program for fitting RGPs. Spectrum 11:37, 1996.

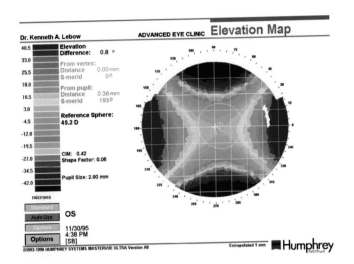

FIG. 24-35. *Elevation map showing relative height differences between a computer-generated reference sphere and the actual corneal curvature. Red or warm zones depict areas above the reference surface, and blue or cool colors depict areas below the reference surface. (CIM = corneal irregularity measure.)*

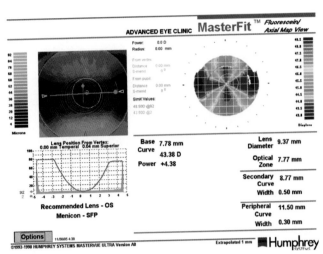

FIG. 24-36. *Simulated fluorescein pattern and axial map of a contact lens placed on the ocular surface demonstrating how a contact lens displaces fluorescein (touch or bearing) in areas coincident with red colors and pools fluorescein (steep or clearance) in areas with blue colors. (SimK = simulated K reading.)*

rescein pattern (Fig. 24-36). This is verified by observing the tear thickness profile on the display. However, axial or curvature maps may not always correlate accurately with clinical fluorescein patterns.

First-generation computerized contact lens fitting nomograms have shown minimal advantages compared to clinical diagnostic fitting procedures.[160,161] Also, errors obtained when measuring the convex surface of ellipsoidal PMMA buttons were sufficiently large to make their use for contact lens fitting questionable.[162] These early fitting systems were limited to applying clinically established manufacturer design recommendations based solely on central corneal curvature and toricity, producing a base curve selection using the same analysis a practitioner had available without the sophistication of corneal mapping.

Contemporary or second-generation contact lens modules use a topographically driven fitting technique to analyze and evaluate the entire CT during initial base curve selection. They calculate suggested posterior lens curves based on a preselected tear layer thickness[163,164] or shape factor (eccentricity), or both.[149] Some systems use a sagittal depth fitting technique,[78] where the software calculates a posterior lens curve beneath an optical zone until a desired tear layer clearance is achieved between the front surface of the cornea and the back surface of the contact lens. Most of these second-generation programs also incorporate some compensation for peripheral corneal flattening into their lens design algorithms.[87] The knowledge of the eccentric-

ity value calculated from videokeratography allows for better prediction of the base curve–to-cornea alignment relationship than was provided by only a central curvature measurement.[165] A study using the Humphrey Systems MasterVue CT software reported 90% base curve selection accuracy and 88% power selection accuracy using this approach.[169] Another study found no significant difference in corneal physiologic response between conventionally derived and computer-designed lenses after 3 months of wear.[166] However, when different instruments' fitting nomograms are compared with identical clinically derived parameters, lens design calculations varied. Even when the same base curve was selected by the topographer, power variations between instruments were as much as a diopter or more.[167] A busy practice can save significant time, however, by using second-generation contact lens fitting programs, especially in the selection of an initial trial lens.[168] Clinically, assistants or practitioners can prefit a patient just by evaluating the simulated fluorescein pattern created on the computer and adjusting the on-screen parameters to achieve an optimum fluorescein fit with a high degree of accuracy.[169] Additionally, second-generation contact lens fitting software should advise practitioners when sufficient corneal toricity is present to warrant the use of toric base or bitoric contact lenses. The simplicity of designing toric lenses in this manner should increase the use of these more complicated contact lenses. Moreover, the application of toric peripheral curves can

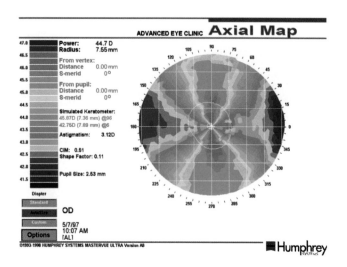

FIG. 24-37. *Axial map of high corneal toricity extending over the entire corneal surface from limbus to limbus. (CIM = corneal irregularity measure.)*

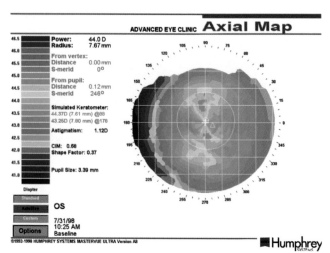

FIG. 24-39. *Axial map of high corneal toricity limited to the central corneal area. (CIM = corneal irregularity measure.)*

be considered when evaluating CT patterns. For example, when corneal toricity extends over the entire corneal surface, the incorporation of toric peripheral curves on a toric base curve helps to stabilize the lens and improve comfort (Fig. 24-37). This software-generated information ensures proper alignment fitting techniques and eliminates the use

of spheric base curve lenses on highly toric corneas, creating marked astigmatic bands (Fig. 24-38). Conversely, when toricity is isolated to the central cornea, not only are toric peripheral curves unnecessary, but often just spheric base curves are required to achieve an alignment fluorescein pattern (Figs. 24-39 and 24-40).

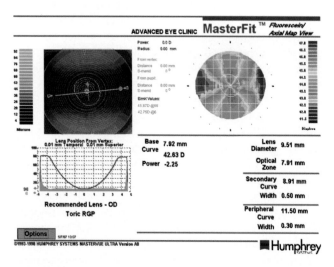

FIG. 24-38. *Simulated fluorescein pattern and axial map of a spheric base curve lens fit for an eye with corneal toricity extending from limbus to limbus, demonstrating a marked with-the-rule bearing pattern. A bitoric lens design is required to achieve a proper base curve–to-cornea fitting relationship. (SimK = simulated K reading.)*

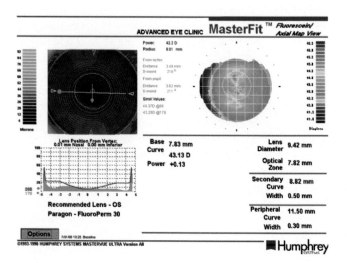

FIG. 24-40. *Simulated fluorescein pattern and axial map of a spheric base curve lens fit for an eye with toricity limited to the central cornea, demonstrating an alignment base curve–to-cornea fitting relationship. (SimK = simulated K reading.)*

Corneal Topography and Contact Lens Complications **501**

Rigid Gas-Permeable Bifocals

No computerized fitting software exists that designs bifocal contact lenses. However, the relative steepness or flatness of the corneal curvature and the location of the apex of the cornea can provide valuable information to aid the practitioner in the lens selection process. Should the corneal apex be centered or superior on the topography map, aspheric bifocal designs are recommended. Conversely, when the corneal apex falls below the geometric center of the cornea, alternating vision lenses appear to be more successful (Fig. 24-41).[170] Combined with the knowledge that aspheric lenses are preferred for steep corneas and alternating designs are preferred for flat corneas, practitioners are now able to select an initial lens design based on the CT.[171]

Preliminary studies mapping the convex surface of aspheric RGP lenses have demonstrated that manufacturing techniques differ for various lenses.[172] These differences are manifest in the overall lens profile (profile map) and represent lenses designed with either mathematically defined conicoid or multispheric posterior surface lens geometry. True aspheric lens geometry manifests a conicoid profile associated with a smaller central apical radius and increased steepness centrally, with a relatively rapid peripheral flattening (Figs. 24-42A and 24-42C). Multispheric posterior lens geometry clearly differs, with progressively flatter concentric or annular spheric zones emanating from a smaller central apical zone (Figs. 24-42B and 24-42D). In the future, computer algorithms may be available to map the anterior corneal surface and compare it to a database of aspheric lens profiles to achieve the ideal fitting relationship and visual performance, thereby simplifying the fitting of this often-complicated lens design.

Soft Toric Lenses

Soft toric contact lens fitting represents another investigational area for the application of CT. To understand which corneas would perform best with soft toric lenses (ocular surface topography) and to evaluate the fit of toric lenses on the eye (over the in situ lens surface), CT can be a valuable adjunct to the fitting and evaluation process. Just as with rigid lens designs, evidence suggests that an understanding of CT aids in the selection and fitting of soft toric lenses. When toricity is limited to the central cornea (see Fig. 24-39), it may be better neutralized by back toric lenses, which enable practitioners to empirically fit lenses to this corneal shape. Toricity that is distributed from limbus to limbus (see Fig. 24-37), however, exhibits significant lens draping, inducing on-eye lens flex-

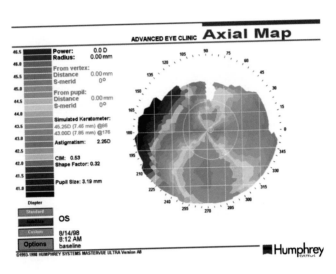

FIG. 24-41. *Axial map demonstrating the inferior placement of the corneal apex (triangle indication), suggesting the use of "alternating design" rigid gas-permeable bifocal contact lenses rather than aspheric or concentric lens designs. (CIM = corneal irregularity measure.)*

ure, and it requires diagnostic lens fitting regardless of lens design.[173] Some reports indicate that soft spheric lenses neutralize corneal toricity,[174] but other studies have demonstrated that fitting spheric soft lenses actually increases corneal toricity on the front lens surface.[175] Regardless, spheric hydrogel lenses of varying center

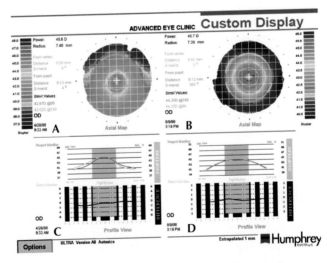

FIG. 24-42. *Custom display demonstrating differences in posterior surface lens geometry (axial maps) and lens profile (profile view) for conicoid (A,C) and multispheric (B,D) aspheric multifocal rigid lenses. (SimK = simulated K reading.)*

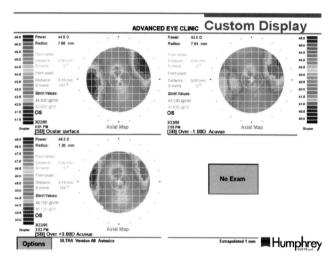

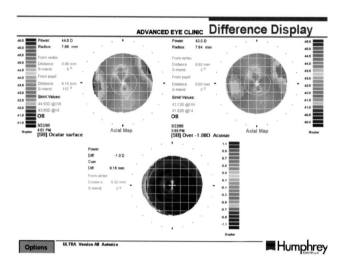

FIG. 24-43. *Custom display, with axial maps of the ocular surface (upper left), over a –1.00 D ACUVUE (Vistakon, Jacksonville, FL) soft lens (upper right) and over a +3.00 D ACUVUE soft lens (lower right), showing that regardless of lens thickness, no masking of corneal toricity exists. (SimK = simulated K reading.)*

FIG. 24-44. *Difference map comparing the ocular toricity with the toricity obtained when a –1.00 D ACUVUE (Vistakon, Jacksonville, FL) lens was mapped over the ocular surface, showing a spheric difference of approximately 1 D (lens power), thus indicating no masking of corneal toricity from this lens. (SimK = simulated K reading.)*

thickness cannot mask corneal toricity in the same sense that RGP lenses provide a sphericalized front surface. Figure 24-43 demonstrates an ocular surface with –1.50 cx 16 (central cornea symmetric astigmatism) and compares it to topography taken on the same eye with a –1.00 D ACUVUE lens (Vistakon, Jacksonville, FL) and +3.00 D lens in place. Regardless of lens thickness (–1.00 D center thickness [ct] = 0.05 mm and +3.00 D ct = 0.15 mm), the CT pattern is identical to the ocular surface, and the measured toricity over the lens surface is virtually identical to that of the ocular surface (–1.00 D shows –1.50 cx 14 and +3.00 D shows –1.62 cx 16). When the corneal surface is compared to the in situ lens surface, a spheric difference map is generated with a power of –1.00 D, showing that the corneal toricity was transferred directly through the lens surface (Fig. 24-44).

In the absence of residual astigmatism, soft toric lenses should neutralize all corneal astigmatism so that the front lens surface appears spheric when a soft toric lens is fit to a cornea with astigmatism. Although soft toric lenses are capable of neutralizing corneal toricity, some patients manifest residual astigmatism on the front surface of a toric soft lens that can interfere with vision.[176] However, if a patient manifests internal astigmatism, the front lens surface should show toricity of an equal amount but opposite in direction to correct for the internal astigmatism. Not withstanding on-eye lens flexure and index of refraction issues, evaluating ocular surface topography and

comparing it with in situ lens surface topography can provide practitioners with a better understanding of lens fit and the optical properties required to correct vision. When difference maps are generated comparing the ocular surface and the in situ lens surface, the total astigmatism should correlate to the manifest refractive astigmatism. The following example presents the basis for using CT to understand how soft lenses fit. Table 24-9

TABLE 24-9. *Summary of Topographic, Refractive, and Contact Lens Data for a Patient*

Ocular surface map	
SimK value	43.00/46.12 (180/90)
Corneal cylinder	–3.12 cx 180
Refraction	–3.00–2.50 cx 180
Internal cylinder	–0.62 cx 90
Contact lens	8.3/–2.50–2.50 cx 170/14.0 CSI toric (Wesley-Jessen, Des Plaines, IL)
In situ contact lens surface map	
SimK value over lens surface	40.25/41.12 (18/108)
On-eye lens cylinder	–0.87 cx 18
Axis shift (on-eye)	Approximately 10 degrees nasal
Difference map	
Sphere power centrally	3.3 D
Cylinder power	Approximately 2.3 D

SimK = simulated K reading.

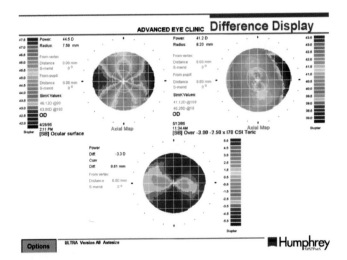

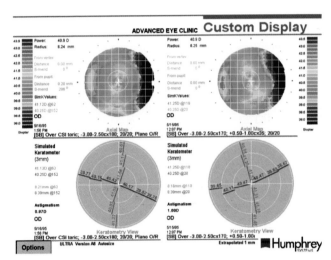

FIG. 24-45. *Difference map comparing the ocular surface with the in situ contact lens surface and the differences generated between the two surfaces. Note that the in situ contact lens surface reduced corneal toricity from 3.00 D to 0.87 D, producing a relative neutralization of the corneal toricity. (SimK = simulated K reading.)*

FIG. 24-46. *Custom display showing axial maps (upper left and right) and keratometry views (lower left and right) of soft toric on-eye lens rotation varying approximately 45 degrees between two soft toric lenses that differ by only 10 degrees in labeled axis. (SimK = simulated K reading.)*

presents the significant topographic, refractive, and contact lens data for a patient. To neutralize the refractive error for this patient, a –3.00 D power is required horizontally and a –5.50 D power vertically. When the SimK of the ocular surface is compared to that of the in situ contact lens surface, the difference generates a contact power of –2.75 D horizontally and –5.00 D vertically. Other than the slight rotation observed in the in situ lens axis (18 degrees instead of 180 degrees), the CT maps confirm the presence of an ideal lens fitting relationship (Fig. 24-45). Moreover, in situ lens rotation can be accurately demonstrated with CT. Figure 24-46 demonstrates two lenses, each with 2.50 D cylinders that vary by only 10 degrees (one at 180 degrees and the other at 170 degrees). Both are significantly rotated in opposite directions, creating an approximate 45-degree difference in position on the eye.

Keratoconus Fitting

Keratoconus, especially in its later stages, represents one of the most difficult contact lens fitting challenges. Using CT provides a rational basis for selecting appropriate trial lenses for these patients[177] from a general quantification of keratoconic types[139] and for specific fitting recommendations. Donshik et al.[161] suggest that in patients with keratoconus, the average flat corneal curvature at the 3.0-mm zone, as measured by the EyeSys videokeratoscope,

appears to be helpful in selecting the initial base curve. Others have suggested that the flattest K reading at the 5-mm zone offers the best initial base curve selection.[178] Regardless, CT provides significantly more information about the cornea in keratoconus.

SUMMARY

The use of the corneal topographer has evolved significantly from a research tool to the standard of care for measuring the corneal surface. CT provides more data about the global shape of the corneal surface, and the incorporation of statistical indices have enabled practitioners to obtain a better understanding of corneal shape and the effect that contact lenses and disease processes have on the cornea. Artificial intelligence programs combined with videokeratoscopy further the capabilities of this technology and help practitioners understand differences between keratoconus, corneal warpage, pellucid marginal degeneration, subclinical keratoconus, and other related conditions. The next generation of contact lens fitting programs will be capable of designing a variety of rigid and soft contact lenses incorporating the effects of on-eye lens flexure and aspheric lens dynamics. Bifocal and keratoconus fitting will become as simple as pushing a button on a software program. Eventually, all keratometers will be replaced with corneal topographers.

REFERENCES

1. Humphreys FJA, Larke JR, Parrish ST: Microepithelial cysts observed in extended contact lens wearing subjects. Br J Ophthalmol 64:888, 1980

2. Zantos SG: Cystic formations in the corneal epithelium during extended wear of contact lenses. Int Contact Lens Clin 10:128, 1983

3. Schoessler JP, Woloschak MJ: Corneal endothelium in veteran PMMA contact lens wearers. Int Contact Lens Clin 8:19, 1981

4. Bonanno JA, Polse KA: Corneal acidosis during contact lens wear: effects of hypoxia and CO_2. Invest Ophthalmol Vis Sci 28:1514, 1987

5. Bonanno JA, Polse KA: Effect of rigid contact lens oxygen transmission on stromal pH in the living human eye. Ophthalmology 94:1305, 1987

6. Kame RT, Herskowitz R: The corneal consequences of hypoxia. In Bennett ES, Grohe RM (eds): Rigid Gas Permeable Contact Lenses. Professional Press, New York, 1986

7. Smelzer G, Ozanics V: Structural changes of corneas of guinea pigs after wearing contact lenses. Am J Ophthalmol 88:543, 1953

8. Levitt AP: Specific gravity and RGP lens performance. Spectrum 11:43, 1996

9. Carney LG: Corneal topography changes during contact lens wear. Contact Lens J 3:5, 1974

10. Carney LG: The basis for corneal shape change during contact lens wear. Am J Optom 52:445, 1975

11. Swarbrick HA: A possible etiology for RGP lens binding (adherence). Int Contact Lens Clin 15:13, 1988

12. Swarbrick HA, Holden BA: Rigid gas permeable lens binding: significance and contributing factors. Am J Optom Physiol Opt 64:815, 1987

13. Rivera RK, Polse KA: Corneal response to different oxygen levels during extended wear. CLAO J 17:96, 1991

14. Young G, Port M: Rigid gas permeable extended wear: a comparative study. Optom Vis Sci 69:214, 1992

15. Mandell RB: Contact Lens Practice, Hard and Flexible Lenses. 2nd ed. p. 167. Thomas, Springfield, IL, 1974

16. Waring GO III, Hannush SB, Bogen SJ, Maloney RK: Classification of corneal topography. p. 42. In Schanzlin DJ, Robin JB (eds): Corneal Topography: Measuring and Modifying the Cornea. Springer-Verlag, New York, 1992

17. Mandell RB, St. Helen R: Mathematical model of corneal contour. Br J Physiol Opt 26:183, 1971

18. Townsley M: New knowledge of the corneal contour. Contacto 14:38, 1970

19. Dingeldein SA, Klyce SD: The topography of normal corneas. Arch Ophthalmol 107:512, 1989

20. Mandell RB: Methods to measure the peripheral curvature. Part I, Photokeratoscopy. J Am Optom Assoc 9:137, 1961

21. Wilson SE, Wang JY, Klyce SD: Quantification and mathematical analysis of photokeratoscopic images. p. 1. In Schanzlin DJ, Robin JB (eds): Corneal Topography: Measuring and Modifying the Cornea. Springer-Verlag, New York, 1992

22. Maeda N, Klyce SD: Videokeratography in contact lens practice. Int Contact Lens Clin 21:163, 1994

23. Szczotka L, Lebow KA, Caroline P, et al: Mapping the future of contact lenses. Contact Lens Spectrum 3:28, 1996

24. Frobin W, Hierholzer E: Rasterstereography: a photogrammetric method for measurement of body surfaces. J Biolog Photog 51:11, 1983

25. Warnicki JW, Rehkopf PG, Curtain DY, et al: Corneal topography using computer analyzed rasterstereographic images. Applied Optics 27:1135, 1988

26. Belin MW, Zloty P: Accuracy of the PAR corneal topography system with spatial misalignment. CLAO J 19:64, 1993

27. Naufal SC, Hess JS, Friedlauder MH, et al: Rasterstereography-based classification of normal corneas—comments. J Cataract Refract Surg 23:143, 1997

28. Arffa RC, Warnicki JW, Rehkopf PC: Corneal topography using rasterstereography. Refract Corneal Surg 5:414, 1989

29. Snook RK: Pachymetry and true topography using the ORBSCAN system. p. 89. In Gills JP, Sanders DR, Thornton SP, et al. (eds): Corneal Topography: The State of the Art. Slack, Thorofare, NJ, 1995

30. Corbett MC, O'Brart DPS, Stultiens BAT, et al: Corneal topography using a new Moiré image-based system. Eur J Implant Ref Surg 7:353, 1995

31. Belin MW: Intraoperative raster-photogrammetry—the PAR corneal topography system. J Cataract Refract Surg (suppl.)19:188, 1993

32. Tennen DG, Keates RH, Montoya C: Comparison of three keratometry instruments. J Cataract Refract Surg 21:407, 1995

33. Koch Dd, Wakil JS, Samuelson SW, et al: Comparison of the accuracy and reproducibility of the keratometer and the EyeSys Corneal Analysis System Model I. J Cataract Refract Surg 18:342, 1992

34. Greivenkamp JE, Mellinger MD, Snyder RW, et al: Comparison of three videokeratoscopes in measurement of toric test surfaces. J Refract Surg 12:220, 1996

35. Varssano D, Rapuano CJ, Luchs LI: Comparison of keratometric values of healthy and diseased eyes measured by the Javal keratometer, EyeSys and PAR. J Cataract Refract Surg 23:419, 1997

36. Pole J, Lowther GE: Comparison of simulated K's as measured by computerized videokeratographers to keratometry measurements. Int Contact Lens Clin 21:180, 1994

37. Heath GG, Gerstman DR, Wheeler WH, et al: Reliability and validity of videokeratoscopic measurements. Optom Vis Sci 68:945, 1991

38. Belin MW, Ratliff CD: Evaluating data acquisition and smoothing functions of currently available videokeratoscopes—Comment in: J Cataract Refract Surg 22:871, 1996

39. Jeandervin M, Barr J: Comparison of repeat videokeratography: repeatability and accuracy. Optom Vis Sci 75:663, 1998

40. Kraff CR, Robin JB: Normal corneal topography. p. 33. In Schanzlin DJ, Robin JB (eds): Corneal Topography: Measuring and Modifying the Cornea. Springer-Verlag, New York, 1992
41. Bogan SJ, Waring GO 3rd, Ibrahim O, et al: Classification of normal corneal topography based on computer-assisted videokeratography. Arch Ophthalmol 108:945, 1990
42. Longanesi L, Cavallini GM, Toni R: Quantitative clinical anatomy of the human cornea in vivo: a morphometric study by ultrasonic pachymetry and computer-assisted topography videokeratoscopy. Acta Anat (Basel) 157:73, 1996
43. Clark BAJ: Mean topography of normal corneas. Aust J Optom 108:539, 1990
44. Clark BAJ: Topography of some individual corneas. Aust J Optom 38:389, 1974
45. Clark BAJ: Variations in corneal topography. Aust J Optom 56:399, 1973
46. Townsley MG: New equipment and methods for determining the contour of the human cornea. Contacto 11:72, 1967
47. Lindsay R, Smith G, Atchison D: Descriptors of corneal shape. Optom Vis Sci 75:156, 1998
48. Bibby MM: Computer-assisted photokeratoscopy and contact lens design—2. Optician 171:11, 1976
49. Waring GO: Making sense of keratospeak II: proposed conventional terminology for corneal topography. Refract Corneal Surg 5:362, 1989
50. Mandell RB, Chiang SC, Lee L: Asymmetric corneal toricity and pseudokeratoconus in videokeratography. J Am Optom Assoc 67:540, 1996
51. Wilson SE, Klyce SD: Screening for corneal topographic abnormalities before refractive surgery. Ophthalmology 101:147, 1994
52. Kraff CR, Robin JB: Topography of corneal disease processes. p. 39. In Schanzlin DJ, Robin JB (eds): Corneal Topography: Measuring and Modifying the Cornea. Springer-Verlag, New York, 1992
53. McDonnell PJ: The Corneal Modeling System. p. 145. In Schanzlin DJ, Robin JB (eds): Corneal Topography: Measuring and Modifying the Cornea. Springer-Verlag, New York, 1992
54. Wilson SE, Lin DT, Klyce SD, et al: Rigid contact lens decentration: a risk factor for corneal warpage. CLAO J 16:177, 1990
55. Smolek MK, Klyce SD, Maeda N: Keratoconus and contact lens–induced corneal warpage analysis using the keratomorphic diagram. Invest Ophthalmol Vis Sci 35:4192, 1994
56. Wilson SE, Lin DT, Klyce SD, et al: Topographic changes in contact lens-induced corneal warpage. Ophthalmology 97:734, 1990
57. Wilson SE, Klyce SD, Husseini ZM: Standardized color-coded maps for corneal topography. Comment in Ophthalmology 101:795, 1994; discussion in Ophthalmology 100:1723, 1993
58. Maeda N, Klyce SD, Smolek MK: Comparison of methods for detecting keratoconus using videokeratography. Arch Ophthalmol 113:870, 1995
59. Novo AG, Pavlopoulos G, Feldman ST: Corneal topographic changes after refitting polymethylmethacrylate contact lens wearers into rigid gas permeable materials. CLAO J 21:47, 1995
60. Phillips CI: Contact lenses and corneal deformation: cause, correlate or co-incidence? Acta Ophthalmol (Copenh) 68:661, 1990
61. Maguire LJ; Lowry JC: Identifying progression of subclinical keratoconus by serial topography analysis. Am J Ophthalmol 112:41, 1991
62. McDonnell PJ: Current applications of the Corneal Modeling System. Refract Corneal Surg 7:87, 1991
63. Parker J, Ko WW, Pavlopoulos G, et al: Videokeratography of keratoconus in monozygotic twins. J Refract Surg 12:180, 1996
64. Doyle SJ, Hynes E, Naroo S, Shah S: PRK in patients with a keratoconic topography picture. The concept of a physiological 'displaced apex syndrome'. Br J Ophthalmol 80:25, 1996
65. Kame RT, Caroline PJ, Hayashida JK, et al: Computerized mapping of corneal contour changes with various contact lenses. Contact Lens Spectrum 4:35, 1989
66. Karabatsas CH, Cook SD: Topographic analysis in pellucid marginal corneal degeneration and keratoglobus. Eye 10(Pt. 4):451, 1996
67. Bogan SJ, Maloney RK, Drews CD, et al: Computer-assisted videokeratography of corneal topography after radial keratotomy. Arch Ophthal 109:834, 1990
68. Lebow KA: Using corneal topography to evaluate the efficacy of orthokeratology fitting. Contacto 39:20, 1996
69. Rabinowitz YS, Yang H, Brickman Y, et al: Videokeratography database of normal human corneas. Br J Ophthalmol 80:610, 1996
70. Maeda N, Klyce SD, Smolek MK, et al: Automated keratoconus screening with corneal topography analysis. Invest Ophthalmol Vis Sci 35:2749, 1994
71. Holladay JT: Understanding Corneal Topography: The Holladay Diagnostic Summary, User's Guide and Tutorial Version 3.30-3.11. EyeSys Technologies, pp. 1–18, 1995
72. Holladay JT: Corneal topography using the Holladay Diagnostic Summary. Comment in: J Cataract Refract Surg 23:143, 1997 Source: J Cataract Refract Surg 23:209, 1997
73. Hersh PR, Shah SI, Holladay JT: Corneal asphericity following exicmer laser photorefractive keratectomy. Summit PRK topography study group. Ophthalmic Surg Laser 27(suppl. 5):S421, 1995
74. Binder PS: Software review: dioptimum. CLAO J 14:188, 1998
75. Smolek MK, Klyce SD: The Tomey technology/computed anatomy TMS-1 videokeratoscope. p. 123. In Gills JP, Sanders DR, Thornton SP, et al. (eds): Corneal Topography: The State of the Art. Slack, Thorofare, NJ, 1995
76. Rabinowitz YS, McDonnell PJ: Computer-assisted corneal topography in keratoconus. Refract Corneal Surg 5:400, 1989

77. Maeda N, Klyce SD, Smolek MK, Thompson HW: Automated keratoconus screening with corneal topography analysis. Invest Ophthalmol Vis Sci 35:2749, 1994

78. Tomey Manual. AutoTopographer (TMS-3) Operator Manual, Version 2.1, 10:8, 1998

79. Smolek MK, Klyce SD: Current keratoconus detection methods compared with a neural network approach. Invest Ophthalmol Vis Sci. 38:2290, 1997

80. Humphrey Atlas Owner's Manual. Rev A PN46940 4:16(1)-16(11), 1998

81. Lebow KA, Grohe RM: Differentiating contact lens–induced warpage from true keratoconus using corneal topography. CLAO J 25(2):114, 1999

82 Dao CL, Kok JH, Brinkman CJ, van Mil CJ: Corneal eccentricity as a tool for the diagnosis of keratoconus. Cornea 13:339, 1994

83. Szczotka LB, Lebow KA: Understanding corneal topography for contact lens fitting. Optom Today July 6:38, 1998

84. Maeda N, Klyce SE, Hamano H: Alteration of corneal asphericity in rigid gas permeable contact lens induced warpage. CLAO J 20:27, 1994

85. Doughman DW: Corneal edema. p. 1. In Duane TD, Jaeger EA (eds): Clinical Ophthalmology. Harper & Row, Philadelphia, 1985

86. Lohman LE: Corneal epithelial response to contact lens wear. CLAO J 12:153, 1986

87. Rom ME, Keller WB, Meyer CJ, et al: Relationship between corneal edema and topography. CLAO J 21:191, 1995

88. Bonanno JA, Polse KA: Hypoxic changes in the corneal epithelium and stroma. p. 21. In Tomlinson A (ed): Complications of Contact Lens Wear. Mosby–Year Book, St. Louis, 1992

89. Bennett ES: Contact lens–induced changes in corneal topography and refractive error. p. 69. In Tomlinson A (ed): Complications of Contact Lens Wear. Mosby–Year Book, St. Louis, 1992

90. Hill JF: A comparison of refractive and keratometric changes during adaptation to flexible and non-flexible contact lenses. J Am Optom Assoc 46:290, 1975

91. Hill JF: Variation in refractive error and corneal curvature after wearing hydrophilic contact lenses. J Am Optom Assoc 46:1136, 1975

92. Herse P, Akakura N, Ooi C: Topographical corneal edema. An update. Acta Ophthalmol (Copenh) 71:539, 1993

93. Erickson P, Comstock TL, Zantos SG: Effects of hydrogel lens transmissibility profiles on local corneal swelling-during eye closure. Optom Vis Sci 73:169, 1996

94. Kohler JE, Flanagan GW: Clinical dehydration of extended wear lenses. Int Contact Lens Clin 12:152, 1985

95. Kame R, Herskowitz R: The corneal consequence of hypoxia. p. 21. In Bennett ES, Grohe RM (eds): Rigid Gas-Permeable Contact Lenses. Professional Press, New York, 1986

96. Rengstorff RH: Corneal curvature and astigmatic changes subsequent to contact lens wear. J Am Optom Assoc 26:996, 1965

97. Hill JF: A comparison of refractive and keratometric changes during adaptation to flexible and non-flexible contact lenses. J Am Optom Assoc 46:290, 1975

98. Harris MG, Sarver MD, Polse KA: Corneal curvature and refractive error changes associated with wearing hydrogel contact lenses. Am J Optom Physiol Opt 52:313, 1975

99. Masnick K: A preliminary investigation into the effects of corneal lenses on central corneal thickness and curvature. Aust J Optom 54:87, 1971

100. Miller JP: Contact lens-induced corneal curvature and thickness changes. Arch Ophthalmol 80:420, 1968

101. Polse KA, Sarver MD, Kenyon E, et al: Gas-permeable hard contact lens extended wear: Ocular and visual response to a 6-month period of wear. CLAO J 13:31, 1987

102. De Rubeis MJ, Shily BG: The effects of wearing the Boston II gas-permeable contact lens on central corneal curvature. Am J Optom Physiol Opt 62:497, 1985

103. Young G, Port M: Rigid gas-permeable extended wear: a comparative clinical study. Optom Vis Sci 69:214, 1992

104. Polse KA, Rivera RK, Bonanno J: Ocular effects of hard gas-permeable-lens extended wear. Am J Optom Physiol Opt 65:358, 1988

105. Kok JH, Hilbrink HJ, Rosenbrand RM, et al: Extended-wear of high oxygen-permeable Quantum contact lens. Int Ophthalmol (Netherlands) 16:123, 1992

106. Bailey NJ, Carney LG: Corneal changes from hydrophilic contact lenses. Am J Optom Arch Am Acad Optom 50:299, 1973

107. Rengstorff RH, Nilsson KT: Long-term effects of extended wear lenses: changes in refraction, corneal curvature and visual acuity. Am J Optom Physiol Opt 62:66, 1985

108. Ruiz-Montenegro J, Mafra CH, Wilson SE, et al: Corneal topographic alterations in normal contact lens wearers. Ophthalmology 100:128, 1993

109. Rengstorff RH: Contact lens–induced corneal distortion. p. 351. In Silbert JA (ed): Anterior Segment Complications of Contact Lens Wear. Churchill Livingstone, New York, 1994

110. Rengstorff RH: The Fort Dix report: longitudinal study of the effects of contact lenses. Am J Optom Arch Am Acad Optom 42:153, 1965

111. Harstein J: Corneal warping due to wearing corneal contact lenses: a report of 12 cases. Am J Ophthalmol 60:1103, 1965

112. Colin J, Sale Y, Malet F, et al: Inferior steepening is associated with thinning of the inferior temporal cornea. J Refract Surg 12:697, 1996

113. Watters GA, Ownes H: Evaluation of mild, moderate and advanced keratoconus using ultrasound pachymetry and the EyeSys videokeratoscope. Optom Vis Sci 75:640, 1998

114. Maeda N, Klyce SD, Hamano H: Alteration of corneal asphericity in rigid gas permeable contact lens induced warpage. CLAO J 20:27, 1994

115. Bennett ES: Keratoconus. p. 297. In Bennett ES, Grohe RM (eds): Rigid Gas-Permeable Contact Lenses. Professional Press, New York, 1986

116. Bron AJ: Keratoconus. Cornea 7:163, 1988

117. Daxer A, Fratzl P: Collagen fibril orientation in the human corneal stroma and its implication in keratoconus. Invest Ophthalmol Vis Sci 38:121, 1997

118. Quantock AJ, Meek KM, Brittain P, et al. Alteration of the stromal architecture and depletion of keratan sulphate proteoglycans in oedematous human corneas: histological, immunochemical and X-ray diffraction evidence. Tissue Cell 23:593, 1991

119. Nauheim JS, Perry HD: A clinicopathologic study of contact lens related keratoconus. Am J Ophthalmol 100:543, 1985

120. Macsai MS, Varley GA, Krachmer JH: Development of keratoconus after contact lens wear. Patient characteristics. Arch Ophthalmol 108:534, 1990

121. Szczotka LB, Thomas J: Comparison of axial and instantaneous videokeratographic data in keratoconus and utility in contact lens curvature prediction. CLAO J 24:22, 1998

122. Klein SA, Mandell RB: Shape and refractive powers in corneal topography. Invest Ophthalmol Vis Sci 36:2096, 1995

123. Rabinowitz YS: Tangential vs. sagittal videokeratographs in the 'early' detection of keratoconus. Am J Ophthalmol 122:887, 1996

124. Salmon TO, Horner DG: Comparison of elevation, curvature, and power descriptors for corneal topography mapping. Optom Vis Sci 72:800, 1995

125. Chan JS, Mandell RB: Alignment effects in videokeratography in keratoconus. CLAO J 23:23, 1997

126. Chan JS, Mandell RB, Burger DS, et al: Accuracy of videokeratoscopy for instantaneous radius in keratoconus. Optom Vis Sci 72:793, 1995

127. Egbalhi F: Keratoconus or pseudokeratoconus? Contact Lens Spectrum 12:30, 1997

128. Baum J: On the location of the cone and the etiology of keratoconus. Cornea 14:142, 1995

129. McMahon TT, Robin JB, Scarpulla KM, et al: The spectrum of topography found in keratoconus. CLAO J 17:198, 1991

130. Caroline PJ, Andre MA, Norman V: Corneal topography in keratoconus. Contact Lens Spectrum 12:36, 1997

131. Owens H, Watters GA: An evaluation of the keratoconic cornea using computerised corneal mapping and ultrasonic measurements of corneal thickness. Ophthalmic Physiol Opt (England) 16:115, 1996

132. Caroline PJ, Norman CW: Corneal topography in the diagnosis and management of keratoconus. p. 75. In Schanzlin DJ, Robin JB (eds): Corneal Topography: Measuring and Modifying the Cornea. Springer-Verlag, New York, 1992

133. Keller PR, Reid PG, van Saarloos PP: Corneal topography bow-tie pattern: artifact of videokeratoscopy? J Cataract Refract Surg 23:1339, 1997

134. Fall HF, Allen AW: Dominantly inherited keratoconus: report of a family. J Genetic Hum 17:317, 1969

135. Rabinowitz YS, et al: Corneal topography in family members of patients with keratoconus using computer-assisted corneal topography analysis. Invest Ophthalmol Vis Sci (suppl.)30:188, 1989

136. Rabinowitz YS, Garbus J, McDonnell PJ: Computer-assisted corneal topography in family members of patients with keratoconus. Arch Ophthalmol 108:365, 1990

137. Rabinowitz YS, Nesburn AB, McDonnell PJ: Videokeratography in the fellow eye in unilateral keratoconus [see comments]. Ophthalmol 100:181, 1993

138. Rabinowitz YS: Keratoconus. Surv Ophthalmol 42:297, 1998

139. McKay T: A Clinical Guide to the Humphrey Corneal Topography System. San Leandro, California, Humphrey Systems, 1998

140. De Beus AM, Brodie SE: Toward intrinsic representations of the corneal surface. (Abstract.) Invest Ophthalmol Vis Sci 35:2197, 1994

141. Hubbe RE, Foulks GN: The effect of poor fixation on computer-assisted topographic corneal analysis. Pseudokeratoconus. Ophthalmol 101:1745, 1994

142. Maguire LJ, Bourne WM: Corneal topography of early keratoconus. Am J Ophthalmol 108:107, 1989

143. Harrison DA, Maguire LJ: Biomicroscopic evidence of keratoconus with an apex power of 45.5 diopters by videokeratoscopy. Am J Ophthalmol 119:366, 1995

144. Bruce AS, Mainstone JC: Lens adherence and postlens tear film changes in closed-eye wear of hydrogel lenses. Optom Vis Sci 73:28, 1996

145. Sevigny J. The Boston lens clinical performance. Int Contact Lens Clin 10:73, 1983

146. Dougal J: Abrasions secondary to contact lens wear. p. 123. In Tomlinson A (ed): Complications of Contact Lens Wear. Mosby–Year Book, St. Louis, 1992

147. Swarbrick HA, Holden BA: Ocular characteristics associated with rigid gas-permeable lens adherence. Optom Vis Sci 73:473, 1996

148. Kenyon E, Polse KA, Mandell RB: Rigid contact lens adherence: incidence, severity and recovery. J Am Optom Assoc 59:168, 1988

149. Karabatsas CH, Cook SD: Topographic analysis in pellucid marginal degeneration and keratoglobus. Eye 10(Pt. 4):451, 1996

150. Edrington TB: Diagnosing and fitting irregular corneas. Spectrum (suppl.)13:3s, 1998

151. Kerns RL: Research on orthokeratology: Part VIII. Results, conclusions and discussion of techniques. J Am Optom Assoc 49:308, 1978

152. Winkler TD, Kame RT: Orthokeratology Handbook. Butterworth–Heinemann, Boston, 1995

153. Coon LJ: Orthokeratology, part II: Evaluating the Tabb method. J Am Optom Assoc 55:409, 1984

154. Joe JJ, Marsden HJ, Edrington TB: The relationship between corneal eccentricity and improvement in visual acuity with orthokeratology. J Am Optom Assoc 67:87, 1996

155. Kerns RL: Research on orthokeratology: Part III, results and observations. J Am Optom Assoc 47:1505, 1976

156. Lebow KA: Orthokeratology. In Bennett ES, Weissman BA (eds): Clinical Contact Lens Practice. Lippincott, Philadelphia, 1991

157. Levy B: Permanent corneal damage in a patient undergoing orthokeratology. Am J Optom Physiol Opt 59:697, 1982

158. Roberts C: A practical guide to the interpretation of corneal topography. Spectrum 13:25, 1998

159. Lebow KA: Fitting Accuracy of an arc step-based contact lens module. Spectrum 12:25, 1997

160. Szczotka LB, Capretta DM, Lass JH: Clinical evaluation of computerized topography software method for fitting rigid gas permeable contact lenses. CLAO J 20:231, 1994

161. Donshik PC, Reisner DS, Luistro AE: The use of computerized videokeratoscopy as an aid in fitting rigid gas permeable contact lenses. Trans Am Ophthalmol Soc 94:135;discussion 143, 1996

162. Douthwaite WA: EyeSys corneal topography measurement applied to calibrated ellipsoidal convex surfaces [see comments]. Br J Ophthalmol 79:797, 1995

163. Soper B, Rhodes L: Fluorescein simulation of the EyeSys Corneal Analysis System. Aust J Optom 4:22, 1994

164. Soper B, Shovlin J, Bennett E: Evaluating a topography software program for fitting RGPs. Spectrum 11:37, 1996

165. Chan JS, Mandell RB, Johnson L, et al: Contact lens base curve prediction from videokeratoscopy. Optom Vis Sci 75:445, 1998

166. Lam AK, Douthwaite WA: Three month study of changes in the cornea after computer-determined and conventionally determined contact lens fitting. Ophthalmic Physiol Opt (England) 14:59, 1993

167. Jeandervin M: Computer-aided contact lens fitting with the corneal topographer. Spectrum 13:21, 1998

168. Szczotka LB: Clinical evaluation of a topographically based contact lens fitting software. Optom Vis Sci 74:14, 1997

169. Szczotka LB, Reinhart W: Computerized videokeratoscopy contact lens software for RGP fitting in a bilateral post-keratoplasty patient: a clinical case report. CLAO J 21:52, 1995

170. Hansen DW: Mapping your way to bifocal fitting success. Spectrum 12:14, 1998

171. Hansen DW: Fitting flat and steep corneas with rgp multifocals. Spectrum 12:19, 1998

172. Lebow KA: Are all aspheric contact lenses created the same? Spectrum 14:31, 1999

173. Aggarwal T, Szczotka L: Utility of corneal topography in soft toric contact lens fitting. Spectrum (World Wide Web Electronic Poster: www.clspectrum.com/) Dec, 1998

174. Harris MG, Lau S, Ma H, Tuan J: Do disposable contact lenses mask astigmatism? Spectrum 10:21, 1995

175. McCarey BE, Amos CF, Taub LR: Surface topography of soft contact lenses for neutralizing corneal astigmatism. CLAO J 19:114, 1993

176. McCarey BE, Amos CF: Topographic evaluation of toric soft contact lens correction. CLAO J 20:261, 1994

177. Rabinowitz YS, Garbus JJ, Garbus C, McDonnell PJ: Contact lens selection for keratoconus using a computer-assisted videokeratoscope. CLAO J 17:88, 1991

178. Wasserman D, Itzkowitz J, Kamenar T, Asbell P: Corneal topographic data: its use in fitting aspheric contact lenses. CLAO J 18:83, 1992

X

Medicolegal Complications

25

Medicolegal Complications of Contact Lens Wear

JOHN G. CLASSÉ AND MICHAEL G. HARRIS

Approximately 40–50% of all malpractice claims involving optometrists arise from the fitting or wear of contact lenses,[1,2] which makes contact lens practice the greatest source of liability claims within optometry. Three major causes exist for this plethora of claims: advances in contact lens technology, an obligation to monitor eye health, and poor patient compliance.[3]

From polymethylmethacrylate to gas-permeable to hydrophilic lenses, from daily wear to extended wear to disposable wear, each improvement in technology has brought a concomitant change in the standard of care. For each contact lens patient, regardless of the lens modality, an unshirkable obligation exists to monitor ocular health, external and internal. As every contact lens practitioner has learned, management of contact lens patients is invariably complicated by poor patient compliance with instructions, warnings, wearing schedules, and lens care regimens.

Two strategies can be used to minimize the risk of clinicolegal problems: (1) establish a highly structured program of examination and management and (2) provide adequate patient education and communication. Because these two strategies require careful record keeping and documentation, they greatly strengthen the defense of any legal claims arising out of contact lens practice.[4]

To describe these two strategies, it is most convenient to divide the discussion into five categories: daily-wear lenses, monovision lenses, extended-wear lenses, disposable lenses, and contact lens prescriptions. Each category has special concerns that merit consideration.

USING A STRUCTURED PROGRAM

A structured contact lens program is built on a foundation of education and communication. Patients must be prepared for their responsibilities as contact lens wearers: If potential risks exist associated with lens wear, patients must be advised of them. Wearing schedules, lens care regimens, and follow-up care must be described, and financial details must be clearly explained.[5] These requirements are best met through the use of printed forms that describe these and other aspects of the relationship between patient and clinician. Although verbal communication remains the primary source of information, forms serve a variety of purposes. They are a printed reference for the patient, they describe the contractual relationship between the parties, and they provide powerful evidence should a legal dispute arise. A structured program is built on the use of forms, which must today be regarded as a *sine qua non* of contemporary contact lens practice.[6–8]

When a patient first enters a contact lens clinic or practice, a general information form, brochure, or handbook should be provided, along with a description of the clinician's policy with respect to the release of contact lens prescriptions (Fig. 25-1). Because prescriptions can easily become a source of discord between patient and clinician, the form, brochure, or handbook should describe the following:

- Components of a contact lens prescription
- When the prescription is provided to patients
- When the prescription expires and is no longer valid

The value of this approach is that it describes how problems are managed before they are encountered, thereby reducing the likelihood of conflict with patients. It also provides needed education about the patient's obligations as a contact lens wearer. The form, brochure, or handbook should discuss the general management of contact lens patients during the fitting period. The actual details of care should be described in a separate fitting agreement.

University Optometric Group
908 19th Street South
Birmingham, AL 35294
(205) 934-5161

Information for Contact Lens Patients

Welcome to our clinic! Before we begin the process of fittting you with lenses, we would like to acquaint you with the specialized care you will receive from our doctors and staff.

Fitting You With Lenses

All contact lens patients must receive a thorough eye health examination before being fitted with lenses. The purpose of this examination is to ensure that you will have the best possible opportunity to enjoy uncomplicated contact lens wear. Because of the nature of the testing that must be performed to assess the health of your eyes, it will be necessary for the actual contact lens fitting to be scheduled as a separate appointment at a later time.

At the conclusion of the eye health examination, however, you will receive a copy of your prescription for spectacles and, if you wish, you may select frames from our dispensary. Because there may be occasions when contact lens wear is not possible, all of our contact lens patients are expected to have a pair of spectacles for use as necessary.

At the contact lens fitting, our contact lens agreement will be explained to you, and you will have an opportunity to ask any questions you may have about our contact lens program before signing the agreement. During the examination, the lenses most appropriate for you will be selected and you will have an opportunity to wear them. The doctor will assess the vision, comfort and quality of fit obtained with the lenses. If for any reason during the fitting you decide that you do not want the lenses, you have no obligation other than payment for the evaluation. If you wish to become a contact lens wearer, you will be required to pay the fee for services and lenses at the conclusion of this visit.

Often we will be able to provide you with lenses from our inventory, enabling you to begin lens wear right away. If we do not have the lenses that have been chosen for you, they will have to be obtained from a laboratory, a process which usually requires less than a week.

Before you will be allowed to begin lens wear, you must receive training from our staff in the insertion and removal of lenses and in their care and maintenance. Proper handling, cleaning and storage of lenses increases lens life and minimizes the risk of complications. If at any time you have questions about the care of your lenses, do not hesitate to ask your doctor or one of our contact lens staff.

Checking On Your Progress

When you begin lens wear you will be scheduled for several followup examinations. The time and frequency of these examinations will be determined by your doctor, based upon the type of lenses and wearing schedule that has been determined to be best for you. In general, patients who wear lenses overnight or on a planned replacement or disposable basis must be seen more frequently than patients fitted with lenses for daily wear only. During these examinations the doctor will evaluate the lens fit, the response of your eyes to lens wear, and how you are progressing as a lens wearer. Occasionally, changes in the lens design or type of lens become necessary. If this occurs, an additional fee will be required, which is described in your contact lens fitting agreement.

Ensuring You Receive Continuing Care

When your doctor has determined that the lens fit and ocular response are satisfactory and that no further followup evaluations are necessary, you will be released from care for a period varying from 3 to 12 months, depending upon the type of lenses and wearing schedule. At this time you will be eligible to receive a copy of your contact lens prescription, which will be valid for one year from the date of issue.

You will also be eligible to enroll in our special continuing care program, which provides eye examinations, emergency consultations, replacement of lost or damaged lenses, and other benefits during the year that follows. The purpose of this program is to ensure that our patients receive the best care and materials, at reasonable cost, without undue delay or difficulty.

Our doctors and staff are dedicated to providing the highest level of professional eye care, and making your experience an enjoyable one is our highest priority. We appreciate that you have trusted us with your vision, and we look forward to serving you.

© 1992 John G. Classé

FIG. 25-1. *Contact lens information form and prescription release policy. (Courtesy of the University of Alabama at Birmingham School of Optometry, Birmingham, AL.)*

DAILY-WEAR PATIENTS

The fitting agreement for a daily-wear patient (Fig. 25-2) should emphasize the patient's obligations as a contact lens wearer.[8] Patients should be informed that a successful fit depends in part on the patient's compliance with instructions for wear, requirements for maintenance of lenses, and scheduled appointments to return for follow-up evaluation.

In addition, the agreement should specify the services and materials to be received, the cost to the patient for these services and materials, and the provisions for lens replacements or changes. Other things to be specified are the manner in which payment must be made, the clinic policy for refunds if a fit is unsuccessful, and the schedule of appointments during the fitting period.[8] The form is signed by the patient and the original is kept by the practitioner; the patient is given a copy.

A fitting agreement provides excellent documentation should a dispute arise between practitioner and patient. It is also usable as evidence should a liability claim occur.

MONOVISION PATIENTS

Monovision patients should be carefully instructed in the wear and use of lenses. A separate fitting agreement may be appropriate for presbyopic patients (Fig. 25-3).[9] The agreement should describe the contact lens options available for the correction of presbyopia (contact lenses for distance and spectacles for near, bifocal contact lenses, or monovision) with particular emphasis on monovision. To satisfy informed consent requirements, the patient must be advised of the reduced stereopsis and visual acuity of monovision and of the significance of these effects while driving a motor vehicle, operating machinery, or performing other potentially hazardous activities.[10]

At the time of fitting, it is advisable to allow the patient to wear the lenses around the office. One should also urge the patient to ride as a passenger in a vehicle before attempting to drive so that the patient can appreciate the effects of monovision on distance acuity, stereopsis, and field of vision. It may be appropriate to apply restrictions to some monovision patients who operate a motor vehicle (e.g., monovision not permitted while driving at night; the patient must wear lenses that provide best distance acuity). A fitting agreement serves as an informed consent document in these cases, establishing that a warning or restriction was discussed with the patient.[9]

If a patient is fitted with monovision lenses to be worn on an overnight basis, the requirements of informed consent are even greater, and the risks of extended wear must also be described.

EXTENDED-WEAR PATIENTS

Because extended-wear patients incur greater risks than daily-wear patients, they present a greater clinical and legal responsibility for contact lens practitioners.[3,11] Care must be taken to select extended-wear patients judiciously, use the appropriate lens care regimen, establish a reasonable wearing schedule, and evaluate patients regularly.

It is estimated that extended-wear patients face a risk of complications that is 10–15 times that of daily-wear patients.[12,13] For this reason, informed consent must be obtained at the time of fitting.[11] A fitting agreement may be modified to explain these risks and to supply the necessary documentation (Fig. 25-4). Among other things, such an agreement should do the following:

- Emphasize the patient's responsibilities as a wearer of overnight lenses.
- Describe the risks in lay terms.
- Describe the symptoms that require immediate examination.
- Provide a schedule of progress checks during the fitting period.
- Limit wearing time to no more than 7 days (i.e., 6 nights) of continuous wear.
- Inform the patient that a return to daily wear may become necessary.
- Inform the patient that lens life is unpredictable and that frequent replacement may become necessary; indeed, that frequent replacement using disposable contact lenses is indicated for most extended-wear lenses.
- Describe the lens care regimen.
- Inform the patient that noncompliance with wear or maintenance requirements or not returning as scheduled for progress checks constitute grounds for termination from lens wear.

Although the U.S. Food and Drug Administration (FDA) has issued a letter stating that extended-wear patients should be permitted no more than 7 days (i.e., 6 nights) of continuous wear,[14] some patients require wear beyond this period. Informed consent, if properly obtained, permits the practitioner to recommend wearing schedules longer than 7 days and provides a defense in the event a legal claim should result from this extended wear of lenses. In such a case, careful documentation of the warning to the patient and of the patient's consent are necessary.[15,16]

As with daily-wear lenses, a number of legal issues pose potential liability problems. These issues may be managed, in part, through the use of a structured program of care. During the fitting period, scheduled progress checks can be used to assess the patient's status and to reinforce

UNIVERSITY OF CALIFORNIA
School of Optometry

Contact Lens Services, Meredith W. Morgan University Eye Center, Berkeley, CA 94720
(510) 642-2020

Contact Lens Services, Tang Center, Berkeley, CA 94720
(510) 643-2020

Contact Lens Services
Information and Policy

July 1, 1998©

INFORMATION ON CONTACT LENS SERVICES

The University of California School of Optometry provides contact lens services for University students, faculty, employees, and the general public. Our primary emphasis is proper patient care and instruction. *All services are provided by optometry students under the supervision of the attending clinical faculty.* These services are made avaiilable in order to provide a contact lens teaching facility for students in Optometry and a contact lens consultation, research and service unit within the University.

The School provides two categories of contact lens services:
(1) Examinations and fitting services, and (2) Extended care services for patients currently wearing contact lenses.

1. Examination and Fitting Services
   A. *Patient Eligibility:* The patient must have had a primary care eye examination within one year prior to obtaining a contact lens examination and fitting. This eye examination can be performed in our Eye Center as part of the contact lens fitting or by an outside eye doctor.
   B. *Services included in the examination and fitting:* A contact lens examination and evaluation will be performed by an optometry student clinician at the time of the first appointment in the Eye Center. Final acceptance as a patient will depend upon the results of this examination. If contact lenses are advisable, tentative lenses will be prescribed and ordered upon the payment of the necessary fee. After the patient's response to the contact lenses has been properly evaluated, the lens prescription will be finalized. If either the attending doctor or the patient decides that the fitting should not be completed, a portion of the fee may be refunded. The following services specific to a contact lens evaluation and fitting are included in the contact lens examination:
     1. Consultation and history
     2. Refraction and vision analysis
     3. Examination for ocular disease or abnormalities
     4. Measurement of eye dimensions
     5. Prediction of lens type and dimensions
     6. Diagnostic lens fitting
     7. Design of lenses
     8. Tentative prognosis
     9. Prescribing and ordering of appropriate tentative lenses
     10. Dispensing and evaluation of tentative lenses
     11. Instructions in lens care and handling
     12. Initial supply of contact lens care products
     13. Evaluation of patient response
     14. Follow-up visits for a period not exceeding 3-6 months
     15. Necessary lens changes in the 3-6 month fitting period
     16. Final contact lenses.

   C. *Fitting Schedule:* Contact lenses are fitted througout the year. The examination takes about 1-1/2 to 2 hours. Subsequent visits may be scheduled for the same day of the week as the original appointment. The time required for these subsequent visits is from 1/2 to 1-1/2 hours. A minimum of 3 follow-up visits are usually required over a 3 month period. Because of the thoroughness of our examination and fitting process, the time involved until dismissal may be longer than that encountered in some private practices.
   D. *Request for Fitting:* Persons who want to be fitted with contact lenses can make an appointment at the University Eye Center Appointment Desk (642-2020) or the Tang Center (643-2020) in person or by telephone. Patient scheduling will be based upon the nature of the patient's visual needs. Patients are generally scheduled within 1 - 2 weeks for an appointment.

2. Extended Care Services
   A. *Patient eligibility:* Extended care services are available for patients fitted at the Eye Center who have passed the 3-6 month fitting period and for patients fitted elsewhere. To be eligible for extended care contact lens services, the patient should have (1) had a primary care eye examination within the past year, and (2) adequate contact lens examination and fitting information on file at the Eye Center. Patients fitted elsewhere should have a referral report sent to the Eye Center by the original practitioner or have a primary care eye examination and a contact lens evaluation at the Eye Center. Referral report forms are available at the Appointment Desk. Emergency services are available without referral reports.
   B. *Extended Care Services Available:*
     1. Examination and evaluation of contact lens patients
     2. Post-fitting examinations and evaluation
     3. Replacement of current contact lens (may be ordered by mail, phone, fax, etc.) Applies only to patients examined at the University Eye Center within the past year who have a successful response to their current contact lenses. Some patients may need to be examined before lenses are ordered. The lens replacement fee includes the required dispensing appointment and one follow-up appointment but does not include the examination or fitting if needed.
     4. Lens adjustments, refinishing, repolishing, inspection, cleaning
     5. Prescription changes (for patients examined at the Eye Center)
     6. Contact lens refittings
     7. Advice and instruction

8. Additional examination and fitting procedures.
9. Emergency Services
C. *Fees:* $25 to $52 per examination (depending on services required). An additional charge will be made for any special services or materials required. Fees must be paid at the time of the visit and before any materials are ordered.
D. *Appointments:* Appointments are available throughout the year. They can be made by appearing at the Appointment Desk, by calling the University Eye Center at 642-2020, or the Tang Center at 643-2020. The number of such appointments available may be limited by the teaching needs of the Eye Center.

3. Additional Information
A. *Parking:* Parking is available on-campus with shuttle service to the University Eye Center. Street parking is available at the Tang Center.
B. *Vision Care Plans:* Many vision care plans and insurance programs provide partial coverage for contact lens services. Contact your individual plan for information.
C. *Contact Lens Prescriptions:* A contact lens prescription can be released only to patients we have fitted after the contact lens examination and fitting have been completed and the patient is wearing contact lenses successfully. Patients who have not been examined in the Eye Center within the past six months may need to be re-examined before a contact lens prescription can be released.

4. Policy
The fee for the contact lens examination and fitting depends on the nature of the patient's visual needs and the type of lenses ordered. The exact fee will be quoted before lenses are ordered. The contact lens examination and fitting fees generally range from $150 - $340, similar to or lower than those encountered in private practice for similar services and materials. Fees may be higher for specialty fittings and lenses. Payment will be expected on the day of the first appointment. If lenses are not prescribed, there is a $52 fee for the examination and evaluation. Additional fees are charged for duplicate or replacement contact lenses and other supplies or services. Fees must be paid in full prior to the ordering of any materials. The $52 evaluation and examination fee is non-refundable.

Most patients are able to wear contact lenses successfully; however, a successful fit cannot be guaranteed. Those who are not successful with the initial pair of lenses ordered may be refitted with additional lenses. Additional fees will apply if additional services or more expensive lenses are needed. Patients who cannot be fitted successfully may be eligible for a partial refund.

If contact lens wear is discontinued for any reason within the initial 60 day fitting period, the refund will not exceed 50% of material and fitting fees. Any refund will be reduced by the cost of additional materials used in an attempt to complete the fitting. No refund is available after the initial 60 day fitting period has ended.

PATIENT INFORMED CONSENT

I am requesting contact lens services at the University of California School of Optometry. These services may include a primary care eye examination, a contact lens examination, evaluation and fitting, and/or extended care services. I will be able to ask any questions I have about the Eye Center's policies and contact lenses prior to the ordering of lenses. I give my permission to the School of Optometry to perform all the tests involved in a primary care eye examination, a contact lens examination, evaluation and fitting, and/or extended care services. I understand that contact lenses have many benefits, but as with any other drug or device, they are not without possible risks. A small percentage of wearers develop potentially serious complications which can lead to permanent eye damage and vision loss.

I agree to follow the advice and instructions given to me by the Eye Center. I will remove my lenses and seek care immediately from the Eye Center, an eye doctor, or a hospital emergency room if I experience any unexplained eye pain, redness, discharge or vision change.

I have read and received a copy of the *Information on Contact Lens Services.* I understand the current policies, including fees and refunds. I agree to pay the fees for the services and materials I receive. I understand my responsibilities as stated in this form and by the Eye Center.

Signed _____
(Patient)

Signed _____ Date _____
(Parent or guardian if parent is a minor)

FIG. 25-2. *Fitting agreement for daily-wear contact lenses. (Courtesy of the University of California School of Optometry, Berkeley, CA.)*

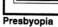

UNIVERSITY OF CALIFORNIA
School of Optometry

Contact Lens Clinic, School of Optometry, Berkeley, California 94720-2020
(510) 642-2020
Contact Lens Services, Tang Center, Berkeley, CA 94720-4300

Presbyopic Contact Lenses
Information, Instructions and Consent Form
December 1995

Presbyopia

Presbyopia occurs in adults when the eyes can no longer focus adequately for near tasks like reading. Presbyopic patients require two different vision corrections, one for distance and one for near tasks. This special vision requirements can be accomplished with bifocal spectacles or reading glasses. Presbyopic vision correction can also be accomplished with contact lenses, alone or in combination with spectacles.

Presbyopic Contact Lenses

Three common methods of correcting presbyopic vision with contact lenses are: Contact lenses for distance vision with separate reading spectacles, monovision contact lenses, and bifocal contact lenses.

Distance Contact Lenses and Reading Glasses

A straight forward way to correct a presbyopic with contact lenses is to prescribe contact lenses for distance vision and reading glasses for near tasks. The advantages are simplicity, precise vision, and lack of visual adaptation. The disadvantage is dependency on a separate pair of glasses for all near tasks. .

Monovision Contact Lenses

Monovision contact lenses provide distance and near vision simultaneously by correcting one eye for distance and the other eye for near. This method requires the fitting of only two single vision contact lenses.

Monovision has several possible disadvantages. First, it is a vision compromise whereby one eye is correct optimally for distance while the other eye is corrected optimally for near. Additionally, monovision may reduce depth perception (stereopsis) for some tasks.

Many presbyopes adapt readily to monovision prescriptions. Potentially dangerous activities, such as driving an automobile, operating machinery or performing other potentially hazardous activities usually require adaptation and supplemental distance contact lens for the near eye or supplemental spectacles for use during these activities and at times when precise vision is necessary.

Bifocal Contact Lenses

Bifocal contact lenses provide each eye with a distance and near correction, similar to bifocal spectacle lenses. The advantage is one prescription for distance and near vision. the disadvantages include the higher cost and greater time involved in fitting these lenses and possible vision compromise. Bifocal contact lenses, like monovision lenses, require an adaptation period. Bifocal patients must follow the same precautions as patients wearing monovision contact lenses.

Presbyopic Contact Lenses Require Special Care

Additional responsibilities and requirements come with presbyopic contact lenses. You must adhere to the recommended lens wear and care procedures and you must return to the Clinic for periodic progress evaluations. We generally require the following progress evaluation schedule:

- 1 week after receiving contact lenses
- 2 weeks after receiving contact lenses
- 4 weeks after receiving contact lenses
- Each 3-6 month period after receiving contact lenses

- *Immediately* if any symptom listed below occurs

It is impossible to determine in advance whether a patient will have a successful response to a presbyopic contact lens correction. Certain personal, visual, physiological, and environmental factors may adversely affect success with contact lenses and may necessitate a change in the type of correction, the recommended wearing schedule, or termination of contact lens wear.

These factors include:

- Poor lens hygiene
- Inability to Unwillingness to return for follow-up visits
- Manual dexterity problems which would prevent daily lens removal, cleaning and   disinfection
- Certain general or ocular health problems
- Severe emotional stress
- Use of certain medications
- Visual requirements
- Inability or unwillingness to follow instructions

The use of contact lenses entails certain risks. A small, but significant, percentage of individuals wearing contact lenses develop potentially serious complications which can lead to permanent eye damage and vision loss.

Symptoms Requiring Immediate Evaluation

If you have any of the following symptoms:

- Eye Pain or Redness
- Watering of the Eye or Discharge
- Cloudy or Foggy Vision
- Decrease in Distance or Near Vision
- Sensitivity to Light

Remove your lenses and call the Clinic immediately.

We will arrange to have your eyes examined as needed. Do not resume wear until advised to do so by us. If you are unable to reach the clinic, call and eye doctor or go to the nearest emergency hospital immediately.

Patient Responsibility

You understand that your cooperation is vital to successful usage of presbyopic contact lenses. You have been instructed in the proper methods of lens care and handling. You understand the importance of adhering to proper lens care procedures and periodic follow-up examinations. You agree to follow the recommended wearing schedule and to keep scheduled appointments. You agree to follow the Clinic's advice for safe contact lens wear as indicated on this form and in your record and will notify the Clinic immediately if any eye or vision problem occurs. If you are unable to reach the Clinic, you will call and eye doctor or go to the nearest emergency hospital immediately.

You understand that presbyopic contact lenses have many benefits, but as with any drug or device, they are not without possible risks. A small percentage of wearers develop serious complications, including corneal ulcers, which can lead to permanent eye damage and vision loss.

You have been told the nature, purpose and benefits of presbyopic contact lenses. You have also been told the possible risks, consequences and side effects of presbyopic contact lenses which are greater than those of spectacles or single vision contact lenses. You know there are feasible alternatives, including reading glasses and bifocal spectacles. You understand your chance of success is less than that of non-presbyopic patients. You may ask any questions you have about the Clinic's policies and contact lenses prior to the ordering of the lenses.

Vision

You understand that presbyopic contact lens corrections (monovision, bifocal contact lenses, or other alternatives) can create a vision compromise that may reduce visual acuity and depth perception for distance and near tasks. You understand that this compromise can create an increased risk when operating a motor vehicle, dangerous machinery or performing other potentially hazardous activities. you have been advised that you should become adapted to your presbyopic contact lenses before attempting any of the above mentioned activities and use a supplemental or alternative vision correction for these activities. You have been offered this correction which may be alternative contact lenses or supplemental spectacles to wear over your presbyoptic contact lenses. you agree to follow the Clinic's instructions about adapting to your presbyoptic contact lenses and will not wear them during hazardous activities until fully adapted.

Before driving a motor vehicle, you should be a passenger in the vehicle to make sure that your vision is satisfactory for operating the vehicle. During the first several weeks of wear (when adaptation is occurring), you should only drive while wearing your presbyopic correction during optimal driving conditions (short trips during daylight hours). After adaptation and success with these activities, you may be able to drive under other conditions (evenings, longer trips) with caution. We recommend you wear supplemental or alternative vision correction during all potential hazardous activities.

Lens Care and Handling Instructions:

Proper care and handling are necessary for successful wear, proper vision, good eye health and normal lens life. You have been instructed in the proper methods of lens care and handling. You have been provided with products to clean, disinfect and store your presbyopic contact lenses. Care for your contact lenses as instructed. If a lens accumulates deposits such as protein, calcium nicotine, etc., which cannot be removed, that lens must be replaced.

Presbyopic patients may have difficulty in handling and caring for their contact lenses because of reduced near vision or dexterity. Lost or damaged lenses resulting accidentally or form mishandling will require lens replacement and re-evaluation. If you have any questions concerning proper lens care and handling, you should call the Clinic or an eye doctor immediately.

You have been fitted with the following kind of presbyopic contact lens correction:

Type of Presbyopic Correction
_____ distance contact lenses and reading glasses
_____ bifocal contact lenses
_____ monovision contact lenses
_____ other

Type of lens
_____ soft contact lenses
_____ rigid gas permeable contact lenses

Your lens cleaner is _____

Your lens disinfectant is _____

Your soaking solution is _____

Your lens wetting solution is _____

Eye drops to use while wearing contact lenses _____

Other _____

Note: These products have been prescribed specifically for you eyes and lenses. Do not change or substitute brands unless you check with us first. Use of improper solutions may result in eye irritation or lens damage.

We advise you to follow the wearing schedule listed below.

Wearing Schedule:

_____

_____

_____

Like any medical device, contact lenses must be monitored on a regular basis. Professional follow-up care is the most important element in successful long term contact lens wear. Regular examination by a licenses eye doctor is necessary to evaluate your visual and ocular response to presbyopic contact lenses. Your appointment schedule for follow-up progress evaluations is:

First _____

Second _____

Third _____

Additional _____

Further examinations will be scheduled will be scheduled as needed and in accordance with the "Progress Evaluation Schedule." You should have a thorough eye-contact lens examination annually or more frequently if advised to do so. *It is important for the health of your eyes and your vision that you follow carefully the schedule recommended by the Clinic for wearing, cleaning, disinfecting, and evaluating your lenses.*

Patient Informed Consent

By signing this consent, I acknowledge that I have read, understood, and received a copy of the "Presbyopic Contact Lenes Information, Instructions, and Consent Form". I have also read, understood, and received a copy of the "Information on Contact Lens Service". I understand the Clinic's current policies, fees and refund schedule.

I understand my responsibilities as stated on this form and by the Clinic. I agree to follow the instructions given to me by the Clinic.

Date _____

Patient Signature (or Legal Guardian) _____

Contact Lenses Dispensed by _____

FIG. 25-3. *Fitting agreement for monovision contact lenses. (Courtesy of the University of California School of Optometry, Berkeley, CA.)*

UNIVERSITY OF CALIFORNIA
SCHOOL OF OPTOMETRY

Contact Lens Services, Optometric Eye Center, Berkeley, CA 94720-2020
(510) 642-2020
Contact Lens Services, Tang Center, Berkeley, CA 94720-4300
(510) 643-2020

EXTENDED WEAR (OVERNIGHT) CONTACT LENS INFORMATION, INSTRUCTION, AND CONSENT FORM

DECEMBER 1, 1995©

EXTENDED WEAR MEANS EXTENDED CARE

The use of extended wear contact lenses has additional responsibilities and requirements. You must adhere to the recommended lens wear and care procedures, and you must return to the Clinic for periodic progress evaluations (see schedule).

We *require* the following Progress Evaluation Schedule:
- 24 hours after receiving extended wear contact lenses
- 3 days after receiving extended wear contact lenses
- 1 week after receiving extended wear contact lenses
- 2 weeks after receiving extended wear contact lenses
- 4 weeks after receiving extended wear contact lenses
- Each 12 week period after receiving extended wear contact lenses

It is impossible to determine in advance whether a patient will have a successful response to extended wear contact lenses. Certain personal, physiological, and environmental factors may adversely affect the success of extended wear contact lenses, and may necessitate a change in the recommended wearing schedule or termination of lens wear. These factors include:
- Poor lens hygiene
- Inability or unwillingness to return for follow-up visits
- Manual dexterity problems which would prevent periodic lens removal and cleaning
- Severe emotional stress
- Use of certain medications
- Inability or unwillingness to follow instructions

The use of extended wear contact lenses is not without risk. A small, but significant, percentage of individuals wearing extended wear lenses develop potentially serious complications which can lead to permanent eye damage and vision loss.

IF YOU HAVE ANY OF THE FOLLOWING SYMPTOMS:
- EYE PAIN OR REDNESS
- WATERING OF THE EYE OR DISCHARGE
- CLOUDY OR FOGGY VISION
- DECREASE IN VISION
- SENSITIVITY TO LIGHT

REMOVE YOUR LENSES AND CALL THE CLINIC IMMEDIATELY. WE WILL ARRANGE TO HAVE YOUR EYES EXAMINED AS NEEDED. DO NOT RESUME WEAR UNTIL ADVISED TO DO SO BY US. IF YOU ARE UNABLE TO REACH THE CLINIC, CALL AN EYE DOCTOR OR GO TO THE NEAREST EMERGENCY HOSPITAL IMMEDIATELY.

PATIENT RESPONSIBILITY

You understand that your cooperation is vital to successful usage of extended wear contact lenses.

You have been instructed in the proper methods of lens care and handling. You understand the importance of adhering to proper lens care procedures and the need for periodic follow-up examinations. You agree to follow the recommended wearing schedule and to keep scheduled appointments. You agree to follow the Clinic's advice for safe extended wear as indicated on this form and in your record. You will notify the Clinic immediately if any eye or vision problem occurs. If you are unable to reach the Clinic you will call an eye doctor or the nearest emergency hospital immediately.

You understand that extended wear contact lenses have many benefits, but as with any other drug or medical device they entail possible risks. The risks of complication with extended wear lenses are 5 to 15 times greater than those with daily wear. Even one night of overnight wear may carry the risk of serious injuries. A percentage of wearers develop serious complications including corneal ulcers which can lead to permanent eye damage and vision loss. You agree to follow the advice and instructions given to you by the Clinic. You will remove your lenses and seek care immediately if you experience any unexplained eye pain, redness, or vision change.

You have been told the nature, purpose and benefits of extended wear contact lenses. You have also been told the possible risks, consequences, and side effects of extended wear contact lenses which are greater than those of daily wear contact lenses. You know there are feasible alternatives, including daily wear contact lenses and spectacles. You understand your chances of success with extended wear contact lenses. You will be able to ask any questions you have about the Clinic's policies and contact lenses prior to the ordering of lenses.

LENS CARE INSTRUCTIONS

Proper care is necessary for successful wear, proper vision, good eye health and normal lens life. You have been instructed in the proper methods of lens care and handling. You have been provided with products to clean, disinfect and store your extended wear lenses. Use them as instructed. You have been fitted with the following kind of extended wear contact lenses:

Type   *Manufacturer/Brand*

☐ soft contact lenses _____

☐ rigid gas permeable contact lenses _____

☐ disposable soft contact lenses _____

Your lens cleaner is _____

Your lens disinfectant is _____

Your soaking solution is _____

Your rinsing solution is _____

Eyedrops to use before sleep and upon waking _____

Other _____

NOTE: **1)** These products have been prescribed specifically for your eyes and lenses. Do not change or substitute brands unless you check with us first. Use of improper solutions may result in eye irritation or lens damage.

2) Patients should wear their lenses no longer than advised. Patients should never wear extended wear lenses for more than 6 consecutive days. Lenses must be left off overnight before lens wear can be resumed. We are advising you to follow the wearing schedule listed below.

WEARING SCHEDULE

_____
_____
_____
_____
_____

Like any medical device contact lenses must be monitored on a regular basis. Professional follow-up care is the most important element in successful long term lens wear. Regular examination by a licensed eye care professional is necessary to evaluate your eyes' response to extended wear lenses. Your appointment schedule for follow-up progress examination is:

First _____

Second _____

Third _____

Fourth _____

Fifth _____

Sixth _____

Additional examinations will be scheduled as needed and in accordance with the "Progress Evaluation Schedule." It is important for the health of your eyes that you carefully follow the schedule recommended by the Clinic for wearing, cleaning, and disinfecting your lenses.

If a lens accumulates deposits such as protein, calcium, nicotine, etc., which cannot be removed, that lens must be replaced. In some instances a lens may become displaced from the eye and get lost or damaged, requiring a replacement.

DISPOSABLE EXTENDED WEAR LENSES

If you are wearing disposable contact lenses, you must remove your lenses and discard them according to the following schedule. Only new lenses should be worn during the next wearing period. Disposable lenses should not be replaced on the eyes after removal. Patients should not wear disposable extended wear lenses for more than 6 consecutive days. We are advising you to follow the wearing schedule listed below:

Remove lenses after _____ days of wear.

Keep lenses off eyes for _____ hours.

Replacement lenses can be worn for _____ days.

You must inspect each new lens carefully and not wear any lens that looks defective. Further you should not wear any lens that doesn't provide proper vision and comfort. If no problems are encountered, repeat the above schedule for _____ weeks at which time a progress evaluation will be scheduled and a new supply of lenses will be dispensed.

PATIENT INFORMED CONSENT

By signing this consent form, I acknowledge that I have read, understood, and received a copy of the "Information on Extended Wear (Overnight) Contact Lenses." I have also read, understood, and received a copy of the "Information on Contact Lens Services." I understand the Clinic's current policies, fees and refund schedule. I understand my responsibilities as stated on this form and by the Clinic. I agree to follow the instructions given to me by the Clinic.

Signature _____
                    Patient

Signature _____
                    Parent or Guardian if patient is a minor

Contact Lenses Dispensed by _____ Date _____

FIG. 25-4. *Fitting agreement for extended-wear contact lenses. (Courtesy of the University of California School of Optometry, Berkeley, CA.)*

the need for immediate evaluation if significant symptoms occur. Once a successful fit is obtained, continuing care can be provided afterward through a prepaid service agreement or planned replacement program.[17-19] At scheduled annual or semiannual examinations, the practitioner can once again evaluate the lens fit, assess eye health, advise the patient as necessary concerning problems, and emphasize the value of following instructions and procedures. A structured program also provides excellent documentation of the care rendered and of any deviations from care on the part of the patient.

DISPOSABLE-WEAR PATIENTS

Because the risk of complications with extended-wear lenses, even if disposable, is greater than with daily-wear lenses, there must be disclosure of this risk at the time of fitting. Ulcerative keratitis is a particular concern because the risk is estimated to be 1.5–14 times that of daily-wear lenses.[20-24] An informed consent agreement provides adequate documentation of the appropriate warning (see Fig. 25-4).[25,26]

Because lenses are usually dispensed in packets containing several months' supply of lenses, a customary legal obligation—inspection and verification of lens parameters—cannot be performed. Once again, informed consent is needed to warn the patient of this fact and to advise the patient of the need for immediate examination should pain, blurred vision, redness, discharge, photophobia, or other serious symptoms occur.[14,15] An informed consent agreement may be used for this purpose and to notify patients if they are to restrict lens wear to daily use only.

The informed consent document should also serve as a fitting agreement, describing the many pertinent requirements of extended wear already discussed. Of particular importance is the schedule of progress checks, which usually provides for reassessment at 3-month intervals.[3] At each progress check, the practitioner must decide whether to issue another supply of lenses, modify the lenses or the wearing schedule, or terminate the patient from disposable lens wear. These options should be described in the informed consent agreement.

The agreement should also describe the cleaning and disinfection of lenses whenever disposable lenses are reworn. One-day disposable lenses should be discarded when removed.

CONTACT LENS PRESCRIPTIONS

Every clinician should establish a policy for the release of contact lens prescriptions. That policy must conform with the requirements of federal and state law, which together regulate the release of patient information, including spectacle and contact lens prescriptions.[27,28]

The U.S. Federal Trade Commission, as part of its "Eyeglasses Rule" proceedings, made it clear that the agency would not attempt to exercise regulatory authority over the release of contact lens prescriptions.[29] Therefore, state law must be consulted.

In 29 states (Table 25-1), a contact lens prescription is defined by law (i.e., statute or optometry board rule or regulation).[27,30,31] If a contact lens prescription is to be released to a patient in any of these states, it must contain the minimum information specified in the state statute or optometry board rule.

The release of contact lens prescriptions is regulated by law in 22 states (see Table 25-1).[27,30,31] These laws must be consulted to determine to whom and the circumstances under which a prescription must be released.

In the other 28 states and the District of Columbia, no statute exists that specifically regulates the release of contact lens prescriptions. However, numerous laws (federal and state freedom-of-information acts, state statutes, and rules or regulations of optometry boards) exist that regulate the release of health care information. Even in states in which no statutory law exists, probably a court decision exists that allows patients the right of access to information contained in the records of health care providers.[32] Therefore, patients (or their legal representatives) generally have the right to inspect or copy their health care records.[32]

But prescription information, if included in a copy of a record, a letter, or other summary of care rendered, or a vial or other container, must be differentiated from an actual prescription, which is an order by a health care provider that must contain certain elements to be valid.[30] A prescription is necessary for a patient to obtain contact lenses from a dispenser who does not have prescription-writing authority (i.e., an optician).

A contact lens prescription should contain information sufficient to enable the patient to obtain the lenses prescribed by the practitioner. Only if the patient obtains the exact lenses fitted can the practitioner be sure that satisfactory comfort, acuity, and physiologic response will continue. For this reason, the prescription should contain the following[28,30]:

- Refractive data
- Lens parameters
- Lens manufacturer
- Lens material or water content
- Reasonable expiration date
- Permissible number of refills

TABLE 25-1. *Release of Contact Lens Prescriptions*

State	State Statute	Optometry Board Rule or Regulation
Alabama	—	630-X-12.03
Arizona	—	R4-21-305
Colorado	Title 12, Art 40, Sec 117	9.00.01
Delaware	—	4.02
Florida	Title XXXII, Chap 468, Sec .012	21Q-3.012
Georgia	Title 31, Chap 12, Sec 12	—
Indiana	Title 16, Art 39, Chap 1, Sec 1	Title 852 IAC 1-5.1-1
Iowa	Title VIII, Chap 147, Sec 108	645-180.9(2)
Louisiana	Title 40, Chap 5, Sec 1299.97	—
Maine	Title 32, Chap 34A, Sec 2417 4, 4A	—
Massachusetts	—	Title 246, Chap 5.00, Sec 5.02(5) (7)
New Hampshire	Title XXX, Chap 327, Sec 25-a	—
New Jersey	Title 52, Chap 17B, Sec 41.31	—
New York	—	29.8 (Board of Education rule)
North Carolina	—	Subchapter 42E, Sec .0100.0103
Ohio	Title 47, Chap 4725, Sec 17	—
Oregon	Title 52, Chap 683, Sec 190	852-01-002
South Dakota	—	20:50:10:02
Vermont	Title 26, Chap 30, Sec 1719	—
Virginia	—	VR 510-01-1, Sec 3.16
Washington	Title 18, Chap 18.195, Sec .030	246-852-010 (Department of Health rule)
Wyoming	Title 33, Chap 23, Sec 101	—

Source: Adapted from JG Classé: Release of contact lens prescriptions: an update. J Am Optom Assoc 68:125, 1997.

- Notation of "no substitutions"
- Limitations on wear (e.g., "daily wear only" or "limited to 6 nights of continuous wear")
- Any special instructions (e.g., "monovision fit")

Contact lens prescription forms should provide for the inclusion of this information (Fig. 25-5).

The completeness of the prescription not only ensures that the patient will obtain the appropriate lenses from another dispenser, it also helps to protect the prescriber if the dispenser makes any substitutions. For example, if a dispenser makes a substitution (without obtaining the permission of the prescriber), and as a result of this substitution the patient has a physical or economic injury, the injury becomes the sole responsibility of the dispenser.

Contact lens practitioners should encourage completeness whenever prescriptions are released to patients or to other eye care providers. If a prescription is released, a copy should always be retained in the patient's record.

STRUCTURED CARE AND LIABILITY

A structured program is used to obtain understanding of instructions, warnings, wearing schedules, lens care reg-

imens, and the necessity for follow-up examinations. Such an educational effort can assist greatly in reducing patient noncompliance with these important aspects of contact lens wear while reducing the opportunity for misunderstanding and conflict between practitioner and patient, particularly with respect to the release of contact lens prescriptions. A structured program is also an excellent means of documenting informed consent when fitting patients with extended-wear lenses.[28] Because of better patient compliance with the obligations of lens wear and owing to periodic opportunities to assess the patient's status, the risk of incurring complications that result in legal action is greatly diminished.

Litigation arising out of contact lens wear is a legitimate concern for contact lens practitioners. Although contact lens practice is a frequent source of professional liability claims, the majority of claims are for minor damages.[1,2] Sizable claims most often result from allegations that the clinician mismanaged a corneal abrasion (especially one that evolved into ulcerative keratitis) or that the contact lens practitioner did not diagnose intraocular disease, such as glaucoma.[33] Such claims allege that the clinician was negligent.

Claims alleging breach of the doctrine of informed consent are less frequent than claims alleging negligence, but it is necessary to review both legal theories before describ-

University Optometric Group
908 19th Street South
Birmingham, AL 35294

Name _____John Smith_____   Record Number ___12345___   Date ___Feb 14, 1994___

Soft Contact Lens Specifications

	Sphere Power	Cylinder Power	Axis	Add or Prism	Base Curve	Lens Diameter	Material or Water Content	Color	Manufacturer
OD									
OS									

Rigid Lens Specifications

	Sphere Power	Cylinder Power	Axis	Add or Prism	Base Curve	2nd Curve Radius	2nd Curve Width	3rd Curve Radius	3rd Curve Width	Lens Diameter	OZ Diameter	Center	Edge	Color	Laboratory or Manufacturer
OD	-4.25				7.38	8.2	.3	11.0	.2	8.8	7.6	.10		Blue	Boston IV
OS	-2.75				7.34	8.2	.3	11.0	.2	8.8	7.6	.12		Blue	Boston IV

This prescription expires on ___Feb 14, 1995___.   Special instructions: Dot right lens

Number of prescription refills: ___1___.

Lens wear limited to: (daily wear only)

~~daily and extended wear~~

Extended wear is limited to no more than _____ consecutive nights.

_____ JB Classé _____ OD
                              License Number S-409

FIG. 25-5. *Contact lens prescription.*

ing the types of situations that have evolved into litigation involving clinicians.

DOCTRINE OF INFORMED CONSENT

Because contact lens practitioners are fiduciaries (like other professionals), patients are owed an affirmative duty of disclosure. This duty requires the clinician to make a full and complete disclosure of pertinent facts related to a recommended procedure so that an informed consent can be obtained from the patient. Not obtaining consent is construed as a breach of this duty.[15,16,34-37]

If a disclosure to the patient occurs, the adequacy of the information provided may be questioned. Two dif-

ferent rules may be applied, depending on the state (Table 25-2).

The oldest and most commonly applied of the two rules, the "professional community" rule, holds that a practitioner must divulge the degree of information that would commonly be provided by a like practitioner acting under the same or similar circumstances.[34] To establish the actual information that should be disclosed, expert testimony is needed. Thus, another practitioner must testify about the information to be provided.

The newer form of the rule, the "reasonable patient" rule, requires the scope of disclosure to be determined by the patient's need to know information that would be material to the ability to make an informed decision.[34] No need exists for expert testimony because the rule is not based on a practitioner's obligation to divulge but instead on the patient's need to know.

Despite these different rules, general agreement exists on the basic requirements of disclosure. Informed consent obligates a practitioner to divulge the following information:

- The inherent and potential risks of treatment
- Alternative methods of treatment
- The anticipated results of treatment

In providing this information to patients, clinicians should observe the following guidelines:

- Known risks of serious injury must be divulged.
- Complicated procedures must be explained in lay terms.
- Minor risks of low incidence do not have to be disclosed.
- A remote possibility of serious injury in a common procedure does not have to be divulged.
- If the risks are known by the patient or the patient asks not to be informed, no disclosure is necessary.

Although informed consent has not been a significant legal problem for optometry, it has been the subject of litigation involving optometrists.[38] It has its widest application in contact lens practice.[4,14,15]

Three potential areas of applicability exist for the contact lens practitioner: not disclosing the risks of a proposed treatment, not disclosing alternatives to therapy, and not disclosing suspicious findings.

Not Disclosing Risks

Because of the known risk of significant complications associated with extended-wear contact lenses[12,13] (e.g., ulcerative keratitis), it is necessary to warn patients of this risk at the time of fitting. Patients do not have to be advised in exact terms (e.g., "a 10–15 times greater risk of ulcerative keratitis exists") unless specific information is requested. During the discussion, the practitioner must make the patient appreciate that because extended wear entails a greater risk of complications—including complications that can permanently affect vision—the program of care is different from daily wear and is organized in a manner that attempts to minimize these risks. If the patient understands the risk and accepts the program of care, informed consent has been obtained and valuable patient education achieved. This same obligation applies to other aspects of contact lens practice, such as fitting patients with monovision or using orthokeratology. A fitting agreement may be used to

TABLE 25-2. *Informed Consent Standards*

Jurisdictions applying the "professional community" standard
    Arizona
    Arkansas
    Colorado
    Delaware
    Florida
    Georgia
    Hawaii
    Idaho
    Illinois
    Indiana
    Kansas
    Maine
    Massachusetts
    Michigan
    Missouri
    Montana
    Nevada
    New Hampshire
    North Carolina
    North Dakota
    South Carolina
    South Dakota
    Virginia
    Wyoming
Jurisdictions applying the "reasonable patient" standard
    Alabama
    Alaska
    California
    Connecticut
    District of Columbia
    Iowa
    Kentucky
    Louisiana
    Maryland
    Minnesota
    Mississippi
    Nebraska
    New Jersey
    New Mexico
    New York
    Ohio
    Oklahoma
    Oregon
    Pennsylvania
    Rhode Island
    Tennessee
    Texas
    Utah
    Vermont
    Washington
    West Virginia
    Wisconsin

Source: Adapted from "Modern status of views as to general measure of physician's duty to inform patient of risks of proposed treatment," 88 ALR 3d 1008.

provide the necessary disclosure and documentation for all these situations.

Alternatives to Therapy

Daily wear of lenses should be described as an alternative when extended wear of lenses is being considered. In some instances, it may even be advisable to fit patients with lenses intended for extended wear (e.g., disposable lenses) but to limit use so that lenses are not worn overnight. It is prudent to warn extended-wear patients that a return to daily wear may become necessary.

For presbyopic patients, in addition to monovision, it is appropriate to describe other contact lens correction options, such as contact lenses for distance and spectacles for near or the use of bifocal or multifocal contact lenses. Of course, spectacles are an option for patients who are considering orthokeratology.

A fitting agreement may be used in all these cases to satisfy disclosure requirements and to provide documentation.

Disclosure of Suspicious Findings

If, during the course of examination, the clinician encounters a suspicious finding, it should be disclosed to the patient. Not doing so can result in liability.

Often, an optometrist performs testing to investigate a suspicious finding before discussing the significance of the finding with the patient. If further testing is required, the patient should be advised of this need, and a recall appointment should be scheduled. Documentation of the communication and the appointment is necessary.

Because of the applicability of informed consent to contact lens practice, optometrists are well advised to incorporate the use of fitting agreements (modified to provide informed consent) into daily practice. These forms are the most time efficient and legally defensible means of satisfying informed consent obligations.

NEGLIGENCE

Negligence is the most common type of liability claim involving contact lens practitioners. Proof of negligence is usually established by presenting evidence from two sources: the record of care and an expert witness.[38]

Because the records of clinicians are subject to scrutiny in professional liability cases,[39] they must be maintained in accordance with professional standards.[40] Documentation of examination findings, diagnoses, and treatment plans (particularly recall and referral appointments) are essential.[41] The problem-oriented record, which is efficient, well organized for episodic care (such as is found in contact lens practice), and accepted by the medical and legal professions, is ideal.[41,42]

The purpose of expert testimony is to provide information that is not normally within the province of a jury of laypeople. Although optometrists customarily serve as expert witnesses in cases alleging injury from contact lenses, ophthalmologists may also be deemed competent to offer testimony.[33,43]

To establish negligence, proof of each of the following is required:

Duty to observe due care. When the doctor-patient relationship is created, the optometrist is required to follow a course of conduct that is intended to minimize the risk of injury to the patient. The practitioner must offer the patient *due care*, which is an obligation to act prudently and to use reasonable levels of knowledge and skill in the diagnosis and treatment of the patient. Proof of the doctor-patient relationship establishes the obligation.

CASE REPORT

A myopic woman in her late 20s was examined by an optometrist for the purpose of being fitted with contact lenses. While evaluating a trial lens through the slit lamp, the optometrist noted a dense vertical line of pigment on the patient's endothelium. Although he recognized the need to perform further testing to rule out the presence of pigmentary glaucoma, the patient had been placed in a time slot for a contact lens fitting. The optometrist dispensed contact lenses to the patient and scheduled her for follow-up the next day, at which time he planned to evaluate her more carefully for glaucoma. The patient did not return the next day, however, and, in fact, did not return until a year had elapsed. At this examination, the optometrist found the patient's cup-to-disk ratio had changed from 0.2 to 0.4, and tonometry readings were 26 and 39 mm Hg. Although he referred the patient to an ophthalmologist for treatment, the patient sued him for negligence and for breach of the doctrine of informed consent, alleging that his not warning her of the presence of a suspicious finding had delayed diagnosis and treatment.[33]

Breach of the standard of care. The duty to provide due care obligates the practitioner to act reasonably, to adhere to an accepted standard of care. Proof of breach of the standard of care is often the most difficult aspect of negligence to prove. It is almost always the most contested aspect of a trial. Expert testimony is needed to determine the conduct that is considered reasonable; if the optometrist's acts (or inaction) fall below this accepted level of conduct, a breach of the duty to provide due care exists.

Actual physical injury. There must be some physical injury to the patient; psychological injury, by itself, is rarely permitted, but it may be claimed if a physical injury also occurs. Eye injury is most commonly determined by loss of acuity, loss of visual field, or impaired ocular motility (i.e., motility with diplopia). The evaluation of ocular injury has been standardized and expert testimony is necessary to determine the extent of injury.[44] Damages may include doctor and hospital bills, lost wages from work, compensation for temporary or permanent impairment, and payment for pain and suffering. Permanent, significant injury to the cornea can result in substantial damages.[45]

Proximate cause. The legal link between the act or failure to act on the part of the optometrist and the resultant injury suffered by the patient is called *proximate cause.* For example, failure to perform a periodic eye health assessment would be the proximate cause of loss of visual field in a contact lens wearer with undiagnosed open-angle glaucoma. Expert testimony is required. Proximate cause can be difficult to establish in some instances, and if it cannot be proved, the negligence claim fails.[46,47]

Negligence claims in contact lens practice are most conveniently discussed by type of lens: daily wear or extended wear.

Daily-Wear Liability Claims

In the United States, approximately 30 million contact lens wearers exist, with approximately 15–20% of these individuals using extended-wear lenses.[48] Because of their greater numbers, daily-wear patients incur more complications and file more liability claims than extended-wear patients do, even though the risk of serious complications is greater for extended-wear patients.

For optometrists, two principal sources of significant claims exist for damages: improper management of contact lens–related corneal abrasions and failure to diagnose anterior or posterior segment disease[33] (a result also reported in a study of liability claims against ophthalmologists[49]). Corneal ulceration with invasion by *Pseudomonas* secondary to a contact lens–related corneal abrasion and undiagnosed open-angle glaucoma are the most likely causes of negligence claims for contact lens practitioners.[33] But other potential liability issues of which optometrists must be aware exist. These are described in order of ascending importance:

- Use of approved materials or solutions in an unapproved manner
- Verification of lenses before dispensing
- Fitting and dispensing of monovision contact lenses
- Delegation of responsibilities to contact lens technicians
- Management of corneal abrasions
- Periodic monitoring of ocular health

Each potential liability issue is illustrated with case reports providing examples of actual claims.

Unapproved Use

Contact lens solutions and materials should be used in the approved manner. Unapproved lenses or solutions require that this fact be communicated to the patient.[14,15] Clinical trials of unapproved lenses or solutions demand disclosure sufficient to satisfy the requirements of the doctrine of informed consent.[34] If approved lenses or solutions are used in an unapproved manner, this fact must also be communicated to patients.

Even if a patient has no injury, a practitioner may become embroiled in a time-consuming legal dispute. If

---

CASE REPORT

A mother took her adolescent son to an ophthalmologist to be fitted with contact lenses. The physician fitted the boy with gas-permeable lenses, and although the lens material had not been approved for extended wear (it was still under FDA investigation), he permitted the lenses to be worn on an extended-wear basis. The mother subsequently learned that the lenses had not been approved for extended wear and called the ophthalmologist, asking for an explanation. After his response, she filed a complaint with the FDA and the state board of medicine, and the physician was forced to defend his conduct before both agencies.[50]

CASE REPORT

A patient examined by an optometrist was prescribed gas-permeable contact lenses with a base curve of 8.2 mm. When the lenses were dispensed to the patient in the office, they became tightly bound to the corneal surface, and the effort to remove the lenses caused the patient considerable difficulty and pain. After the optometrist succeeded in removing the lenses, he found that they had a base curve of 7.2 mm. Although his assistant customarily verified contact lens parameters before dispensing, no documentation existed that an inspection had been performed in this case. The patient subsequently consulted a physician, who told her that her corneas had been scarred by the lenses. The patient sued the optometrist for her injuries, alleging negligence for not inspecting the lenses and verifying that they met the specifications ordered.[2]

---

an ocular injury does result from unapproved use of a lens or solution, the claim is very difficult to defend because the doctrine of informed consent demands a warning if an experimental product is being used.[14,15] Any unapproved use of a product should be described to the patient, and documentation of permission should be retained in the patient's record. For contact lenses, a fitting agreement is an excellent means of providing this documentation.

Verification of Lenses
Inspection and verification of lenses must be performed before or at the time of dispensing.[50] This obligation may be fulfilled by physical inspection or by verification while the lens is on the eye. Not performing this obligation can result in liability.

Although the parameters of rigid contact lenses can be verified easily by measurement with instruments, such as lensometers and radiuscopes, a soft lens is not so easily inspected. An adequate evaluation of soft lenses may be conducted while the lens is on the eye, however, through examination with the slit lamp, over-refraction, keratometry, and measurement of acuity. When a lens is inspected, the individual providing the verification should note in the record that this responsibility has been fulfilled.

Monovison Lenses
Monovision patients should be carefully instructed in the wear and use of their lenses. Because vision is altered in a manner that may not be readily understandable to patients, it is preferable to allow a trial period of wear while the patient is in the office. Owing to informed consent requirements, it is appropriate to warn the patient about the use of monovision while driving a motor vehicle, operating machinery, or performing other potentially hazardous activities.[9,10] Not providing an adequate warning, especially concerning the operation of a motor vehicle, can create liability.[51]

A fitting agreement can be used to describe the contact lens options available to presbyopic patients and to communicate the limitations of a monovision fit.[9,10] The agreement serves as an informed consent document in these cases, providing written evidence that a warning or restriction was discussed with the patient.[9,10]

Contact Lens Technicians
Duties are frequently delegated to contact lens technicians. If they perform these duties negligently, the employer is legally responsible for any resulting damages under the doctrine of *respondeat superior*.[52]

CASE REPORT

A presbyopic physician who had never before worn contact lenses was changed from spectacles to monovision contact lenses by an optometrist. Less than a week after receiving the lenses, the physician left for vacation, and, while driving a van, he was involved in an accident when he misjudged the vehicle's position on the road at a curve and ran off the highway, causing injury to himself and the vehicle. He instituted legal action against the optometrist, alleging that he had not been adequately warned of the reduced acuity and stereopsis of a monovision fit. The optometrist had no written documentation to support his discussion of the risks of wear with the patient (Thomas Morgan, JD, personal communication).

CASE REPORT

A daily-wear soft contact lens patient returned as scheduled to his optometrist for a progress evaluation. During the examination, a contact lens technician mistakenly rinsed the lenses with a cleaning solution before returning them to the patient. When she inserted the lenses in his eyes, he suffered an intense chemical keratitis; the corneal injury required treatment and caused considerable pain and discomfort. He filed a lawsuit, alleging that the optometrist was liable for the assistant's negligence.[53]

Because many duties in contact lens practice, such as the ordering, verification, and dispensing of contact lenses, are delegated to assistants, liability can be created for the optometrist even though the assistant committed the negligence. An employer is responsible for the acts or omissions of employees that occur while employees are acting within the line and scope of their duties, and any negligence committed by an employee may be imputed to the employer.[52] Therefore, contact lens assistants should be adequately educated, trained, and supervised to ensure that they are acting in compliance with standards of care intended to protect the patient from an unreasonable risk of injury.

Management of Abrasions

Complications of lens wear, especially abrasions severe enough to require antibiotic therapy, must be managed in accordance with a medical standard of care.[54,55] Not complying with medical standards results in liability.

If treatment is instituted, use of a broad-spectrum antibiotic sensitive to *Pseudomonas* is generally required (e.g., tobramycin, ciprofloxacin), without patching, along with follow-up within 24–48 hours and assessment of the patient's progress at 3–5 days after injury.[54,56] If medical therapy cannot be provided, timely referral must be arranged. Abrasions that lead to ulceration are an important source of anterior segment liability claims against optometrists.[55]

Monitoring of Ocular Health

Not monitoring ocular health is a major cause of large liability claims in the daily-wear population.[33] The most common cause of claims is failing to diagnose open-angle glaucoma.[57]

Open-angle glaucoma, ocular tumors, and retinal detachments do occur in contact lens wearers, and patients must be seen on a periodic basis for the purpose of conducting an eye health examination. Because patients do not always keep follow-up appointments, it may be appropriate to contact patients who have suspicious findings, require care, or are in need of further disposition. No-show appointments should be documented in the patient's record, as should efforts to reschedule patients after missed appointments.

If a patient is referred for treatment, it is preferable to schedule the appointment with the selected practitioner at a specific date and time. The practitioner and date should be documented in the patient's record of care. Such

---

CASE REPORT

A patient fitted with daily-wear soft lenses returned for evaluation, complaining of discomfort in one eye. The practitioner's slit-lamp examination revealed a superficial stippling of the cornea and a "depression" at the limbus; the eye was slightly injected, but acuity was $^{20}/_{20}$. The patient was instructed to cease lens wear, given a broad-spectrum antibiotic (an aminoglycoside), and instructed to return the next day for a follow-up examination. Over the course of a week, the "depression" resolved but the stippling persisted and the patient's acuity decreased to $^{20}/_{25}$. The practitioner instructed the patient to continue the antibiotic therapy, but after another week, the stippling remained and visual acuity had dropped to $^{20}/_{30}$. After the practitioner decided to continue with the antibiotic therapy, the patient consulted another clinician, who referred her to a medical center clinic. Cultures revealed *Herpes simplex*, but despite treatment, the best acuity that could be obtained in the eye was $^{20}/_{100}$. A lawsuit was filed against the first practitioner, alleging negligent diagnosis and treatment.[33]

CASE REPORT

A myopic man in his 20s consulted an optometrist because of problems with his contact lens fit. The optometrist changed the parameters of the lenses, obtaining satisfactory comfort and acuity. During the course of the examination, the optometrist measured the patient's intraocular pressures by noncontact tonometry and found them to be between 25 and 30 mm Hg. Because the patient had signed a prepaid service agreement, requiring a follow-up examination in 6 months, the optometrist did not advise the patient of the significance of the elevated intraocular pressure; he planned to repeat tonometry at the 6-month evaluation. However, the patient moved out of town before the 6 months had elapsed and did not return for follow-up; 2 years later he was diagnosed as having reduced visual acuity and visual field secondary to pigmentary glaucoma. He filed a lawsuit against the optometrist, alleging negligence in not diagnosing the glaucoma.[58]

an approach provides optimum care while affording the best defense against a legal claim.

LIABILITY FOR EXTENDED-WEAR PATIENTS

Well-publicized studies underwritten by the Contact Lens Institute have reported that the incidence of ulcerative keratitis is approximately five times greater for wearers of extended-wear soft lenses than for wearers of daily-wear soft lenses.[12] If soft lenses are worn overnight, the risk of incurring ulcerative keratitis is estimated to be 10–15 times higher than for daily wear.[13] The relative risk increases with accumulated overnight wear, becoming approximately 5% greater with each consecutive night of wear without removal.[13] These risks are clearly significant and obligate a clinician not only to inform patients of the greater likelihood of complications associated with extended wear but also to manage patients in a manner that will minimize them. Therefore, the care of extended-wear patients entails legal obligations not encountered with daily-wear patients.

Extended-wear patients can comply with wearing schedules and lens maintenance requirements and still encounter serious complications.[59] The most dreaded complication, of course, is infectious keratitis. Traumatic injury to the corneal epithelium, often by a fingernail or lens, is a common cause of infection that leads to ulceration.[60] Another important cause of corneal compromise is overnight edema, loss of epithelial adhesion, and resultant susceptibility of the corneal surface to even minimal trauma.[61,62] Under these circumstances, the cornea is uniquely vulnerable to the risk of infection by *Pseudomonas*.[60,63]

It is estimated that more than 50% of the cases of ulcerative keratitis occurring in extended-wear soft contact lens patients are caused by *Pseudomonas*.[65] Because it is also estimated that 70,000 cases of contact lens–related ulcerative keratitis occur annually in the United States, the opportunity for misdiagnosis and litigation is significant.[66] For this reason, the care of extended-wear patients poses a unique liability risk for contact lens practitioners.

Liability claims involving the care of extended-wear patients can be divided into five categories: inappropriate patient selection, inadequate instruction of the patient, improper wearing schedule, improper management of contact lens–related ocular complications, and inadequate monitoring of ocular health.

Each potential source of liability is illustrated by the use of case reports describing actual negligence claims.

CASE REPORT

A man who had worn daily-wear lenses for 3 years was fitted with extended-wear lenses. Ten months later, he telephoned and requested replacement lenses, which were sent to him by mail. Nearly a year afterward, he had corneal ulcers in both eyes. He filed a lawsuit, alleging that the lenses had been negligently prescribed, that he had been inadequately warned about the risks of extended wear, and that he had not received an examination after receiving the replacement lenses sent by mail.[64]

CASE REPORT

A woman with mildly dry eyes was fitted with extended-wear lenses by an optometrist, and on the first evening of overnight wear, she awoke at 3:00 AM with extreme pain in one eye. She removed the lens, but the persistent pain prompted her to be examined the next day by the optometrist, who found a significant area of epithelial loss in the affected eye. Her symptoms did not diminish by the following day, so the optometrist referred her to an ophthalmologist. She continued to experience severe pain, and after a week of unsuccessful treatment, she was hospitalized with a corneal infection that a culture determined was caused by *Pseudomonas*. She ultimately filed a lawsuit against the optometrist, the ophthalmologist, and the manufacturer of the lenses. Her claim against the optometrist alleged not only that he had breached the doctrine of informed consent in not warning her of the potential risks of extended wear but also that he had not properly managed the corneal abrasion.[70]

Inappropriate Patient Selection

Patients with obvious physical contraindications to extended wear, such as reduced tear breakup time, significant allergies, a history of chronic lid infections, or dry eye, should be eliminated as candidates for extended wear.[67] Patients with a documented history of noncompliance with instructions, wearing schedules, or lens care regimens also should not be considered for extended wear.[68] Young patients who do not have the maturity to deal with the demands of extended wear are similarly a poor choice for this contact lens modality.[69]

If a marginal candidate for extended wear wants to be fitted with lenses, the practitioner should provide an assessment of risk, using written agreements to document informed consent. If the patient understands the potential risks of extended wear and agrees to the conditions imposed by the practitioner to ensure that these risks are minimized, the practitioner has satisfied the requirements of informed consent.[14,15] If a complication ensues, the practitioner has a defense to a resulting legal claim. If a marginal patient is fitted without adequate communication and documentation, however, liability may result.

Inadequate Instruction of the Patient

Patients must be afforded an adequate opportunity to learn lens removal and insertion techniques, lens care regimens, and proper management of common problems of wear. Training of patients is often delegated to assistants, who must possess the knowledge and skill necessary to instruct patients in these techniques. Not providing adequate instruction, if it is the cause of an injury to the patient, can create liability.

Of particular importance are instructions on lens cleaning and disinfection. At follow-up examinations, patients should be questioned about lens care techniques, and deviations from accepted procedures should be identified and corrected. A pattern of inadequate care should be documented in the patient's record, and, if appropriate, termination of wear should be recommended or instituted.

Improper Wearing Schedule

Although extended-wear lenses were first approved by the FDA for up to 30 days of continuous wear, it soon

CASE REPORT

A young woman was examined by an optometrist, who prescribed extended-wear contact lenses. She returned a few days later to pick up the lenses and to receive instructions on their handling, care, and maintenance. The optometrist's son, who worked in the office, provided the information; the patient did not see the practitioner. While wearing the lenses, the patient had an eye infection that caused serious injury to one of her corneas. She subsequently filed a lawsuit against the optometrist, alleging that she had received inadequate instructions about disinfecting the lenses and that the instructions had been provided by an untrained and unlicensed person.[71]

533

A 15-year-old boy purchased a pair of extended-wear contact lenses from an optical shop. Although he wore the lenses "in compliance with the instructions given," after 3 weeks of wear, one eye became red and painful, allegedly developing a corneal ulcer that, despite treatment, caused decreased visual acuity in the eye. He filed a lawsuit against the optical shop, its parent company, and the lens manufacturer, alleging that the lenses were an unreasonably dangerous product, that they would cause injury even if worn as instructed, and that advertising stating that the lenses were safe for 30 days of continuous wear created an unreasonable risk of injury because it was not accompanied by a warning of the inherent risks of extended wear.[73]

---

became apparent that such prolonged wearing times were inappropriate. Numerous lawsuits resulted, with many of them alleging that the lenses were an unsafe product.[72]

Because of this rash of product liability lawsuits, many practitioners reduced wearing schedules for extended-wear lenses. Prompted by reports of these complications, in 1990 the FDA issued a warning that advised practitioners to restrict continuous wear to no more than 6 consecutive nights.[74] For this reason, patients should be placed on wearing schedules that comply with the FDA directive. In rare cases (e.g., stroke), it may be impossible for the patient to regularly insert and remove lenses, thus necessitating wear for extended periods. If the benefits outweigh the risks, and if the patient gives an informed consent to the extended wearing schedule, the practitioner has complied with legal requirements.[14,15] The discussion of risks and benefits and the patient's decision to proceed with a longer wearing schedule should be carefully documented.

Improper Management of Contact Lens–Related Complications

The most serious complication of extended wear is a corneal ulcer. Not managing this condition properly and in a timely manner can lead to significant injury and, consequently, to significant damages.[57]

A corneal ulcer requires timely care to prevent permanent corneal injury. The clinician must decide whether to manage the patient by direct therapeutic intervention (where permitted) or to refer for specialized treatment (as may be required for a *Pseudomonas* ulcer on the line of sight). If treatment is instituted, a culture should be taken to identify the causative organism and a broad-spectrum antibiotic sensitive for *Pseudomonas* should be prescribed.[75] Once the causative organism has been identified, fortified antibiotics are necessary, and subconjunctival, sub-Tenon's capsule, or intravenous drug delivery may be required in particularly resistant cases.[56,76,77] Practitioners should be prepared to provide

---

CASE REPORT

An optometrist fitted an attorney with extended-wear contact lenses. After the first night of wear, no complications were noted, and she was scheduled for a routine 3-day progress check. Because of professional responsibilities, she did not return for evaluation until a week had passed, however, and at this examination, she complained of irritation in one eye. The optometrist found a small corneal abrasion in the affected eye and prescribed a topical antibiotic (which was not an aminoglycoside), instructing the patient to discontinue lens wear, use the drug overnight, and return the next day. Although the patient did not return as scheduled, she used the antibiotic for almost a week, but continued pain and discomfort caused her to consult another practitioner. A 2 × 3–mm corneal ulcer was found. Cultures revealed that the causative agent was *Pseudomonas*, necessitating that she be hospitalized for treatment. After recovery, the patient sued the optometrist for negligence, alleging that he did not explain the potential seriousness of the injury to her and that he used an inappropriate drug for treatment.[33]

CASE REPORT

A myopic 22-year-old woman was fitted with contact lenses by an ophthalmologist. On numerous occasions over the course of a decade, the patient returned for evaluation, expressing complaints about her vision that the physician assumed were related to contact lens wear. It was not until the patient was 32 years old that the physician performed tonometry for the first time. Testing revealed markedly elevated intraocular pressure, and an assessment of the patient's visual field determined that it was reduced to 5 × 10 degrees. The patient filed a lawsuit against the ophthalmologist, alleging that not testing her for open-angle glaucoma constituted negligence.[80]

---

management in accordance with a medical standard of care; not doing so may result in liability.[33]

Inadequate Monitoring of Ocular Health

Patients must receive periodic eye health assessments. This responsibility must not be neglected, and practitioners must avoid the temptation to reduce contact lens care to a series of progress checks. As litigation has proved, contact lens wearers may experience retinal detachments, ocular tumors, glaucoma, and other diseases,[57] and careful assessment of the anterior and posterior segment of the eye should be performed at reasonable intervals.

Although no absolute requirements exist to determine the frequency with which eye health assessments should be performed, clinical practice guidelines suggest that 1 or 2 years, depending on patient age and condition, should be appropriate (Table 25-3).[78,79] Even so, clinical judgment must always be exercised in making this determination.

SUMMARY

A contact lens practitioner can take steps to minimize the risk of liability (see Table 25-3). If a practitioner adopts a structured program of care, complies with informed consent requirements, documents care adequately, and acts promptly and appropriately when complications are encountered, the risk of litigation is significantly reduced. At the same time—and not incidentally—the quality of care is enhanced. The end result is an improved contact lens practice for patient and practitioner.

TABLE 25-3. *Steps to Minimize the Risk of Litigation*

1. Use a structured program for contact lens patients; document care with printed fitting agreements.
2. Discuss the effects of monovision before fitting presbyopic patients with lenses; allow the patient to adapt to wear before attempting potentially hazardous tasks.
3. Obtain an informed consent from the patient if unapproved materials or solutions are used; also obtain consent for unapproved use of approved materials or solutions.
4. Inspect and verify all lenses before dispensing.
5. Adequately educate, train, and supervise contact lens assistants.
6. Discuss risk and obtain an informed consent before fitting a patient with extended-wear lenses.
7. Select patients for extended wear in accordance with accepted clinical guidelines.
8. Recommend an overnight wearing schedule that is appropriate for the patient; do not exceed 6 nights of continuous wear except when justified by clinical circumstances.
9. Document patient noncompliance with instructions, wearing schedules, lens care, or recall instructions.
10. Inform patients fitted with disposable lenses that individual lenses cannot be inspected before wear.
11. If contact lens–related complications occur, manage them promptly and in accordance with a medical standard of care, particularly corneal abrasions.
12. Periodically evaluate the ocular health of contact lens patients.
13. Describe your policy for the release of contact lens prescriptions at the outset of the doctor-patient relationship.
14. When a contact lens prescription is released, make certain it is accurate and complete; retain copies of all prescriptions provided to patients.

REFERENCES

1. Scholles JR. A review of professional liability claims in optometry. J Am Optom Assoc 57:764, 1986
2. Scholles JR. Malpractice: watch your step. Rev Optom 123:26, 1986
3. Smith SK: Patient noncompliance with wearing and replacement schedules of disposable contact lenses. J Am Optom Assoc 67:160, 1996
4. Classé JG: Avoiding liability in contact lens practice. Optom Clin 4:1, 1994
5. Farkas P: Integrating disposable or planned replacement lenses into contact lens practice. Optom Clin 4:61, 1994
6. Classé JG: Contractual considerations in contact lens practice. J Am Optom Assoc 57:220, 1986
7. Classé JG: Legal Aspects of Optometry. Butterworth, Stoneham, MA, 1989, 373
8. Classé JG, Harris MG: Contracts for contact lens patients. Optom Management 24:48, 1988
9. Harris MG: Informed consent for presbyopic contact lens patients. J Am Optom Assoc 61:717, 1990
10. Harris MG, Classé JG: Clinicolegal considerations in monovision. J Am Optom Assoc 59:491, 1988
11. Classé JG, Harris MG: Liability and extended wear contact lenses. J Am Optom Assoc 58:848, 1987
12. Schein OD, Glynn RJ, Poggio EC, et al: The relative risk of ulcerative keratitis among users of daily wear and extended wear soft contact lenses. N Engl J Med 321:777, 1989
13. Poggio EC, Glynn RJ, Schein OD, et al: The incidence of ulcerative keratitis among users of daily-wear and extended-wear soft contact lenses. N Engl J Med 321:779, 1989
14. Harris MG, Dister RE: Legal consequences of the FDA's 7 day extended wear letter. J Am Optom Assoc 61:212, 1990
15. Harris MG, Dister RE: Informed consent in contact lens practice. J Am Optom Assoc 58:230, 1987
16. Harris MG, Dister RE: Informed consent for extended wear patients. Optom Clin 1:33, 1991
17. Classé JG: Legal Aspects of Optometry. Butterworth, Stoneham, MA, 1989; 373
18. Freeman MI, Davis RA: Programmed replacement and disposables put practitioners in control. Cont Lens Spectrum 7(4)Part II:5, 1991
19. Ritzer JA: Service agreement strategies for 21st century survival. Optom Management 25:29, 1989
20. Kaye DB, Hayashi MN, Schenkein JB: A disposable contact lens program, a preliminary report. CLAO J 14:33, 1988
21. Marshall EC: Disposable vs. non-disposable contact lenses—the relative risk of ocular infection. J Am Optom Assoc 63:28, 1992
22. Buehler PO, Schein OD, Stamler JF, et al: The increased risk of ulcerative keratitis among disposable soft lens users. Arch Ophthalmol 110:1555, 1992
23. Dunn JP Jr, Mondino BJ, Weissman BA, et al: Corneal ulcers associated with disposable hydrogel contact lenses. Am J Ophthalmol 108:113, 1989
24. Matthews TD, Frazer DG, Minassian DC, et al: Risks of keratitis and patterns of use with disposable contact lenses. Arch Ophthalmol 110:1559, 1992
25. Classé JG, Snyder C, Benjamin WJ: Documenting informed consent for patients wearing disposable lenses. J Am Optom Assoc 60:215, 1989
26. Classé JG, Harris MG: Disposable lenses don't dispose of your legal responsibilities. Optom Management 25:78, 1989
27. Classé JG, Harris MG: Doctor, I want a copy of my . . . . Optom Management 25:19, 1989
28. Classé JG: Management of contact lens prescriptions. Optom Clin 4:93, 1994
29. CFR Part 456. Federal Register 57(85):18822, May 1, 1992
30. Harris MG, Classé JG: Contact lens prescriptions: a clinicolegal view. J Am Optom Assoc 59:732, 1988
31. Classé JG: Release of contact lens prescriptions: an update. J Am Optom Assoc 68:125, 1997
32. Rosoff AJ: Informed Consent: A Guide for Health Care Providers. Rockville, MD, Aspen, 1981, 21
33. Classé JG: A review of 50 malpractice claims. J Am Optom Assoc 60:694, 1989
34. Classé JG: Legal Aspects of Optometry. Butterworth, Stoneham, MA, 1989, 295
35. Classé JG: Informed consent and contact lens practice. J Am Optom Assoc 67:132, 1996
36. Harris MG: Informed consent for contact lens practice. J Br Contact Lens Assoc 17:119, 1993
37. Harris MG: Keep presbyopic contact lens wearers informed. Contact Lens Spectrum 8:50, 1993
38. Harris MG, Gold AR, Classé JG: A review of five recent cases of significance for optometrists. J Am Optom Assoc 59:964, 1988
39. Scholles JR: Documentation and recordkeeping in clinical practice. J Am Optom Assoc 57:624, 1986
40. Classé JG: Legal Aspects of Optometry. Butterworth, Stoneham, MA, 1989, 215
41. Classé JG: Recordkeeping and contact lens practice. Optom Clin 4:69, 1994
42. American Optometric Association: Scope of Practice: Patient Care and Management Manual. American Optometric Association, St. Louis, 1986
43. Classé JG: Liability and the primary care optometrist. J Am Optom Assoc 57:926, 1986
44. American Medical Association: Guides to the Evaluation of Permanent Impairment. 2nd ed. American Medical Association, Chicago, 1984, 141
45. *In re Bourne,* 566 So 2d 147 (La App 1990)
46. Classé JG: The eye-opening case of *Keir v United States.* J Am Optom Assoc 60:471, 1989
47. Classé JG: A dark victory. Optom Economics 1:44, 1990
48. Herman CL: An FDA study of US contact lens wearers. Cont Lens Spectrum 2:89, 1987
49. Bettman JW: Seven hundred medicolegal cases in ophthalmology. Ophthalmology 97:1375, 1990
50. Classé JG: Legal Aspects of Optometry. Butterworth, Stoneham, MA, 1989, 373

51. Harris MG: Monovision and driving: elude getting sued. Rev Optom 129:69, 1992

52. Classé JG: Legal Aspects of Optometry. Butterworth, Stoneham, MA, 1989, 285

53. Classé JG: How your helper can help you get sued. Optom Management 16:61, 1980

54. Catania LJ: Management of corneal abrasions in an extended wear contact lens population. Optom Clin 1:123, 1991

55. Classé JG: Liability for the treatment of anterior segment eye disease. Optom Clin 1:1, 1991

56. Silbert JA: A review of therapeutic agents and contact lens wear. J Am Optom Assoc 67:165, 1996

57. Classé JG: Standards of Practice for Primary Eyecare. Anadem, Columbus, OH, 1998

58. Classé JG: Standards of care when diagnosing or treating the glaucomas. Optom Clin 1:193, 1991

59. Weissman B, Donzis P, Hoft R: Keratitis and contact lens wear: a review. J Am Optom Assoc 58:799, 1987

60. Koidan-Tsiligranni A, Alfonso E, Forster RK: Ulcerative keratitis associated with contact lens wear. Am J Ophthalmol 108:64, 1989

61. Madigan MD, Holden BA, Kwok LS: Extended wear of contact lenses can compromise corneal epithelial adhesion. Curr Eye Res 6:1257, 1987

62. Holden BA, Mertz GW, McNally JJ: Corneal swelling response to contact lenses worn under extended wear conditions. Invest Ophthalmol Vis Sci 24:218, 1983

63. Connor C: Microbiological aspects of extended wear. Optom Clin 1:79, 1991

64. *Cousineau v. Barnes-Hind, Inc.*, 697 So2d 367 (La App 1997)

65. Baum J, Panjwani N: Adherence of *Pseudomonas* to soft contact lenses and cornea: mechanism and prophylaxis. In Cavanaugh HD (ed): The Cornea: Transactions of the World Congress on the Cornea III. Raven, New York, 1988, 301

66. Benjamin WJ: Assessing the risks of extended wear. Optom Clin 1:13, 1991

67. McMonnies CW, Ho A: Patient history and screening for dry eye conditions. J Am Optom Assoc 58:296, 1987

68. Chun NW, Weissman BA: Compliance in contact lens wear. Am J Optom Physiol Optics 64:274, 1987

69. Harris MG: Compliance and soft contact lens wear. Int Cont Lens Clin 15:143, 1988

70. *Beaman v Schwartz*, 738 SW 2d 632 (Tenn App 1986)

71. *Menaugh v Resler Optometry, Inc.*, 799 SW2d (1991)

72. *Otis v Bausch & Lomb, Inc.*, 532 NYS 2d 933 (1988)

73. News review: patient sues Sterling, B&L. Rev Optom 122:3, 1985

74. Dister RE, Harris MG: Legal consequences of the FDA's seven day extended wear letter. J Am Optom Assoc 61:212, 1990

75. Silbert J: Complications of extended wear. Optom Clin 1:95, 1991

76. Abbott RL, Abrams MA: Bacterial corneal ulcers. p. 8. In Duane TD (ed): Clinical Ophthalmology. Vol. 4. Harper & Row, Hagerstown, MD, 1986

77. Liesegang TJ: Bacterial and fungal keratitis. p. 217. In Kaufman HE, Barron BA, McDonald MB, Waltman SR (eds): The Cornea. Churchill Livingstone, New York, 1988

78. American Optometric Association: Comprehensive Adult Eye and Vision Examination. American Optometric Association, St. Louis, 1994

79. American Optometric Association: Pediatric Eye and Vision Examination. American Optometric Association, St. Louis, 1994

80. *Helling v Carey*, 83 Wash 2d 514, 519 P 2d 981 (1974)

Appendix

Cornea and Contact Lens Research Unit*
Grading Scales

---

*Cornea and Contact Lens Research Unit (CCLRU) School of Optometry, University of New South Wales, Australia.

CCLRU ⊚ GRADING SCALES

Cornea and Contact Lens Research Unit, School of Optometry, University of New South Wales

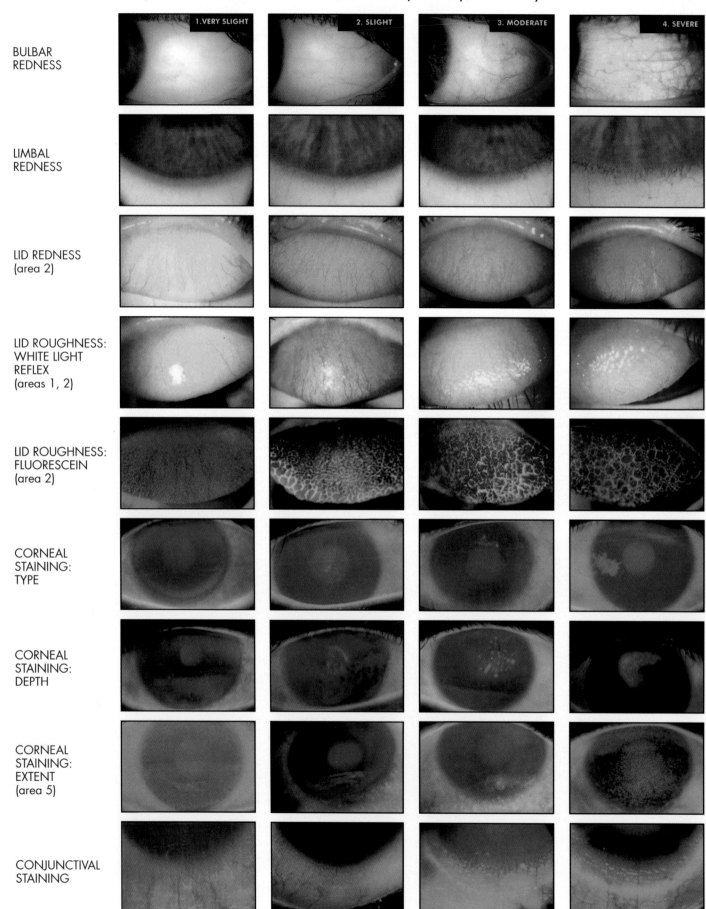

1. VERY SLIGHT · **2. SLIGHT** · **3. MODERATE** · **4. SEVERE**

BULBAR REDNESS

LIMBAL REDNESS

LID REDNESS (area 2)

LID ROUGHNESS: WHITE LIGHT REFLEX (areas 1, 2)

LID ROUGHNESS: FLUORESCEIN (area 2)

CORNEAL STAINING: TYPE

CORNEAL STAINING: DEPTH

CORNEAL STAINING: EXTENT (area 5)

CONJUNCTIVAL STAINING

Sponsored by an Educational Grant from Johnson & Johnson VISION PRODUCTS, INC

CCLRU 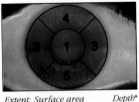 GRADING SCALES

APPLICATION OF GRADING SCALES

- Patient management is based on how much the normal ocular appearance has changed.
- In general, a rating of slight (grade 2) or less is considered within normal limits (except staining).
- A change of one grade or more at follow up visits is considered clinically significant.

PALPEBRAL CONJUNCTIVAL GRADES

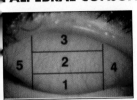

- The palpebral conjunctiva is divided into five areas to grade redness and roughness.
- Areas 1, 2 and 3 are most relevant in contact lens wear.

ADVERSE EFFECTS WITH CONTACT LENSES

CLPC CONTACT LENS PAPILLARY CONJUNCTIVITIS
Inflammation of the upper palpebral conjunctiva

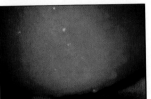

Signs:
- Redness
- Enlarged papillae
- Excess mucus

Symptoms:
- Itchiness
- Mucus strands
- Lens mislocation
- Intolerance to lenses

INFILTRATES
Accumulation of inflammatory cells in corneal sub-epithelial stroma.
Inset: high magnification view

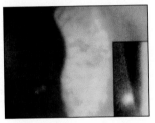

Signs:
- Whitish opacity (focal) or grey haze (diffuse)
- Usually confined to 2-3mm from limbus
- Localised redness

Symptoms:
- Asymptomatic or scratchy, foreign body sensation
- Redness, tearing and photophobia possible

CLARE CONTACT LENS ACUTE RED EYE
An acute corneal inflammatory episode associated with sleeping in soft contact lenses

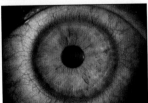

Signs:
- Unilateral
- Intense redness
- Infiltrates
- No epithelial break

Symptoms:
- Wakes with irritation or pain
- Photophobia
- Lacrimation

CORNEAL STAINING GRADES

- Staining assessed immediately after single instillation of fluorescein using cobalt blue light and wratten 12 (yellow) filter over slit lamp objective.
- The cornea is divided into five areas. The type, extent and depth of staining are graded in each area.

Type
1 Micropunctate
2 Macropunctate
3 Coalescent macropunctate
4 Patch

Extent: Surface area	*Depth**
1 1-15%	1 Superficial epithelium
2 16-30%	2 Deep epithelium, delayed stromal glow
3 31-45%	3 Immediate localised stromal glow
4 > 45%	4 Immediate diffuse stromal glow

*Based on penetration of fluorescein and slit lamp optic section

EROSION
Full thickness epithelial loss over a discreet area

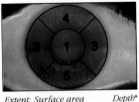

Signs:
- No stromal inflammation
- Immediate spread of fluorescein into stroma

Symptoms:
- Can be painful
- Photophobia
- Lacrimation

CLPU CONTACT LENS PERIPHERAL ULCER
Round, full thickness epithelial loss with inflamed base, typically in the corneal periphery which results in a scar. Insets: with fluorescein, scar

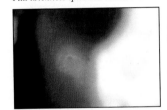

Signs:
- Unilateral, "white spot"
- Localised redness
- Infiltrates
- Post healing scar

Symptoms:
- Varies from foreign body sensation to pain
- Lacrimation and photophobia may occur

INFECTED ULCER
Full thickness epithelial loss with stromal necrosis and inflammation, typically central or paracentral

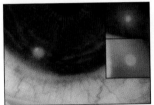

Signs:
- Intense redness
- "White patch" (raised edges)
- Infiltrates
- Epithelial and stromal loss
- Anterior chamber flare
- Conjunctival & lid edema

Symptoms:
- Pain, photophobia
- Redness, mucoid discharge
- ↓VA (if over pupil)

POLYMEGETHISM

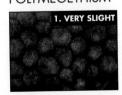
1. VERY SLIGHT

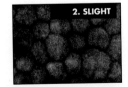
2. SLIGHT

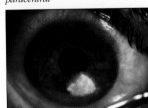
3. MODERATE

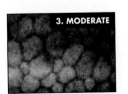
4. SEVERE

VASCULARIZATION

Vessel extension beyond translucent limbal zone is recorded (mm)

STROMAL STRIAE and FOLDS

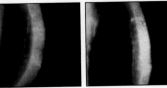

One striae = 5% edema
One fold = 8% edema
(each additional striae or fold indicates 1% more edema)

Record number observed

MICROCYSTS and VACUOLES

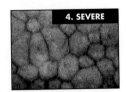

Located in epithelium. Identified by side showing brightness

Microcysts   reversed

Vacuoles   unreversed

Record number observed

Sponsored by an Educational Grant from *Johnson & Johnson* VISION PRODUCTS, INC

Index

Note: Page numbers followed by *f* refer to illustrations; page numbers followed by *t* refer to tables.

Narcissus lens design for, 457, 457f
Wesley-Jessen opaque lens design for, 455–456, 455f
Wesley-Jessen prosthetic lens design for, 456, 456f, 457f
sectoral, 455
Histamine
in giant papillary conjunctivitis, 138
in inflammation, 113–115, 115f, 117f
HIV. *See* Human immunodeficiency virus (HIV) infection.
Homatropine
in fungal keratitis, 267
in herpes zoster ophthalmicus, 216
Hordeolum (stye), 185–186, 186f
in staphylococcal blepharitis, 175, 175f
Human immunodeficiency virus (HIV) infection, 218–222, 240–241
Candida infection and, 222
conjunctival microvasculopathy with, 220, 221f
contact lens disinfection in, 222–223
contact lens wear in, 219, 222
dry eye in, 219, 219f
herpes simplex keratitis with, 220
herpes zoster virus infection with, 219–220, 220f
Kaposi's sarcoma and, 221, 221f
microsporidia infection with, 220
molluscum contagiosum infection with, 220
opportunistic infections with, 219–220, 220f
precautions against, 222–223
Pseudomonas infection and, 222
superficial punctate keratitis in, 213, 214f
Hybrid lenses. *See* SoftPerm lens.
Hydrogel lenses
adherence of, 81f, 88–89, 88f
adrenochrome staining of, 443
annular tinted contact lens syndrome with, 339, 339t
arcuate staining with, 82, 83f
bacterial keratitis with, 230
for bandage application, 17, 430, 431
chlorhexidine effects on, 443
corneal infiltrates with, 122–123
corneal topography for, 501–503, 502f, 502t, 503f
corneal vascularization with, 96–97, 97f, 100, 101, 124–125, 124f, 125f
corneal warpage syndrome and, 338–339, 339t
decentration of, 81
defects in, 82
discoloration of, 442–443
disposable, 293–297
carefree characteristics of, 295
categories of, 294
hypoxia with, 295
imperfections in, 296
infection with, 296–297
inflammation with, 295–296
oxygen transmissibility of, 295
drug delivery with, 436–437

dry eye with, 3, 13, 15–16, 18. *See also* Dry eye; Keratoconjunctivitis sicca.
epinephrine effects on, 443
epithelial pits with, 77
epithelial splitting with, 83, 83f
extended-wear, 273–300
acute red eye with, 273–275, 276f, 288
aging of, 294–295
case report of, 273–275
corneal hypoxia with, 277–285
acidosis and, 284
critical oxygen transmissibility and, 280–281, 280t, 281t
edema and, 278–280, 278f, 279f
endothelial effects of, 283–285, 285f
epithelial effects of, 281–283, 282f, 283f
oxygen supply and, 277
stromal effects of, 283
corneal infection with, 291–293
critical oxygen transmissibility of, 280–281, 280t, 281t
deposits on, 294
vs. disposable lenses, 293–297
inflammation with, 285–291, 286f, 287f
papillary conjunctivitis with, 289–291, 290f
patient care compliance for, 297–299
peripheral ulcers with, 276f, 277f, 288–289
solution sensitivities of, 294–295
ulcerative bacterial keratitis and, 232–233
keratoconjunctivitis sicca with, 204–207
for keratoconus, 378–379, 366ff, 379f
limbal hyperemia with, 102
mechanical corneal staining with, 82, 82f, 83f
myopic creep with, 339
after penetrating keratoplasty, 411–412
peripheral corneal staining with, 76–77, 78f, 78t
after refractive surgery, 398–399
replacement frequency for, 339
rifampin effects on, 443
rippling effect of, 338–339
sodium fluorescein staining of, 70
sorbic acid effects on, 442
superior limbic keratoconjunctivitis with, 153
tear film evaporation with, 13
Hydrogen peroxide, 156–157, 157t
for adenovirus disinfection, 217
epitheliopathy with, 85, 86f
for herpes simplex virus disinfection, 215
for herpes zoster disinfection, 216
toxicity of, 156–157, 157t
Hydrops, corneal, in keratoconus, 360, 360f
Hydroxypropyl cellulose, in keratoconjunctivitis sicca, 201
Hypersensitivity reactions. *See also* Corneal inflammation.
chlorhexidine-induced, 154
in giant papillary conjunctivitis, 114–115, 115f, 138–139
papain-induced, 158
preservative-induced, 84–85, 84f, 85f